Tough Calls in Acute Neurology

Tough Calls in Acute Neurology

Edited by
Alejandro A. Rabinstein, M.D.

Assistant Professor of Clinical Neurology
Cerebrovascular Division, Department of Neurology
University of Miami School of Medicine
Attending Consultant
Neuroscience Intensive Care Unit
Jackson Memorial Hospital
Miami, Florida

Eelco F. M. Wijdicks, M.D., Ph.D., F.A.C.P.

Chair, Division of Critical Care Neurology
and Professor of Neurology
Mayo Clinic College of Medicine
Attending Consultant, Neurological/Neurosurgical Intensive Care Unit
St. Mary's Hospital
Rochester, Minnesota

With 39 Contributing Authors

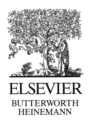

ELSEVIER
BUTTERWORTH
HEINEMANN

Amsterdam Boston London New York Oxford Paris Philadelphia
San Diego San Francisco Singapore Sydney Tokyo

ELSEVIER
BUTTERWORTH
HEINEMANN

The Curtis Center
170 S Independence Mall W 300E
Philadelphia, Pennsylvania 19106

TOUGH CALLS IN ACUTE NEUROLOGY   0–7506–7466–0
Copyright © 2004 Elsevier Inc. All rights reserved.

Notice

Neurology is an ever-changing field. Standard safety precautions must be followed, but as new research and clinical experience broaden our knowledge, changes in treatment and drug therapy may become necessary or appropriate. Readers are advised to check the most current product information provided by the manufacturer of each drug to be administered to verify the recommended dose, the method and duration of administration, and contraindications. It is the responsibility of the licensed prescriber, relying on experience and knowledge of the patient, to determine dosages and the best treatment for each individual patient. Neither the publisher nor the authors assume any liability for any injury and/or damage to persons or property arising from this publication.

The Publisher

Library of Congress Cataloging-in-Publication Data

Tough calls in acute neurology / [edited by] Alejandro A. Rabinstein, Eelco F.M. Wijdicks.
     p. ; cm.
   Includes index.
   ISBN 0-7506-7466-0
   1. Neurology—Decision making. 2. Neurological errors. I. Rabinstein, Alejandro A. II. Wijdicks, Eelco F. M., 1954-
   [DNLM: 1. Nervous System Diseases—therapy. 2. Acute Disease. 3. Evidence-Based Medicine. 4. Nervous System Diseases—diagnosis. WL 140 T722 2004]
   RC346.3.T68 2004
   616.8—dc22

                                                                              2004043626

Acquisitions Editor: *Susan Pioli*
Developmental Editor: *Joan Ryan*
Publishing Services Manager: *Joan Sinclair*
Project Manager: *Cecelia Bayruns*

Printed in the United States of America

Last digit is the print number: 9 8 7 6 5 4 3 2 1

Contents

Contributing Authors

Henry E. Aryan, M.D.
Neurosurgeon, University of California, San Diego, School of Medicine;
Neurosurgeon, University of California,
San Diego, Medical Center, San Diego, California

Mustafa K. Başkaya, M.D.
Resident, Department of Neurological Surgery,
University of Miami School of Medicine;
Jackson Memorial Hospital, Miami, Florida

James L. Bernat, M.D.
Professor of Medicine (Neurology), Dartmouth Medical School,
Hanover; Neurologist, Dartmouth-Hitchcock Medical Center,
Lebanon, New Hampshire

José Biller, M.D.
Professor of Neurology and Neurosurgery, Loyola University Stritch School of
Medicine; Associate Chairman, Department of Neurology,
Loyola University Medical Center, Maywood, Illinois

Valérie Biousse, M.D.
Associate Professor of Ophthalmology and Neurology,
Emory University School of Medicine, Atlanta, Georgia

Christopher J. Boes, M.D.
Assistant Professor of Neurology, Mayo Clinic College of Medicine;
Consultant, Department of Neurology, Mayo Clinic,
Rochester, Minnesota

Ian Bone, M.B., Ch.B., F.R.C.P., F.A.C.P.
Honorary Professor of Clinical Neurology,
University of Glasgow; Consultant Neurologist,
Institute of Neurological Sciences, Southern General Hospital,
Glasgow, Scotland, United Kingdom

Cecil O. Borel, M.D.
Associate Professor of Anesthesiology and Surgery (Neurosurgery),
Duke University School of Medicine; Chief, Otolaryngology, Head, Neck,
Neurology, and Offsite Anesthesia and Medical Director, Neurosciences Intensive
Care Unit, Duke University Medical Center, Durham, North Carolina

Louis R. Caplan, M.D.
Professor of Neurology, Harvard Medical School;
Chief, Cerebrovascular Disease, Beth Israel Deaconess Medical Center,
Boston, Massachusetts

Ji Y. Chong, M.D.
Clinical Stroke Fellow, Columbia University College of Physicians and Surgeons;
Assistant Attending, Department of Neurology,
Columbia-Presbyterian Medical Center, New York, New York

Carmen D. Cirstea, M.D.
Department of Neurology, Boston University School of Medicine,
Boston, Massachusetts

Aaron A. Cohen-Gadol, M.D.
Senior Neurosurgery Resident, Mayo Clinic,
Rochester, Minnesota

Marek Czosnyka, Ph.D., D.Sc.
Affiliated Lecturer, Department of Neurosurgery,
University of Cambridge Clinical School; Director of Neurophysics,
Neurosurgical Unit, Addenbrooke's Hospital, Cambridge,
United Kingdom

Robert G. Feldman, M.D.*
Professor of Neurology, Boston University School of Medicine,
Boston, Massachusetts

Steven J. Frucht, M.D.
Assistant Professor of Neurology, Columbia University College of
Physicians and Surgeons; Assistant Attending, Department of Neurology,
Columbia-Presbyterian Medical Center, New York, New York

Osvaldo Fustinoni, M.D.
Professor of Neurology, Buenos Aires University School of Medicine;
Chief, Cerebrovascular Diseases, Department of Neurology, Instituto de
Neurociencias, Buenos Aires, Argentina

Peter J. Goadsby, M.D., Ph.D., D.Sc.
Wellcome Senior Research Fellow and Professor of Clinical Neurology,
Headache Group, Institute of Neurology; Consultant Neurologist,
The National Hospital for Neurology and Neurosurgery,
London, United Kingdom

*Deceased

Ricardo A. Hanel, M.D.
Neuroendovascular Fellow, Department of Neurosurgery,
State University of New York at Buffalo, Millard Fillmore Hospital,
Buffalo, New York

Roberto C. Heros, M.D.
Professor, Co-Chairman, and Director of Neurological Surgery, University of
Miami School of Medicine, Miami, Florida

Andrew Jea, M.D.
Department of Neurological Surgery, University of Miami School of Medicine,
Miami, Florida

Stanley H. Kim, M.D.
Neurosurgeon/Neurointerventionist, St. David's Medical Center, Austin, Texas

Jawad F. Kirmani, M.D.
Endovascular Surgical Neuroradiology Fellow, Department of Neurology,
University of Medicine and Dentistry of New Jersey, Newark, New Jersey

William E. Krauss, M.D.
Assistant Professor of Neurosurgery, Mayo Clinic College of Medicine,
Rochester, Minnesota

Claudia F. Lucchinetti, M.D.
Associate Professor of Neurology, Mayo Clinic, Rochester, Minnesota

Cormac O. Maher, M.D.
Chief Resident of Neurosurgery, Mayo Clinic, Rochester, Minnesota

Edward M. Manno, M.D.
Assistant Professor of Neurology, Mayo Clinic; Medical Director,
Neurological and Neurosurgical Intensive Care Unit, Saint Mary's Hospital,
Rochester, Minnesota

Lawrence F. Marshall, M.D.
Professor and Chair, Division of Neurological Surgery, Chief of Neurosurgery,
University of California at San Diego School of Medicine, La Jolla, California;
Professor and Chief, Division of Neurological Surgery, University of California at
San Diego Medical Center, San Diego, California

Warren P. Mason, M.D.
Assistant Professor of Medicine, University of Toronto Faculty of Medicine; Staff
Physician, Department of Medicine, Princess Margaret Hospital, Toronto, Canada

Stephan A. Mayer, M.D.
Associate Professor of Clinical Neurology and Neurosurgery,
Columbia University College of Physicians and Surgeons; Director,
Neuro-ICU, Columbia-Presbyterian Medical Center,
New York Presbyterian Hospital, New York, New York

David L. McDonagh, M.D.
Fellow, Department of Anesthesiology,
Duke University Medical Center, Durham,
North Carolina

Nancy J. Newman, M.D.
Leo Delle Jolley Professor of Ophthalmology,
Professor of Neurology, and Instructor in
Neurological Surgery, Emory University School of Medicine; Director,
Department of Neuro-Ophthalmology, Emory Eye Center,
Atlanta, Georgia

Alejandro A. Rabinstein, M.D.
Assistant Professor of Clinical Neurology, Cerebrovascular Division,
Department of Neurology, University of Miami School of Medicine,
Attending Consultant, Neuroscience Intensive Care Unit, Jackson Memorial
Hospital, Miami, Florida

Adnan I. Qureshi, M.D.
Professor of Neurology and Neurosciences and Director of
Cerebrovascular Program and Stroke Center, University of Medicine and
Dentistry – New Jersey Medical School; Endovascular/Stroke Attending,
Department of Neurology and Neurosciences, University Hospital,
Newark, New Jersey

Daniel S. Sax, M.D.
Emeritus Professor of Neurology, Boston University School of Medicine,
Boston, Massachusetts; Neurologist and Director, EEG Lab,
Gifford Medical Center, Randolph, Vermont

David Schiff, M.D.
Associate Professor of Neurology, Neurosurgery, and
Medicine and Co-Director of Neuro-Oncology Center,
University of Virginia Health System, Charlottesville, Virginia

Magdy H. Selim, M.D., Ph.D.
Assistant Professor of Neurology, Harvard Medical School;
Attending Physician, Department of Neurology,
Beth Israel Deaconess Medical Center, Boston, Massachusetts

Mark E. Shaffrey, M.D.
Professor and Vice-Chairman of Neurosurgery, University of
Virginia Health System, Charlottesville, Virginia

Joseph I. Sirven, M.D.
Associate Professor of Neurology, Mayo Clinic, Scottsdale, Arizona

Brian G. Weinshenker, M.D.
Professor of Neurology, Mayo Clinic and Foundation; Consultant Neurologist,
Saint Mary's Hospital; Rochester Methodist Hospital, Rochester, Minnesota

Eelco F. M. Wijdicks, M.D., Ph.D., F.A.C.P.
Chair, Division of Critical Care Neurology and Professor of Neurology,
Mayo Clinic College of Medicine; Attending Consultant,
Neurological/Neurosurgical Intensive Care Unit,
Saint Mary's Hospital, Rochester, Minnesota

Andrew R. Xavier, M.D.
Clinical Instructor in Neurosciences, University of
Medicine and Dentistry – New Jersey Medical School;
Endovascular Fellow, Department of Neurosciences,
University Hospital, Newark, New Jersey

Preface

Acutely ill neurological patients are complex to manage, and most physicians have a hard time of it. Choosing between several therapeutic options is less academic, and decisions are sometimes based on prior single cases that went well. Comprehensive literature reviews or guiding principles are not readily available in acute neurological conditions, and in most general neurology texts they have blended into the background. Thus, the confrontation with these patients is a hard nut to crack ("tough call"). We felt a monograph of topic reviews was needed.

Tough Calls in Acute Neurology is a collection of criticisms. One could quibble with the choice of the topics but we felt it was reasonably across the board. Each chapter includes reflection on entrenchment of ideas and how a certain view of a problem has gained validity. Wherever appropriate, authors try to pinpoint when certain myths were born and how they have been repeated over the years. Not only are these pros and cons presented, but also every chapter ends with a practical section summarizing the current state of the art and a reasonable approach. (It is evidenced-based medicine with a practical twist.)

Tough Calls in Acute Neurology has a clear focus on clinical problems with difficult decision making. This often occurs in less common disorders but also occur in straightforward day-to-day clinical conditions. Each chapter includes an archetypal case *(the patient)* not infrequently presenting in the emergency department. Usually it is a major problem that would in most cases prompt the attending physician to consult other physicians or even call other institutions for guidance. In the next section *(the problem)*, the 3–5 most important questions and dilemmas concerning care are formulated. In the following section the available literature *(the evidence)* is discussed and areas where we are agnostic are emphasized. Evidence to support management is presented somewhere in between the opinion of the "éminence grise" (now called quality of evidence category C grade III) and the comprehensive statistical analysis of the Cochrane project. This section is followed by a section in which the author can voice his opinion and discuss management, allowing a narrative style *(the pros and cons)*. The chapter ends with practical concluding remarks *(the main points)*.

We hope it is a useful text for neurologists, neurosurgeons, neurointensivists, emergency physicians, and fellows in these specialties. If this book is received well, it would energize us to edit "tougher calls" and "the toughest calls" as the next volumes.

Alejandro A. Rabinstein, M.D.
Eelco F. M. Wijdicks, M.D.

Acknowledgments

Our sincere thanks to the authors of the chapters who had to tolerate our prodding to make the deadline, which often seemed like a moving target. We are grateful to Raquel J.S. Nelson for her wonderful editorial assistance and patience. We admire our wives (Carlota and Barbara) for their support. We thank Susan Pioli for believing in this unusual project.

PART I
Tough Calls in Clinical Diagnosis

Chapter 1
Found Comatose

Alejandro A. Rabinstein

It is a scene all too familiar. A patient is rolled into the critical section of the emergency room manually ventilated by an Emergency Medical Services worker. No signs of trauma are evident. Vital signs seem stable, pupils are symmetric and responsive to light, yet the patient is comatose. Emergent brain computed tomography (CT) is unremarkable. Blood is drawn for routine analyses, but the initial laboratory results are unremarkable. The neurologist is called in for emergency consultation.

Those of us meeting this clinical problem should have a clear algorithm in mind in order to quickly assess the situation. History is often unavailable, localizing signs can be absent, sedation may have been administered during intubation, and vital signs may become unstable. Discovery of the cause of coma in a patient found unresponsive may be life-saving. Thus, it is not an overstatement to say that finding the cause of coma in these patients is a challenge. There are usually several high-priority questions that demand immediate answers.

■ The Patient

A 38-year-old man was brought to the emergency room after he became acutely unresponsive and collapsed to the ground while being questioned by the security staff in a train station. The patient was not carrying any identification but had a ticket in his possession stamped 1 hour prior to hospital arrival.

Physical examination revealed a blood pressure of 135/75 mmHg, pulse of 85 beats per minute,

respiratory rate of 18 breaths per minute, and temperature of 37° Celsius. The patient was unresponsive. He had been intubated for airway protection without use of sedation prior to arrival of the neurology consultant. The pupils were symmetric, 3 mm in diameter, and not reactive to light. There was skew eye deviation, with the left eye lower than the right. Oculocephalic reflexes were abolished and cold-caloric testing elicited no response. Corneal reflexes were absent. There were no facial movements to pain. The gag reflex was absent, but the cough reflex could be elicited by deep suction, and the patient was overbreathing the ventilator. Motor exam showed flaccid tetraplegia with no response to noxious stimuli. Deep tendon reflexes were hypoactive in the upper extremities and absent in the lower extremities. There was no response to plantar stimulation. There was no resistance to neck flexion. General examination was essentially unremarkable.

There was no response to the administration of naloxone and flumazenil. An emergent CT of the brain without contrast was unremarkable. A 12-lead electrocardiogram was normal. No alterations in cardiac rhythm were seen on telemetry monitoring. Arterial blood gases showed pH 7.46, Pco_2 35 mmHg, bicarbonate 24 mg/dL, and adequate oxygenation (Po_2 116 mmHg with an inspired oxygen fraction of 0.3). Serum electrolytes, renal function tests, anion gap (4 mmol/L), and calculated osmolality (284 mOsm/kg) were normal. Complete blood count and liver enzymes were also unremarkable. CPK was elevated (450 U/L) with a normal troponin I. Urine analysis was negative including ketones, acetaminophen, and salicylate levels. Drugs of abuse were undetectable on a urine toxicology screen. Serum ethanol level was 20 mg/dL.

A CT angiography of the brain showed a patent basilar artery without evidence of thrombosis. In addition, an emergency MRI of the brain showed no evidence of restricted diffusion.

In an attempt to further delineate the source of the coma, additional chemistry studies were ordered. A measured osmolality at 337 mOsm/L was discordant with the calculated osmolality of 284 mOsm/L (osmolal gap = 53) suggesting a nonethanol alcohol intoxication. Gas chromatography demonstrated an isopropanol (IPA) level of 2870 µg/mL with an acetone level of 1230 µg/mL. Lactic acid was also elevated (3.3 mg/dL). Repeat testing 7 hours later showed an IPA level of 2000 µg/mL and an acetone level of 1910 µg/mL. Forty hours after admission, the IPA level had decreased to 54.4 µg/mL and the acetone level was 5235 µg/mL. The measured osmolality peaked at 358 mOsm/kg 7 hours after admission. There was never any abnormality of the serum HCO_3 level or anion gap; CPK increased to a maximum of 453 U/L 7 hours after admission. Renal function tests remained normal throughout the course of the intoxication.

Hemodialysis was not initiated given incipient signs of patient recovery and the reassuring decline in the IPA level. Over the next 48 hours the patient progressively recovered neurological function, and he was successfully extubated 84 hours after admission. On follow-up clinical examination, there was no evidence of persistent neurological deficit. When his identity became available, we learned that the patient was homeless and had a history of multiple hospitalizations for paranoid schizophrenia. At that time, the patient confirmed that he had ingested a nonquantifiable amount of rubbing alcohol with suicidal intention. He was subsequently transferred from the intensive care unit to the psychiatric service.

■ The Problem

- Is the patient ventilating well and maintaining adequate blood pressure?
- Is the patient really comatose?
- Is there structural damage to the brain or other vital organs?

- Have I considered all treatable life-threatening diagnoses?

■ The Evidence

Assessing Ventilatory and Hemodynamic Status

Comatose patients are often intubated to protect their airway and ensure appropriate oxygen exchange. Any question about the safety of the airway should prompt immediate intubation. Pooling of respiratory secretions with absent gag and cough reflexes and abnormal breathing patterns, other than Cheyne-Stokes, are typical indications. Arterial blood gases must be obtained as soon as the patient arrives at the emergency room. They provide information on the status of gas exchange and may be diagnostic in cases of profound acid-base disturbances from toxic or acute metabolic derangements. Relying solely on pulse oximetry is not sufficient in these situations. Mechanical ventilation is necessary when gas exchange is poor (presence of hypoxia or hypercapnia). Measurement of arterial blood pressure, palpation of peripheral pulses, and assessment of the color and temperature of the extremities are rudimentary but fairly dependable indicators of circulatory sufficiency. Fluid resuscitation should be instituted emergently if the systolic blood pressure is below 90 mmHg. Vasopressors should be infused early when fluid treatment fails to achieve rapid recovery of normal blood pressure. All comatose patients should be monitored with cardiac telemetry since various causes of coma can also produce potentially fatal arrhythmias.

Recognizing States Mimicking Coma

Coma is a state of unresponsiveness in which the patient lies with eyes closed and cannot be aroused even by noxious stimuli.[1] Spontaneous movements are absent and, at most, only primitive reflex responses can be elicited. Several conditions may mimic coma and their recognition depends on keeping a high index of suspicion.

Patients with *locked-in syndrome* are fully conscious, yet totally unable to communicate except through blinking and vertical eye movements (so-called de-efferented state). All other voluntary movements are abolished, including those depending on innervation by lower cranial nerves ("paralysis from the nose down"). Destructive lesions of the basis pontis interrupting the corticospinal and corticobulbar pathways are responsible for this syndrome[2] but spare the peripherally located auditory tracts and dorsally located ascending sensory tracts. Patients can feel pain and hear conversations. *Generalized muscle paralysis* due to neuromuscular blocking drugs or an acute neuromuscular disease (such as acute inflammatory demyelinating polyradiculoneuropathy or myasthenia gravis) can present similarly.

Patients with *catatonia* may be rigid, mute, and appear unresponsive to environmental stimuli. However, these patients typically maintain their eyes open and have preserved optokinetic and vestibuloocular responses. Waxy flexibility, catalepsy, posturing, and grimacing are relatively common. It is mostly seen in major psychiatric disorders but may also be caused by structural damage.[3]

Assessment of Structural Damage to the Brain

In the emergency setting, the main goals of the neurological examination of comatose patients are distinguishing between structural, physiological, and metabolic cerebral disorders. Brain imaging can complement a neurological examination in the evaluation of comatose patients.

Simple inspection of the patient often provides valuable information to the trained observer. Body posture, head position, spontaneous movements, and pattern of breathing should be carefully observed. The level of responsiveness is then graded according to the type of stimulus needed to arouse the patient. Describing the stimulus used and the response obtained reduces ambiguity in the interpretation of the clinical notes. The Glasgow Coma Scale (Table 1-1)[4] is the most widely used tool to gauge the level of consciousness in daily practice. Although originally designed for use in patients with traumatic brain injury, this time-honored scale has been adopted in the care of patients with any form of impaired level of consciousness. Ideally, the scores for each of the three components of the scale—eye opening, verbal response, and motor response—should be recorded and not only the sum score.

Table 1-1. Glasgow Coma Scale

Activity/Response	Score[*]
Eye opening (E)	
Spontaneous	4
After verbal stimulus	3
After painful stimulus	2
None	1
Verbal response (V)	
Oriented	5
Confused	4
Inappropriate but recognizable words	3
Incomprehensible sounds	2
None	1
Best motor response (M)	
Obeys verbal commands	6
Localizes painful stimulus	5
Withdraws to painful stimulus	4
Abnormal flexion posturing	3
Abnormal extensor posturing	2
None	1

[*]Score may be reported by separate components (preferable) or as a total sum score.

The Pupils

Assessment of pupillary symmetry and light reactivity is crucial in comatose patients. A fixed, dilated pupil may signal compression or stretching of the third cranial nerve produced by an expanding intracranial mass. Horizontal displacement of the midbrain or medial temporal lobe, or downward distortion of the brainstem, may be responsible for this physical finding.[5] Differential loss of innervation of a segment of the papillary sphincter may cause the pupil to lose its round configuration; this appearance should not lead the examiner to dismiss the anisocoria as "congenital" or "secondary to eye surgery or previous eye damage." Transient unilateral mydriasis with loss of pupillary light reactivity has been reported after nebulizations with anticholinergic drugs, likely due to inadequate sealing of the oral mask and asymmetric condensation of the mist on the eyelids.[6] Extensive mesencephalic destruction causes bilateral mydriatic nonreactive pupils. However, similar pupils may be found in extreme cases of drug overdose with tricyclic antidepressants, carbamazepine, cocaine, or amphetamines, and after using large doses of atropine for cardiac resuscitation.[7] Anxiety, pain, and sympathomimetic agents may provoke pupillary dilatation, but in those cases light reactivity is spared.

Pontine tegmental lesions characteristically produce pinpoint pupils. Light reaction is preserved, but it often takes a sharp eye (or better the use of magnifying lenses) and a strong light source to recognize this subtle reaction. Opiate overdose can also cause pinpoint pupils; in those instances intravenous naloxone (0.4 to 2 mg) reverses the abnormality. Lesser degrees of bilateral miosis are seen after barbiturate intoxication and have been reported in cases of metabolic derangements, such as nonketotic hyperosmolar hyperglycemia.[8] Unilateral miosis is most often part of Horner's syndrome. It may be caused by lesions at any level of the sympathetic pathway from the hypothalamus to the plexus surrounding the internal carotid artery.

The Eye Position and Movements

Abnormal positions of the resting eyes typically reflect structural brain damage and may have great localizing value. Horizontal conjugate gaze deviation away from a paralyzed side is indicative of a large hemispheric lesion involving the frontal center for eye movements. Conjugate deviation toward the paralyzed side reflects unilateral pontine damage. Exceptions to these rules may occur with thalamic and upper brainstem lesions causing deviation of the eyes to the opposite side ("wrong-way" deviation). Also, hemispheric lesions may trigger seizures during which the eyes are forced toward the opposite side of the lesion; associated nystagmoid eye jerks may be easily missed. Mesencephalic tectum damage may manifest by downward gaze, paralysis of elevation, and convergence-retraction nystagmus (Parinaud's syndrome). Forced downward deviation of the eyes may also be seen in thalamic lesions extending into the dorsal midbrain. Meanwhile, upward deviation is less localizing and is often seen after diffuse hemispheric damage following cardiac resuscitation. Skew deviation is highly indicative of brainstem dysfunction, the higher eye often pointing to the side of the lesion. Disconjugate resting eyes may reflect paralysis of individual extraocular muscles or pre-existent tropia or phoria.

Spontaneous eye movements are less helpful to the localization efforts and may be seen after intoxications and metabolic derangements. Roving eye movements are seen after bilateral hemispheric damage and indicate that the brainstem has not been severely injured. Ping-pong movements (conjugate movements from side to side every few seconds) and periodic alternating nystagmus (side to side movements every few minutes) typically occur after bihemispheric or vermis damage. Ocular bobbing (rapid movement down, slower upward return) indicates damage to the pontine tegmentum. Ocular dipping (slow downward movement followed by rapid return to the meridian) is not uncommon after severe diffuse anoxic insults. The localizing value of blinking is not well defined. Rhythmic blinking in a comatose patient, however, should raise suspicion for subtle status epilepticus but can also be seen with postanoxic coma.

Horizontal oculocephalic (doll's eyes) reflexes denote sparing of the ocular motor nerves and the ocular movement pathways in the tegmentum of midbrain and pons. Similarly, vertical head tilting may be used to check the integrity of the upper brainstem structures. In patients with suspected or documented neck injuries and any time the oculocephalic reflexes cannot be elicited, oculovestibular reflexes should be tested by irrigating ice water in each ear. Asymmetric failure to elicit these reflexes is a reliable sign of structural brainstem damage. Uncovering internuclear ophthalmoplegia certifies damage to the medial longitudinal fasciculus. Meanwhile, bilateral absence of these reflexes implies brainstem dysfunction but not necessarily irreversible destruction, since this finding can be seen in cases of hypothermia and drug intoxications (most notably with anticonvulsants and sedatives). Corneal reflexes are typically lost in deep stages of coma of any cause. Unilateral loss of corneal reflex may be due to lesions either in the contralateral hemisphere or the ipsilateral brainstem.

The Neck

Resistance to passive neck flexion but not to other neck movements as a sign of meningeal irritation can be present in comatose patients with meningitis or subarachnoid hemorrhage. This sign may disappear when patients progress to flaccidity and absent motor response. Neck rigidity in all directions of head movement may be observed in patients with antipsychotic drug reactions, or merely advanced degenerative disease of the cervical spine.

The Breathing Pattern

Cheyne-Stokes respiration (*CRS*) occurs after bilateral hemispheric dysfunction. The isolated brainstem respiratory centers presumably become more sensitive to changes in CO_2, leading to the characteristic regularly alternating periods of hyperpnea and apnea. Frequently observed in metabolic coma, CRS is usually not an ominous sign. Its presence does not demand endotracheal intubation if the airway remains patent and the arterial gases are normal or only show respiratory alkalosis. Conversely, the more irregular *cluster breathing* (sometimes referred to as "short-cycle CRS") and *apneustic breathing* (pauses of several seconds in full inspiration) typically imply low pontine damage from basilar artery occlusion or impending herniation of posterior fossa lesions calling for immediate intervention. *Biot breathing*, essentially characterized by its chaotic nature, is classically considered a sign of medullary involvement and a prelude to *agonal breathing.*

Central neurogenic hyperventilation is a rather infrequent sign. Extreme hyperventilation occurs with diencephalic herniation but is most frequently caused by underlying systemic conditions such as metabolic acidosis, early respiratory failure, salicylate overdose, or end-stage liver failure.

In isolation, the breathing pattern has limited localizing value. However, changes of breathing pattern over time may indicate progression to herniation in patients with expanding intracranial masses. Several caveats need to be considered when assessing respiration in mechanically ventilated patients. Respiratory drive is very depressed in markedly hypocarbic patients (as seen with iatrogenic or therapeutic hyperventilation, or with certain intoxications). Conversely, spontaneous breaths may deceivingly seem to occur in apneic patients when the ventilator is set with a very sensitive flow trigger.

The Limb Movements

When present, spontaneous movements should be observed in detail. Subtle twitching of the mouth or fingers may be the only clinical evidence of subtle status epilepticus. Asymmetric or preferential movements may represent seizures or hemiparesis. Myoclonic jerks, complex repetitive movements, and various dystonic postures may be seen in such disparate situations as emergence from sedation (most notably with propofol), liver or renal failure, and anoxia. Unfortunately, these abnormal movements are fairly often misinterpreted as seizures, misleading the diagnostic plan and prompting unwarranted treatment with anticonvulsants. Myoclonic status epilepticus predicts grim prognosis after cardiac arrest.[9]

Motor responses to pain should be subsequently evaluated. Appropriate localization and withdrawal are markers of less severe coma and indicate potential for good recovery. Use of inadequate painful stimulus is one of the most common pitfalls in the examination of comatose patients. Contrary to general belief, rubbing the sternum is much less effective than pressing on the patient's temporomandibular joints. Traditional teaching dictates that abnormal *flexion* (*decorticate*) and *extensor* (*decerebrate*) *posturing* indicate rostrocaudal progression of structural neuraxis damage. However, clinical experience not infrequently defies this aphorism. Not only may abnormal posturing fail to follow the expected progression, but also it may occur with metabolic and toxic disorders. Also, mechanical ventilation may trigger posturing in certain patients, especially those with central autonomic imbalance. Flaccid unresponsiveness may indicate extensive lower brainstem destruction but it may also be seen in patients with extreme neuromuscular weakness (such as Guillain-Barré syndrome) or concomitant high cervical injury.

The Herniation Syndromes

Hemispheric mass lesions produce coma by brain tissue shifts. In his seminal study using CT scans to measure the degree of brain shift, Ropper concluded that early depression of consciousness correlates better with lateral brain displacement.[5] Nonetheless, as the pressure from the mass increases, downward herniation through the opening of the tentorium ensues. Plum and Posner[1] recognized two different syndromes due to transtentorial herniation:

1. Uncal Syndrome. Lateral and downward shift of the inferomedial temporal lobe causes early compression of the oculomotor nerve resulting in ipsilateral fixed mydriasis. The upper midbrain gets pushed against the opposite free edge of the tentorium; the ensuing contusive lesion is known as Kernohan's notch and its most incipient clinical expression is an ipsilateral Babinski sign. Unilateral abnormal posturing may be present before bilateral signs appear.

2. Central Syndrome. Central downward pressure results in early diencephalic and bilateral upper midbrain involvement. Initially impairment of consciousness may not be associated with any pupillary abnormalities. Shortly after, bilateral mid-position nonreactive pupils, abnormal posturing, and Babinski signs become manifest.

In clinical practice, the distinction between these two syndromes is at times far from clear and the clinical course may not follow traditional descriptions.[10] Also, both syndromes coalesce as rostrocaudal progression of the herniation occurs leading to bilateral extensor posturing, loss of brainstem reflexes, irregular breathing with increasing frequency of apneic periods, and finally brain death.

Infratentorial structural lesions may also produce coma by direct involvement or indirect compression of the brainstem. Herniation may occur transtentorially (upward shift) or more commonly transforaminally (downward migration of the cerebellar tonsils through the foramen magnum). In the latter case, sudden medullary compression results in respiratory arrest and cardiocirculatory collapse. Intermittent raises in intracranial pressure in patients with posterior fossa masses precipitate episodes of bilateral extensor posturing often confused with seizures ("cerebellar fits").

The General Examination

Assessment of the vital signs is a crucial first step. Hypothermia, when pronounced (i.e., < 32°C), may be responsible for the coma. In other less severe cases, it may tell us that the patient has been unconscious and exposed to cold for some time. Other causes of low body temperature in coma include sedative overdose (barbiturates, benzodiazepines), opioids, neuroleptics, hypoglycemia, Addisonian crisis, myxedema, and Wernicke's encephalopathy. After trauma, it may be due to cervical spinal cord injury resulting in autonomic dysreflexia.

Hyperthermia should always raise suspicion of meningitis or encephalitis and prompt lumbar puncture if there is associated meningismus or brain imaging fails to display the cause of the coma. However, one must be aware that fever may occur after various intracranial catastrophes, such as massive pontine hemorrhage, poor-grade subarachnoid hemorrhage, and severe traumatic brain injury. Actually, the presence of fever is a predictor of poor prognosis in these cases and may exacerbate brain damage; thus, body temperature must be lowered aggressively. Hyperthermia can also be observed in patients intoxicated with amphetamines, cocaine, phencyclidine, and other psychedelics (salicylates, tricyclic antidepressants). Both hypo- and hyperthermia can be seen with sepsis and systemic sources of infection should be appropriately investigated.

Hypertension is very prevalent among patients with acute structural central nervous system lesions. It is presumably driven by a dramatic increase in the central release sympathetic mediators. The combination of hypertension and bradycardia may indicate ongoing herniation (Cushing's reflex). When brain imaging is normal, severe hypertension may hint at intoxication with amphetamines, cocaine, hallucinogens, or other drugs with sympathomimetic action. Extreme hypertension may result in hypertensive encephalopathy, a diagnosis that should be substantiated by the presence of bilateral papilledema. This entity is rare, and it is ill advised to settle for this diagnosis before a thorough evaluation, even when very high blood pressure values are documented. Hypotension, especially when associated with tachycardia, is suggestive of sepsis. Low blood pressure is common in patients poisoned with sedative hypnotics, neuroleptics, opioids, tricyclic antidepressants, lithium, and organophosphates. In trauma patients, it demands immediate fluid resuscitation and should lead to an emergent search for internal vessel or visceral rupture.

It is worth re-emphasizing that heart rate and rhythm should be monitored with cardiac telemetry. Until the cause of coma is identified, every comatose patient should be considered to be at high risk for life-threatening arrhythmias.

Skin inspection may be very rewarding to the discriminating examiner. Signs of otherwise occult trauma may become apparent. Periorbital and retroauricular ecchymoses (known as "raccoon eyes" and Battle's sign respectively) indicate skull base fractures. Subtle axillary and conjunctival petechiae may be the only physical signs pointing to underlying fat embolism in patients with long bone fractures. A careful search for needle marks over the trajectory of superficial veins must always be part of the skin examination. Jaundice may denote advanced liver failure, and cherry-red coloration indicates carbon monoxide poisoning. Dark discoloration is typical of Addison's disease. A petechial or purpuric rash may be the clue to the diagnosis of meningococcal meningitis. Fairly nonspecific macular rashes with limited petechial components can be seen in cases of viral meningitis and encephalitis (including West Nile virus), Rocky Mountain spotted fever, *Streptococcus pneumoniae*, and *Staphylococcus aureus*. Thrombotic thrombocytopenic purpura can also be diagnosed on the basis of the skin appearance. Profuse diaphoresis, especially when combined with copious respiratory secretions, diarrhea, and fasciculations, is highly suggestive of organophosphate poisoning. Extremely dry skin and mucosal surfaces may signal intoxications with antihistamine or anticholinergic drugs and can also be seen in uremia. Skin bullae in pressure areas suggest prolonged immobility and are typical of alcohol, barbiturate, or opioid intoxication.

A traditional practice, smelling the patient's breath odor should not be forgotten. Distinctive odors in comatose patients include the odor of alcohol, the rotten-fruit odor of diabetic ketoacidosis, the urine-like odor of uremia, the musty or fishy fetor hepaticus, the garlic-like odor of pesticide poisoning, the onion-like odor of paraldehyde, and the bitter-almond odor of cyanide intoxication.

Table 1-2 summarizes some of the most useful physical signs to differentiate between coma from structural and diffuse brain disease.

Our patient had disconjugate gaze, absent pontomesencephalic reflexes, and no response to pain. Despite a normal CT scan of the brain, further brain imaging seemed reasonable given the presence of the findings on examination.

Recognizing Treatable Life-Threatening Diseases

Initial diagnostic efforts should be focused on excluding diseases that may be fatal unless specific

Table 1-2. Physical Findings Useful in the Differential Diagnosis of Structural Versus Diffuse Causes of Coma

Supratentorial structural lesion
Initial contralateral focal cerebral signs
Depression of consciousness usually progressive
Subsequent signs of brainstem involvement
  Ipsilateral corticospinal signs
          and
  Unilateral fixed dilated pupil   = Uncal herniation
       or
  Bilateral fixed mid-position pupils   = Central herniation
          followed by
  Rostrocaudal progression of deficits

Infratentorial structural lesion
Initial signs of brainstem dysfunction
Depression of consciousness usually sudden
Pattern of weakness less predictable
Early loss of pontomesencephalic reflexes
Early changes in respiratory pattern

Diffuse brain disorder
Initial changes in content and level of consciousness
Motor signs usually symmetric
Pupillary light reflex typically spared
Abnormal breath odor
Acute skin rash
Early ventilatory changes

treatment is emergently provided. These include herniating lesions amenable to surgical decompression, hydrocephalus, basilar artery thrombosis, meningitis or brain abscess, acute renal failure, intoxications and poisonings requiring hemodialysis, CO inhalation, cyanide toxicity, hypoglycemia, diabetic ketoacidosis, nonketotic hyperosmolar coma, pituitary apoplexy, Addison's crisis, myxedema, and sepsis.

In our case, certain intoxications, endocrine disorders, and, most notably, acute basilar artery thrombosis were possible. Further evaluation was pressingly needed to exclude those diagnostic alternatives.

Causes of Coma with Normal Brain CT

A normal brain CT excludes most structural causes of coma, but there are a few notable exceptions. *Acute basilar artery occlusion*, especially when embolic, may present with sudden coma.[11–13]

Initially, brain CT may be totally unremarkable, and the correct diagnosis depends on the physical findings and maintaining a high level of suspicion in patients with sudden unexplained coma. In patients with acute basilar artery occlusion, coma results from infarction of the brainstem reticular formation or bilateral damage of the dorsomedial thalami as it occurs in the "top of the basilar" syndrome.[14] Various brainstem signs may be present. In comatose patients, the most telling findings are usually those involving the eye positions and movements. Internuclear ophthalmoplegia, one-and-a-half syndrome, ocular bobbing, Parinaud's syndrome, and different degrees of skew deviation may be present according to the level and extension of the ischemic lesion. When the damage is so severe as to render the patient comatose, tetraplegia with bilateral Babinski signs is typically present. However, asymmetries in motor response to pain may be informative. A history of initial hemiparesis (herald hemiparesis), especially when fluctuating, or brainstem signs (transient or permanent) before the patient became comatose is highly suggestive of basilar thrombosis.[15] In suspected cases, the brain CT should be carefully examined for the presence of a hyperdense basilar artery sign; this may be the only detectable abnormality on CT and its presence may portend poor outcome.[16,17] The prognosis of basilar artery occlusion is ominous if recanalization is not achieved promptly.[18,19] Intra-arterial thrombolysis, sometimes combined with mechanical clot disruption, may be effective even up to 48 hours after symptom onset,[19] and it should always be attempted unless extensive brainstem damage is already visible on MRI. In centers where intra-arterial treatment is not available, intravenous thrombolysis should be attempted especially if it may be administered within 3 hours of symptom onset.[20] Emergency stenting to treat acute basilar artery occlusion is also a promising alternative in specialized centers.[21]

Nonconvulsive status epilepticus is another potential cause of sudden coma with normal brain CT scan. However, this condition presents more commonly with fluctuating level of consciousness, sometimes lasting for days before the diagnosis is made. Previous history of epilepsy and convulsive seizure at onset are usually present.[22] Coma from nonconvulsive status epilepticus may occur more frequently in acutely ill hospitalized patients.[23,24]

In those cases, attention to subtle clinical signs, such as twitching of one corner of the mouth or a single finger, may signal the diagnosis. Careful observation of the eyes may reveal the presence of nystagmoid jerks. Final diagnosis depends on the demonstration of continuous seizure activity on bedside electroencephalogram.

Fulminant meningitis and encephalitis may also be responsible for coma in the absence of visible abnormalities on brain CT scan. In rapidly deteriorating patients, the diagnosis may only become apparent when purulent meninges are noted during necropsy. Presence of fever and meningeal signs are useful clinical signs but they may be absent. Elderly patients with meningitis may be afebrile, and their neck stiffness may be difficult to distinguish from cervical osteoarthritis. When present, a recent history of febrile illness, confusion, or agitation may be useful clues. Papilledema may be observed in patients with fulminant meningitis. The skin should be carefully inspected for the presence of telling rashes. When in doubt, it is always safer to perform a lumbar puncture and start intravenous antibiotics emergently.[25] Use of dexamethasone before or at the time of infusion of antibiotics is beneficial in patients with severe bacterial meningitis.[26]

Although often associated with diffuse cerebral edema, *anoxic-ischemic brain injury* may present with a normal initial CT scan. This diagnosis should be strongly considered in patients found comatose with evidence of acute myocardial ischemia or arrhythmias on electrocardiogram. However, since only supportive treatment can be provided in these cases, other more treatable diagnoses should be excluded before the diagnosis of anoxic brain injury is established. Hypothermia initiated immediately after cardiac resuscitation may be of value in reducing brain damage,[27,28] but its value in other patients with brain anoxia has not been established. Diffusion-weighted MRI may show extensive areas of restricted fluid motion especially throughout the cortex in comatose patients with brain anoxia and otherwise normal brain imaging.[29]

Various *acute metabolic disorders* may cause acute coma. They include hypoglycemia, diabetic coma (ketotic or nonketotic hyperosmolar), uremia, hepatic coma, extreme thyroid dysfunction (thyrotoxicosis, myxedema),[30,31] Addison's crisis, severe hypercapnia, severe acidosis, profound hyponatremia, hypercalcemia[32] or hypocalcemia,[33] thiamine deficiency (Wernicke's encephalopathy), and sepsis. Blood testing in patients with coma should therefore include measurement of glucose and electrolytes, serum osmolality, renal, liver, and thyroid function, and arterial blood gases. When adrenal insufficiency is suspected, early morning cortisol level should be measured. Thiamine injection should be routinely administered to patients with acute unexplained coma; even when thiamine deficiency is not responsible for the coma, the administration of glucose to malnourished patients may precipitate Wernicke's encephalopathy.[34] In patients responding to thiamine, the diagnosis of Wernicke's encephalopathy may then be confirmed by testing blood transketolase activity, which is markedly decreased in patients with thiamine deficiency. Table 1-3 summarizes remarkable

Table 1-3. Diagnostic Features of Common Metabolic Causes of Coma

Metabolic Disorder	History and Physical Features	Laboratory Findings
Hypoglycemia	Initial restlessness, sweating, flushing. Then pallor, shallow breathing, seizures. Focal signs may be present	Hypoglycemia (< 40 mg/dL) Low CSF glucose
Diabetic ketoacidosis	Background of diabetes Preceding polyuria, polydipsia, polyphagia. Possible infection. Hyperventilation with Kussmaul breathing pattern Rotten-fruit breath odor Extracellular volume contraction	Hyperglycemia, acidosis, glucosuria Ketonemia, ketonuria
Diabetic nonketotic hyperosmolality	Typically elderly patients with diabetes type 2 Triggers: dehydration, infection, medications Severe volume contraction	Glycemia > 600 mg/dL Serum osm > 320 mOsm/L No ketones
Uremia	Initial apathy, confusion, asterixis. Then seizures, myoclonus Pale, dry skin with uremic "frost". Possible oligoanuria Hypertension Hyperventilation Urine-like breath odor	Elevated serum BUN and creatinine Anemia Metabolic acidosis Hypocalcemia Hyperphosphatemia Abnormal urinary sediment
Liver failure	Initial sleep changes, confusion, stupor, asterixis Triggers: GI hemorrhage, protein load, infection Jaundice, ascites, spider angiomata	Elevated blood ammonia Abnormal PT/PTT Low platelet count High bilirubin Triphasic waves on EEG
Adrenal failure	Initial fatigue, confusion, stupor Hypotension, tachycardia, fever pallor. Skin hyperpigmentation Triggers: infection, surgery, trauma	Hypoglycemia Low Na, high K, high Ca Mild metabolic acidosis Low AM cortisol and low response to cosyntropin
Myxedema	Progressive fatigue, lethargy Delayed reflexes Hypothermia. Bradycardia. Ileus. Dry skin, "dough" edema	Elevated TSH
Thiamine deficiency (Wernicke's encephalopathy)	Initial diplopia, ataxia, confusion. Then ophthalmoplegia Background of alcoholism or malnutrition.	Reduced blood transketolase activity
Hyponatremia	Initial lethargy, confusion, delirium Asterixis, myoclonus, seizures	Serum Na < 110 mEq/L
Hypercalcemia	Initial confusion, lethargy Skin tenting, polyuria, dehydration, constipation	Serum Ca > 14 mg/dL

diagnostic features of the most common causes of metabolic coma.

Intentional or unintentional poisoning is probably the most common cause of coma presenting to the emergency department. Numerous drugs and toxins can produce central nervous system depression (Table 1-4). Clues from the history supporting the suspicion of a toxicological diagnosis include previous suicidal attempts, a background of major depression or bipolar disorder, and empty medication bottles or drug paraphernalia found at the scene. Progression from delirium to coma is also suggestive of intoxication. Carbon monoxide poisoning should always be suspected when the patient was found comatose in a closed, nonventilated space.

The physical and laboratory findings of the most frequently encountered causes of toxic coma are

Table 1-4. Diagnostic Features of Common Toxic Causes of Coma

Toxin	History and Physical Features	Laboratory Findings
Carbon monoxide	Patient found in closed space Headache, confusion, agitation Seizures Cherry-red skin (very late) Cardiovascular collapse	Carboxyhemoglobin Metabolic acidosis Elevated CK, myoglobinuria
Cyanide	Exposure to sodium nitroprusside Headache, confusion, agitation Bitter-almond breath odor Cardiovascular instability	High RBC or plasma cyanide level Anion gap metabolic acidosis Elevated lactic acid Decreased AVO$_2$ difference
Ethanol	Confusion, agitation, delirium Ataxia, nystagmus, dysarthria Tremors Alcohol breath odor	Elevated serum ethanol
Atypical alcohols:* Methanol Ethylene glycol Isopropyl alcohol	Blindness and breath odor (M) Crystalluria (EG) Hematemesis (IPA)	Large osmolal gap Severe anion gap metabolic acidosis (M and EG) Hypoglycemia, high CK with no acidosis (IPA)
Salicylate	Tinnitus, confusion, delirium, seizures Hyperpnea and tachypnea Dehydration Hyperthermia	Acid-base disorders (respiratory alkalosis, anion gap metabolic acidosis, or mixed) Elevated serum salicylate
Anticholinergics: Antihistamines Belladonna alkaloids Benztropine Trihexyphenidyl	Dry, flushed skin. Dry mucosas. Hyperthermia. Mydriasis. Tachycardia. Ileus. Urinary retention Delirium. Myoclonus. Seizures.	EKG with QRS widening and QT$_c$ prolongation Drug levels when available
Cholinergics: Organophosphates Sarin gas	Cramps. Excessive secretions. Miosis. Diarrhea. Bronchoconstriction. Hypertension. Tachycardia. Fasciculations. Weakness. Seizures. Delirium.	Low cholinesterase activity in RBC
Sedative hypnotics: Benzodiazepines Barbiturates Chloral hydrate	Confusion, lethargy, ataxia With barbiturates: hypotension, respiratory, depression, hypothermia, fixed pupils Withdrawal seizures (BDZ, barbiturates) Response to flumazenil (BDZ)	Drug levels when available Urinary toxic screen (BDZ)

Table 1-4. *Continued*

Toxin	History and Physical Features	Laboratory Findings
Opioids	Lethargy. Pinpoint reactive pupils.	Urinary toxic screen (BDZ)
	Hypothermia. Hypotension.	Drug levels when available
	Respiratory depression	
	Urinary retention	
	Response to naloxone	
Stimulants	Hypervigilance, paranoia, agitation	Urinary toxic screen
Sympathomimetics:	Mydriasis. Tremulousness. Seizures	Respiratory alkalosis
Amphetamines	Diaphoresis. Hyperthermia	Hyperglycemia
Cocaine	Hypertension	May cause elevated CK, renal failure
Methylphenidate	Tachycardia, rapid arrhythmias	
Theophylline		
Psychedelics:	Delirium with profound agitation	Blood levels when available
LSD	Florid hallucinations	PCP level in gastric juice
Mescaline	Dilated pupils	
PCP	Hyperreflexia	
	Tachycardia. Hyperthermia.	
Antidepressants:		
Tricyclics	Anticholinergic syndrome	Blood levels
MAO inhibitors	Drowsiness, ataxia, seizures	Blood levels
	Hypertensive crisis	
Neuroleptic agents	Dystonia, akathisia, rigidity	Drug levels when available
Butyrophenones	Miosis. Hypotension	May cause elevation of CK,
Phenothiazines	Neuroleptic malignant syndrome (hyperthermia,	renal failure
	extreme rigidity, autonomic instability)	
	Anticholinergic signs	
Lithium	Lethargy, tremulousness, weakness	Blood level
	Clonus. Ataxia. Seizures	Hypernatremia
	Polyuria, polydipsia	

*See also Table 1-6.

CK, creatinine kinase; RBC, red blood cells; M, methanol; EG, ethylene glycol; IPA, Isopropyl alcohol; BDZ, benzodiazepines.

presented in Table 1-4. Blood tests indicating liver or renal insufficiency should alert the clinician to the patient's higher susceptibility to the effects of drugs and toxins. Close scrutiny of the electrocardiogram may reveal abnormalities that are characteristic, though never pathognomonic, of certain intoxications. The most notable is the QT prolongation seen after poisoning with tricyclic antidepressants; not only does this finding have diagnostic value, but it also carries great importance for management since it may lead to torsades de pointes and subsequent life-threatening ventricular fibrillation.[35]

Careful assessment of the acid-base balance is of utmost relevance in cases of possible toxic coma. Anion gap metabolic acidosis in the absence of ketosis, lactic acidosis, renal failure, or sepsis should prompt investigations to exclude poisoning with cyanide, carbon monoxide, methanol, ethylene glycol, salicylates, or toluene. Respiratory acidosis is less distinctive, occurring after intoxications with any central nervous system depressant (such as opioids, sedatives, or barbiturates). Identification of cyanide and carbon monoxide intoxications is particularly important since specific and potentially life-saving treatments are available for these conditions. Respiratory alkalosis typically occurs after theophylline and less severe salicylate intoxications. A more complete differential diagnosis of coma according to the findings on arterial blood gases is provided in Table 1-5. Patients should also be evaluated for the presence

Table 1-5. Differential Diagnosis of Coma According to the Findings on Arterial Blood Gases

Anion gap metabolic acidosis
Ketoacidosis (diabetes, starvation)
Lactic acidosis (sepsis, shock, seizures, adrenal failure, toxins, Wernicke's encephalopathy, carbon monoxide, cyanide, paraldehyde)
Uremia
Salicylates
Ethylene glycol
Methanol
Toluene

Metabolic alkalosis
Hyperglycemic nonketotic coma
Lithium

Respiratory acidosis
Barbiturates
Benzodiazepines
Opioids
Organophosphates
Tricyclic antidepressants
Primary hypercapnia (restrictive or obstructive lung disease, upper airway disorder, sleep apnea)

Respiratory alkalosis
Salicylates
Sympathomimetics
Anticholinergics
Diencephalic herniation
Autonomic storms
Liver failure
Hypoxia

of an osmolal gap (difference between measured and calculated osmolality). A large osmolal gap is found after poisoning with ethanol, ethylene glycol, methanol, and isopropanol. Mild elevations in osmolal gap may occur with uremia (osmolal gap < 20 mOsm)[36] and to a lesser degree with severe lactic acidosis, sepsis, or ketoacidosis (osmolal gap < 15 mOsm).[37]

While a positive toxicologic screen may be helpful—although it does not necessarily prove that the drug found is responsible for the coma—a negative screen has minimal value.[38] Many potent toxins are not detectable on routine laboratory screens used in the emergency department. Quantitative levels of specific suspected drugs or toxins (e.g., cyanide, carbon monoxide by way of carboxyhemoglobin, various anticonvulsants, barbiturates, lithium, ethanol, theophylline, salicylate,

digoxin, etc.) are much more informative and may be diagnostic. However, the clinician should always interpret the results in the individual clinical context to avoid being misled by inaccurate or unrelated information.

Isopropanol (isopropyl alcohol, IPA) is a readily available agent found in rubbing alcohol cleaning agents and antifreeze products which may be responsible for serious intoxications when ingested as a substitute for ethanol by alcoholics or with suicidal intentions.

After oral ingestion, IPA undergoes complete absorption within 30 minutes to 2 hours.[39,40] IPA is metabolized via liver alcohol dehydrogenase to acetone which is then cleared largely by the kidneys.[41,42] IPA intoxication typically does not produce acidosis and may frequently remain unsuspected after baseline laboratory testing as illustrated in our case. Its diagnosis hinges on the presence of an osmolal gap.[39] An osmolal gap greater than 15 mOsm/kg suggests intoxication with atypical alcohols (in the absence of ethanol) and should prompt further investigation using gas chromatography to identify methanol, IPA, or ethylene glycol. Typical clinical manifestations such as visual changes with methanol and crystalluria with ethylene glycol (Figure 1-1) may also help in the differential diagnosis. Distinctive features of alcohol intoxications are displayed in Table 1-6 and in Figure 1-2.

Of 27 cases of IPA intoxication reported in the literature, 5 were fatal.[40,43] Neurological manifestations ranged from altered mental status with ataxia to profound coma.[40,44] Associated systemic signs included severe hypotension, respiratory failure, rhabdomyolysis, gastritis, and hypoglycemia.[39,40,45]

Identification of severe IPA intoxication may allow early intervention with hemodialysis, which is 40 to 50 times more effective in removing IPA and acetone than urinary excretion.[45,46] Otherwise, the treatment should be focused on supporting vital functions and preventing complications.

■ The Pros and Cons

Our patient had sudden coma of unclear cause. He was intubated, afebrile, hemodynamically stable, and well ventilated and oxygenated. His neurological exam was remarkable for skew eye deviation, absent pontomesencephalic reflexes, and no response

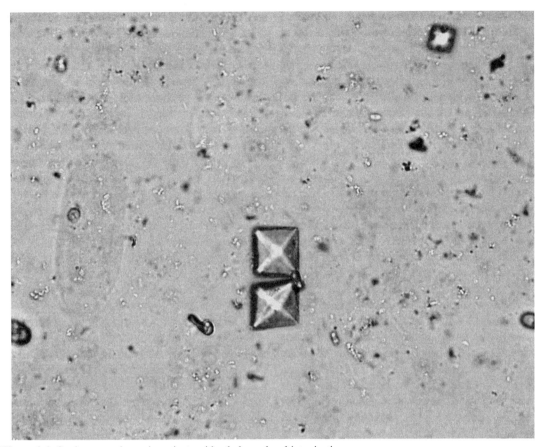

Figure 1-1. Oxalate crystal seen in patients with ethylene glycol intoxication.

Table 1-6. Distinctive Features of Alcohol Intoxications

Feature	ETOH	Methanol	Ethylene Glycol	IPA
Clinical finding	Ataxia	Blindness	Crystalluria	Hematemesis
Distinctive breath odor	Yes	Yes	No	Yes
Hypoglycemia	Yes	No	No	Yes
High CK	Yes	No	No	Yes
Metabolic acidosis	Mild	Severe	Severe	None
Anion gap	Moderate	Large	Large	Slight or none
Ketones	Acetoacetic	Ketobutyric	Acetone	Hydroxybutyrate
Osmolar gap	Yes	Yes	Yes	Yes
Metabolites	Hydroxybutyrate	Formic acid	Glycolic acid Oxalic acid	Acetone

ETOH, ethanol; IPA, isopropyl alcohol; CK, creatinine kinase.

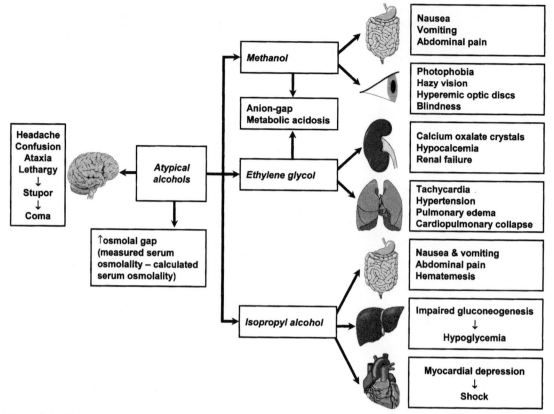

Figure 1-2. Clinical manifestations of intoxication with atypical alcohols.

to pain. CT scan of the brain was normal. Basic laboratory studies were unrevealing except for very mild elevation of creatinine kinase.

At this juncture, it was essential to focus the subsequent diagnostic workup to exclude treatable life-threatening conditions. Basilar artery occlusion was possible given the history of sudden coma and the presence of skew eye deviation on examination. In cases of suspected basilar artery occlusion, catheter cerebral angiography not only provides definitive diagnostic information but also makes recanalization treatment possible. However, this procedure is invasive, labor-intensive, and lengthy. While the first two disadvantages are of relatively minor significance when confronted with the severity of the diagnosis in question, saving time is fundamental when other dangerous conditions need to be excluded emergently if the angiography is nondiagnostic. Noninvasive angiography

using MR or CT technology can reliably exclude basilar artery occlusion. Yet if such occlusion is present, emergent catheterization is necessary for intra-arterial thrombolysis and mechanical clot disruption. Use of MR angiography may be combined with diffusion-weighted imaging and thus provide additional information on the extension of ischemic damage.[37]

Nonconvulsive status epilepticus was not supported by history or examination in our patient. The onset of coma was witnessed and there had been no convulsive movements. No subtle twitching movements were noticed on examination. Still, the diagnosis was possible and could only be totally excluded by electroencephalography.

There were no features suggestive of meningitis or encephalitis. Onset was more sudden than would be expected with a central nervous system infection. Body temperature was normal and the neck was supple. There was no leukocytosis. We considered that lumbar puncture was not emergently indicated.

Normal baseline laboratory results excluded most life-threatening metabolic disorders, although formal testing for endocrine abnormalities had not been performed. Toxic causes of coma deserved careful consideration. The detection of a large osmolal gap suggested the possibility of alcohol intoxication. In the absence of acidosis, IPA was the most likely culprit. Once the intoxication was confirmed by gas chromatography, the major decision was whether to dialyze the patient. We decided to forgo hemodialysis in light of the incipient signs of clinical recovery and the rapid decline in measured serum osmolality and IPA level.

■ **Main Points**

- When evaluating an unresponsive patient, the first priority is to stabilize ventilation, gas exchange, and hemodynamic status; treat seizures; provide comfort; and treat injuries.
- Conditions simulating coma should always be considered and rapidly excluded.
- The main goals of the initial neurological examination of a comatose patient are distinguishing between structural brain lesions and diffuse cerebral disorders and identifying signs of brain herniation.
- When developing a list of differential diagnoses, emphasis should be focused on conditions that lead to persistent morbidity or mortality when left untreated.
- The presence of focal neurological signs does not necessarily imply that the coma is due to a structural lesion.
- In comatose patients with negative brain CT, consider basilar artery thrombosis, nonconvulsive status epilepticus, fulminant meningitis or encephalitis, anoxic-ischemic brain damage, intoxications, and acute metabolic derangements.
- Careful assessment of the acid-base balance is essential when assessing a diffuse cerebral disorder. However, normal arterial blood gases do not exclude certain intoxications.
- Screen for the presence of an osmolal gap (measured serum osmolality – calculated serum osmolality) on any patient with unexplained coma. A large osmolal gap (> 20 mOsm) is highly suggestive of intoxication with alcohols, even in the absence of metabolic acidosis.

Acknowledgment

Part of this case example has been published as a clinical note.[47]

■ **References**

1. Plum F, Posner JB. *Diagnosis of Stupor and Coma,* 3rd ed. Philadelphia, FA Davis, 1982.
2. Dehaene I, Martin JJ. "Locked-in" syndrome: a clinico-pathological study of two cases. *Eur Neurol* 1976; 14:81–89
3. Carroll BT, Anfinson TJ, Kennedy JC, Yendrek R, Boutros M, Bilon A. Catatonic disorder due to general medical conditions. *J Neuropsychiatry Clin Neurosci* 1994;6:122–133.
4. Teasdale G, Jennett B. Assessment of coma and impaired consciousness: a practical scale. *Lancet* 1974;2:81–84.
5. Ropper AH. Lateral displacement of the brain and level of consciousness in patients with an acute hemispheral mass. *N Engl J Med* 1986;314:953–958.
6. Helprin GA, Clarke GM. Unilateral fixed dilated pupil associated with nebulised ipratropium [letter]. *Lancet* 1986;2:1469.
7. Cordova S, Lee R. Fixed, dilated pupils in the ICU: another recoverable cause. *Anesth Intensive Care* 2000;28:91–93.
8. Boutros G, Insler MS. Reversible papillary miosis during a hyperglycemic episode: case report. *Diabetologia* 1984;27:50–51.
9. Wijdicks EF, Young GB. Myoclonus status in comatose patients after cardiac arrest. *Lancet* 1994;343:1642–1643.
10. Ropper AH, Shafran B. Brain edema after stroke: clinical syndrome and intracranial pressure. *Arch Neurol* 1984;41:26–29.
11. Kubik C, Adams R. Occlusion of the basilar artery: a clinical and pathological study. *Brain* 1946;69:73–121.
12. Archer CR, Horenstein S. Basilar artery occlusion: clinical and radiological correlation. *Stroke* 1977;8(3):383–390.
13. Chase TN, Moretti L, Prensky AL. Clinical and electroencephalographic manifestations of vascular lesions of the pons. *Neurology* 1968;18:357–368.
14. Sato M, Tanaka S, Kohama A. "Top of the basilar" syndrome: clinico-radiological evaluation. *Neuroradiology* 1987;29:354–359.

15. Fisher CM. The "herald hemiparesis" of basilar artery occlusion. *Arch Neurol* 1988;45:1301–1303.

16. Ehsan T, Hayat G, Malkoff MD, Selhorst JB, Martin D, Manepalli A. Hyperdense basilar artery: an early computed tomography sign of thrombosis. *J Neuroimaging* 1994;4:200–205.

17. Castillo M, Falcone S, Naidich TP, Bowen B, Quencer RM. Imaging in acute basilar artery thrombosis. *Neuroradiology* 1994;36:426–429.

18. Devuyst G, Bogousslavsky J, Meuli R, Moncayo J, de Freitas G, van Melle G. Stroke or transient ischemic attacks with basilar artery stenosis or occlusion: clinical patterns and outcome. *Arch Neurol* 2002;59:567–573.

19. Brandt T, von Kummer R, Muller-Kuppers M, Hacke W. Thrombolytic therapy of acute basilar artery occlusion: variables affecting recanalization and outcome. *Stroke* 1996;27:875–881.

20. Grond M, Rudolf J, Schmulling S, Stenzel C, Neveling M, Heiss WD. Early intravenous thrombolysis with recombinant tissue-type plasminogen activator in vertebrobasilar ischemic stroke. *Arch Neurol* 1998;55:466–469.

21. Spreer J, Els T, Hetzel A, Arnold S, Klisch J, Huppertz HJ, Oehm E, Schumacher M. Primary stenting as emergency therapy in acute basilar artery occlusion. *Neuroradiology* 2002;44:791–795.

22. Drislane FW. presentation, evaluation, and treatment of nonconvulsive status epilepticus. *Epilepsy Behav* 2000;1:301–314.

23. Dennis LJ, Claassen J, Hirsch LJ, Emerson RG, Connolly ES, Mayer SA. Nonconvulsive status epilepticus after subarachnoid hemorrhage. *Neurosurgery* 2002;51:1136–1143.

24. Chow KM, Wang AY, Hui AC, Wong TY, Szeto CC, Li PK. Nonconvulsive status epilepticus in peritoneal dialysis patients. *Am J Kidney Dis* 2001;38:400–405.

25. Quagliarello VJ, Scheld WM. Treatment of bacterial meningitis. *N Engl J Med* 1997;336:708–716.

26. de Gans J, van de Beek D; European Dexamethasone in Adulthood Bacterial Meningitis Study Investigators. Dexamethasone in adults with bacterial meningitis. *N Engl J Med* 2002;347:1549–1556.

27. Bernard SA, Gray TW, Buist MD, Jones BM, Silvester W, Gutteridge G, Smith K. Treatment of comatose survivors of out-of-hospital cardiac arrest with induced hypothermia. *N Engl J Med* 2002;346:557–563.

28. Hypothermia after Cardiac Arrest Study Group. Mild therapeutic hypothermia to improve the neurologic outcome after cardiac arrest. *N Engl J Med* 2002;346:549–556.

29. Singhal AB, Topcuoglu MA, Koroshetz WJ. Diffusion MRI in three types of anoxic encephalopathy. *J Neurol Sci* 2002;196:37–40.

30. Jordan RM. Myxedema coma: pathophysiology, therapy, and factors affecting prognosis. *Med Clin North Am* 1995;79:185–194.

31. Howton JC. Thyroid storm presenting as coma. *Ann Emerg Med* 1988;17:343–345.

32. Ziegler R. Hypercalcemic crisis. *J Am Soc Nephrol* 2001;12(Suppl 17):S3–9.

33. Post SS. Hyperphosphatemic hypocalcemic coma caused by hypertonic sodium phosphate (fleet) enema intoxication. *J Clin Gastroenterol* 1997;24:192.

34. Wallis WE, Willoughby E, Baker P. Coma in the Wernicke-Korsakoff syndrome. *Lancet* 1978;2:400–401.

35. De Ponti F, Poluzzi E, Cavalli A, Recanatini M, Montanaro N. Safety of nonantiarrhythmic drugs that prolong the QT interval or induce torsade de pointes: an overview. *Drug Saf* 2002;25:263–286.

36. Sklar AH, Linas SL. The osmolal gap in renal failure. *Ann Intern Med* 1983;98:481–482.

37. Schelling JR, Howard RL, Winter SD, Linas SL. Increased osmolal gap in alcoholic ketoacidosis and lactic acidosis. *Ann Intern Med* 1990;113:580–582.

38. Osterloh JD. Utility and reliability of emergency toxicologic testing. *Emerg Med Clin North Am* 1990;8:693–723.

39. Monaghan MS, Ackerman BH, Olsen KM, Farmer C, Pappas AA. The use of delta osmolality to predict serum isopropanol and acetone concentrations. *Pharmacotherapy* 1993;13:60–63.

40. Zaman F, Pervez A, Abreo K. Isopropyl alcohol intoxication: a diagnostic challenge. *Am J Kidney Dis* 2002;40:E12.

41. Natowicz M, Donahue J, Gorman L, et al. Pharmacokinetic analysis of a case of isopropanol intoxication. *Clin Chem* 1985;31:326–328.

42. Gaudet MP, Fraser GL. Isopropanol ingestion: case report with pharmacokinetic analysis. *Am J Emerg Med* 1989;7:297–299.

43. Adelson L. Fatal intoxication with isopropyl alcohol. *Am J Clin Pathol* 1962;38:144–151

44. Rich J, Scheife RT, Katz N, Caplan LR. Isopropyl alcohol intoxication. *Arch Neurol* 1990;47:322–324.

45. Abramson S, Singh AK. Treatment of the alcohol intoxications: ethylene glycol, methanol and isopropanol. *Curr Opin Nephrol Hypertens* 2000;9:695–701.

46. Rosansky SJ. Isopropyl alcohol poisoning treated with hemodialysis: kinetics of isopropyl alcohol and acetone removal. *J Toxicol Clin Toxicol* 1982;19:265–271.

47. Muller-Kronast N, Rabinstein AA, Voung L, Forteza AM. Isopropanol intoxication mimicking basilar artery thrombosis. *Neurology* 2003;61:1456–1457.

Chapter 2
Acute Neuro-ophthalmological Conditions

Valérie Biousse and Nancy J. Newman

Patients with neurological and neurosurgical diseases commonly present to the emergency room with neuro-ophthalmological symptoms and signs. A brief neuro-ophthalmological evaluation may allow immediate recognition of neurological or neurosurgical emergencies. The neuro-ophthalmic examination in the emergency room should include the measurement of visual acuity with a near card (using the patient's reading glasses), color vision testing (with a red cap), confrontation visual field (with your fingers and a red cap), orbital and lid evaluation looking for ptosis, lid retraction, proptosis, pupil evaluation (in the dark and in the light, near reaction, relative afferent pupillary defect), corneal sensitivity, extraocular movements (versions, oculocephalic maneuvers, cross cover, nystagmus), examination of the external aspect of the eye with a penlight and a direct ophthalmoscope (red eye, cornea, cataract, etc.), and dilated funduscopy with a direct ophthalmoscope.[1,2] Most patients are usually very sensitive to any change in their visual function and this chapter will address the most commonly presenting signs.

■ Acute Visual Loss

The Patient

A 75-year-old man came to the emergency room with acute visual loss in his right eye. He had awoken that morning with severely decreased vision.

Over the past 2 days, he had repeated episodes of transient visual loss of his right eye lasting a few seconds. His past medical history included hypertension. He denied ocular pain or headaches. His neurological and general examinations were normal. Neuro-ophthalmological examination in the emergency room showed visual acuity of "count fingers" in the right eye and 20/30 in the left eye with a near card (and the patient's reading glasses). Pupils were round, equal, and reactive to light; there was a dense right relative afferent pupillary defect. Extraocular movements were full in both eyes. The anterior segments of both eyes appeared normal with a penlight. Corneal sensation was intact OU. Intraocular pressure was normal in both eyes (as assessed by the doctor's fingers). Confrontation visual field was full in the left eye. Dilated funduscopic examination was normal in the left eye and showed optic nerve swelling in the right eye, suggestive of anterior ischemic optic neuropathy (Figure 2-1). An erythrocyte sedimentation rate (ESR) obtained in the emergency room was 89 mm/hr, raising suspicion for giant cell arteritis as the cause of the ischemic optic neuropathy. The patient was admitted and treated with intravenous methylprednisolone (250 mg every 6 hours) during 3 days, then prednisone 1 mg/kg/day. A right temporal artery biopsy was performed 2 days later and confirmed the diagnosis of giant cell arteritis. The patient's vision did not improve, but his left eye remained normal.

The Problem

- What diagnostic tests are helpful in giant cell arteritis?
- When should corticosteroid therapy start?
- What is the value of temporal artery biopsy?

The Evidence

When a patient complains of visual loss, it is of foremost importance to determine whether the visual loss involves one eye or both eyes. Indeed, bilateral visual loss is rarely due to a lesion involving both eyes at the same time (Table 2-1). More often, it is related to a lesion involving the intracranial visual pathways such as the chiasm or retrochiasmal visual pathways (Table 2-2).[1,2] Unilateral visual loss is most often secondary to ocular diseases. It can be transient or permanent (Tables 2-3, 2-4). The diagnosis of unilateral visual loss relies mostly on the ophthalmological examination. Optic nerve pallor takes 4 to 6 weeks to develop after initial injury, and therefore is not seen in emergency. Multiple retinal or optic nerve diseases can be associated with neurological and neurosurgical emergencies. The diagnosis of unilateral optic nerve disease relies mostly on the finding of a relative afferent pupillary defect, and of optic disc swelling if the anterior portion of the optic nerve is involved, such as in this patient (see Figure 2-1). Acute visual loss in the elderly should prompt a presumptive diagnosis of giant cell arteritis (GCA), even without prominent systemic symptoms. Indeed, up to 25 percent of patients with visual loss from GCA do not have any systemic symptoms.[3] Because GCA can strike the fellow eye within hours or days after visual loss, the diagnosis of GCA is urgent and should be suspected in the emergency room in any elderly patient presenting with acute visual loss. Visual loss in GCA is most often due to anterior ischemic optic neuropathy, sometimes associated with retinal or choroidal ischemia (Figure 2-2).[4–6] Anterior ischemic optic neuropathy preceded by episodes of transient visual loss is highly suggestive of GCA. In GCA, if the optic nerve in the second eye becomes infarcted, it will do so within 48 hours in one-third of untreated patients and within

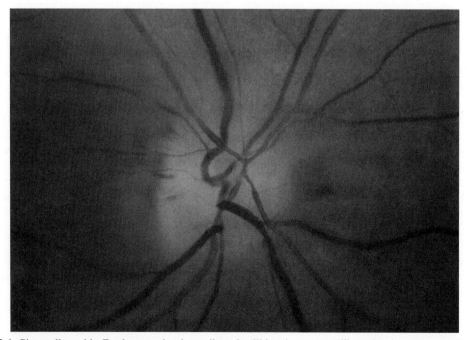

Figure 2-1. Giant cell arteritis. Funduscopy showing unilateral pallid optic nerve swelling related to acute anterior ischemic optic neuropathy in a patient with giant cell arteritis.

Table 2-1. Visual Loss—Differential Diagnosis

Bilateral (persistent when the patient closes either eye)
Ocular
  Transient visual obscuration (bilateral optic nerve head swelling)
  Hyperglycemia
  Bilateral ocular disease such as cataracts
  Bilateral hypertensive or diabetic retinopathy
  Bilateral optic neuropathy
Intracranial visual pathways
  Bitemporal homonymous hemianopia (chiasm)
  Homonymous hemianopia (retrochiasmal visual pathways)
  Bilateral homonymous hemianopia or cerebral blindness (bilateral occipital lobes)

Unilateral (disappears when the patient closes the affected eye)
Ocular disease
Optic neuropathy

Table 2-2. Acute Cerebral Blindness—Differential Diagnosis

Bilateral occipital infarction
Superior sagittal venous sinus thrombosis
Cerebral hypoxia
Dural fistula
Occipital arteriovenous malformation
Head trauma
Hypertensive encephalopathy
Eclampsia
Cyclosporine/Tacrolimus toxicity
Carbon monoxide intoxication
Mitochondrial encephalopathy, lactic acidosis, stroke-like episodes (MELAS)
Progressive multifocal leukoencephalopathy
Migraine

Table 2-3. Transient Monocular Visual Loss—Differential Diagnosis

Vascular ("amaurosis fugax")
  Retinal ischemia
    Central and branch retinal arteries
    Central and branch retinal veins
  Choroidal ischemia
    Posterior ciliary arteries
  Optic nerve ischemia
    Posterior ciliary arteries
  Ocular ischemia
    Ophthalmic artery
  ? Migraine
Optic nerve head swelling
Anomalous disk
  Disk drusen
  Congenital disk anomalies
Optic nerve compression (orbital mass)
Uhthoff's phenomenon
Lacrimal disorders (dry eyes)
Keratoconus
Corneal edema
Hyphema
Intermittent angle closure glaucoma
Serous retinal detachment

The Pros and Cons

one week in another one-third. Involvement of the second eye after one month is rare.[3] Erythrocyte sedimentation rate (ESR) and C-reactive protein (CRP) remain important diagnostic tests. In less than 10 percent of patients, ESR is low or normal, but CRP is elevated in most of those patients.[4–6] GCA is exquisitely sensitive to corticosteroids which should be started immediately to prevent involvement of the other eye. The diagnosis of GCA relies on a positive temporal artery biopsy, which should be performed within 2 weeks of starting corticosteroids.[3]

High-dose corticosteroid treatment rarely restores vision but usually prevents involvement of the other eye. One study found visual loss in 9 of 91 patients while on corticosteroids but usually within the first week after initiation of therapy.[7] In this study, deterioration was less common in patients treated with intravenous methylprednisolone. Current regimens employ prednisone 1–1.5 mg/kg/day or a loading dose with intravenous methylprednisolone 1–2 g/day for 3 days followed by prednisone 1–1.5 mg/kg/day. Neuro-ophthalmologists tend to use the latter, although there is no trial supporting the use of high-dose intravenous corticosteroids in

Table 2-4. Painful Transient Monocular Visual Loss—Differential Diagnosis

Giant cell arteritis
Internal carotid artery dissection
Ocular ischemic syndrome
Intermittent angle closure glaucoma
? Migraine

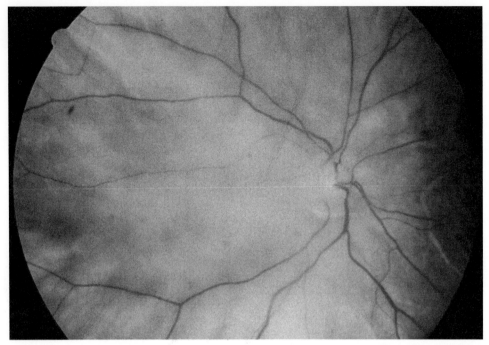

Figure 2-2. Giant cell arteritis. Funduscopy showing retinal and choroidal ischemia in a patient with giant cell arteritis.

patients with visual loss from GCA. Anecdotal case reports suggest a higher rate of visual recovery with high-dose intravenous methylprednisolone than with PO prednisone alone.[3] However, steroids should be used with caution in elderly patients with high risk of complications such as vascular events and osteoporosis. Tapering corticosteroids is mostly considered when ESR and CRP remain consistently low typically 2 weeks after initiation of therapy. One protocol followed patients every 2 to 3 weeks until prednisone reached 40 mg and monthly after that for 3 months.

The Main Points

- Presume that all elderly patients with acute visual loss could have GCA and examine them promptly.
- The diagnosis of GCA should be suspected in all elderly patients with anterior ischemic optic neuropathy and visual acuity worse than 20/200, previous episodes of transient monocular visual loss (Figure 2–3), and systemic symptoms such as jaw claudication, headache,

scalp tenderness, anorexia, weight loss, fatigue, and elevated ESR or CRP.
- Anemia or elevated platelet count should raise suspicion of this inflammatory syndrome even in the setting of a normal sedimentation rate.[8,9] CRP is often elevated prior to the sedimentation rate and should be monitored.[3]

■ Acute Ptosis

The Patient

A 48-year-old woman came to the emergency room with a 2-day history of droopiness of the left upper eyelid (Figure 2-4). Her past medical history was unremarkable. Neurological and general physical examinations were normal. Neuro-ophthalmological examination showed visual acuity of 20/20 OU with a near card (and the patient's reading glasses). Pupils were round, equal, and reactive to light; there was no relative afferent pupillary defect. There was 2 mm ptosis of the left upper eyelid. Extraocular movements were limited in all directions of gaze in both eyes. During examination the

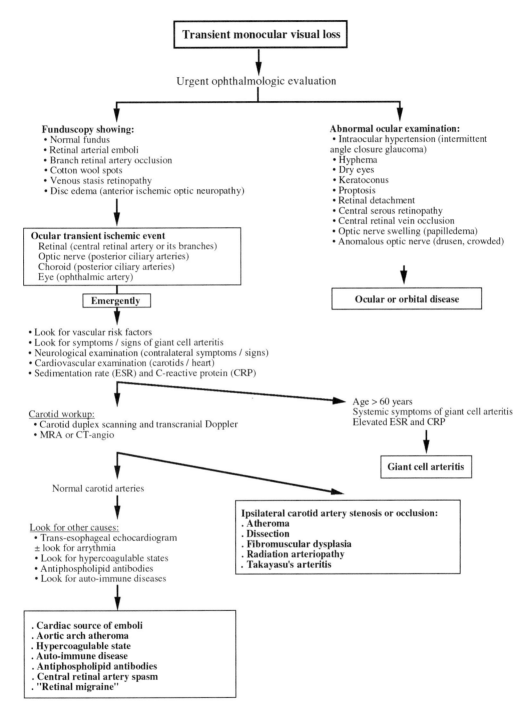

Figure 2-3. Diagram showing the management of transient monocular visual loss.

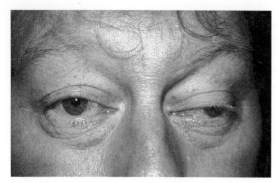

Figure 2-4. Myasthenia gravis. Bilateral asymmetric ptosis in a patient with myasthenia gravis. Note the right ptosis that appears when the left upper lid is elevated. The eye movements are limited in all directions of gaze.

patient complained of intermittent binocular horizontal diplopia. With sustained upgaze, the left ptosis worsened and she developed a 2 mm ptosis in the right eye. After 5 minutes of rest, her ptosis improved dramatically and her diplopia resolved. Corneal sensation was intact OU. The anterior segments of both eyes appeared normal with a penlight. The eyes were soft and symmetric (with the doctor's fingers). Confrontation visual fields were full in both eyes. Dilated funduscopic examination was normal in both eyes. The patient was diagnosed with presumed ocular myasthenia gravis. Her review of system was negative for shortness of breath, voice changes, dysphagia, proximal limb weakness, or fatigue with exercise. Acetylcholine receptor antibodies were obtained and a chest CT was ordered to rule out a thymoma. The patient was scheduled to see a neurologist 2 weeks later. Over the following days she developed persistent diplopia with worsening of her ptosis. One week later, she presented again to the emergency room with respiratory distress and dysphagia.

The Problem

- How to diagnose ocular myasthenia and differentiate it from other causes of diplopia (e.g., third nerve palsy)?
- Is there a role of corticosteroids in ocular myasthenia?

The Evidence

A unilateral or bilateral ptosis of more than 1–2 mm may be secondary to a lesion involving the lid levator muscle (senile ptosis, myopathies), the neuromuscular junction (myasthenia), or the oculomotor nerve (third cranial nerve). The neuro-ophthalmological evaluation allows a clinical topographic diagnosis of the lesion, and helps determine which studies should be obtained. New onset ptosis should alert the clinician to look for a third nerve palsy. When the ptosis covers the visual axis, patients do not complain of diplopia and careful examination should look for ocular motor paresis and anisocoria. A common cause of "mild ptosis," usually 2 mm or less, is Horner's syndrome, in which the palpebral fissure is reduced. Pupillary examination showing anisocoria with the smaller pupil ipsilateral to the ptosis confirms the diagnosis of Horner's syndrome. Ocular myopathies are rarely seen in emergent consultation. Ocular myasthenia is not a therapeutic emergency, unless the patient has symptoms and signs suggestive of systemic myasthenia, such as respiratory distress or dysphagia. The diagnosis of ocular myasthenia is usually made clinically and then confirmed by an edrophonium (Tensilon) test. Ancillary tests such as acetylcholine receptor antibodies, electromyogram, and chest CT do not need to be obtained emergently. However, although about 75 percent of patients with myasthenia gravis initially present with ocular signs, about 60 percent of these patients eventually develop other signs and symptoms suggesting systemic myasthenia.[10] In general, patients with only ocular manifestations at onset who go on to develop systemic manifestations do so within 2 years.[10]

The Pros and Cons

Whether to systematically treat patients with pure ocular myasthenia with agents such as corticosteroids that may reduce the rate of systemic myasthenia remains debated. Indeed, a few studies have suggested that oral prednisone prescribed as soon as the diagnosis of ocular myasthenia is made, in addition to anticholinesterase drugs, may prevent or delay the development of systemic symptoms.[10] It should be kept in mind that muscle weakness frequently worsens before improving when steroids are initiated.

The Main Points

- When you see a patient with ptosis, always carefully check the pupils in the dark and in the light. An ipsilateral mydriasis is suggestive of third nerve palsy; an ipsilateral miosis is suggestive of Horner's syndrome.
- Myopathies and myasthenia are very rarely associated with pain, whereas a third nerve palsy and Horner's syndrome may be painful.
- When suspecting myasthenia, carefully look for systemic symptoms, which may change your immediate management. Patients with pure ocular myasthenia are rarely corrected by anti-cholinesterase agents alone. Corticosteroids are often helpful in the treatment of diplopia.

■ Diplopia

The Patient

A 52-year-old woman came to the emergency room with a 2-day history of right orbital pain associated with droopiness of the right upper eyelid (Figure 2-5A). Her past medical history was remarkable for systemic hypertension. When she opened her right eye her vision was normal, but she saw double. Neurological and general examinations were unremarkable. Neuro-ophthalmological examination showed visual acuity of 20/40 OD and 2/30 OS with a near card (and the patient's reading glasses). Pupils were round. The left pupil was reactive to light, but the right pupil was only moderately reactive; there was no relative afferent pupillary defect. There was partial ptosis of the right upper eyelid. Extraocular movements were normal in the left eye. In the right eye, only abduction was intact (see Figure 2-5A). Corneal sensation was normal OU. The anterior segments of both eyes appeared normal with a penlight. The eyes were soft and symmetric (with the doctor's fingers). Confrontation visual fields were full in both eyes. Dilated funduscopic examination was normal in both eyes. The patient was diagnosed with a right third nerve palsy with pupil involvement, most likely secondary to a compressive lesion. A MRI and MRA of the brain were immediately obtained in the emergency room and showed a right posterior communication artery aneurysm (see Figure 2-5B).

A conventional angiogram was performed, during which the aneurysm was coiled. Follow-up one week later showed normal pupils. The patient's diplopia resolved within 6 weeks.

The Problem

- How can diplopia be easily and reliably assessed?
- What are urgent causes of diplopia?

The Evidence

Patients with diplopia usually present emergently. The first step is to confirm that the diplopia is binocular (i.e., the diplopia resolves when the patient closes either eye). Monocular diplopia is due to an ocular problem (e.g., refractive error, cataract, macular edema), and it is not an emergency.[2] Binocular diplopia occurs as a result of ocular misalignment and is secondary to abnormal extraocular movements. There are multiple causes of ocular misalignment, such as diseases involving the muscles themselves (thyroid disease), the neuromuscular junction (myasthenia), cranial nerve palsies (third, fourth, and sixth), or internuclear or supranuclear abnormalities. The identification of the muscle responsible for the diplopia and recognition of signs suggestive of an orbital syndrome (visual loss, proptosis, redness, pain), ptosis, pupillary abnormalities, disc edema, and other neurological symptoms and signs, all help to localize the lesion.[2] Third nerve palsies may indicate a neurosurgical emergency such as intracranial aneurysm or pituitary apoplexy.[11,12] Sixth nerve palsies can be associated with raised intracranial pressure. The association of a sixth nerve palsy with an ipsilateral Horner's syndrome localizes the lesion to the cavernous sinus and may reveal a cavernous sinus aneurysm.[12] Isolated fourth nerve palsy is rarely an emergency. Most often, the diplopia is secondary to a decompensation of a congenital fourth nerve palsy, which may occur at any age. It may also result from minor head trauma.[12] Diplopia can also result from multiple ocular motor nerve palsies such as from Miller-Fisher syndrome, the prognosis of which mostly depends on whether the acute polyradiculopathy generalizes.[12] Supranuclear

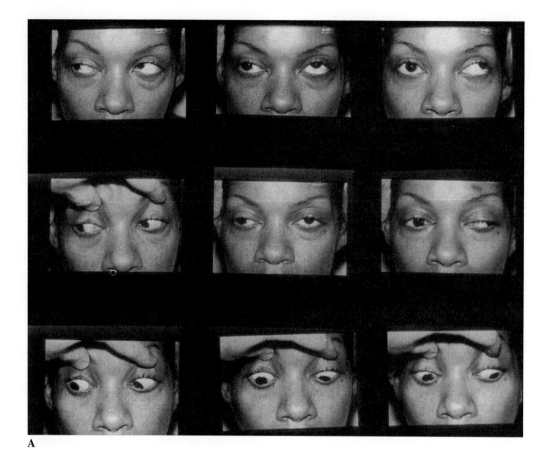

A

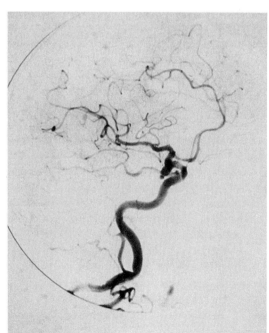

B

Figure 2-5. Third nerve palsy. Right third nerve palsy with mydriasis (A). Angiogram (B) showing a right posterior communication artery aneurysm.

motility disorders are often emergencies since they could be associated with lesions affecting the brainstem. Vertical gaze palsies such as seen in the dorsal midbrain syndrome (Parinaud's syndrome) may indicate pineal or third ventricle tumors, sometimes associated with obstructive hydrocephalus. Internuclear ophthalmoplegia is associated with brainstem lesions. Skew deviation may result from any lesion involving the vestibular pathways in the brainstem. Horizontal gaze palsies are usually associated with an ipsilateral peripheral facial palsy and occur with pontine lesions at the level of the sixth nerve nucleus. Rarely, thalamic lesions produce an esotropia (thalamic esotropia).

In a patient with isolated third nerve palsy, careful evaluation of the extraocular muscles and the pupils dictates the management (Figure 2-6). In younger patients, a compressive lesion should always be excluded by neuroimaging, regardless of the clinical presentation. In patients older than 50 years, mydriasis is always concerning and neuroimaging should be obtained in the emergency room. The pupillary fibers are located at the periphery of the third nerve in the subarachnoid space.

Therefore, compression of the third nerve will typically cause ipsilateral mydriasis as well as paresis involving all or part of the extraocular muscles innervated by the third nerve.[13] The most threatening neurological emergencies responsible for isolated third nerve palsies are intracranial aneurysms (posterior communicating artery, superior cerebellar artery, and basilar artery) and pituitary apoplexy. Because of their anatomical location, pupillary fibers are usually spared in patients with ischemic third nerve palsy, who present with pupil-sparing complete third nerve palsies. When not all extraocular muscles innervated by the third are involved, a compressive lesion should be suspected, even if the pupil is spared (see Figures 2-5 and 2-6).[11,12]

The Pros and Cons

The most debated topic is when to obtain a conventional angiogram to document or exclude an aneurysm in a patient with an isolated third nerve palsy (see Figure 2-6). Although very sensitive, MRA or CT-angio cannot definitely exclude a

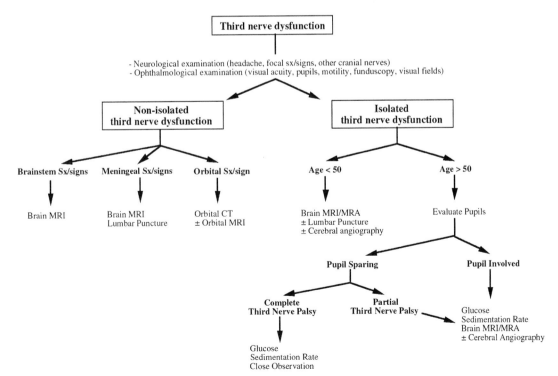

Figure 2-6. Diagram showing the management of third nerve palsy.

small intracranial aneurysm.[14–20] When the clinical suspicion of intracranial aneurysm is high in a patient with a third nerve palsy, a conventional angiogram must be ordered emergently.

The Main Points

- Beware of compression from an aneurysm when a third nerve palsy is partial—even when the pupil is spared. The "rule of the pupil" applies only if the patient has a complete third nerve palsy (i.e., all muscles innervated by the third nerve are affected) (see Figure 2-6).[13,17,19]
- A patient with pupil-sparing complete third nerve palsy must be seen in follow-up to verify that the pupil remains normal, since mydriasis may be delayed for a few days in patients with compressive third nerve palsy.

■ Anisocoria

The Patient

A 28-year-old woman presented to the emergency room with a 5-day history of pain over her right face. The morning of the fifth day, she noticed that her left pupil was larger than her right. Her past medical history was remarkable for migraine without aura. Neurological and general examinations were unremarkable. Neuro-ophthalmological examination showed visual acuity of 20/20 OU. The right palpebral fissure was 2 mm smaller than the left. Pupils were round and reactive to light. There was anisocoria, with the left pupil larger than the right. The anisocoria was exacerbated in the dark, suggesting decreased dilatation of the right pupil (Figure 2-7A). There was no relative afferent pupillary defect. There was no proptosis. Extraocular movements were full in both eyes. Corneal sensation was intact OU. The anterior segments of both eyes appeared normal with a penlight. The eyes were soft and symmetric (with the doctor's fingers). Confrontation visual fields were full in both eyes. Dilated funduscopic examination was normal OU. The anisocoria was believed to reflect a right Horner's syndrome, implicating a lesion along the right sympathetic pathways. The

absence of other neurological symptoms and signs, and the association with pain, was highly suggestive of a spontaneous dissection of the ipsilateral internal carotid artery. This was confirmed by a MRI/MRA of the brain and circle of Willis obtained in the emergency room (Figure 2-7B). The MRA of the circle of Willis showed severely decreased signal in the right middle cerebral artery, suggesting poor blood flow (Figure 2-7C). Because of the high risk of hemodynamic cerebral infarction, the patient was admitted and bedrest was ordered. She was monitored with transcranial Doppler, and discharged 5 days later after normalization of the blood flow in the right middle cerebral artery. She was anticoagulated for 3 months and recovered without complication. At 3-month follow up, repeat MRI and MRA showed recanalization of the right internal carotid artery.

The Problem

- How to evaluate mydriasis and miosis in the emergency room?
- What imaging studies are required?

The Evidence

When a patient presents with anisocoria, the first step is to determine which pupil is abnormal by evaluating the pupil size in the dark and in the light. If the large pupil does not constrict well in the light (anisocoria worse in the light than in the dark), it is the mydriatic pupil that is abnormal; if the small pupil does not dilate well in the dark (anisocoria worse in the dark than in the light), it is the miotic pupil that is abnormal. Other neurological symptoms and signs besides anisocoria could further localize the lesion as a Horner's syndrome (ipsilateral mild ptosis in the eye with the small pupil), a third nerve palsy (ipsilateral ptosis and ocular dysmotility in the eye with the big pupil), or an Adie's pupil (isolated pupillary mydriasis frequently with an intact near response).[2] The most important cause of mydriasis is a third nerve palsy. Mydriasis in the setting of a third nerve palsy suggests third nerve compression. In a patient with altered mental status and mydriasis, temporal herniation should be suspected. Intracranial aneurysms (typically of the

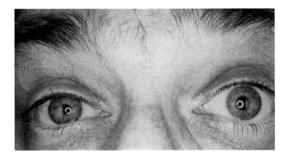
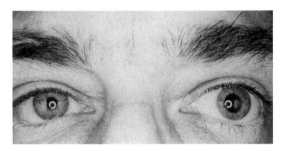
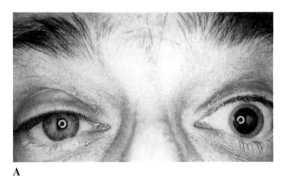

A

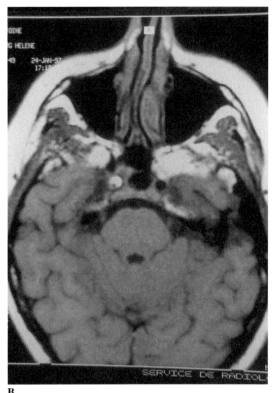

B

Figure 2-7. Horner's syndrome. (A) In the light, there is a mild anisocoria with the right pupil being smaller than the left (top). In the dark (middle), the amount of anisocoria increases and the right pupil does not dilate, confirming the diagnosis of right Horner's syndrome. 45 minutes after putting 2 drops of hydroxyamphetamine in both eyes (bottom), the left pupil dilates while the right does not, suggesting a lesion involving the third-order neuron of the right sympathetic pathway (pericarotid sympathetic fibers). The T1-weighted axial brain MRI (B) shows a hyperintense signal consistent with a right internal carotid artery dissection. The MRA of the circle of Willis (C) demonstrates a decreased signal in the right middle cerebral artery suggesting poor flow distal to the dissection.

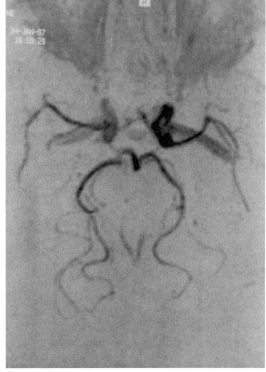

C

posterior communicating, superior cerebellar, or basilar arteries), and pituitary apoplexy are two examples of neurological emergencies that may present with third nerve palsy. In these cases, the mydriasis is not isolated and is associated with at least a slight ptosis and abnormal extraocular movements.[11] Adie's pupil is a cause of isolated mydriasis. The pupil does not react to light but does constrict slowly when the patient looks at a near target (accommodation). Dilute pilocarpine 1 percent (1/10) constricts the abnormal pupil while it has no effect on the normal pupil (denervation hypersensitivity).[1,2] Pharmacological mydriasis (mydriatic drops, scopolamine patch, nebulizers) is isolated and the pupil shows either no or only partial constriction with pilocarpine 1 percent (which provokes a tight miosis in the normal eye).[1,2] Traumatic mydriasis is common after blunt trauma, and results from tears in the iris sphincter muscle.[1,2] A unilateral miosis is either pharmacological (pilocarpine commonly prescribed in glaucoma patients) or related to a Horner's syndrome.[1,2] Two causes of isolated Horner's syndrome are neurological emergencies: internal carotid artery dissections and cavernous sinus aneurysms.[21] In both cases, Horner's syndrome is secondary to involvement of the pericarotid sympathetic fibers (third order) and is usually associated with pain.

Up to 60 percent of patients with internal carotid artery dissections present with isolated painful Horner's syndrome. These patients are at high risk of cerebral infarction that develops within 2 weeks after the painful Horner's syndrome in 80 percent of cases and may occur as late as one month later. After one month the risk of cerebral infarction is extremely low.[22,23]

The Pros and Cons

The proper treatment of cervical artery dissections is not known. While there are no trials evaluating the optimal management of these patients, most experts treat patients with cervical artery dissections with heparin, then warfarin for at least 3 months.[22,23] We strongly recommend that all patients with isolated painful Horner's syndrome and suspected carotid dissection be admitted emergently and treated with heparin when seen within 2 to 3 weeks after the onset of the Horner's syndrome.

When they are seen more than one month after the onset of the Horner's syndrome they may be treated as outpatients with antiplatelet agents.

The Main Points

- Determine the cause of anisocoria before imaging the patient in the emergency room. The noncontrast CT scan of the brain often obtained in the emergency room for any patient with anisocoria is useless in most instances. It will miss the most emergent causes of third nerve palsy and Horner's syndrome. Furthermore, a patient with third nerve palsy or isolated mydriasis does not always need to be imaged; on the other hand, an intracranial aneurysm must not be missed. The appropriate imaging has to be carefully chosen in the setting of an emergency (see Figure 2-6).
- A painful acute Horner's syndrome is due to a carotid dissection until proven otherwise. However, in some cases of Horner's syndrome (painless or chronic), imaging can be delayed until a neuro-ophthalmologist can localize the lesion with hydroxyamphetamine (hydroxyamphetamine does not dilate pupils with third-order neuron Horner's syndrome).

■ Proptosis

The Patient

A 78-year-old woman presented to the emergency room with a one-week history of redness of her right eye. Over the past 2 days, her right eye felt as if "it was coming out of her head." She also heard a whooshing sound that kept her from sleeping. One month prior to her visit to the emergency room, she had fallen and hit her head. She was seen by her primary physician and had a normal examination at that time. Her past medical history was unremarkable. In the emergency room, neurological and general examinations were unrevealing. Neuro-ophthalmological examination showed visual acuity of 20/60 OU with a near card (and the patient's reading glasses). Pupils were round, equal, and reactive to light. There was no relative afferent pupillary defect. There was no ptosis, but there was 3 mm of proptosis of the right eye (Figure 2-8A). The right eye was red with chemosis and dilatation of the episcleral vessels, which were tortuous (Figure 2-8B). The cornea was clear and the patient had a mild cataract in both eyes. Extraocular movements were full in the left eye. In the right eye there was an almost complete ophthalmoplegia. Corneal sensation was intact OU. The left eye was soft, but the right eye felt harder (with the doctor's fingers). Confrontation visual fields were full in both eyes. Dilated funduscopic examination was normal in the left eye. In the right eye the veins were dilated, and there were flame-shaped retinal hemorrhages (Figure 2-8C). Intraocular pressure measured later by an ophthalmologist was 32 mmHg OD and 17 mmHg OS. The association of proptosis, redness, dilatation of the episcleral blood vessels, ophthalmoplegia,

dilatation of the retinal veins with retinal hemorrhages, elevated intraocular pressure, and pulsatile tinnitus was highly suggestive of a carotid cavernous fistula. The CT scan of the head obtained in the emergency room with thin cuts through the orbits showed a dilated superior orbital vein on the right (Figure 2-8D). This patient had a post-traumatic direct carotid cavernous fistula that was confirmed by conventional angiogram.

The Problem

- Which disorders presenting with acute proptosis should be emergently excluded to avoid permanent loss of ocular function?
- What imaging modalities (and special views) are required?

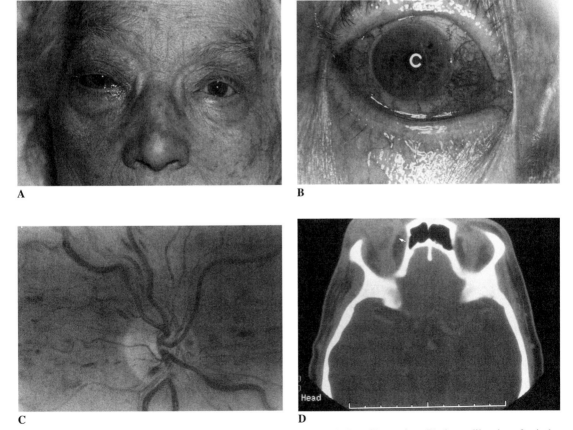

A   B

C   D

Figure 2-8. Post-traumatic direct carotid cavernous fistula. (A) External view. Closer view (B) shows dilatation of episcleral vessels that are arterialized. Funduscopy (C) shows venous dilatation and mild disk edema. Orbital CT (D) shows dilatation of the right superior orbital vein (arrow).

The Evidence

Unilateral or bilateral proptosis indicates an orbital process. The most common cause of unilateral or bilateral proptosis is Graves' disease. It may be secondary to a space-occupying lesion in the orbit such as an orbital mass, orbital hemorrhage, or orbital inflammation/infection, or to orbital congestion (decreased venous drainage) such as in carotid cavernous fistulas or in cavernous sinus thrombosis.[1,2,24,25] It is important to look for signs showing the severity of the orbital syndrome, such as corneal exposure, visual loss, or optic neuropathy (relative afferent pupillary defect and disc edema).[2,24,25] The finding of retinal hemorrhages and pulsatile tinnitus is suggestive of carotid cavernous fistula.[22,23] Other orbital processes such as orbital infections (orbital cellulitis), orbital inflammation (orbital pseudotumor, sarcoidosis, Wegener disease), or orbital masses (tumors, varix) are most often unilateral.

Carotid cavernous fistula is rarely a life-threatening condition. However, visual function may be compromised.[2,22,23] Patients should be evaluated emergently by an ophthalmologist to detect and manage conditions altering the visual prognosis such as corneal exposure, intraocular hypertension, and retinal hemorrhages. Permanent treatment of the carotid cavernous fistula (endovascular or surgical) is followed by a progressive improvement of the ocular disease.[22,23] Optic atrophy from persistently elevated intraocular pressure and corneal opacities are the most common causes of permanent visual loss.[22,23]

The Pros and Cons

Patients with orbital syndrome often have dramatic symptoms and commonly present to the emergency room. The differential diagnosis is wide and emergent orbital imaging is of greatest importance. Orbital CT and orbital MRI are both very useful; they both provide the same kind of information as long as they are obtained with contrast, focus on the orbits (a brain CT or MRI do not study the orbits well enough), show both axial and coronal views, have bone windows if a CT is ordered, and fat suppression images if a MRI is obtained.

The Main Points

- Look for a cranial and orbital bruit in every patient with an orbital syndrome.
- Carotid cavernous fistulas may be difficult to diagnose, and the finding of a dilated superior ophthalmic vein on the orbital CT is very suggestive of this diagnosis (see Figure 2-8D).
- Remember that the most common cause of proptosis (even unilateral) is Graves' disease, which can develop without any symptoms suggestive of thyroid disease and with normal thyroid function.
- The most common cause of orbital syndrome in children is orbital cellulitis, which is a life-threatening condition.[24]

■ Acute Ocular or Orbital Pain

The Patient

A 78-year-old man presented to the emergency room with a 2-week history of pain over his left eye. The pain was dull, constant, and had been getting worse over the past week. The pain improved slightly when he was lying down. He experienced episodes of dimming of his vision in the left eye when he looked at bright lights and when he stood up in the morning. His past medical history was remarkable for multiple vascular risk factors, including systemic hypertension, hypercholesterolemia, and tobacco use. He was treated for coronary artery disease and peripheral artery disease. In the emergency room, neurological examination was unremarkable. Neuro-ophthalmological examination showed visual acuity of 20/30 OD and 20/80 OS with a near card (and the patient's reading glasses). Pupils were round and reactive to light. There was no relative afferent pupillary defect. There was no ptosis or proptosis. Extraocular movements were full in both eyes. Corneal sensation was intact OU. The anterior segment of the right eye appeared normal with a penlight. In the left eye, the episcleral arteries were dilated and there were abnormal vessels on the iris (Figure 2-9A). The eyes were soft and symmetric (with the doctor's fingers). Confrontation visual fields were full in both eyes. Dilated funduscopic examination was normal in the right eye, and showed dot-blot retinal

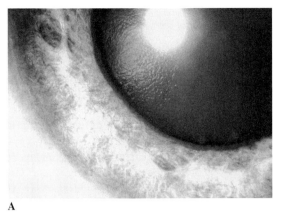
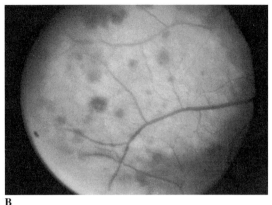

A   B

Figure 2-9. Ischemic ocular syndrome. View of the anterior segment of the left eye (A) showing the iris neovascularization. Dilated funduscopy (B) reveals multiple retinal dot-blot hemorrhages and dilatation of the veins consistent with
venous stasis retinopathy.

hemorrhages in the mid-periphery of the retina in
the left eye (Figure 2-9B). These findings were
suggestive of ocular ischemic syndrome with pain,
neovascularization of the iris, and venous stasis
retinopathy. Evaluation showed an occlusion of
the left internal carotid artery and tight stenosis of
the right internal carotid artery. The sedimentation rate was 14 mm/hr. He was then evaluated
by an ophthalmologist, who confirmed the ocular
findings. Intraocular pressure was 12 mmHg OU.
The patient underwent laser pan photocoagulation of his left retina with subsequent regression of
his iris neovascularization and improvement of
his pain.

The Problem

- What does the neurologist need to know about
  causes of orbital pain?
- What are the urgent available ophthalmological
  therapies?

The Evidence

Ocular and orbital pain are most often secondary
to ocular diseases involving the anterior segment of the eye (e.g., corneal erosions, dry eyes,
uveitis).[1] Less commonly, pain results from elevated intraocular pressure (glaucoma) or ocular

hypotony (choroidal detachment). In these cases,
the eye may be red and visual acuity is decreased.[1]
Ocular and orbital pain may also be referred pain
associated with carotid artery disease such as cervical artery dissections (Table 2-5), cavernous
sinus lesions, cluster headache, or migraine.
Ischemic ocular syndrome and giant cell arteritis are emergencies to consider in any elderly
patient presenting with pain. An evaluation in the
emergency room specifically looking for ocular
abnormalities (including intraocular pressure),
hypo- or hyperesthesia in the trigeminal distribution, proptosis and extraocular movement abnormalities, and Horner's syndrome should always be
performed in patients presenting with ocular or
orbital pain.[1,2]

Table 2-5. Ocular Manifestations of Carotid
Lesions

Asymptomatic retinal emboli
Transient monocular visual loss
Central and branch retinal artery occlusion
Ophthalmic artery occlusion
Episcleral artery dilatation
Venous stasis retinopathy
Ocular ischemic syndrome
Horner's syndrome
Ocular motor syndrome
Referred pain

This patient's pain is related to his ocular ischemic syndrome and is secondary to chronic hypoperfusion of the eye and orbital contents. The most effective treatment would be to reperfuse the eye, but such surgical intervention is rendered difficult by the patient's underlying conditions. Moreover, reperfusion of the eye is associated with a high risk of ocular hypertension and neovascular glaucoma.[26-28]

The Pros and Cons

Although it is accepted that reperfusion of the eye and orbit is the most effective way to treat patients with ischemic ocular syndrome, it is not always done because of the surgical risk. Indeed, most patients have severe bilateral carotid disease, and may require extracranial-intracranial bypass when the ipsilateral internal carotid artery is occluded. Furthermore, the visual function only rarely improves even after revascularization of the eye.[28] Symptomatic treatment and pan retinal laser photocoagulation should be performed to prevent neovascular glaucoma in all patients, especially when revascularization is planned.[27]

The Main Points

- Ocular ischemic syndrome is always associated with severe, diffuse vascular disease.
- These patients are at very high risk of cerebral ischemia and coronary artery disease. Prompt diagnosis may not preserve their visual function but may reduce mortality.

■ Disk Edema

The Patient

A 13-year-old boy was sent to the emergency room with the diagnosis of "bilateral optic nerve swelling." His past medical history was unremarkable. He had been complaining of malaise and headaches for approximately 3 weeks. He had vomited twice and was thought to have a viral illness. He was seen by an ophthalmologist because of the recent onset of "floaters." In the emergency room,

neurological and general examinations were unremarkable. He was irritable and poorly cooperative. Neuro-ophthalmological examination showed visual acuity of 20/20 OU. Pupils were round, equal, and reactive to light; there was no relative afferent pupillary defect. There was no ptosis or proptosis. Extraocular movements were normal in the left eye. There was an esotropia in primary position with a mild right abduction deficit (Figure 2-10A). Corneal sensation was intact OU. The anterior segments of both eyes appeared normal with a penlight. The pressure of the eyes was soft and symmetric (as assessed by the doctor's fingers). Confrontation visual fields were full in both eyes. Dilated funduscopic examination showed bilateral optic disk swelling suggestive of papilledema in the setting of normal visual acuity (Figure 2-10B). The association of papilledema, unilateral sixth nerve palsy, headache, and vomiting was suggestive of raised intracranial pressure. A CT scan of the brain with contrast obtained in the emergency room was unremarkable. A lumbar puncture showed elevated opening pressure with normal CSF contents. His symptoms dramatically improved after the lumbar puncture. A MRI and MRV of the brain showed evidence of right lateral venous sinus thrombosis (Figure 2-10C). A coagulation workup was negative. He was anticoagulated for 3 months, without recurrence of his symptoms. His papilledema resolved and formal visual fields remained full.

The Problem

- How to assess acute disk edema?
- What is the most logical evaluation in these patients?

The Evidence

Disk edema is nonspecific and may be associated with any optic neuropathy. When occurring in the setting of visual loss, disk edema results from an optic neuropathy such as ischemic optic neuropathy or anterior optic neuritis. When visual acuity is normal and disk edema is bilateral, the most likely cause for disk edema is raised intracranial pressure (i.e., papilledema).[2] When disk edema is mild, it may be difficult to differentiate true disk edema

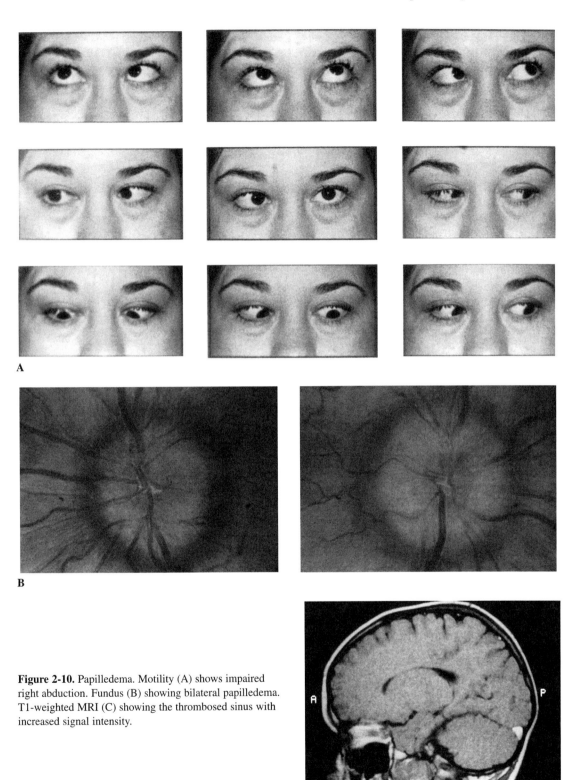

Figure 2-10. Papilledema. Motility (A) shows impaired right abduction. Fundus (B) showing bilateral papilledema. T1-weighted MRI (C) showing the thrombosed sinus with increased signal intensity.

from pseudo-disk edema associated with disk drusen, small crowded optic nerves, and congenital anomalies.[2] This patient had optic nerve swelling suspected to be related to papilledema (i.e., raised intracranial pressure). Such patients should have emergent imaging of the brain to rule out intracranial masses or hydrocephalus. A good-quality head CT with contrast is appropriate in the emergency room, but a MRI/MRV of the brain will eventually be required to refine the diagnosis and rule out cerebral venous sinus thrombosis. A diagnostic algorithm is proposed in Figure 2-11.

Cerebral venous sinus thrombosis commonly presents as isolated raised intracranial pressure.[29] Because of the risk of visual loss associated with chronic raised intracranial pressure and the risk of cortical venous thrombosis and subsequent cerebral venous infarction, its treatment is an emergency.

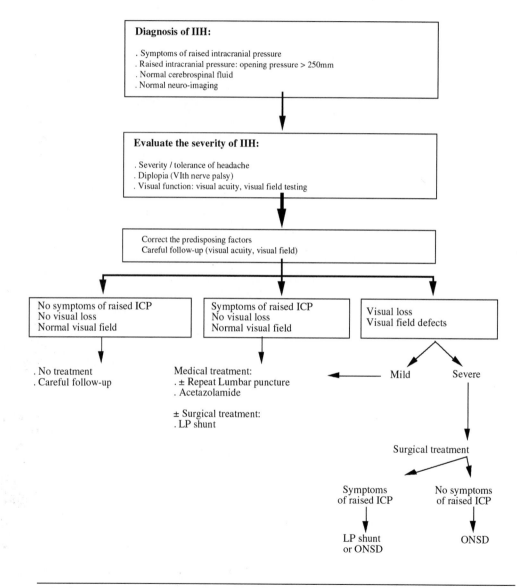

ICP: intracranial pressure
LP shunt: lumboperitoneal shunt
ONSD: optic nerve sheath decompression

Figure 2-11. Diagram showing the management of papilledema related to benign idiopathic intracranial hypertension (IIH).

The lumbar puncture performed as part of the workup of a patient with papilledema and normal neuroimaging improves the patient's symptoms dramatically by decreasing the intracranial pressure.

Even when the diagnosis of venous thrombosis is made by MRI before a lumbar puncture is performed, always consider performing a lumbar puncture before the patient is started on anticoagulants. The lumbar puncture is the fastest and most efficient way to decrease the intracranial pressure and improve the patient's headache and papilledema, thereby preventing visual loss. Rarely, persistent visual loss from chronic raised intracranial pressure in a patient with cerebral venous thrombosis may require surgery such as CSF shunting or optic nerve sheath fenestration.[29] Anticoagulation is likely beneficial, and the risks, even when intracerebral hematomas emerge, remain low.[30] If recanalization is documented, anticoagulation can be discontinued if no underlying coagulopathy is found after a few months. When thrombus remains organized, long-term management is uncertain.

The Main Points

- Consider cerebral venous thrombosis in patients with papilledema and "normal" neuroimaging.
- The diagnosis of venous thrombosis is difficult to make on MRI and a MRV is often necessary.[29]
- Although the treatment of cerebral venous thrombosis remains debated, there is evidence that anticoagulation is safe and effective.[29,30]
- Anticoagulation is needed in patients with cerebral venous thrombosis even when they present with isolated raised intracranial pressure.

■ References

1. Liu GT, Volpe NJ, Galetta SL, eds. *Neuro-Ophthalmology: Diagnosis and Management.* Philadelphia, WB Saunders, 2001.
2. Miller NR, Newman, NJ, eds. *Walsh and Hoyt's Clinical Neuro-Ophthalmology,* 5th ed. Philadelphia, Williams & Wilkins, 1999.
3. Hayreh SS, Podhajsky PA, Zimmerman B. Ocular manifestations of giant cell arteritis. *Am J Ophthalmol* 1998;125:509–520.
4. Gonzalez-Gay MA, Garcia-Porrua C, Llorca J, Llorca J, Hajeer AH, Branas F, Dababneh A, Gonzalez-Louzao C, Rodrigues-Gil E, Rodriguez-Ledo P, Ollier WE. Visual manifestations of giant cell arteritis: trends and clinical spectrum in 161 patients. *Medicine (Baltimore)* 2000;9:283–292.
5. Gordon LK, Levin LA. Visual loss in giant cell arteritis. *JAMA* 1998;280:385–386.
6. Hayreh, SS. Acute ischemic disorders of the optic nerve: pathogenesis, clinical manifestations, and management. *Ophthalmol Clin North Am* 1996;9:407–442.
7. Hayreh SS, Zimmerman B. Visual deterioration in giant cell arteritis patients while on high doses of corticosteroid therapy. *Ophthalmology* 2003;110:1204–1215.
8. Liozon E, Jauberteau-Marchan MO, Ly K, Loustaud-Ratti V, Soria P, Vidal E. Giant cell arteritis with low erythrocyte sedimentation rate: comments on the article by Salvarani and Hunder. *Arthritis Rheum* 2002;47:692–694.
9. Smetana GW, Shmerling RH. Does this patient have temporal arteritis? *JAMA* 2002;287;92–101.
10. Kupersmith MJ, Moster M, Bhuiyan S, Warren F, Weinberg H. Beneficial effects of corticosteroids on ocular myasthenia gravis. *Arch Neurol* 1996;53:802–806.
11. Biousse V, Newman NJ. Third nerve palsies. *Semin Neurol* 2000;20:55–74.
12. Newman NJ. Third-, fourth-, and sixth-nerve palsies and the cavernous sinus. In Albert DM, Jakobiec FA, eds. *Principles and Practice of Ophthalmology*, 2nd ed. Philadelphia, WB Saunders, 2000:3992–4028.
13. Jacobson DM. Pupil involvement in patients with diabetes-associated oculomotor nerve palsy. *Arch Ophthalmol* 1998;116:723–727.
14. Bederson JB, Awad IA, Wiebers DO, Piepgras D, Haley EC Jr, Brott T, Hademenos G, Chyatte D, Rosenwasser R, Caroselli C. Recommendations for the management of patients with unruptured intracranial aneurysms: a statement for healthcare professionals from the Stroke Council of the American Heart Association. *Circulation.* 2000;102:2300–2308.
15. Friedman JA, Piepgras DG, Pichelmann MA, Hansen KK, Brown RD, Wiebers DO. Small cerebral aneurysms presenting with symptoms other than rupture. *Neurology* 2001;57:1212–1216.
16. Hutchinson PJ, Kirkpatrick PJ. What is the most sensitive non-invasive strategy for the diagnosis of intracranial aneurysms? *J Neurol Neurosurg Psychiatry* 2001;71:289.
17. Jacobson DM, Trobe JD. The emerging role of magnetic resonance angiography in the management of patients with third cranial nerve palsy. *Am J Ophthalmol* 1999;128:94–96.
18. Okahara M, Kiyosue H, Yamashita M, Nagatomi H, Hata H, Saginoya T, Sagara Y, Mori H. Diagnostic accuracy of magnetic resonance angiography for cerebral aneurysms in correlation with 3D-digital subtraction

angiographic images: a study of 133 aneurysms. *Stroke* 2002;33:1803–1808.

19. Trobe JD. Managing oculomotor nerve palsy. *Arch Ophthalmol* 1998;116:798.

20. White PM, Teadsale E, Wardlaw JM, Easton V. What is the most sensitive non-invasive imaging strategy for the diagnosis of intracranial aneurysms? *J Neurol Neurosurg Psychiatry* 2001;71:322–328.

21. Keane JR. Oculosympathetic paresis: Analysis of 100 hospitalized patients. *Arch Neurol* 1979;36:13–16.

22. Biousse V, Touboul PJ, D'Anglejan-Chatillon J, Lévy C, Schaison M, Bousser MG. Neuro-ophthalmological manifestations of internal carotid artery dissections: a series of 146 patients. *Am J Ophthalmol* 1998;126: 565–577.

23. Biousse V, Mendicino M, Simon D, Newman NJ. The ophthalmology of intracranial vascular abnormalities. *Am J Ophthalmol* 1998;125:527–544.

24. Dudim A, Othman A. Acute orbital swelling: evaluation and protocol. *J Pediatr Emerg Care* 1996;12:16–21.

25. Kennerdell JS, Dresner SC. The nonspecific orbital inflammatory syndromes. *Surv Ophthalmol* 1984;29: 93–103.

26. Biousse V. Carotid disease and the eye. *Curr Opin Ophthalmol* 1997;8:16–26.

27. Malhotra R, Gregory-Evans K. Management of ocular ischaemic syndrome. *Br J Ophthalmol* 2000;84: 1428–1431.

28. Mizener JB, Podhajsky P, Hayreh SS. Ocular ischemic syndrome. *Ophthalmology* 1997;104:859–864.

29. Biousse V, Bousser MG. Cerebral venous thrombosis. *Neurologist* 1999;5:326–349.

30. Stam J, de Bruijn S, de Veber G. Anticoagulation for cerebral sinus thrombosis. *Stroke* 2003;34: 1054–1055.

Chapter 3

Generalized Convulsive Status Epilepticus

Joseph I. Sirven

Status epilepticus (SE) is a medical emergency because effective treatment can avoid its high morbidity and mortality. Most importantly, early treatment implementation is essential to avert a poor response to therapy and to reduce secondary neuronal damage from continuous seizure activity. Improved understanding of the pathophysiological processes involved in the origin and perpetuation of seizure activity and the results of recent prospective randomized trials have resulted in the adoption of new therapeutic approaches. The best management of refractory SE remains undetermined and termination of SE becomes increasingly more difficult over time. One aspect of refractory SE management is whether treatments that consume a large amount of financial and emotional resources are justified. In certain situations, physicians may question each new treatment and simply suggest to stop care. There are major differences between patients with favorable prognostic etiology such as where antiepileptic drug (AED) withdrawal is the culprit, in which case all possible therapies should be employed, and others, such as SE from hypoxia or other catastrophic cause, where withdrawal of care is more compassionate and realistic. How to meet these challenges is the focus of this chapter.

■ The Patient

A 64-year-old Caucasian woman has a history of longstanding primary generalized epilepsy. She had been recently evaluated for concurrent myoclonus, tremor, and ataxia associated with cerebellar atrophy. The patient had been on phenytoin for more than two decades and the cerebellar atrophy was attributed to long-term phenytoin use. The patient was transitioning to valproic acid; however, her husband mistakenly withdrew phenytoin abruptly. The patient now presents to the emergency room after being lethargic and unable to respond for more than 24 hours. The ER physician witnesses four generalized tonic-clonic seizures. The patient receives up to 10 mg of lorazepam and 20 mg/kg of fosphenytoin in the emergency room. The patient is unresponsive after treatment, and it is assumed that her seizures have terminated.

An electroencephalogram (EEG) is performed to assess therapeutic response and demonstrates ongoing generalized convulsive status epilepticus (SE) (Figure 3-1). The patient has a phenytoin serum level of 25 mg/dL after intravenous bolus administration; therefore, a 15 mg/kg dose of phenobarbital is administered. This intervention leads to a burst suppression pattern on the EEG (Figure 3-2) but is subsequently followed by a return of the ongoing status epilepticus. The patient is intubated for airway protection and ventilation. A computed tomography (CT) of the brain is normal. Lumbar puncture is performed showing 16.5 white blood cells per cm^3 (81 percent neutrophils), total protein of 119 mg/dL, glucose 65 mg/dL (serum glucose 101 mg/dL), 45,000 erythrocytes per cm^3, and no evidence of xanthochromia.

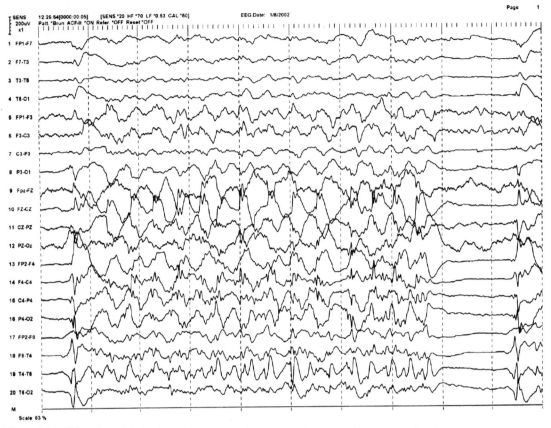

Figure 3-1. EEG performed in the intensive care unit shows generalized convulsive status epilepticus. Note continuous seizure activity.

Gram stain, bacterial, viral, and fungal cultures are negative. Herpes simplex polymerase chain reaction is negative.

Phenobarbital is supplemented to a serum level of 50 mg/dL, phenytoin is maintained at a serum level of 25 mg/dL, and, due to lack of any effect, parenteral valproic acid is administered to a serum level of 80 mg/dL. Despite the polypharmacy used to terminate SE, the patient's EEG continues to demonstrate episodic ongoing seizure activity after 48 hours of treatment. Because of the refractory nature of the seizures, the patient is then anesthetized with pentobarbital in an attempt to stop the seizures. The pentobarbital is maintained and titrated to nearly complete suppression of the EEG for approximately one week with attempts to wean off the drug every 48 hours. However, the ongoing status epilepticus persists. Other anesthetic agents (propofol and

midazolam) are utilized to terminate SE with no particular benefits noted.

After two weeks of unsuccessful therapy, SE persists on EEG and the patient remains unresponsive. Magnetic resonance imaging of the brain is performed revealing increased T2 signal and diffusion abnormalities in the anterior and mesial temporal lobes, insular cortex, and cingulate gyrus bilaterally. The MRI results are attributed to edema from ongoing seizures. All antiepileptic drugs are maintained (phenobarbital, phenytoin, and valproic acid) at supratherapeutic levels.

Six weeks after SE began, compassionate use of epilepsy surgery, namely, corpus callosotomy versus vagus nerve stimulation, is entertained. A vagus nerve stimulator is placed to serve as an adjunct to the AEDs already being administered. Approximately 3 weeks later, the patient begins to awaken and

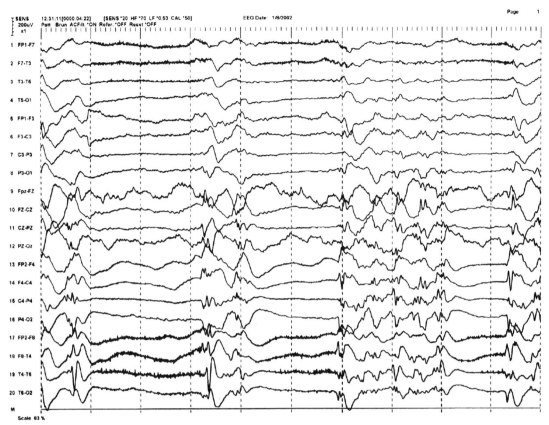

Figure 3-2. EEG demonstrating the burst suppression pattern after initiation of treatment.

ongoing seizure activity is no longer seen on EEG. The patient is eventually discharged to a rehabilitation facility with a tracheostomy approximately 3 months after her admission. Later, she is able to return home but with significant short-term memory loss and word-finding difficulties. MRI of the brain 2 months after the episode revealed bilateral temporal lobe atrophy and persistent signal abnormality in the mesial areas (Figure 3-3).

■ The Problem

- Which is the appropriate first-line agent for management of SE?
- What is the role of EEG in the management of refractory SE? What degree of EEG suppression is necessary for SE termination? How does one interpret periodic EEG abnormalities after SE?

- Which are the best agents for the management of refractory SE?
- What are the indications and appropriate timing of invasive interventions such as resective surgery or implantation of a vagal nerve stimulator?

■ The Evidence

Pharmacological Management

Rapid treatment of SE is crucial in order to prevent neurological and organ injury, which requires immediate diagnosis. To be effective for SE, a drug should have intravenous formulation, rapid distribution to the brain, and no significant adverse effects. Currently available drugs are discussed below.

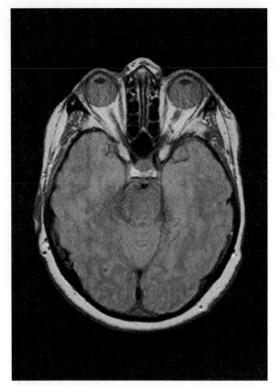

Figure 3-3A. MRI performed within the first 3 days of status epilepticus.

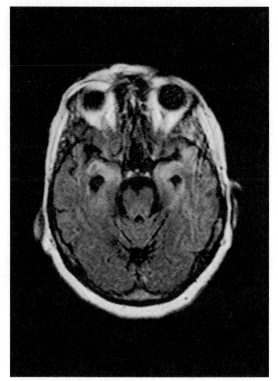

Figure 3-3B. MRI performed after 2 months of therapy. Note the remarkable signal change with marked temporal lobe atrophy.

Benzodiazepines (BZD)

The BZDs are one of the most efficacious classes of drugs for the treatment of SE. This section will review the pharmacology of the three most commonly used BZDs for SE: diazepam, lorazepam, and midazolam. All three compounds work by enhancing GABAergic inhibition by binding to the BZD-GABA and barbiturate receptor complex.

Diazepam (Valium). Diazepam is considered one of the drugs of choice for first-line management of SE (level of evidence I, randomized controlled trial [RCT]).[1–4] It enters the brain rapidly due to its high lipid solubility, but 15–20 minutes after entering the brain, it redistributes to other areas of the body, reducing its clinical effect.[4,5] Despite its fast distribution half-life, the elimination half-life is approximately 24 hours. Thus, sedative effects potentially could accumulate with repeated administration. A typical dose of 5–10 mg will terminate seizures of any type in about 75 percent of patients.[2,3,6] Adverse effects include respiratory

suppression, hypotension, sedation, and local tissue irritation. Hypotension and respiratory suppression may be potentiated by the coadministration of other AEDs, particularly barbiturates. Diazepam may also be given intramuscularly and rectally (Diastat).[7] Despite its pharmacokinetic and adverse effect limitations, diazepam remains important among abortive drugs due to its rapid and broad-spectrum effect.

Lorazepam (Ativan). Lorazepam has emerged as the preferred BZD for acute management of SE (level of evidence I, RCT). Lorazepam differs from diazepam in two important respects. It is less lipid-soluble than diazepam, with a distribution half-life of 2–3 hours versus 15 minutes for diazepam. Therefore, it should have a longer duration of clinical effect.[4] Lorazepam also binds the GABAergic receptor more tightly than diazepam, which also should explain a longer duration of action. Its anticonvulsive effects last from 6 to 12 hours and the typical intravenous dose is from 4 to 8 mg. It also has a broad spectrum of efficacy, terminating seizures in 75–80 percent of cases.[6] Its adverse effects are identical to those of diazepam. Therefore, lorazepam is the first choice for acute seizure management due to longer duration of action than diazepam.

Midazolam (Versed). Midazolam is rarely used as a first-line drug for SE in the United States due to its short half-life. A continuous infusion of midazolam may be used to treat refractory SE.[8] When used for this purpose, its loading dose is 0.2 mg/kg and should be repeated at 0.2–0.4 mg/kg boluses every 5 minutes until seizures stop, up to a maximum loading dose of 2 mg/kg. The initial rate of continuous infusion is 0.1 mg/kg/hr with a dose range between 0.05 and 2 mg/kg/hr. The half-life of midazolam is 1.5 to 3.5 hours initially, but with prolonged use its half-life may increase to several days. SE can stop in less than one hour with a duration of effect of minutes to hours and a duration of sedation from minutes to days. Side effects include marked hypotension, development of tolerance, and tachyphylaxis.

Phenytoin (Dilantin)

Phenytoin is one of the most effective drugs for treating acute seizures and SE (level of evidence A, RCT). However, due to serious potential side effects, continuous cardiac and blood pressure monitoring are recommended during infusion. Arrhythmias and hypotension have been reported, particularly in patients over the age of 40 years. These are likely related to the rate of administration and the propylene glycol vehicle used as diluent. Additionally, local irritation, phlebitis, and dizziness may accompany intravenous administration. Thus, despite its efficacy and long duration of action, there are a number of potential problems to be considered when using intravenous phenytoin.

Fosphenytoin (Cerebyx)

Fosphenytoin received FDA approval for use in 1996. It is a prodrug of phenytoin that is completely converted to phenytoin following parenteral administration. Because it is water-soluble, adverse events related to propylene glycol do not occur. Like phenytoin, fosphenytoin is useful in treating acute partial and generalized tonic-clonic seizures. Fosphenytoin is converted to phenytoin in 8 to 15 minutes.[9–11] It is metabolized by the liver and has a half-life of 14 hours. The dose, concentration, and infusion rate of IV fosphenytoin are expressed as phenytoin equivalents (PE). The initial dose of fosphenytoin is 15 to 20 mg PE/kg, and it can be infused at a rate as high as 150 mg PE/min for an infusion time three times faster than IV phenytoin. Intramuscular doses can also be given but levels are not therapeutic for 30 minutes.[12]

Adverse effects unique to fosphenytoin include perineal paresthesias and pruritus, both related to a high rate of administration.[13] Fosphenytoin is not associated with local irritation as is phenytoin. Cardiac arrhythmias and hypotension have not been significant problems with intramuscular dosing, but intravenous dosing has been associated with hypotension. Continuous cardiac and blood pressure monitoring remains necessary for patients receiving intravenous fosphenytoin. Because the cost of fosphenytoin is high, it is not available on some hospital formularies.[1] Nevertheless, if fosphenytoin is available, it should be used preferentially over phenytoin.

Phenobarbital

In most traditional protocols, phenobarbital is typically used after a BZD or phenytoin has failed to control SE. The usual loading dose is 15–20 mg/kg at 100 mg/min. High-dose phenobarbital is sedating, making airway protection and aspiration a major concern, and patients are usually intubated and mechanically ventilated during and following infusion. Intravenous phenobarbital is also associated with systemic hypotension. Although phenobarbital can be loaded fairly rapidly, infusion of a full therapeutic dose may take 30 minutes. Parenteral phenobarbital is diluted in 60–80 percent propylene glycol. Propylene glycol toxicity is associated with a number of complications including renal failure, myocardial depression, and seizures.[2,5] These limitations relegate phenobarbital to those cases that failed to respond to other agents and explain the growing resistance to using barbiturates.

Valproate (Depacon)

The FDA approved this parenteral compound for use in 1997.[14] Depacon has a broad spectrum of efficacy and may be useful for absence or myoclonic SE. Parenteral valproate is used primarily for rapid loading or as a substitute when oral therapy is impossible. Sinha and Naritoku were able to load valproate doses of 15 mg/kg intravenously at a rate of 50 to 100 mg/min (approximately 5 minute infusion) without significant changes in blood pressure or pulse.[14] Adverse effects include local irritation, gastrointestinal distress, and lethargy. However, significant sedation, hypotension, and cardiac abnormalities have not been reported. The FDA has not approved this drug specifically for treatment of SE.

Pentobarbital

Pentobarbital is used primarily in the treatment of refractory status epilepticus. Typically, a loading dose of 10 mg/kg is initially infused at a rate of up to 100 mg/min.[1,15,16] Then, 5 mg/kg boluses are repeated until seizures stop. The maximum bolus rate is 25–50 mg/min and should be based primarily on blood pressure recordings. Continuous dosing ranging between 0.5 and 5 mg/kg/hr is typically titrated by continuous EEG monitoring. The half-life of intravenous pentobarbital is 15–60 hours. Side effects include prolonged coma that may last days after stopping the infusion, hypotension (often requiring vasopressor support), myocardial depression, immune suppression, and ileus. For many physicians, pentobarbital is now the ultimate last-resort drug.

Propofol

Propofol, a GABA agonist, is a phenolic compound with anticonvulsant properties. This drug is utilized strictly in the management of refractory SE requiring medication-induced coma.[1,17–20] It is completely unrelated to barbiturates, opioids, and benzodiazepines. Continuous intravenous propofol is loaded at 1 mg/kg and boluses should be repeated every 3–5 minutes until seizures stop, up to a maximum loading dose of 10 mg/kg. Continuous infusion rates are 2 mg/kg/hr, with a dose range between 1 and 15 mg/kg/hr. Time to SE termination is seconds to minutes, and duration of sedation is between 5 and 10 minutes. Adverse effects associated with propofol include a large lipid load (up to 3000 calories/day), occasional pancreatitis, and reports of multiorgan failure secondary to acidosis in children with certain enzymatic defects. Propofol can also be proconvulsant and myoclonus can occur during its induction and withdrawal.

Other Treatments

Numerous other agents or therapies have been reported in the literature as case series for refractory SE. These have included thiopental, lidocaine, paraldehyde, desflurane, isoflurane etomidate, ketamine, immunotherapy with methylprednisolone, and intravenous immunoglobulin.[1,19–23] Therapies such as electroconvulsive therapy, vagus nerve stimulation, thalamic deep brain stimulation, and surgical resections such as temporal lobectomy, corpus callosotomy, and multiple subpial transections have been attempted. Lastly, nearly all AEDs, either in an oral solution or delivered via nasogastric tube, have been used in SE. Most case reports mention the use of carbamazepine, levetiracetam, topiramate, and gabapentin.

Choice of AED

Although there is no ideal drug to treat SE, a number of considerations influence the choice of AED for this condition. Table 3-1 summarizes dosing, pharmacology, and adverse effects of drugs used for SE and refractory SE. Comparative studies of SE treatments are few, but consensus has emerged concerning initial medications. Most authors agree that lorazepam or diazepam should be initiated first, followed by fosphenytoin or phenytoin (level of evidence I, RCTs). The evidence for these choices is summarized below. Table 3-2 lists randomized controlled trials performed in SE.

Diazepam versus Lorazepam

A randomized double-blind trial compared intravenous lorazepam and diazepam as first-line treatment for all types of SE. Seventy-eight patients received either 10 mg of diazepam or 4 mg of lorazepam intravenously injected over 2 minutes. There was no significant difference in efficacy between the drugs due to the small number of enrolled patients. Seizures were terminated in 58 percent of diazepam- and 78 percent of lorazepam-treated patients.[6] There was no significant difference in latency of action. Diazepam had a median latency of 2 minutes versus a median latency of 3 minutes with lorazepam. There were no notable differences between treatment groups in types of seizures treated.

Table 3-1. Antiepileptic Drugs Used in Status Epilepticus

Drug	Loading Dose	Maintenance Dose	Route of Metabolism	% Protein Binding	Adverse Effects
Diazepam	10–20 mg	None	Hepatic	>90	Respiratory depression, hypotension, sialorrhea
Lorazepam	4–8 mg	None	Hepatic	90	Same as diazepam
Phenytoin	18–20 mg/kg at 50 mg/min	5 mg/kg/day	Hepatic	70	Cardiac depression, hypotension
Fosphenytoin	18–20 mg PE/kg at 150 mg PE/min	None	Hepatic	70	Cardiac depression, hypotension, paresthesias
Phenobarbital	20 mg/kg at 100 mg/min	1–4 mg/kg/hr	Hepatic	50–60	Respiratory depression
Pentobarbital	2–10 mg/kg	0.5–5 mg/kg/hr	Hepatic	59–63	Hypotension, respiratory depression
Midazolam	0.2 mg/kg	0.05–2 µg/kg/min	Hepatic	96	Hypotension, respiratory depression
Propofol	1 mg/kg	1–15 mg/kg/hr initially, then 1–3 mg/kg/hr	Hepatic	97–98	Respiratory depression, hypotension, lipemia, acidosis

PE, Phenytoin equivalent.

Adverse effects were nearly identical for both drugs. Thus, both drugs are acceptable as first-line treatment, but lorazepam may be preferable due to longer duration of therapeutic effect (level of evidence I, RCT).

More recently, a landmark randomized, double-blind trial comparing diazepam, lorazepam, and placebo administered by paramedics out of the hospital was published.[4] Of 205 enrolled patients, both lorazepam and diazepam terminated SE faster than placebo, and lorazepam was more successful than diazepam in stopping SE (termination rates of 59 percent with lorazepam, 43% with diazepam and 21% with placebo). Rates of respiratory or circulatory complications after the study treatment was administered were 10.6 percent for the lorazepam group, 10.3 percent for the diazepam group, and 22.5 percent for the placebo group. The investigators concluded that benzodiazepines are safe and effective when administered by paramedics for out-of-hospital status epilepticus in adults. These results also suggest that lorazepam is likely a better therapy than diazepam (level of evidence I, RCT).[4]

Table 3-2. Summary of Randomized Controlled Trials (RCT) in Status Epilepticus

RCT (PI, Year)	Drug Comparison	Patients	Conclusion
Leppik 1983[6]	Lorazepam versus diazepam for SE	County Emergency Room patients ($N=78$)	No statistical differences between both drugs for SE efficacy
Treiman 1998[3]	Diazepam versus phenytoin versus phenobarbital for overt and subtle SE	Veteran patients ($N=518$)	Lorazepam was best for first-line treatment of overt SE
Alldredge 2001[4]	Lorazepam versus diazepam versus placebo	Out-of-hospital patients in metropolitan San Francisco ($N=205$)	Both diazepam and lorazepam are better than placebo for out-of-hospital SE. Lorazepam may be better therapy than diazepam.

PI, principal investigator.

VA Cooperative Study

The Veterans' Administration cooperative study compared response rates to four different treatments in 384 patients with overt SE and 134 patients with subtle (not clinically noticeable) SE.[3] The four regimens consisted of 0.15 mg/kg diazepam followed by 18 mg/kg phenytoin, 0.1 mg/kg lorazepam, 15 mg/kg phenobarbital, or 18 mg/kg phenytoin. For overt SE, the highest response was found with lorazepam (64.9 percent), followed by phenobarbital (58.2 percent), diazepam with phenytoin (55.8 percent), and finally phenytoin monotherapy (43.6 percent).

Subtle SE, a designation of uncertain clinical relevance, had significantly lower response rates to all treatments. Phenobarbital had the highest response rate at 24.2 percent, followed by lorazepam (17.9 percent), diazepam plus phenytoin (8.3 percent), and phenytoin monotherapy (7.7 percent). The authors found no statistically significant differences between treatments for either overt or subtle SE. There were also no differences between the treatments with respect to recurrence during the 12-hour study period, incidence of adverse reactions, or outcome at 30 days. The dramatic drop in response rate between early and late SE emphasizes

the importance of early treatment of SE. The authors concluded that lorazepam is easiest to use among all first-line agents in SE (level of evidence A, RCT).[3]

Recommendations of the Epilepsy Foundation of America's Working Group on Status Epilepticus

In 1993, the EFA committee on the treatment of convulsive SE published guidelines and a treatment protocol.[22] The SE treatment protocol was based on a literature review, expert reviewers, and a professional advisory board. There is agreement that a medical protocol should be adopted that is uniformly applied to all in need of treatment. The use of such a protocol leads to improved competence and efficiency, which in turn may be associated with favorable outcomes. However, there is no consensus with regard to the safety and efficacy of the recommended protocol.[21] Table 3-3 outlines the author's preference for management of SE.

The committee also made special mention of treatment of pediatric SE. They noted that drug efficacy is similar in adults and children, but children may tolerate more rapid intravenous administration than older patients (level of evidence V, expert opinion). Despite the existence of rectal preparations, intravenous drug administration is the

Table 3-3. Sample Protocol for Status Epilepticus Management

Time: 0 minutes
Keep patent airway, monitor gas exchange, and start nasal oxygen prongs.
Start intravenous catheter with isotonic saline at a low infusion rate.
Inject 50 ml of 50 percent glucose IV and 100 mg of thiamine IV or IM.
Administer lorazepam 0.1–0.15 mg/kg IV (2 mg/min).
Send sample serum for evaluation of electrolytes, blood urea nitrogen, glucose level, complete blood count, drug screen, and anticonvulsant levels, check arterial blood gas values.
Call EEG laboratory to start recording as soon as feasible.
If seizures persist, administer fosphenytoin 18 mg PE/kg IV (150 mg/min), with an additional 7 mg PE/kg if seizures continue.

Time: 20–45 minutes (if seizures persist)
Pentobarbital, midazolam and propofol should be used with no proven preference.
Begin pentobarbital infusion 5 mg/kg IV initial dose, then push until seizures have stopped using EEG monitoring; continue pentobarbital infusion at 1–5 mg/kg/hr. Slow infusion rate every 4–6 hours to determine if seizures have stopped, using EEG guidance. Monitor blood pressure and respiration carefully. Support blood pressure with pressors if needed.
or
Begin midazolam at 0.2 mg/kg, then at a dose of 0.75–10 µg/kg/min titrated to EEG monitoring.
or
Begin propofol at 1–2 mg/kg loading followed by 2–10 mg/kg/hr. Adjust maintenance dose on the basis of EEG monitoring.

route of choice in the pediatric group (level of evidence V, expert opinion). Although these guidelines are helpful, more studies are needed to address whether this protocol is applicable to pediatric patients and to address the role of newer drugs such as fosphenytoin, rectal diazepam, and parenteral valproic acid in the treatment of SE.

The Value of the EEG

While overt convulsive SE is readily diagnosed, the EEG can establish the diagnosis in less obvious circumstances. Studies have found that 8–37 percent of patients with altered consciousness and unclear diagnosis had nonconvulsive SE when EEG was performed.[24–26] One study showed that EEG led to a diagnosis of subtle SE in 37 percent of patients with altered consciousness whose diagnoses were in doubt.[24] A surprising number of patients had no clinical signs of SE, and the EEG was crucial in establishing the diagnosis. Moreover, the EEG can confirm that an episode of SE has ended, particularly when questions arise about the possibility of recurrent subtle seizures. In one of these studies, investigators monitored patients for at least 24 hours after clinical signs of generalized convulsive SE had ended.[26] In nearly half of their patients, the EEG continued to demonstrate electrographic seizures, which often had no clinical correlate.[26] Thus, when SE patients do not rapidly and completely recover, monitoring with EEG for at least 24 hours after an episode of SE seems advisable to ensure that recurrent seizures are not missed.

Two of the most problematic debates with regards to EEG are (1) to what degree of EEG suppression should refractory SE be managed, and (2) how does one interpret and treat (or not treat) the finding of periodic epileptiform discharges (PEDs). It is common teaching that burst suppression pattern on EEG should be the goal of management in SE, and therapy should be titrated to this endpoint. However, there is little evidence that burst suppression or isoelectric patterns are required for the termination of SE. Seizure control can be achieved in many patients with a background of continuous slow activity. On the other hand, there are patients who continue to exhibit seizure activity despite burst suppression patterns, and rendering the patient isoelectric is required to control SE. One systematic review found that titrating therapy to

background suppression was associated with a lower frequency of breakthrough seizures as compared with simply suppressing seizures.[17] However, EEG suppression was associated with a higher frequency of hypotension.

PEDs can be seen as an initial manifestation of SE or alternatively in the aftermath of SE. There is controversy regarding the interpretation and significance of these findings. Some authors have found that PEDs are associated with increased focal blood flow on SPECT and increased metabolism on FDG-PET, arguing that PEDs are an ictal phenomenon.[27] Others classify PEDs as postictal or a marker of injury or encephalopathy.[28] Whether these EEG patterns should be treated as SE remains problematic. There are anecdotal reports of favorable outcome in some patients whose PEDs were treated, yet other reports have found treating this pattern to be harmful in the critically ill or older adults. To date, there is no consensus opinion as to whether to treat PEDs as one of the electrographic manifestations of SE.

Refractory SE

One of the most debated issues in SE is how to choose between certain anesthetic agents when SE fails to respond to a benzodiazepine, phenytoin, or phenobarbital. There are no randomized comparative studies of treatments for refractory SE. These studies may be difficult to orchestrate because the total number of eligible patients may be small. This is expected as a result of a generally favorable initial response and exclusion of patients with myoclonus status epilepticus. Three choices seem to have emerged as the most popular alternatives: pentobarbital, midazolam, and propofol. Because of the side-effect profile of high-dose barbiturate infusions, propofol and midazolam have become increasingly favored. There is very little comparative data between these medications. One small study[18] compared 8 patients on propofol to 6 on pentobarbital and found that propofol was associated with faster termination of SE. However, nearly all of the patients ultimately died. Claassen and colleagues recently published a systematic review of pentobarbital, propofol, and midazolam.[17] They found that, compared with midazolam or propofol, pentobarbital was associated with a lower frequency of short-term treatment failure and breakthrough seizures. Yet pentobarbital was also associated with a higher incidence of clinically significant hypotension. The authors concluded that pentobarbital or any continuously infused anesthetic titrated to EEG suppression is the most effective strategy. Nevertheless, prospective randomized trials would be needed in order to clarify this issue. Moreover, outcome measures for these trials need to transcend simply reporting SE termination by also assessing survivability, post-SE quality of life, and neuroprotection.

■ The Pros and Cons

Current evidence suggests that the first-line agent in the management of SE should be a benzodiazepine preferably delivered as soon as SE is recognized. Thus, similar to the public health measures in place for cardiac care in the community with omnipresent cardiac defibrillators available in public spaces and jetliners, some form of accessible benzodiazepine should be available for rapid termination of SE by both the lay public and health professionals. The problem that arises is the cost of such measure and the appropriate delivery vehicle because intravenous access is not practical. Buccal, sublingual, or subcutaneous, administration would be preferable.

Initial treatment in our case was the appropriate use of lorazepam rapidly followed by phenytoin (titrated to supratherapeutic levels of 25 mg/dL). However, when seizures failed to stop after these interventions, the management becomes more empirical since there are no randomized controlled data to help guide treatment decisions. Following our protocol, we decided to use phenobarbital and then parenteral valproic acid while maintaining supratherapeutic serum levels of anticonvulsants. There is a growing tendency among neurointensivists to opt for using continuous infusion of propofol or midazolam immediately after lorazepam and phenytoin in patients with persistent SE. The efficiency of this treatment approach remains to be established but offers the advantage of avoiding the complications so often encountered with barbiturates.

The next crucial aspect of our case was the choice of medication for stopping SE refractory to all other treatments. Pentobarbital was our initial choice, and we titrated this agent to achieve complete suppression of EEG background as much as the patient could hemodynamically tolerate. However, when the EEG continued to demonstrate ictal discharges, we kept dosing the patient with boluses. We also attempted other agents including midazolam and propofol. Switching to other agents is an intuitive and perhaps an incorrect decision. Consistency may be the best option in the scenario of refractory SE, if one is going to suppress the EEG to stop SE. Remaining with one agent is the soundest advice, particularly when there are no randomized trials to suggest efficacy of one agent over another.

The degree of EEG suppression is another controversial point, which has been often addressed. We chose to suppress the EEG background as much as possible and did not settle for a burst suppression pattern when it became clear that our patient had seizures through this pattern. In order to best achieve this goal, we used pentobarbital. Criticisms to this approach are the risk of cardiovascular instability and committing the patient to a long recovery because of the long half-life of pentobarbital. Midazolam and propofol are acceptable alternatives in light of the absence of scientific evidence to choose one drug over another. Table 3-4 summarizes the history and arguments for the major agents commonly used for RSE. Interestingly, the literature reflects that, depending on the specialists treating RSE (either epileptologist, intensivist, or anesthesiologist), their approach appears to closely mirror their own specialty. For instance, intensivists and anesthesiologists will advocate use of an anesthetic/hypnotic agent,[17–21,23,30–32] whereas an epileptologist will likely suggest a known AED such as phenobarbital or pentobarbital[1,15,16] or surgery.[33] A recent survey in Austria, Germany, and Switzerland revealed a lack of any consensus, and overall preference for phenobarbital.[34] Consequently, a consensus between various specialties that manage RSE is needed in order to determine which treatment yields the best clinical outcome.

A perplexing aspect of refractory SE is that the EEG, although necessary to monitor treatment, can become confusing even to the most experienced experts. Continuous EEG monitoring often reveals periodic patterns that may be misinterpreted as ictal. Stimulation, arousals, mechanical artifacts, and medication effects all have an impact on the EEG and it is a concern that patients may be overtreated due to EEG misinterpretation. Moreover, when anesthetic agents are tapered off

Table 3-4 History and Arguments for and Against Agents for Refractory Status Epilepticus (RSE)

Agent	History of its Introduction for RSE Treatment	Pros	Cons
Midazolam	Crisp 1988 (case report)[29] Kumar and Bleck 1992 (7 cases)[30] Claassen 2001 (33 cases)[23]	GABAergic Favorable hemodynamics Faster recovery from sedative-hypnotic effects	Unclear why a benzodiazepine (BZD) would benefit a condition that inherently has already failed another BZD Tachyphylaxis Breakthrough seizures Expensive
Pentobarbital	Rashkin 1987 (9 cases)[31] Lowenstein 1988 (8 cases)[16]	GABAergic Effective EEG suppression ? Neuroprotective	Hemodynamic intolerance Prolonged sedation Prolonged respiratory suppression with pneumonia risk
Propofol	Wood 1988 (case report)[32] Stecker 1998 (8 cases)[18] Prasad 2001 (14 cases)[21]	GABAergic Effective EEG suppression	Can be proconvulsant upon induction and withdrawal Metabolic acidosis, renal failure Expensive

and an individual emerges from coma, one may often observe transient patterns that can be misconstrued as ictal. Clinical correlation will help clarify the situation.

The most controversial aspect of this case was the use of surgery, clearly done as a form of compassionate care. The MRI changes (Figure 3-3B) were ominous and spurred our team to aggressive action. There is no clear evidence to support the use of surgery or vagus nerve stimulation in SE. Many experts may question this particular choice and rightfully so. However, when faced with a desperate situation in a patient without a terminal underlying lesion, resorting to experimental measures is the only option. We believe that surgical intervention allowed a speedier withdrawal from anesthetic agents. As our case illustrates, one should take the etiology of SE under consideration. If favorable prognosis is possible (e.g., in cases of alcohol or AED withdrawal), treatment should be continued and all possible alternatives should be explored. There is much to be said about this argument when some patients can have a reasonable recovery after weeks of seizures.

■ The Main Points

- Early treatment initiation is paramount to achieve successful termination of SE.

- Use EEG immediately to monitor termination of seizures.
- Transient patterns on EEG and PEDs are not hard indications for additional bolus or using other AEDs.
- When dealing with refractory SE, be consistent with your choice of anesthetic agent to control SE, regardless of whether you use pentobarbital, midazolam, or propofol.
- Titrate treatment to suppression of the EEG background, aiming at seizure-free tracings.
- Consider aggressive management such as surgery or vagus nerve stimulation after persistent medical management of refractory SE has failed in patients with no underlying catastrophic CNS disease.

■ References

1. Lowenstein DH, Alldredge BK. Status epilepticus. *N Engl J Med* 1998;338:970–976.
2. Shaner MD, McCurdy S, Herring M, Gabor A. Treatment of status epilepticus: a prospective comparison of diazepam and phenytoin versus phenobarbital and optional phenytoin. *Neurology* 1988;38:202–207.
3. Treiman D, Meyers PD, Walton NY, Collins JF, Colling C, Rowan AJ, Handforth A, Faught E, Calabrese VP, Uthman BM, Ramsay RE, Mamdani MB. A comparison of four treatments for generalized convulsive status

epilepticus. Veterans Affairs Status Epilepticus Cooperative Study Group. *N Engl J Med* 1998; 339:792–798.

4. Alldredge BK, Gelb AM, Isaacs SM, Corry MD, Allen F, Ulrich S, Gottwald MD, O'Neil N, Neuhaus JM, Segal MR, Lowenstein DH. A comparison of lorazepam, diazepam, and placebo for the treatment of out-of-hospital status epilepticus. *N Engl J Med* 2001;345:631–637.

5. Ramsay RE, Hammond EJ, Perchalski RJ, Wilder J. Brain uptake of phenytoin, phenobarbital and diazepam. *Arch Neurol* 1979;36:535–539.

6. Leppik IE, Derivan AT, Homan RW, Walker J, Ramsay RE, Patrick B. Double-blind study of lorazepam and diazepam in status epilepticus. *JAMA* 1983;249: 1452–1454.

7. Camfield CS, Camfield PR, Smith E, Dooley JM. Home use of rectal diazepam to prevent status epilepticus in children with convulsive disorders. *J Child Neurol* 1989;4:125–126.

8. Parent JM, Lowenstein DH. Treatment of refractory generalized status epilepticus with continuous infusion of midazolam. *Neurology* 1994;44:1837–1840.

9. Allen FH, Runge RW, Legarda S, et al. Safety, tolerance and pharmacokinetics of fosphenytoin in status epilepticus. *Epilepsia* 1995;36(Suppl 4): 90–94.

10. Browne TR, Kugler AR, Eldon MA. Pharmacology and pharmacokinetics of fosphenytoin. *Neurology* 1996;46:S3–S7.

11. Ramsay RE, DeToledo J. Intravenous administration of fosphenytoin: options for the management of seizures. *Neurology* 1996;46:S17–S19.

12. Uthman BM, Wilder BJ, Ramsay RE. Intramuscular use of fosphenytoin: an overview. *Neurology* 1996; 46:S24–S28.

13. Eldon MA, Loewan GR, Voightman RE, Koup JR, et al. Pharmacokinetics and tolerance of fosphenytoin and phenytoin administration intravenously to healthy subjects. *Can J Neurol Sci* 1993;20:5810.

14. Sinha S, Naritoku D. Intravenous valproate is well tolerated in unstable patients with status epilepticus. *Neurology* 2000;55;722–724.

15. Yaffe K, Lowenstein DH. Prognostic factors of pentobarbital therapy for refractory generalized status epilepticus. *Neurology* 1993;48:895–900.

16. Lowenstein DH, Aminoff MJ, Simon RP. Barbiturate anesthesia in the treatment of status epilepticus. *Neurology* 1988;38:395–400.

17. Claassen J, Hirsch LJ, Emerson RG, Mayer SA. Treatment of refractory status epilepticus: pentobarbital, propofol, or midazolam: a systematic review. *Epilepsia* 2002;43:146–153.

18. Stecker MM, Kramer TH, Rapps EC. Treatment of refractory status epilepticus with propofol: clinical and pharmacokinetic findings. *Epilepsia* 1998;39:18–26.

19. Manno EM. New management strategies in the treatment of status epilepticus. *Mayo Clin Proc* 2003;78:508–518.

20. Lawn ND, Wijdicks E. Status epilepticus: a critical review of management options. *Can J Neurol Sci* 2002;29:206–215.

21. Prasad A, Worrall BB, Bertram E, Bleck T. Propofol and midazolam in the treatment of refractory status epilepticus. *Epilepsia* 2001;42:380–386.

22. Dodson WE, DeLorenzo RJ, Pedley TA, et al. The treatment of convulsive status epilepticus: recommendations of the Epilepsy Foundation of America's Working Group for Status Epilepticus. *JAMA* 1993;270:854–859.

23. Claasen J, Hirsch LJ, Emerson RC. Continuous EEG monitoring and midazolam infusion for nonconvulsive refractory status epilepticus. *Neurology* 2001;57: 1036–1042.

24. Privitera M, Hoffman M, Moore JL, Jester D. EEG detection of nontonic-clonic status epilepticus in patients with altered consciousness. *Epilepsy Res* 1994;18:155–166.

25. Towne AR, Waterhouse EJ, Boggs JG, Garnett LK, Brown AJ, Smith JR Jr, DeLorenzo RJ. Prevalence of nonconvulsive status epilepticus in comatose patients. *Neurology* 2000;54:340–345.

26. DeLorenzo RJ, Waterhouse EJ, Towne AR, Boggs JG, Ko D, DeLorenzo GA, Brown A, Garnett L. Persistent nonconvulsive status epilepticus after the control of convulsive status epilepticus. *Epilepsia* 1998;39: 833–840.

27. Assal P, Papazyan JP, Slosman DO, Jallon P, Goerres GW. SPECT in periodic lateralizing epileptiform discharges: a form of partial status epilepticus? *Seizure* 2001;10:260–265.

28. Handforth A, Cheng JT, Mandelken MA, Treiman DT. Markedly increased mesiotemporal lobe metabolism in a case with PLEDs: further evidence that PLEDs are a manifestation of partial SE. *Epilepsia* 1994; 35:876–881.

29. Crisp CB, Gannon R, Knauft F. Continuous infusion of midazolam hydrochloride to control status epilepticus. *Clin Pharmacol* 1988;7:322–324.

30. Kumar A, Bleck TP. Intravenous midazolam for the treatment of refractory status epilepticus. *Crit Care Med* 1992;20:483–488.

31. Rashkin MC, Young C, Penovich P. Pentobarbital treatment of refractory status epilepticus. *Neurology* 1987;37:500–503.

32. Wood PR, Brown GP, Pugh S. Propofol infusion for the treatment of status epilepticus. *Lancet* 1988;27:480–481.

33. Ma X, Liporace J, O'Connor MJ, Sperling MR. Neurosurgical treatment of medically intractable status epilepticus. *Epilepsy Res* 2001;46:33–38.

34. Holtkamp M, Masuhr F, Harms L, Einhäupl KM, Meierkord H, Buchheim K. The management of refractory generalised convulsive and complex partial status epilepticus in three European countries: a survey among epileptologists and critical care neurologists. *J Neurol Neurosurg Psychiatry* 2003;74:1095–1099.

Chapter 4
Movement Disorder Emergencies

Steven J. Frucht

Most physicians do not think of a movement disorder as an emergency. Although mostly true, there are clinical scenarios in which patients present with a movement disorder evolving over hours to days that could lead to fatality if not diagnosed and treated appropriately. The severity of symptoms and signs usually prompts patients to seek immediate medical attention. In other circumstances, these patients are often unexpectedly encountered in the emergency room or, against all expectation, as hospital consults.

Although a continuum exists, this chapter will discuss the five major categories of movement disorder emergencies—acute parkinsonism, dystonia, chorea, tics, and myoclonus—illustrated by brief vignettes. Management strategies presented here are based on the best available data in the literature, but also on personal encounters with these very sick patients.

■ Acute Parkinsonism

Acute parkinsonism is diagnosed when extrapyramidal signs occur over hours to days. It may be difficult to recognize. It is often a manifestation or complication of a toxin or systemic illness. A rapid and often dramatic response to dopaminergic drugs is typically seen.

The Patient

Case 1: A 9-year-old boy with relapsed leukemia involving the central nervous system received cytosine arabinoside and methotrexate via an implanted Omaya reservoir. Three weeks after his last infusion, he was brought to the emergency department in "a state of acute immobility." On examination, he was unable to move any body part except his eyes, but could communicate by answering yes/no codes with his eyes. Prominent cogwheel rigidity was present in all limbs. He was diagnosed with acute parkinsonism, and one tablet of carbidopa/levodopa 25/100 was given by nasogastric tube. One hour later, he was able to open and close his hand slowly. The dose was gradually increased to two tablets three times per day and his condition improved over several weeks, to the point that he was able to sit unassisted, feed himself, and walk with assistance. Over the ensuing months his condition improved, although moderate parkinsonism remained. An 18-fluorodopa PET scan (Figure 4-1) revealed extensive damage to the presynaptic dopaminergic projection to the striatum, and follow-up MRIs showed bilateral cystic necrosis of the substantia nigra.

Case 2: A 52-year-old woman with stage IV breast cancer received gemcitabine as part of an experimental protocol. Two weeks later she developed a 3 Hz resting tremor of the right leg, facial masking, and a slow gait. She was restless and pacing. To treat her symptoms of akathisia, levodopa was begun and gradually increased to 1500 mg per day. Over several months her symptoms improved and the dose of levodopa was reduced, although not eliminated.

The Problem

- What is the most common cause of acute parkinsonism?

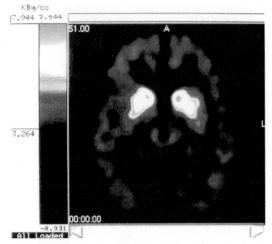

Figure 4-1. Fluorodopa PET scan (sagittal image through the striatum of Case 1). Normal uptake of flourodopa should be robust throughout the caudate (small star) and putamen (big star); however, in this case, uptake is nearly absent in the putamen and diminished in the caudate bilaterally.

- What is the differential diagnosis in rapid-onset dystonia-parkinsonism?
- When should a structural lesion be considered?
- When should one start treatment with levodopa?

The Evidence

Toxins can produce an acute parkinsonian state, and there are many. Well-known toxins are MPTP (1-methyl-4-phenyl-1,2,3,6-tetrahydropyridine) organophosphate pesticides, carbon monoxide, carbon disulfide, cyanide, and methanol.[1] The last four are similar in that parkinsonism is accompanied by severe encephalopathy. Carbon monoxide, carbon disulfide, and cyanide typically produce pallidal necrosis, while methanol usually targets the putamen. Clinical parkinsonism following exposure to these agents is typically without tremor. Acute and reversible parkinsonism has been reported following organophosphate pesticide intoxication. Five patients developed parkinsonism following exposure to a household organophosphate pesticide. All patients spontaneously recovered after they were removed to a pesticide-free environment. Three were treated with levodopa without improvement, and 2 improved before levodopa was administered.[2]

Parkinsonism may occur following infection with viruses that target the substantia nigra. Von Economo described three forms of acute encephalitis lethargica: the somnolent-ophthalmoplegic form (with stupor, external ophthalmoplegia and oculogyric crises), the akinetic-mute form (acute parkinsonism with stupor and mutism), and the hyperkinetic form (akathisia, dyskinesias, and visual hallucinations [Figure 4-2]). The virus responsible for encephalitis lethargica has never been discovered. Sporadic cases of illnesses strikingly similar to encephalitis lethargica still occur, usually following Japanese B encephalitis or infection with measles, coxsackie B2 (Figure 4-3), Western equine, poliomyelitis, cytomegalovirus, HIV, or influenza A. Japanese B encephalitis is the most common cause of endemic encephalitis in Southeast Asia, and the virus can selectively infect the substantia nigra producing parkinsonism.[3] Helpful clinical features of encephalitis lethargica in distinguishing it from other forms of encephalitis include parkinsonism (either acute or delayed), oculogyric crisis, alterations in sleep cycle, ocular or pupillary changes, hyperkinetic movements, and respiratory disturbances.[4] The cerebrospinal fluid in encephalitis lethargica is usually abnormal, with lymphocytosis, elevated protein, and oligoclonal bands.[5] Treatment is supportive and most patients are treated empirically with acyclovir. The response of parkinsonism to dopaminergic stimulation may be incomplete or limited by side effects.

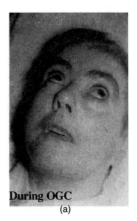
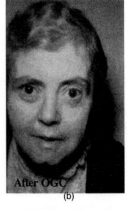

During OGC (a)   After OGC (b)

Figure 4-2. A woman with postencephalitic parkinsonism is shown during (left) and after (right) an oculogyric crisis. Typical dystonic posture of the head, with upward and lateral deviation of the eyes, is seen during the crisis.

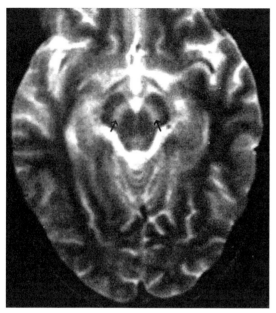

Figure 4-3. A T2 sagittal MRI of a patient with coxsackie virus infection selectively involving the substantia nigra (arrows).

Blunt et al. described 2 patients with encephalitis lethargica who responded rapidly and dramatically to treatment with intravenous methylprednisolone.[6]

The two cases presented illustrate acute parkinsonism as a rare complication of treatment for cancer. The differential diagnosis of a patient who presents with acute immobility and retained arousal also includes pontine infarct (the "locked-in" syndrome), acute motor axonal neuropathy, and disorders of the neuromuscular junction. Acute parkinsonism may occur secondary to cerebral injury or because of chemical or mechanical effects on the nigrostriatal pathway. Lockman et al. reported 5 patients who developed a profound akinetic rigid state following bone marrow transplantation. MRI of the brain revealed leukoencephalopathy, and 4 of 5 patients treated with high-dose methylprednisolone experienced a complete recovery.[7] Three patients were reported who developed a similar syndrome after undergoing treatment with high-dose cytosine arabinoside, cyclophosphamide, total body irradiation, and amphotericin B.[8] Other patients have been reported to develop parkinsonism shortly after receiving chemotherapy. These patients differ in that MRI imaging was normal and their symptoms responded to levodopa. Paclitaxel,[9] cytosine arabinoside,[10] cyclophosphamide and

etoposide,[11] vincristine and adriamycin,[12] and CHOP (cyclophosphamide, doxorubicin, vincristine, and prednisolone[13]) are reported triggers. The response to levodopa and tendency to recover spontaneously suggests a reversible presynaptic inhibition of the nigrostriatal pathway.

Mechanical compression of the nigrostriatal pathway is an extremely rare but potentially reversible cause of acute parkinsonism. In reports published prior to the development of CT scanning, compression of the midbrain was reported to cause parkinsonism.[14,15] Several groups have reported acute or subacute parkinsonism as a presenting sign of aqueductal stenosis. Parkinsonism was typically responsive to both levodopa and ventricular shunting, and recurred during shunt failure.[16–20] It is worthwhile to obtain a head MRI to rule out structural causes of parkinsonism if any features of the clinical presentation or examination are atypical, or if the patient is under the age of 40.

The Pros and Cons

The most critical decision when facing a patient with acute parkinsonism is whether or not to begin treatment with levodopa. The argument against treating with levodopa is that early treatment could potentially engender dyskinesias and motor fluctuations, which might be permanent. There is also a theoretical argument that levodopa could be toxic to damaged dopamine neurons in the substantia nigra. These caveats must be weighed against the pressing need to improve motor performance in patients with severe parkinsonism. Acute parkinsonism due to carbon monoxide, carbon disulfide, and cyanide is poorly responsive to levodopa.

The Main Points

- Tremor may be absent in patients with acute parkinsonism, and the presence of cogwheel rigidity may be the only clue.
- Some patients with structural parkinsonism manifest symptoms of increased intracranial pressure or tectal compromise.
- Drug-induced acute parkinsonism with white matter changes on MRI may respond to treatment with steroids.

- Patients with severe acute parkinsonism should be treated with levodopa, particularly when speech, swallowing, and respiration are involved.

■ Neuroleptic Malignant Syndrome

Neuroleptic malignant syndrome (NMS) is an underappreciated medical emergency. The diagnosis should be considered in any patient who presents with acute parkinsonism and fever. Estimates of the incidence of NMS vary widely, but it is certainly not rare.[21]

The Patient

A 42-year-old man with familial dementia with Lewy bodies was afflicted with an upper respiratory infection that interfered with his ability to take his daily doses of carbidopa/levodopa (every 2 hours) on time. Within 2 days, he developed fever, severe immobility, and soon lapsed into a coma. Creatine kinase was elevated (2000 mU/ml). He was treated with oral levodopa, and recovered within 2 weeks. At a follow-up visit 3 months later, his parkinsonism was back to baseline.

The Problem

- What is the best way to manage neuroleptic malignant syndrome after discontinuation of the offending medication?
- What are the distinctive features of similar, almost indistinguishable, syndromes such as parkinsonism, hyperpyrexia syndrome, and lethal catatonia?

The Evidence

NMS may affect patients of any age and either sex, and may occur in children.[22] Systemic risk factors for NMS include exhaustion, agitation, and dehydration. Certain patients may be more susceptible to NMS, for example those with central nervous system involvement from HIV.[23,24] Any drug with affinity for the D2 dopamine receptor can precipitate NMS, including the antiemetic prochlorperazine and the anesthetic agent droperidol. There is evidence that rapid increases in neuroleptic dose and exposure to high-potency long-acting neuroleptics increase the risk of NMS. Clinical features required for a diagnosis of NMS include exposure to dopamine blockers or withdrawal of dopaminergic stimulation, parkinsonism, and fever. Secondary criteria include autonomic instability, change in mental status, and elevation of creatine kinase. However, NMS may occur without alterations in mental status, without elevations in creatine kinase, and without profound autonomic instability. NMS typically lasts 5 to 10 days and carries significant morbidity and mortality. Patients are best managed in the intensive care unit, where they require supportive care, hydration, temperature regulation, and correction of electrolyte abnormalities.

The offending neuroleptic should be immediately discontinued (quite obvious but not always done!). If a patient with NMS is currently taking medications with dopaminergic agonist properties (such as amantadine), these drugs should not be discontinued as this may aggravate the syndrome. Most patients with NMS are treated with a dopaminergic agent, either a dopamine agonist or levodopa. These drugs can only be administered via the GI tract, usually by nasogastric tube. If gastrointestinal motility is impaired, subcutaneous lisuride is an option,[25] although this preparation is not available in the United States. Dantrolene, a peripherally acting muscle relaxant, has also been used in NMS. For patients who develop NMS and require treatment of psychotic symptoms, electroconvulsive therapy (ECT) has been shown to effectively terminate NMS and control psychosis.[26]

In the 1970s and early 1980s, neurologists would occasionally admit patients with Parkinson's disease to the hospital in order to withdraw them from dopaminergic medications (a "levodopa holiday"). This practice was abandoned following reports of a potentially lethal syndrome reminiscent of NMS.[27,28] Better known as the parkinsonism-hyperpyrexia syndrome,[29] it is clinically indistinguishable from NMS and probably occurs due to central dopamine deficiency. The parkinsonism-hyperpyrexia syndrome is illustrated by the case presented. Friedman et al.[27] reported 3 patients with advanced Parkinson's disease who developed fever, rigidity, autonomic instability, and elevations in creatine kinase several days after withdrawal from levodopa. One patient died and 2 recovered, but only after levodopa was reintroduced. With the advent of bilateral subthalamic nucleus stimulation for advanced Parkinson's disease, similar presentations have occurred when stimulators were accidentally turned off.[30] Although levodopa holidays have been abandoned, this syndrome may occur in patients with Parkinson's disease even if they do not discontinue their medications. Simpson and Davis[31] reported a patient who developed parkinsonism-hyperpyrexia following withdrawal of amantadine. The syndrome has also been reported in the premenstrual period[32] and as a fatal complication of a severe "off" state.[33] Kuno and colleagues reviewed their experience with 19 patients with Parkinson's disease who developed the syndrome,[34] including 7 who continued their medications. Among the latter, parkinsonism-hyperpyrexia developed exclusively between the months of May and August, suggesting that heat and dehydration may be predisposing factors.

A patient may present with symptoms and signs of NMS (parkinsonism, fever, and obtundation) even though there is no history of exposure to dopamine-blocking drugs. In fact, patients were reported with a syndrome indistinguishable from NMS long before neuroleptics were available. Known as lethal catatonia, this condition is now principally reported in Europe and Asia. It usually begins with intense agitation, catatonia, stereotypies, psychosis, and autonomic instability. It lasts an average of 8 days, and temperatures may climb as high as 110°F. This is followed by severe parkinsonism, stupor, and eventual death. In a review of published reports of lethal catatonia, Mann et al.[35] identified 292 cases, and the mortality in this series was 60 percent. 31 percent of patients did not display agitation or psychosis, instead presenting directly with a catatonic syndrome indistinguishable from NMS. Lethal catatonia may occur following stroke, and with a diencephalic tumor, encephalitis, Cushing's disease, or Wernicke's encephalopathy.

The Pros and Cons

The practice of withdrawing levodopa should *never* be performed in patients with Parkinson's disease because of the risk of engendering the parkinsonism-hyperpyrexia syndrome. Parkinson patients who become psychotic are often admitted to the hospital, and in such settings, the dose of levodopa can usually be halved, with the addition of an atypical neuroleptic such as quetiapine or clozapine. In a sense, NMS is an iatrogenic form of lethal catatonia, and it may be difficult to distinguish the two if information about the patient is limited. Several reports suggest that lethal catatonia is best treated with ECT.[36]

The Main Points

- Neuroleptic malignant syndrome should be suspected in any patient with alteration in mental status with fever (could be low grade) and rigidity. Elevation in creatine kinase is not required for diagnosis.
- Patients with advanced Parkinson's disease and prominent motor fluctuations are predisposed to develop the parkinsonism-hyperpyrexia syndrome when dopaminergic drugs are suddenly withdrawn. Treatment with bilateral subthalamic nucleus stimulation may also precipitate this entity.

■ Acute Laryngeal Dystonia Causing Stridor

When evaluating patients with laryngeal dystonia in the office, neurological findings may be subtle. Signs of laryngeal dysfunction such as hoarseness and dysarthria are usually absent. Daytime stridor is a particularly ominous complaint with a mean survival of less than one year without treatment.[37] Dystonia may affect the vocal cords or laryngeal muscles, triggering acute upper airway obstruction. This catastrophe is most commonly seen during acute dystonic reactions from neuroleptics.

The Patient

Case 1: A 62-year-old man with multiple system atrophy presented for a routine office visit complaining of a change in his sleeping pattern. He reported that his breathing became labored and high-pitched when his levodopa wore off. His wife described episodes in which he made a high-pitched noise while breathing at night.

Videofluoroscopy of his vocal cords revealed moderate paresis of the vocal cord abductors, with stridor. He subsequently required a tracheostomy.

Case 2: A 25-year-old schizophrenic man walked into the emergency room pointing to his throat. Within one minute of arrival, he developed retrocollic and severe opisthotonic posturing that closed his airway. Endotracheal intubation was impossible. Emergent intravenous access was obtained and 50 mg of diphenhydramine were administered, with resolution of acute dystonia and airway closure. It was later learned that he had received a depot preparation of haloperidol.

The Problem

- How do we recognize acute laryngeal dystonia?
- How is stridor best quickly treated?

The Evidence

Acute respiratory compromise is rare in patients with parkinsonism with the exception of Shy-Drager syndrome. Shy-Drager patients are at increased risk for sudden death due to upper airway obstruction. Increased snoring at night may be followed by stridor, typically intermittent and nocturnal. With time, stridor occurs during the day, and the patient may develop sleep apnea.[38] Shy-Drager may present as snoring or stridor in the absence of any other evidence of neurological dysfunction.[39–41] Snoring and stridor occur in Shy-Drager syndrome because of dysfunction of the posterior cricoarytenoid muscles, the sole abductors of the vocal cords. An autopsy study of 3 such patients did not reveal neuronal loss within the nucleus ambiguus,[42] suggesting that abductor dysfunction does not result from denervation. As a result of selective abductor paresis, the vocal cords remain in an adducted position. The degree of snoring and stridor correlate with the extent of paresis.[43] It is prudent to question the bed partners of all patients with parkinsonism about nocturnal snoring and stridor. A history of either complaint should prompt an immediate referral to an otolaryngologist for fiber optic laryngoscopy. Patients with evidence of even partial abductor paresis are at high

risk for sudden death,[44] and the definitive treatment is tracheostomy. One patient with this syndrome was treated successfully with surgical lateralization of the vocal cord.[45] Nasal continuous positive air pressure at night can successfully treat nocturnal stridor and apnea in patients who choose not to undergo tracheostomy.[46]

Laryngeal muscles may be affected in patients with tardive dyskinesia.[47] Flaherty and Lahmeyer were the first to suggest that sudden death following treatment with phenothiazines might occur from acute laryngeal dystonia.[48] Acute laryngeal dystonia following exposure to neuroleptics has been reported in 9 cases.[49] Six patients were young men (under age 30), and all episodes of laryngospasm occurred within 8 days of initiating treatment. Most patients received only a modest dose, suggesting that there may be individuals with a heightened susceptibility to develop acute dystonia. Three of these events occurred in the early morning hours. Immediate treatment with intravenous diphenhydramine in doses ranging from 25 to 62.5 mg was life-saving.

Botulinum toxin injection of the vocal cord adductors is an effective treatment for chronic upper airway obstruction due to adductor dystonia. Feve et al.[47] reported a patient exposed to neuroleptics who developed intermittent complete upper airway obstruction secondary to dystonia of the thyroarytenoid muscles (the muscles that adduct the vocal cords). Injection of 5 units of botulinum toxin into the thyroarytenoids produced immediate and dramatic improvement in his breathing. A similar patient with X-linked dystonia-parkinsonism also benefited from botulinum toxin injections.[50] The largest series of patients with laryngeal dystonia causing stridor was reported by Marion et al.[51] They also observed involuntary activity of the thyroarytenoid muscles and striking improvement with botulinum toxin. Botulinum toxin injection offers a safe and effective treatment for this potentially life-threatening problem.

The Pros and Cons

The decision to perform a tracheostomy on a patient with multiple system atrophy is difficult. While tracheostomy offers the best chance to prevent sudden death from asphyxiation, patients are still at risk for sudden death from autonomic instability and cardiac arrhythmias. Patients with Shy-Drager syndrome who have minimal extrapyramidal signs are the best candidates for this procedure.

The Main Points

- Sudden death may occur with acute laryngeal dystonia or stridor.
- One should question all patients with multiple system atrophy and their bed partner about nighttime snoring or stridor, or any change in respiratory pattern.
- Any history of such change should prompt a referral to an otolaryologist and consideration of tracheostomy.
- Prompt use of intravenous diphenhydramine can be life-saving for patients with acute laryngeal dystonia.

■ Double Hit: Concomitant Neurological Disorders

Marked deterioration in Parkinson's disease may have other neurological causes, and complications of dystonia can occur. Chronic movement disorders naturally fluctuate, and it is routine for patients (especially patients with advanced Parkinson's disease) to have periods where their symptoms are not optimally controlled. Usually, adjusting medication dosing or schedule corrects the problem; however, there are several caveats and extrapyramidal signs could worsen with medical illness.

The Patient

Case 1: A 55-year-old man with advanced Parkinson's disease and motor fluctuations presented for a routine outpatient visit. His wife reported that over the last 3 weeks his walking had become slower, and over the last week he had required a wheelchair. A cursory examination attributed his gait difficulty to worsening parkinsonism, and he was referred for evaluation for possible implantation of bilateral subthalamic nucleus stimulators. Fortunately, a closer examination revealed brisk reflexes and upgoing toes, and a cervical MRI

confirmed a high cervical cord compression from a prolapsed disc. After surgical decompression he recovered to his baseline status.

Case 2: A 40-year-old woman with severe dystonia was treated in the past with bilateral thalamotomies and maintained on high-dose anticholinergics, baclofen, and diazepam. On a routine office visit, she was noted to have a reduction in muscle tone in her extremities and her dystonia seemed improved. Two weeks later, she presented to an outside institution with acute cervical cord compression from an unrecognized cervical disc. She was successfully treated with emergency cervical decompression and recovered.

The Problem

- What are other possible neurological explanations for worsening in Parkinson's disease and dystonia?
- Which tests may be diagnostic?

The Evidence

It is not uncommon for urinary tract infections to present as a deterioration of parkinsonism, particularly in men who may not complain of frank dysuria. Urine analysis and blood cultures can be diagnostic. Marked deterioration in parkinsonism has been reported in several patients with subdural hematomas,[52,53] and prompt recognition with surgical evacuation of hemorrhage reduces additional morbidity. The first case illustrates the difficulty in recognizing acute neurological syndromes in patients who are followed in chronic care clinics, particularly when there is a tendency to attribute any deterioration to the underlying neurological illness. MRI of the cervical spine led to the correct diagnosis.

Patients with severe dystonia are at increased risk for compression of the spinal cord, plexus, or peripheral nerves. This is particularly true for patients with dystonic-athetoid cerebral palsy who are at increased risk for cervical myelopathy from continuous movements of the neck. Hirose and Kadoya[54] reported 4 such patients with an average age of 33 who developed severe spondylotic myelopathy. Degenerative changes were worst at the C3–C4 level and all 4 patients recovered following anterior decompression.

There is virtually no literature on the appropriate management of patients with severe, generalized dystonia who develop intractable scoliosis. The major concern after spine surgery in these patients is that continued dystonic contractions may disrupt the hardware or even cause it to protrude through the skin. Our approach is to refer patients who develop severe scoliosis from generalized dystonia for implantation of bilateral globus pallidus stimulators.

The Main Points

- In a patient with Parkinson's disease and worsening of mobility, cervical cord compression should be considered.
- Acute urosepsis may superficially mimic deteriorating Parkinson's disease.
- Patients with severe torticollis and generalized dystonia patients with retrocollic posturing are at risk for cervical cord compression. Neurologists need to maintain a high index of suspicion for this condition to avoid potential major morbidity.

■ Dystonic Storm

Dystonic storm, continuous unremitting generalized dystonic spasms, is probably more common than the scarcity of reports in the literature would suggest. Affected patients usually have an underlying history of dystonia, and dystonic spasms evolving into a flurry are often triggered by systemic illness. Patients in a so-called dystonic storm must be treated in an intensive care unit, but even with aggressive treatment, the prognosis of this disorder may be ominous.

The Patient

Case 1: A 13-year-old boy was transferred from another institution in dystonic storm. Severe, continuous dystonic movements had begun one week after a respiratory illness. Despite treatment with high-dose anticholinergics and baclofen, dystonic movements persisted and were severe enough to prevent him from sitting up or eating. He was admitted to the intensive care unit and treated with high-dose diazepam. Dystonic storm persisted, and he eventually was successfully treated with intrathecal baclofen.

Case 2: An 8-year-old boy presented to clinic with a history of episodes of severe dystonic movements. During one of these episodes, severe involuntary opisthotonus threw him to the floor. He was febrile (38.5°C), and his creatine kinase was 5500 mU/ml. He was admitted to the intensive care unit and treated with intravenous fluids and sedation with lorazepam. Creatine kinase level quickly decreased. He subsequently underwent implantation of bilateral globus pallidus stimulators with good control of his dystonia and resolution of the episodes of dystonic crisis.

The Problem

- What is the most effective management of dystonic storm?
- What are the major additional medical concerns?

The Evidence

Continuous dystonic movements are a frightening experience. Patients sweat profusely, are febrile, become unable to control posture, and lack the ability to take sufficient fluid and food by mouth. Hyperthermia, fluid loss, and respiratory compromise due to a combination of muscle spasm and fatigue may follow. Two patients who developed rhabdomyolysis from severe dystonic spasms have been reported.[55,56] Dystonic spasms may be resistant to treatment with anticholinergics, baclofen, benzodiazepines, dopamine blockers, or dopamine depleters,[57] and patients often require sedation and paralysis to stop the movements. Manji et al.[57] reported 12 patients with dystonic storm and suggested that the combination of benzhexol, tetrabenazine, and pimozide was often effective in patients who were refractory to other treatments. At least one patient with dystonic storm has been successfully treated with intrathecal baclofen,[58] and there may be a role for bilateral pallidal stimulation for certain intractable patients.

The Main Points

- Dystonic storm is a complex neurological and medical disorder.
- Patients need to be in the intensive care unit in order to prevent fluid loss and rhabdomyolysis.
- Patients often require large doses of sedating medications in order to terminate the dystonia.
- Bilateral globus pallidus stimulator implantation is a drastic but in some patients an effective solution to this problem.

■ **Oculogyric Crisis**

Oculogyric crisis, first described in patients with encephalitis lethargica (see Figure 4-2), is a form of acute dystonia. It takes its name from the tendency of the eyes to deviate, although eye movements are only part of the syndrome. Sacks and Kohl[59] elegantly summarized the panoply of disturbances in postencephalitic crises

> …among the common accompanying symptoms we have observed in oculogyric crises are the following: opisthotonus and generalized rigidity, intense terror or rage, thalamic pain and anguish, multiple autonomic symptoms (sometimes accompanied by conspicuous tachycardia and hypertension), hypervigilance, extreme motor urge, akathisia, complex reiterative movements and ticking, forced gasping and gagging, loud phonation, tachyphemia and tachypraxis, pallilalia and verbigeration, obsessional and sometimes delusional remuneration, and—in all crises—some degree, and in the worst crises a profound degree, of catalepsy and/or block.

The Patient

Case 1: A 92-year-old woman presented with a 2½ year history of episodes occurring every 3 days, characterized by dystonic posturing, myoclonus, gaping mouth, tachypnea and gasping, obsessional thoughts, and tachycardia. Each episode lasted 4 to 8 hours, at which point she would fall asleep exhausted. Episodes resolved with withdrawal of levodopa and treatment with benztropine 0.5 mg three times daily.

Case 2: A 26-year-old man with juvenile parkinsonism was maintained on levodopa with marked motor fluctuations. Pergolide was begun in an attempt to minimize fluctuations. Soon after starting it, he developed oculogryric crises, characterized by dystonic posturing of the right arm, retrocollis, and painful upward and lateral deviation of the eyes. He was able to look down for brief periods only. 25 mg of intravenous diphenhydramine terminated the attack, and pergolide was withdrawn.

The Problem

- Which drugs cause oculogyric crises?
- Should structural lesions be sought?

The Evidence

Oculogyric crises are most commonly seen following exposure to neuroleptics, and crises may occur as acute or tardive phenomena.[60–62] The incidence of oculogyric crises in patients treated with chronic neuroleptics may be as high as 10 percent,[62] and in one report of 24 children accidentally exposed to haloperidol, 14 of them developed oculogyric crises.[63] Tetrabenazine,[64] gabapentin,[65] domperidone,[66] carbamazepine,[67] and lithium carbonate[68] have all been reported to trigger oculogyric crises. Sacks et al.[69] reported that levodopa initially suppressed crises in postencephalitic patients, although it later enhanced their severity and intensity. Oculogyric crisis may occur in patients with dopa-responsive dystonia, and in one such patient, treatment with levodopa eliminated both dystonia and crises.[70] There are also credible reports of oculogyric crises associated with structural brain lesions, such as bilateral paramedian thalamic infarction,[71] herpes encephalitis, cystic glioma of the posterior third ventricle,[72] and as the initial manifestation of Wilson's disease.[73]

Regardless of their cause, acute oculogyric crises can be terminated with injection of intravenous anticholinergics or diphenhydramine (25–50 mg). Diphenhydramine is readily available in hospital emergency rooms and is probably the treatment of choice for this condition. Oral clonazepam may be effective for patients with chronic neuroleptic-induced oculogyric crises that are resistant to anticholinergics.[74]

The Pros and Cons

Anticholinergics should be immediately administered to any patient with oculogyric crisis. After resolution of the crisis, a detailed history and physical examination may indicate which patients must have brain imaging to exclude a possible structural lesion. Imaging may be superfluous in patients with previous history of a well-defined parkinsonian syndrome and recent exposure to a known trigger. But MRI should be considered in any case with atypical features or unclear cause for the crisis.

The Main Points

- Oculogyric crises are commonly a result of neuroleptic agents, but several acute structural lesions have been reported.
- Intravenous diphenhydramine (25–50 mg IV) is the treatment choice.
- Lorazepam may be considered in recalcitrant cases.

■ Pseudodystonia

Pseudodystonia, conditions that mimic dystonia, includes four disorders that may present as emergencies: infectious torticollis, neoplastic torticollis, atlantoaxial rotatory subluxation (AARS), and localized tetanus.

The Patient

An 8-year-old boy who was in good health woke up one morning with a fixed laterocollis. There was no variation in neck posture throughout the day, and his neck remained fixed in sleep. There was no history of trauma and he was otherwise well. An MRI of the brain and cervical cord showed only tilt of the neck, but a CT scan of the neck with fine cuts through C1 to C3 showed AARS with the dens displaced posterior and to the left protruding into the foramen magnum, and the anterior arch of C1 displaced downwards and rotated to the right. He underwent a curative open reduction, followed by 3 months in a halo head ring and jacket.

The Problem

- What conditions may underlie acute torticollis in a child?
- What is the appropriate imaging modality?

The Evidence

Acute infectious torticollis is rare but has been reported in epidemics in eastern and northern China.[75] After a prodrome of fever and malaise, patients develop acute torticollis accompanied by protrusion of the tongue, opening or closing of the mouth, and deviation of the mandible. The etiology is unknown although a viral cause has been postulated. Torticollis occurs more commonly as a sequel to infectious or inflammatory processes of the head or neck. Known as Grisel's syndrome, torticollis may follow nonspecific pharyngitis, tonsillitis or adenoiditis, retropharyngeal or tonsillar abscess, mastoiditis or otitis media, cervical adenitis, acute rheumatic fever, parotitis, syphilitic pharyngeal ulcer, or influenza.[76]

Torticollis is a rare presentation of spinal cord tumor. Visudhiphan et al.[77] reported 4 children with spinal cord tumors (two astrocytomas, one neuroblastoma, and one epidural sarcoma) in which torticollis was a prominent presenting sign—in one case, torticollis preceded other neurological signs by one month. Shafrir and Kaufman[78] reported a disaster in an infant with congenital torticollis due to a spinal cord astrocytoma. Chiropractic manipulation prior to correct diagnosis triggered a respiratory arrest and quadriplegia due to tumor necrosis.

AARS is an uncommon but potentially devastating cause of acute torticollis in children. A child typically presents with acute head tilt, contralateral neck rotation and mild neck flexion, and the muscles of the neck may appear loose. Children are especially prone to this condition due to the increased laxity of spinal ligaments and the degree of freedom of their C1–C2 vertebrae. Three clinical signs help distinguish AARS from other causes of torticollis: (1) the spinous process of C2 may be palpable in the same direction as the head rotation; (2) the sternocleidomastoid on the same side of the head rotation may be taut; (3) the patient may be unable to rotate the neck past midline.[79] It is worth noting that the trauma needed to produce AARS can be slight, and that it may occur spontaneously without trauma.[80]

The Pros and Cons

Bredenkamp and Maceri[81] reviewed their experience with 26 children who presented to the emergency room with acute nontraumatic torticollis, and proposed guidelines for the management of acute torticollis in children. All children presenting with acute nontraumatic torticollis should be assumed to have an inflammatory head and neck process. Initial management should include cervical immobilization. CT or MRI imaging is necessary to delineate the atlantoaxial joint, and has the added benefit of identifying space-occupying lesions in the neck (i.e., plain radiographs are inadequate).

The Main Points

- All patients with acute or persistent torticollis must be assumed to harbor a nontraumatic AARS until proven otherwise.
- Young children with acute nontraumatic torticollis could harbor an infection in the soft tissue space and should be evaluated in the emergency room with appropriate urgent imaging.
- Delineation of the atlantoaxial joint with CT or MRI imaging is mandatory.
- All children with torticollis, even those with "congenital torticollis," should have a neurological and radiological evaluation before any physical therapy is instituted.
- Axial traction is not helpful after one month, and atlantoaxial fusion is necessary, at the cost of limited range of motion of the cervical spine.

■ Acute Chorea

Hemiballism-hemichorea is one of the most dramatic acute hyperkinetic movement disorders. Causes are multiple, including toxic, immunological, infectious, structural, and metabolic disorders.

The Patient

A 72-year-old woman in good health presented to the emergency room with acute generalized chorea. Chorea was so severe that she was unable to eat or walk, and she required protective railings to reduce skin abrasions. Her blood sugar was 450 mg/dL and an MRI revealed bilateral high signal on T1-weighted images in the striatum. Movements were well controlled with 150 mg of tetrabenazine.

The Problem

- What are the main diagnostic considerations in chorea and hemiballism?
- What are the most effective pharmacological agents to suppress chorea and hemiballism?

The Evidence

Early studies correlated hemiballism with lesions in the subthalamic nucleus; however, in a review of 21 patients with hemiballism, only 5 had an identifiable lesion in the subthalamic nucleus.[82] Hemiballism has been reported in association with an ipsilateral chronic subdural hematoma,[82] and in 4 patients as a manifestation of subcortical white matter ischemia.[83,84] Hemiballism may be the first sign of nonketotic hyperglycemia.[85,86] High signal lesions are seen in the striatum on T1-weighted MRI images, and the disorder usually remits with correction of hyperglycemia. Severe dyskinesias have been noted after withdrawal from clozapine,[87] so-called "withdrawal-emergent" dyskinesias.

Most patients with severe hemiballism require treatment. In a small series of patients reported,[82] haloperidol was the most successful drug to suppress ballistic movements followed by reserpine and clonazepam. Olanzapine[88] and clozapine[89] have also been reported to control the movement disorder in single cases.

Harbord and Kobayashi[90] reported two patients with cerebral palsy who developed severe ballism during a febrile illness with, in one case, a several-fold elevation in creatine kinase. Two similar patients with recurrent episodes of chorea were later reported.[91] It is also important to consider other reversible causes of severe chorea, such as phenytoin intoxication[92] and antiphospholipid antibodies.[93]

The Pros and Cons

Neuroleptics will usually suppress hemiballism-hemichorea, and since the disorder is often transient, a short course of treatment can be used. This helps minimize exposure to D2-receptor blockers and reduces the risk of tardive dyskinesias. Tetrabenazine, a dopamine depletor and blocker, can be considered because it does not risk engendering tardive movements. In centers where tetrabenazine is not available, it is reasonable to use standard neuroleptics such as haloperidol to control severe chorea. The risk of engendering a tardive syndrome from a short course of a typical neuroleptic is outweighed by the need to control chorea in this setting. This is particularly because respiratory difficulties may occur due to diaphragm dyskinesias causing ineffective inspiration.[94]

The Main Points

- Tetrabenazine, haloperidol, clonazepam, or olanzapine may mute hemiballism.
- Withdrawal dyskinesias can be severe enough to require feeding with a percutaneous gastrostomy tube.[95,96] Reinstituting the neuroleptic is an appropriate strategy in these patients.
- Tardive dyskinesias may constitute an emergency due to severe respiratory and diaphragmatic dyskinesias.

■ Tic Emergencies

Tic status refers to patients with the following clinical features: (1) continuous tics that cannot be voluntarily suppressed for more than several seconds; and (2) tics that present a personal risk to the patient, including those that interfere with the ability to appear in public, to sit in a classroom, or to work. A patient with a history of tics will typically experience an exacerbation and present to the office or the emergency room. Vocal tics include sniffing, throat clearing, coughing, random sounds, or formed words. Coprolalia is the most distressing

symptoms of Tourette's and is fortunately not common.[97] Loud vocal tics and coprolalia are completely intolerable for school-age children.

The Patient

Case 1: A 55-year-old man with a history of obsessive-compulsive disorder and mild tics presented to the emergency room with a severe exacerbation of vocal tics. He could not suppress continuous vocal tics (squeaks and grunts) and was in danger of losing his job. Treatment with tetrabenazine 25 mg three times per day resolved his tics.

Case 2: An 11-year old boy with Tourette's syndrome was brought by his parents to clinic. Two days prior, he began to have screaming tics that were so loud that neighbors four houses down the street called the police to complain. A short course of risperidone controlled his vocal tics without recurrence.

Case 3: A 15-year-old young man with Tourette's syndrome was well controlled with pimozide. After a respiratory infection, he developed continuous vocal groaning tics that could not be controlled with increasing doses of pimozide. He was unable to attend school due to his tics. Treatment with tetrabenazine (75 mg per day) resolved his vocal tics. However, he became so anxious about returning to school that he developed a severe psychogenic movement disorder, requiring hospitalization.

The Problem

- What type of tic disorders are concerning?
- What are the therapeutic options?

The Evidence

Swedo and colleagues[98] were the first to describe children with an acute syndrome that they called PANDAS (pediatric autoimmune neuropsychiatric disorders associated with streptococcus). These patients present at age 6 or 7 with acute dramatic tics or obsessive-compulsive symptoms following group A β-hemolytic streptococcus infection. Symptoms wax and wane with time, often triggered by further streptococcal infections or episodes of pharyngitis. PANDAS represents only a small subset of patients who present with tics. Although some neurologists have reservations about this entity, others argue that it is important to identify these patients as treatment with plasma exchange or intravenous immunoglobulin rapidly and dramatically improves both obsessive-compulsive symptoms and tics.[99]

Most patients with malignant vocal tics receive a trial of neuroleptics, although these agents are often ineffective or only partially effective. Several reports have described dramatic benefit from injection of botulinum toxin into the thyroarytenoid muscles.[100–102] Botulinum toxin improved not only the vocal tics but also the premonitory urge to tic. Side effects of mild hoarseness were tolerable. Other types of tics also respond to treatment with botulinum toxin injection.[103,104] The advantage of this treatment is that it specifically targets the body part involved by the tic, and it limits the duration and dose of dopaminergic blockade. The psychological stress triggered by malignant vocal tics is great and should not be underestimated.

Tics may occasionally be severe enough to cause additional neurological disease. Goetz and Klawans[105] described 2 patients who developed compressive neuropathies from severe motor tics. Violent neck tics are the most worrisome motor tic because they may accelerate cervical myelopathy. At least 3 patients with this syndrome have been reported.[106,107] Violent neck tics should thus be treated as an emergency and may be treated effectively with botulinum toxin injection.[107]

The Pros and Cons

Medications that may exacerbate tics should be discontinued, particularly stimulants such as methylphenidate.[108] Most patients with severe motor or vocal tics require treatment with a dopamine depleting agent such as tetrabenazine, although a short course of haloperidol or pimozide may be successful. Once a neuroleptic has been started, other tic medications such as clonazepam or clonidine can be substituted (see the discussion of malignant vocal tics). Tic status may occur in adults, and it can impose tremendous psychological and financial burdens for patients and their families.

The Main Points

- Violent or continuous tics often constitute emergencies that demand acute treatment with a dopamine receptor blocker or tetrabenazine.
- Although PANDAS is infrequent and controversial, its treatment with plasmapheresis or intravenous immunoglobulin has, in some cases, yielded dramatic clinical benefits.

■ Acute Myoclonus

Myoclonus (or startle) may be seen in two movement disorder emergencies that should be recognized early.

The Patient

Case 1: A 28-year-old man began taking paroxetine for depression. Three weeks later he became confused, developed a low-grade fever, and was admitted to the intensive care unit. Prominent myoclonus in the legs was accompanied by diaphoresis, tachycardia, and rigidity. Treatment with cyproheptadine was begun, and he recovered within 48 hours.

Case 2: Neurological consultation was requested for a newborn infant afflicted with recurrent apneic episodes. Marked flexor spasms, severe increase in truncal tone, and lack of habituation to repeated nose tapping were evident. Exaggerated startle to monitors in the intensive care unit triggered apneic episodes lasting as long as 45 seconds. Treatment with clonazepam markedly improved clinical signs of hyperexplexia and apneic episodes resolved.

The Problem

- Which myoclonus syndromes warrant immediate intervention?
- Can we reliably distinguish NMS from serotonin syndrome?

The Evidence

One important syndrome is due to a disorder arising from an increase in biological activity of serotonin.[109–111] The serotonin syndrome is mediated by 5-HT1A receptors located in the brainstem.[111] Any drug or combination of drugs that increases serotonergic transmission (by inhibiting metabolism, direct receptor activation, inhibition of reuptake, or increased substrate supply) can precipitate the syndrome. Serotonin-specific reuptake inhibitors, tryptophan, the combination of monoamine oxidase inhibitors and meperidine, clomipramine, and MDMA ("ecstasy") are well-documented triggers. In a review of 100 cases of serotonin syndrome, confusion (51 percent), hyperthermia (45 percent), diaphoresis (45 percent), tachycardia (36 percent), hypertension (35 percent), agitation (34 percent), and coma (29 percent) were the most common cognitive and autonomic symptoms. Myoclonus (58 percent) was the most common neurological sign, often accompanied by hyperreflexia (52 percent), rigidity (51 percent), tremor (43 percent), and ataxia (40 percent). The presence of myoclonus more likely suggests serotonin syndrome rather than neuroleptic malignant syndrome, although it is often not possible to distinguish the two syndromes on clinical grounds (Table 4-1). Unlike NMS, the serotonin syndrome often resolves within 24 hours.

Patients should be managed in an intensive care unit. Propanolol, diphenhydramine, chlorpromazine, diazepam, and methysergide have been used to treat patients with serotonin syndrome. Cyproheptadine, a histamine-1 receptor blocker with 5-HT1A antagonist properties, reverses clinical signs within hours.[112] Electroconvulsive therapy is a feasible option in some patients.[113]

Table 4-1 Some Distinguishing Features of Neuroleptic Malignant Syndrome and Serotonin Syndrome

Neuroleptic Malignant Syndrome	Serotonin Syndrome
Onset in days to weeks	Onset in minutes to hours
Improves in days (average 9 days)	Improves in < 24 hours
Hyperthermia > 90%	Hyperthermia 46%
Muscle rigidity > 90%	Muscle rigidity 49%
Increased CK > 90%	Increased CK 18%
Hyperreflexia rare	Hyperreflexia 55%
Myoclonus rare	Myoclonus 57%

Hyperexplexia, better known as startle disease, is a rare autosomal dominant disorder that has been linked to mutations in the glycine receptor gene. It typically presents immediately after birth with exaggerated startle and sustained profound generalized muscle spasms. When untreated, neonates may experience sleep myoclonus, delay in development, regurgitation, and even apneic spells that can be fatal.[114–118] It is critical to recognize its presence in the neonatal period. All family members of affected patients should be carefully examined. This disorder can be recognized at the bedside by tapping the infant on the nose, which typically produces facial twitching, head extension, and a generalized flexor spasm.[119] This should be done when the parents are *not* at the bedside, and if an abnormal startle is engendered it should only be done once, as these patients do not habituate to peripheral stimuli and apnea may result. There are patients with hypereplexia who do not show this characteristic response to nose tapping.[117] A severe startle reaction can be truncated by holding the infant by the head and legs and forcibly flexing the trunk. This presumably activates a spinal reflex that terminates the spasm, and is clinically useful for obvious reasons. Treatment with clonazepam (0.1–0.2 mg/kg/day) effectively diminishes the startle response and also treats apnea.[116]

The Main Points

- In practice it can be difficult to differentiate neuroleptic malignant syndrome from the serotonin syndrome.
- When in doubt, it is prudent to treat these patients with dopamine repletion and cyproheptadine, and the time course of clinical improvement helps determine the likely diagnosis.
- All family members of patients with proven hypereplexia should be screened for the condition, and women of childbearing potential should be informed to facilitate recognition.

■ References

1. Watts R, Koller WC. *Movement Disorders*. New York, McGraw-Hill, 1997.

2. Bhatt MH, Elias MA, Mankodi AK. Acute and reversible parkinsonism due to organophosphate pesticide intoxication: five cases. *Neurology* 1999;52:1467–1471.

3. Pradhan S, Pandey N, Shashank S, Gupta RK, Mathur A. Parkinsonism due to predominant involvement of substantia nigra in Japanese encephalitis. *Neurology* 1999;53:1781–1786.

4. Rail D, Scholtz C, Swash M. Post-encephalitic parkinsonism: current experience. *J Neurol Neurosurg Psychiatry* 1981;44:670–676.

5. Howard RS, Lees AJ. Encephalitis lethargica: a report of four recent cases. *Brain* 1987;110:19–33.

6. Blunt SB, Lane RJ, Turjanski N, Perkin GD. Clinical features and management of two cases of encephalitis lethargica. *Mov Disord* 1997;12:354–359.

7. Lockman LA, Sung JH, Krivit W. Acute parkinsonian syndrome with demyelinating leukoencephalopathy in bone marrow transplant recipients. *Pediatr Neurol* 1991;7:457–463.

8. Mott S, Packer R, Vezina LG, Kapur S, Dinndorf PA, Conry JA, Pranzatelli MR, Quinones RR. Encephalopathy with parkinsonian features in children following bone marrow transplantations and high-dose amphotericin-B. *Ann Neurol* 1995;37:810–814.

9. Bower JH, Muenter MD. Temporary worsening of parkinsonism in a patient with Parkinson's disease after treatment with paclitaxel for a metastatic grade IV adenocarcinoma. *Mov Disord* 1995;10:681–682.

10. Luque FA, Selhorst JB, Petruska P. Parkinsonism induced by high-dose cytosine arabinoside. *Mov Disord* 1987;2:219–222.

11. Fleming DR, Mangino PB. Parkinsonian syndrome in a dialysis-supported patient receiving high-dose chemotherapy for multiple myeloma. *South Med J* 1997;90:364–365.

12. Boranic M, Raci F. A parkinson-like syndrome as side effect of chemotherapy with vincristine and adriamycin in a child with acute leukemia. *Biomedicine* 1979;31:124–125.

13. Howell SJL, Sagar HJ. A progressive parkinsonian syndrome developing after chemotherapy and radiotherapy for non-Hodgkin's lymphoma. *Mov Disord* 1994;9:373–374.

14. Oliver L. Parkinsonism due to midbrain compression. *Lancet* 1959;2:817–819.

15. De Vera Reyes JA. Parkinsonian-like syndrome caused by posterior fossa tumor. *J Neurosurg* 1970;33:599–601.

16. Brazin ME, Epstein LG. Reversible parkinsonism from shunt failure. *Pediatr Neurol* 1985;1:306–307.

17. Jankovic J, Newmark M, Peter P. Parkinsonism and acquired hydrocephalus. *Mov Disord* 1986;1:59–64.

18. Shahar E, Lambert R, Hwang PA, Hoffman HJ. Obstructive hydrocephalus-induced parkinsonism. I. Decreased basal ganglia regional blood flow. *Pediatr Neurol* 1988;4:117–119.

19. Curran T, Lang AE. Parkinsonian syndromes associated with hydrocephalus: case reports, a review of the literature, and pathophysiologic hypotheses. *Mov Disord* 1994;9:508–520.

20. Zeidler M, Dorman PJ, Ferguson IT, Bateman DE. Parkinsonism associated with obstructive hydrocephalus due to idiopathic aqueductal stenosis. *J Neurol Neurosurg Psychiatry* 1998;64:657–659.

21. Caroff SN, Mann SC. Neuroleptic malignant syndrome. *Med Clin North Am* 1993;77:185–202.

22. Numa A. Neuroleptic malignant syndrome in children. *Med J Austr* 1991;155:417–419.

23. Factor SA, Podskalny GD, Barron KD. Persistent neuroleptic-induced rigidity and dystonia in AIDS dementia complex: a clinico-pathological case report. *J Neurol Sci* 1994;127:114–120.

24. Gabellini AS, Pezzoli A, De Massis P, Casadei G, Grillo A, Sacquegna T. Neuroleptic malignant syndrome in an AIDS patient: clinical and pathological findings. *Ital J Neurol Sci* 1994;15:293–295.

25. Rodriguez ME, Luquin MR, Lera G, Delgado G, Salazar JM, Obeso JA. Neuroleptic malignant syndrome treated with subcutaneous lisuride infusion. *Mov Disord* 1990;5:170–172.

26. Addonizio G, Susman VL. ECT as a treatment alternative for patients with symptoms of neuroleptic malignant syndrome. *J Clin Psychol* 1987;48:102–105.

27. Friedman JH, Feinberg SS, Feldman RG. A neuroleptic malignant-like syndrome due to levodopa therapy withdrawal. *JAMA* 1985;15:2792–2795.

28. Sechi G, Tanda F, Mutani R. Fatal hyperpyrexia after withdrawal of levodopa. *Neurology* 1984;34:249–251.

29. Granner MA, Wooten GF. Neuroleptic malignant syndrome or parkinsonism hyperpyrexia syndrome. *Semin Neurol* 1991;11:228–235.

30. Hariz MI, Johansson F. Hardware failure in parkinsonian patients with chronic subthalamic nucleus stimulation is a medical emergency. *Mov Disord* 2001;16:166–168.

31. Simpson DM, Davis GC. Case report of neuroleptic malignant syndrome associated with withdrawal from amantadine. *Am J Psychiatry* 1984;141:796–797.

32. Mizuta E, Yamasaki S, Nakatake M, Kuno S. Neuroleptic malignant syndrome in a parkinsonian woman during the premenstrual period. *Neurology* 1993;43:1048–1049.

33. Pfeiffer RF, Sucha EL. "On-off"-induced lethal hyperthermia. *Mov Disord* 1989;4:338–341.

34. Kuno S, Mizuta E, Yamasaki S. Neuroleptic malignant syndrome in parkinsonian patients: risk factors. *Eur Neurol* 1997;38(Suppl):56–59.

35. Mann SC, Caroff SN, Bleier HR, et al. Lethal catatonia. *Am J Psychiatry* 1986;143:1374–1381.

36. Ghaziuddin N, Alkhouri I, Champine D, Quinlan P, Fluent T, Ghaziuddin M. ECT treatment of malignant catatonia NMBS in an adolescent: a useful lesson in

delayed diagnosis and treatment. *J ECT* 2002; 18:95–98.

37. Silber MH, Levine S. Stridor and death in multiple system atrophy. *Mov Disord* 2000:15:699–704.

38. Hanson DG, Ludlow CL, Bassich CJ. Vocal fold paresis in Shy-Drager syndrome. *Ann Otol Rhinol Laryngol* 1983;92:85–90.

39. Martinovits G, Leventon G, Goldhammer Y, Sadeh M. Vocal cord paralysis as a presenting sign in the Shy-Drager syndrome. *J Laryngol Otol* 1988;102:280–281.

40. McBrien F, Spraggs PD, Harcourt JP, Croft CB. Abductor vocal fold palsy in the Shy-Drager syndrome presenting with snoring and sleep apnoea. *J Laryngol Otol* 1996;10:681–682.

41. Wu T, Chen C, Ro L, Chen S, Tang L. Vocal cord paralysis as an initial sign of multiple system atrophy in the central nervous system. *J Formos Med Assoc* 1996;95:804–806.

42. Bannister R, Gibson W, Michaels L, Oppenheimer DR. Laryngeal abductor paralysis in multiple system atrophy. *Brain* 1981;104:351–368.

43. Isozaki E, Naiot A, Horiguchi S, Kawamura R, Hayashida T, Tanabe H. Early diagnosis and stage classification of vocal cord abductor paralysis in patients with multiple system atrophy. *J Neurol Neurosurg Psychiatry* 1996;60:399–402.

44. Munschauer FE, Loh L, Bannister R, Newsom-Davis J. Abnormal respiration and sudden death during sleep in multiple system atrophy with autonomic failure. *Neurology* 1990;40:677–679.

45. Kenyon GS, Apps MCP, Traub M. Stridor and obstructive sleep apnea in Shy–Drager syndrome treated by laryngofissure and cord lateralization. *Laryngoscope* 1984;94:1106–1108.

46. Iranzo A, Santamaria J, Tolosa E. Continuous positive air pressure eliminates nocturnal stridor in multiple system atrophy. *Lancet* 2000;356:1329–1330.

47. Feve A, Angelard B, Fenelon G, Logak M, Guillard A, Lacau Saint-Guily J. Postneuroleptic laryngeal dyskinesias: a cause of upper airway obstructive syndrome improved by local injections of botulinum toxin. *Mov Disord* 1993;8:217–219.

48. Flaherty JA, Lahmeyer HW. Laryngeal-pharyngeal dystonia as a possible cause of asphyxia with haloperidol treatment. *Am J Psychiatry* 1978;135:1414–1415.

49. Koek RJ, Pi EH. Acute laryngeal dystonic reactions to neuroleptics. *Psychosomatics* 1989;30:359–364.

50. Lew MF, Shindo M, Moskowitz CB, Wilhelmsen KC, Fahn S, Waters CH. Adductor laryngeal breathing dystonia in a patient with Lubag (X-linked dystonia-parkinsonism syndrome). *Mov Disord* 1994; 9:318–320.

51. Marion M, Klap P, Perrin A, Cohen M. Stridor and focal laryngeal dystonia. *Lancet* 1992;339:457–458.

52. Wiest RG, Burgunder JM, Krauss JK. Chronic subdural haematomas and parkinsonian syndromes. *Acta Neurochir* 1999;141:753–758.

53. Chou SM, Gutmann L. Deteriorating parkinsonism and subdural hematomas. *Neurology* 2001;57:1295.

54. Hirose G, Kadoya S. Cervical spondylotic radiculomyelopathy in patients with athetoid-dystonic cerebral palsy: clinical evaluation and surgical treatment. *J Neurol Neurosurg Psychiatry* 1984;47:775–780.

55. Paret G, Tirosh R, Ben-Zeev B, Vardi A, Brandt N, Barzilay Z. Rhabdomyolysis due to hereditary torsion dystonia. *Pediatr Neurol* 1995;13:83–84.

56. Vaamonde J, Narbona J, Weiser R, Garcia MA, Brannan T, Obeso JA. Dystonic storms: a practical management problem. *Clin Neuropharmacol* 1994;17:344–347.

57. Manji H, Howard RS, Miller DH, et al. Status dystonicus: the syndrome and its management. *Brain* 1998; 121:243–252.

58. Dalvi A, Fahn S, Ford B. Intrathecal baclofen in the treatment of dystonic storm. *Mov Disord* 1998; 13:611–612.

59. Sacks OW, Kohl M. L-dopa and oculogyric crises. *Lancet* 1970;2:215–216.

60. Sherman S, Dussik KT, Lever PG. Oculogyric crisis induced by phenothiazine drugs. *Dis Nerv Syst* 1960;21:333–334.

61. FitzGerald PM, Jankovic J. Tardive oculogyric crises. *Neurology* 1989;39:1434–1437.

62. Sachdev P. Tardive and chronically recurrent oculogyric crises. *Mov Disord* 1993;8:93–97.

63. Yoshida I, Sakaguchi Y, Matsuishi T, et al. Acute accidental overdosage of haloperidol in children. *Acta Paediatr* 1993;82:877–880.

64. Burke RE, Reches A, Traub MM, Ilson J, Swash M, Fahn S. Tetrabenazine induces acute dystonic reactions. *Ann Neurol* 1985;17:200–202.

65. Reeves AL, So EL, Sharbrough FW, Krahn LE. Movement disorders associated with the use of gabapentin. *Epilepsia* 1996;37:988–990.

66. Shafrir Y, Levy Y, Ben-Amitai D, Nitzan M, Steinherz R. Oculogyric crisis due to domperidone therapy. *Helv Paediatr Acta* 1985;40:95.

67. Gorman M, Barkley GL. Oculogyric crisis induced by carbamazepine. *Epilepsia* 1995;36:1158–1160.

68. Sandyk R. Oculogyric crisis induced by lithium carbonate. *Eur Neurol* 1984;23:92–94.

69. Sacks OW, Kohl M, Schwartz W, Messeloff C. Side-effects of l-dopa in postencephalitic parkinsonism. *Lancet* 1970;2:1006.

70. Lamberti P, de Mari M, Iliceto G, Caldarola M, Serlenga L. Effect of l-dopa on oculogyric crises in a case of dopa-responsive dystonia. *Mov Disord* 1993;8:236–237.

71. Kakigi R, Shibasaki H, Katafuchi Y, Iyatomi I, Kuroda Y. The syndrome of bilateral paramedian thalamic infarction associated with oculogyric crisis. *Clin Neurol* 1986;26:1100–1105.

72. Heimburger RF. Positional oculogyric crises. *J Neurosurg* 1988;69:951–953.

73. Lee MS, Kim YD, Lyoo CH. Oculogyric crisis as an initial manifestation of Wilson's disease. *Neurology* 1999;52:1714–1715.

74. Horiguchi J, Inami Y. Effect of clonazepam on neuroleptic-induced oculogyric crisis. *Acta Psychiatr Scand* 1989;80:521–523.

75. Neng T, Yi C, Xiu-Bao Z, Zhi-Jiao Q. Acute infectious torticollis. *Neurology* 1983;33:1344–1346.

76. Berry DS, Moriarty RA. Atlantoaxial subluxation related to pharyngitis: Grisel's syndrome. *Clin Pediatr* 1999;38:673–675.

77. Visudhiphan P, Chiemchanya S, Somburanasin R, Dheandhanoo D. Torticollis as the presenting sign in cervical spine infection and tumor. *Clin Pediatr* 1982;21:71–76.

78. Shafrir Y, Kaufman BA. Quadriplegia after chiropractic manipulation in an infant with congenital torticollis caused by a spinal cord astrocytoma. *J Pediatr* 1992;120:266–269.

79. Subach RB, McLaughlin MR, Albright L, Pollack IF. Current management of pediatric atlantoaxial rotatory subluxation. *Spine* 1998;23:2174–2179.

80. Grogaard B, Dullerud R, Magnaes B. Acute torticollis in children due to atlanto-axial rotatory fixation. *Arch Orthop Trauma Surg* 1993;112:185–188.

81. Bredenkamp JK, Maceri DR. Inflammatory torticollis in children. *Arch Otolaryngol Head Neck Surg* 1990;116:310–313.

82. Dewey RB, Jankovic J. Hemiballism-hemichorea. *Arch Neurol* 1989;46:862–867.

83. Fukui T, Hasegawa Y, Seriyama S, Takeuchi T, Sugita K, Tsukagoshi H. Hemiballism-hemichorea induced by subcortical ischemia. *Can J Neurol Sci* 1993;20:324–328.

84. Piccolo I, Defanti CA, Soliveri P, Volonte MA, Cislaghi G, Girotti F. Cause and course in a series of patients with sporadic chorea. *J Neurol* 2003;150:429–435.

85. Lee B, Hwang S, Chang G. Hemiballismus-hemichorea in older diabetic women: a clinical syndrome with MRI correlation. *Neurology* 1999;52:646–648.

86. Oerlemans WGH, Moll LCM. Non-ketotic hyperglycemia in a young woman, presenting as hemiballism-hemichorea. *Acta Neurol Scand* 1999;100:411–414.

87. Ahmed S, Chengappa KNR, Naidu VR, Baker RW, Parepally H, Schooler NR. Clozapine withdrawal-emergent dystonias and dyskinesias: a case series. *J Clin Psychiatry* 1998;59:472–477.

88. Safirstein B, Shulman L, Weiner WJ. Successful treatment of hemichorea with olanzapine. *Mov Disord* 1999;14:532–533.

89. Bashir K, Manyam BV. Clozapine for the control of hemiballismus. *Clin Neuropharmacol* 1994;17:477–480.

90. Harbord MG, Kobayashi JS. Fever producing ballismus in patients with choreoathetosis. *J Child Neurol* 1991;6:49–52.

91. Beran-Koehn MA, Zupanc ML, Patterson MC, Olk DG, Ashklog JE. Violent recurrent ballism associated with infections in two children with static encephalopathy. *Mov Disord* 2000;15:570–574.

92. Krishnamorthy KS, Zalneraitis EL, Young RSK, Bernad PG. Phenytoin-induced choreoathetosis in infancy: case reports and a review. *Pediatrics* 1983;72:831–834.

93. Okun MS, Jummani RR, Carney PR. Antiphospholipid-associated chorea and ballism in a child with cerebral palsy. *Pediatr Neurol* 2000;23:62–63.

94. Faheem AD, Brightwell DR, Burton GC, Struss A. Respiratory dyskinesias and dysarthria from prolonged neuroleptic use: tardive dyskinesia? *Am J Psychiatry* 1982;139:517–518.

95. Samie MR, Dannenhoffer MA, Rozek S. Life-threatening tardive dyskinesia caused by metoclopramide. *Mov Disord* 1987;2:125–129.

96. Ovsiew F, Meador KJ, Sethi K. Verapamil for severe hyperkinetic movement disorders. *Mov Disord* 1998;13:341–344.

97. Goldenberg JN, Brown SB, Weiner WJ. Coprolalia in younger patients with Gilles de la Tourette syndrome. *Mov Disord* 1994;9:622–625.

98. Swedo SE, Leonard HL, Garvey M, et al. Pediatric autoimmune neuropsychiatric disorders associated with streptococcal infections: clinical description of the first 50 cases. *Am J Psychiatry* 1998;155:264–271.

99. Perlmutter SJ, Leitman SF, Garvey MA, et al. Therapeutic plasma exchange and intravenous immunoglobulin for obsessive-compulsive disorder and tic disorders in childhood. *Lancet* 1999;354:1153–1158.

100. Scott BL, Jankovic J, Donovan DT. Botulinum toxin injection into vocal cord in the treatment of malignant coprolalia associated with Tourette's syndrome. *Mov Disord* 1996;11:431–433.

101. Salloway S, Stewart CF, Israeli L, Morales X, Rasmussen S, Blitzer A, Brin MF. Botulinum toxin for refractory vocal tics. *Mov Disord* 1996;11:746–748.

102. Trimble MR, Whurr R, Brookes G, Robertson MM. Vocal tics in Gilles de la Tourette syndrome treated with botulinum toxin injections. *Mov Disord* 1998;13:617–619.

103. Jankovic J. Botulinum toxin in the treatment of dystonic tics. *Mov Disord* 1994;9:347–349.

104. Kwak CH, Hanna PA, Jankovic J. Botulinum toxin in the treatment of tics. *Arch Neurol* 2000;57:1190–1193.

105. Goetz CG, Klawans HL. Gilles de la Tourette syndrome and compressive neuropathies. *Ann Neurol* 1980;8:453.

106. Brill CB, Hartz WH, Mancall EL. Cervical disc herniation in the Gilles de la Tourette syndrome. *Ann Neurol* 1981;9:311.

107. Krauss JK, Jankovic J. Severe motor tics causing cervical myelopathy in Tourette's syndrome. *Mov Disord* 1996;11:563–566.

108. Lowe TL, Cohen DJ, Detlor J, Kremenitzer MW, Shaywitz BA. Stimulant medications precipitate Tourette's syndrome. *JAMA* 1982;247:1729–1731.

109. Mills KC. Serotonin syndrome. *Am Fam Phys* 1995;52:1475–1482.

110. Sternbach H. The serotonin syndrome. *Am J Psychiatry* 1991;148:705–713.

111. LoCurto MJ. The serotonin syndrome. *Emerg Med Clin North Am* 1997;15:665–675.

112. Graudins A, Stearman A, Chan B. Treatment of the serotonin syndrome with cyproheptadine. *J Emerg Med* 1998;16:615–619.

113. Nisijima K, Nibuya M, Kato S. Toxic serotonin syndrome successfully treated with electroconvulsive therapy. *J Clin Psychopharmacol* 2002;22:338–339.

114. Cioni G, Biagionin E, Bottai P, Castellacci AM, Paolicelli PB. Hyperexplexia and stiff-baby syndrome: an identical neurological disorder? *Ital J Neurol Sci* 1993;14:145–152.

115. Gherpelli JLD, Nogueira AR, Troster EJ, et al. Hyperexplexia, a cause of neonatal apnea: a case report. *Brain & Develop* 1995;17:114–116.

116. Nigro MA, Lim HCN. Hyperexplexia and sudden neonatal death. *Pediatr Neurol* 1992;8:221–225.

117. Scarcella A, Coppola G. Neonatal sporadic hyperexplexia: a rare and often unrecognized entity. *Brain & Develop* 1997;19:226–228.

118. Kurczynski TW. Hyperexplexia. *Arch Neurol* 1983;40:246–248.

119. Shahar E, Brand N, Uziel Y, Barak Y. Nose tapping test inducing a generalized flexor spasm: a hallmark of hyperexplexia. *Acta Paediatr Scand* 1991;80:1073–1077.

Chapter 5
The Febrile, Agitated, Immunosuppressed Patient

Ian Bone

There is little more daunting to the neurologist than to co-manage the critically ill, immunocompromised patient. Such individuals are liable to a host of clinical problems, many neurological. It requires the exploration of the complex history of the primary illness, awareness of the possible variety of atypical and opportunistic infections, and knowledge of the side effects of specific drugs. The increasing sophistication in the management of systemic disease with more widespread application of immunosuppressive agents ensures that the neurologist will continue to see an increasing number of such cases as an integral part of multidisciplinary teams.

Patients become immunocompromised as the result of an immunodeficiency that can simply be divided into *primary* and *secondary* types. Primary immunodeficiency results from an inherent defect in the constituents of the immune system or its products and is rarely encountered in adult neurological practice. Secondary immunodeficiency is *acquired* and due to a breakdown in the components of the immune response. The commonest predisposing factors resulting in secondary or acquired immunodeficiency are *malnutrition, loss of humoral or cellular components* (e.g., nephrotic syndrome), *tumors, irradiation or cytotoxic drugs, systemic disorders* (e.g., diabetes), or *infections* (including, most notably, the human immunodeficiency virus [HIV]). In practice, the neurologist most frequently encounters the immunocompromised individual in patients with *acquired immunodeficiency*

syndrome (AIDS) or following *radical immunosuppression* or *chemotherapy*. These consults are thus usually requested by infectious diseases, oncology, or organ transplant services. It is important herein in this chapter to review how to deal with febrile, confused, immunosuppressed patients.

■ The Patient

Case 1

A 42-year-old man with a history of chronic myeloid leukemia (CML) was diagnosed with blast transformation. He had pancytopenia, fever, and massive splenomegaly. Bone marrow aspirate showed almost total replacement with blast cells and cytogenetic analysis demonstrated Philadelphia translocation with trisomy for chromosomes 7 and 11. He was treated with 2 courses of ADE (daunorubicin, cytarabine, etoposide) chemotherapy. Marrow regeneration was compatible with chronic-phase CML. Given his poor prognosis, allogenic bone marrow transplant was offered. In preparation for a matched unrelated transplant, he underwent total body irradiation plus conditioning with cyclophosphamide and antilymphocytic globulin. Donor marrow was reinfused uneventfully. He then immediately became febrile and was treated empirically with antibiotics, antifungals, ganciclovir (for CMV prophylaxis), and acyclovir with an apparent response. He was discharged on cyclosporin A, methylprednisolone, acyclovir, ganciclovir, fluconazole, diuretics, and antihypertensive agents.

Within a few days his neutrophil count rose and liver function also deteriorated. Graft rejection or "graft versus host disease" (GVHD) was considered. He was given antilymphocytic globulins (following a normal liver MRI) and a course of amphotericin B to cover for possible fungal infection. Renal function worsened, but later recovered after discontinuation of amphotericin B. His donor was CMV positive, and whilst there was no evidence that the patient himself had this infection, he completed a full course of ganciclovir and had CMV PCR monitored thereafter. He briefly displayed skin changes, which, along with his disturbed liver function, were considered compatible with acute GVHD that was treated with a "standard salvage" of high-dose steroids and antithymocyte globulin (ATG). Over the following 2 months he was closely monitored and required platelet and blood transfusions. He was treated with cyclosporin A, and reducing doses of methylprednisolone.

He was emergently readmitted 4 months after his marrow transplant. He had become agitated, confused, and febrile over several days and had developed generalized tonic-clonic seizures immediately prior to admission. Examination in the emergency room showed him to be confused with a Glasgow coma score (GCS) of 14, a left visual field defect, and left extensor plantar response. CT scan of the brain revealed multiple cerebral lesions (Figure 5-1). A lumbar puncture was performed. Pyrimethamine and sulphadiazine were administered in conjunction with fosphenytoin.

His initial response to treatment was poor. He remained "encephalopathic" but without further seizures. Amphotericin B was added to the regimen. PCR in CSF was negative for toxoplasma, TB, *Aspergillus*, and JC virus. MRI scan was performed (Figure 5-2) and showed no radiological improvement compared with the previous CT, with peripheral contrast enhancement of the left temporal lesion. In the absence of clinical and radiological response to antitoxoplasmosis treatment, stereotactic biopsy was performed. It showed reactive changes without any diagnostic features. Finally, toxoplasma serology revealed IgM antibodies indicating acute infection. Over the next 2 to 3 weeks there was a sustained improvement on continuing antitoxoplasmosis therapy. He developed right lower lobe pneumonia due to staphylococcus and beta-hemolytic streptococcus. Hematological evaluation, using molecular diagnostic techniques, confirmed a successful transplant with a 100 percent complement of donor cells.

The patient remained alert with no new focal neurological deficits. He then developed an acute abdomen and became confused, febrile, hypotensive, and unarousable. Despite appropriate resuscitative measures the patient died a few days later (6 months after his bone marrow transplant).

The necropsy revealed a perforated ileum with peritonitis due to EBV-driven B-cell lymphoma affecting the small bowel and liver. The brain was infected by *Aspergillus* with abscess formation (Figure 5-3). There were incidental splenic and renal infarcts and aortic valve vegetations.

The final diagnoses were CML presenting with blast transformation, matched unrelated bone marrow transplantation complicated with acute GVHD, toxoplasmosis, disseminated B-cell lymphoma (with involvement of ileum, lung, liver, and bone marrow), and fungal brain abscesses (*Aspergillus*).

Case 2

A 64-year-old woman presented with a 4-month history of diplopia and several weeks' history of slurring of speech, heaviness of the legs, and generalized weakness. She had a history of hypertension and vitamin B_{12} deficiency. On examination, she was noted to have fatigability resulting in diplopia, dysarthria, and proximal upper and lower limb weakness. Laboratory investigations revealed positive acetylcholine receptor antibodies, a decremental response with increased jitter on EMG, and a normal CT of anterior mediastinum. A diagnosis of myasthenia gravis was made and she was started on pyridostigmine, azathioprine 100 mg, and prednisolone 60 mg daily with potassium replacement and alendronate for osteoporosis prevention. Prednisolone was slowly reduced over the next 2 months to 30 mg on alternate days with excellent clinical response.

She was next admitted in a confused state. She was febrile and reported a history of recent generalized vesicular rash. Generalized tonic-clonic seizures ensued. Glasgow coma score (GCS) was 9.

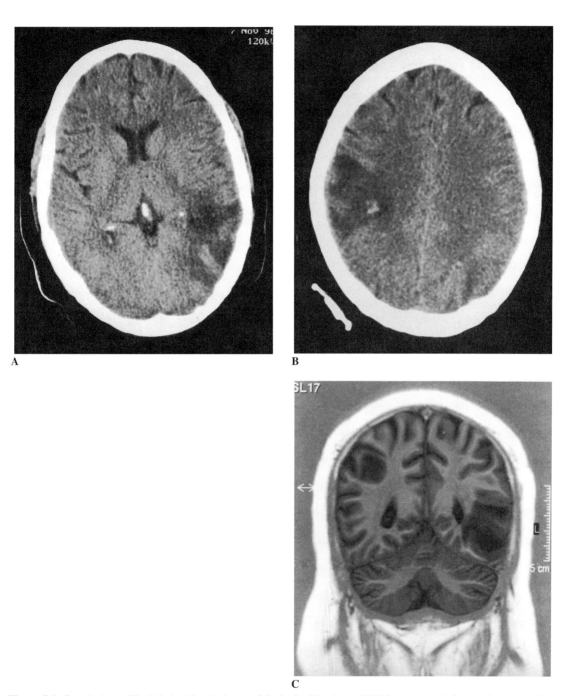

Figure 5-1. Case 1. Aspergillosis in both hemispheres of the brain. Unenhanced CT demonstrates left posterior temporal (A) and right parietal (B) wedge-shaped low-density areas consistent with infarction. Hemorrhagic changes are present within these areas bilaterally. (C) Unenhanced coronal T1-weighted image shows these two areas of infarction.

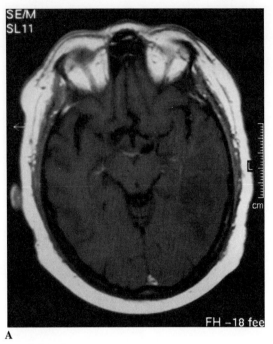
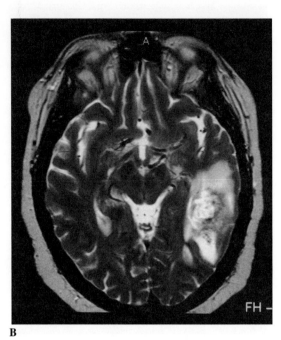

A   **B**

Figure 5-2. Case 1 continued. (A) Axial post-contrast T1-weighted image shows subtle peripheral enhancement of the left temporal lesion. (B) Axial T2-weighted image reveals areas of low signal consistent with hemosiderin indicating hemorrhage within the temporal lesion.

She had forced gaze deviation to the right, reduced left limb movements, and intermittent left-sided focal seizures. She was commenced on broad-spectrum antibiotics and imaged immediately. MRI showed multiple scattered white matter changes on T2-weighted sequences (Figure 5-4). Laboratory examination revealed white blood cell count of 3800 per mm^3 with lymphocytes 0.66, erythrocyte sedimentation rate of 2 cm/hr, C-reactive protein < 10 IU, and normal biochemistry panel. Chest X-ray showed left lower lobe collapse. CSF protein was 145 mg/dL, white cell count 345 (90 percent lymphocytes), and glucose 3.5 mmol/L (serum 4.6 mmol/L). EEG displayed diffuse slowing (2–3 Hz).

After a history of contact with chickenpox was obtained, acyclovir was started. The clinical diagnosis of varicella zoster encephalitis was made. She became increasingly confused and agitated. Sudden episodes of hypoxia required intubation, mechanical ventilation and transfer to the ICU. CSF PCR was positive for varicella zoster virus, confirming the suspected clinical diagnosis. Improvement was slow with repeated seizures refractory to anticonvulsants. She was successfully weaned from ventilation, but she remained dependent, with left hemiplegia and impaired arousal.

The Problem

- What is the specific CNS syndrome?
- What is the time relation between onset of immunosuppression and the development of the neurological syndrome?
- What evidence is there of infection outside the CNS?
- What are the most likely infectious agents that can be anticipated?
- What specific drug treatments should be used in these patients?
- Are there any noninfectious causes that could account for the fever?
- What are the yields of diagnostic tests and what are their limitations?

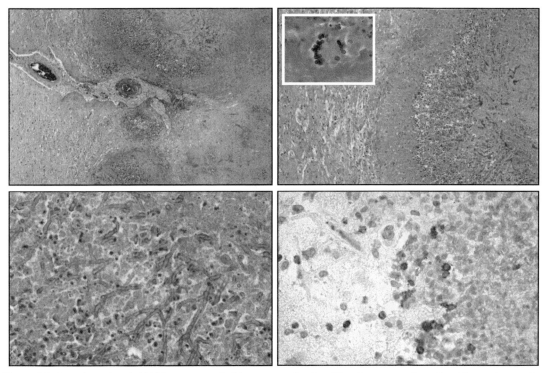

Figure 5-3. Case 1 continued. (A) The cortex and white matter related to this sulcus are partly replaced by an abscess that has also extended into the overlying meninges (H&E × 37). (B) Interface between abscess (right) and normal brain tissue (left). The wall of the abscess consists of necrotic tissue external to which are macrophages, some multinucleated giant cells (inset), and an astrocytic response. (H&E × 90; inset, H&E × 360). (C) Within the abscess are septate hyphae of a fungus that has been identified as *aspergillus* (PAS × 230). (D) The immune response at the edge of the abscess contains only a limited number of T-lymphocytes (immunohistochemistry CD3 × 230).

■ The Evidence

Critical neurological illness in the immunocompromised patient and the neurological complications of organ transplantation have been the subject of recent reviews.[1–4] These advocate approaching such problems in a thoughtful, logical manner in order to narrow the myriad diagnostic possibilities. There are no systematic reviews, Cochrane or otherwise, to guide us in the evaluation of the febrile agitated immunosuppressed patient. Therefore, an evidence-based approach to evaluation and treatment of these patients is challenging. Although a "scattergun" approach, throwing every conceivable investigation and therapy at the patient, should be typically strongly discouraged, it may be unavoidable in this group of high-risk patients. During evaluation of febrile immunosuppressed patients, the following five points should be kept in mind:

1. Multiple organisms may infect multiple organs.
2. Infections that are uncommon in the immunocompetent may occur.
3. The clinical picture is often compounded and confused by organ failure/rejection and increased sensitivity to medication.
4. Clinical presentations of discrete syndromes (e.g., meningitis) may be more indolent, with fewer clinical signs than in the immunocompetent.
5. Diagnostic tests are often less sensitive and imaging may be nonspecific.

The immunocompromised state derives from disease, immunosuppressant therapy, or chemotherapy. Each may affect a different component of the immune system and thus produce a specific repertoire

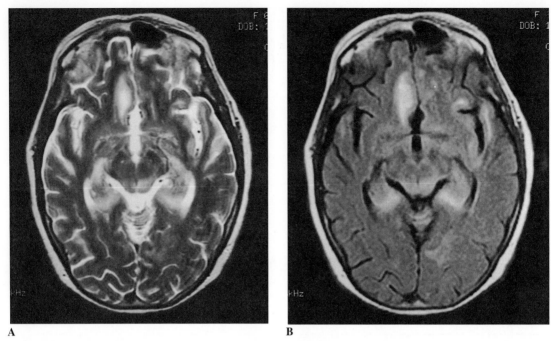

A   B

Figure 5-4. Case 2. Herpes simplex encephalitis. (A) Axial T2-weighted image. (B) Axial FLAIR image. High-signal change is present in the anterior part of the right cingulated gyrus, the left insula and adjacent opercula, and in the isthmus of the cingulated gyri bilaterally. High signal also extends into the adjacent tectal region of the midbrain.

of opportunistic infections that are characteristic of the underlying immune disorder. One approach has been to categorize patterns of infection in relation to specific disorders and immune defects[5] (Table 5-1). However, at second glance, with the overlapping of clinical syndromes, the utility of this guide becomes less practical.

In *HIV infection*, loss of CD4[+] T-lymphocytes results in deficient cellular immunity. The risk of opportunistic infection and lymphoma increases as the degree of immunosuppression worsens. The severity of the immunocompromised state is a reflection of the absolute CD4 count. Recently, the use of highly active antiretroviral therapy (HAART) has resulted in a decline in both morbidity and mortality among those with advanced disease.[6] In particular, there has been a dramatic reduction in the incidence of opportunistic infections such as cytomegalovirus, *Mycobacterium avium*, and *Pneumocystis carinii*.[7] Recent studies[8,9] have addressed these changing patterns of neurological disease in AIDS due to the widespread use of HAART. They demonstrate a relative decline in AIDS-related primary CNS lymphoma (PCNSL),

no significant alteration in the incidence of toxoplasma encephalitis, and a slight increase in cases of progressive multifocal leukoencephalopathy (PML). A shift to a minimally invasive approach to diagnosis with increased reliance on PCR-based assays was noted. While toxoplasmosis was initially responsible for most neurological morbidity, the introduction of prophylaxis[10] has already resulted in a significant change in the incidence of this opportunistic infection.[11] The dramatic increase in the prevalence of PCNSL in the general population noted from the 1970s onwards can be ascribed, almost in its entirety, to HIV infection.[12] However, Ammassari et al.[8] have convincingly shown a relative decline in the risk of all focal brain lesions attributable to HAART despite improved diagnostic sensitivity thanks to advances in brain imaging technique. The multicenter AIDS Cohort Study[9] (1990–1998) studied the impact of the introduction of HAART in 1996 on the incidence rates of HIV dementia, opportunistic infections, and PCNSL. Although incidence rates for infections dropped, the proportion of cases of HIV dementia with CD4 counts above 200 increased.

Table 5-1. Infections in the Immunocompromised Patient

Immune Defect	Neutropenia	Humoral	Cellular
Causes	Hematological malignancy HSCT (early) Organ transplant Cytotoxics/Steroids Diabetes	Hematological malignancy HSCT (late) Lymphoma Myeloma	Organ transplant Lymphoma Immunosuppresant drugs
Syndromes	Meningitis Encephalitis Abscess Rhinocerebral	Meningitis Encephalitis Abscess Rhinocerebral	Meningitis Encephalitis Abscess Rhinocerebral
Organisms	Enterobacteria *Pseudomonas* *Aspergillus* *Staphylococcus*	Enterobacteria *Strep. pneumoniae* *H. influenza* Measles	*Listeria* *Candida* *Aspergillus* *V. zoster* *H. simplex* CMV *Cryptococcus* *Nocardia* Murcomycosis Toxoplasma PML

This table is adapted from Boerman and Kullberg (1997).[5] This table or modifications of it appear in many review articles on infection in the immunocompromised. What it tells us is that a specific disorder of immunity does not result in an absolutely predictable list of potential causes. There is considerable overlap between causes and organisms. Also, a single condition may breach the immune defenses at more than one site. What we do learn, however, is that disordered cellular immunity is associated with the greatest diversity of potentially causal organisms. HSCT, hematopoietic stem cell transplantation.

Whereas evolving resistance to HAART may again change disease patterns,[13] the CNS complications seem well characterized, have become less prevalent, and patients rarely present to neurologists these days with hitherto undiagnosed AIDS. Early HIV infection may still pose diagnostic problems. Both aseptic meningitis and acute encephalopathy can occur at the time of seroconversion.[14] The encephalopathy is associated with mild CSF changes and is self-limited, though more aggressive forms occur with white matter changes, resembling multiple sclerosis on MRI.[15]

Solid organ transplantation (liver, kidney, lung, heart, pancreas, or combinations) is available for increasing numbers of patients despite major donor shortage. Surgical advances, improved intra- and postoperative care, and more selective immunosuppressive agents have resulted in dramatic improvements in survival. Drugs currently used include cyclosporine, tacrolimus, OKT3 (an anti-T-lymphocytic monoclonal antibody), azathioprine, corticosteroids, antithymocyte globulin (ATG), and antilymphocyte globulin (ALG). These drugs have specific mechanisms of action and their side effects have been reviewed in detail elsewhere.[16] With individual variations, they prevent CD4-mediated graft rejection, induce leukopenia, and inhibit antibody formation. Overall, by reducing the number of episodes of rejection that would necessitate additional courses of immunosuppressive therapy, these drugs have paradoxically diminished the frequency of life-endangering infections.[17]

Cyclosporine is universally the most commonly used immunosuppressant in transplantation. Neurological complications occur in 10–20 percent of patients, but renal toxicity remains the most concerning long-term side effect. High serum levels, magnesium deficiency (< 1.3 mEq/L), hypertension, concomitant steroid usage, and antibiotic use appear to enhance the risk of toxicity.[1] Cyclosporin-associated encephalopathy presents with confusion, agitation, depressed level of consciousness, seizures, reduced vision, or cortical blindness.[18] Magnetic resonance imaging may show the appearance of a posterior leukoencephalopathy. Withdrawal of cyclosporine will result in an excellent outcome, but failure to recognize toxicity can lead to permanent disability. OKT3 may produce an aseptic meningitis, akinetic mutism, blepharospasm, and delirium,[19] or acute encephalopathy with cerebral edema.[20]

The use of corticosteroids has dramatically increased in recent years along with their clinical indications. Steroids play an important role in organ transplantation as well as in a host of autoimmune and inflammatory disorders. Their effect on healing, neurophil, lymphocyte, and monocyte-macrophage function predisposes recipients to infection. Infections associated with steroid use have been extensively reviewed.[21] Early pyogenic infection is commonest; viral reactivation or primary infection, fungal and parasitic infections occur less frequently. Acyclovir and ganciclovir prophylaxis (for suspected HSV, VZV, or CMV) is considered in transplant patients, and tuberculin test positive patients on long-term steroids should receive prophylaxis with isoniazid for 6 months.

The infectious complications of solid organ transplants (SOTs) have been recently reviewed.[16] The incidence of infection is determined by opportunity (exposure plus the degree of immunosuppression) and will vary from one unit to the next. The donor organ should not be neglected as a potential source of infection in the recipient,[22] and the risk of transplantation-related infection must be minimized by appropriate presurgical screening. Bacterial, fungal, viral, and protozoal infections may all be derived from the allograft. In the immediate postoperative period, wounds, central lines, and catheters are all potential sources of hazard.[23] In these patients, the time course is of value in predicting causal pathogens. Three epochs of time are important: the first month, months 2–6, and 6 months and beyond.[24] Early infections are similar to those in the immunocompetent postoperative patient; they are usually bacterial, and the transplanted organ is especially at risk. In the middle period, patients are maximally immunosuppressed and vulnerable to intracellular pathogens (CMV, cryptococcus, toxoplasma, or reactivation of latent infection [*Mycobacterium tuberculosis*]). After 6 months, the degree and duration of immunosuppression and how this is titrated with recurrent episodes of threatened rejection assumes importance as risks

among individuals diverge. High-risk patients continue to be prone to opportunistic infections (fungi, protozoa, viruses), and low-risk patients are more susceptible to bacteria and endemic viral infections.

Prophylactic antibacterial treatment has been shown to reduce dramatically the incidence of infections within the first month, especially in renal recipients.[25] The causes and incidence of bacterial infection vary with the organ transplanted, occurring in up to 50 percent of liver transplant patients.[26] Lung transplant patients, not surprisingly, have the highest incidence of bacterial pneumonia (40 percent); in fact, this complication is the major cause of early postoperative death.[27] Heart and heart-lung transplant patients seem at greatest risk from *Legionella* infection.[28] *Listeria* is the commonest bacterial cause of CNS infection in all SOT patients, presenting with meningitis, meningoencephalitis, or brain abscess.[29] Fungal infections are also very much organ-dependent. *Candida* infection occurs after one month and originates from endogenous sources, mainly skin or gastrointestinal tract. *Candida* accounts for the majority of fungal infections in liver patients, being invasive and often involving the CNS. Risk is associated with duration of the procedure, time in intensive transplant unit, renal failure, and concomitant recent or active CMV infection.[30] *Aspergillus* preferentially affects heart and heart-lung recipients,[31] with mortality approaching 100 percent when the CNS is involved.[30] Disseminated infection is common because the organism is angioinvasive. Reactivation of *Mycobacterium tuberculosis* infection usually occurs late after SOT.[32] Although infrequent, it may be difficult to diagnose and results in allograft loss in 27 percent of those cases diagnosed and treated.[33]

Herpes viruses infections (HSV-1, HSV-2, VZV, EBV, CMV) may in themselves further reduce cell-mediated immunity and heighten the risk of additional opportunistic infections. During periods of depressed cell-mediated immunity, reactivation of latent infection takes place. Reactivation of VZV generally occurs late.[34] Also primary infection can occur, with widespread dissemination and often life-threatening CNS involvement. Nearly 50 percent of allograft recipients develop symptomatic CMV infection in the intermediate period.[35] This occurs in up to 17 percent of liver transplant patients, though it rarely specifically involves the CNS.

Toxoplasmosis frequently results from primary infection from the allograft of a seropositive donor. Whilst seroconversion is common (60 percent of cardiac recipients), symptomatic disease develops in less than half.[36] When encephalitis occurs, early diagnosis and treatment is typically associated with a good outcome.

Fever in SOT patients is common and requires an extensive search for infection. Yet noninfectious causes of fever also need to be considered. Fischer et al.[37] have reviewed in detail both infectious and noninfectious causes such as allograft rejection, drug fever, and thromboembolic disease. This study is of especial value for its detailed account of these noninfective causes.

SOT may also be associated with presurgical organ failure manifesting as an encephalopathy or confusional state.[38–40] Immediate perioperative encephalopathy is most likely metabolic, hypoxic-ischemic, or drug-related[2] and must be distinguished from infection in the early postoperative phase. Clues to the presence of these noninfective encephalopathies can be found by meticulous scrutiny of the results of laboratory tests and detailed examination of drug charts.

Hematopoietic stem cell transplantation (HSCT) is utilized in a variety of bone marrow failure states, in the management of hematological malignancy, and occasionally in the therapy of solid tumors (e.g., neuroblastoma and testicular cancer). Infections are commonplace especially where myeloablative or conditioning procedures are involved.[41] Again, three epochs can be identified: the pre-graft, and the early and late post-graft phases. Each phase is similarly associated with different potential infective agents.

In the pre-graft phase there is loss of effective phagocytosis due to destruction of normal hematopoiesis through the conditioning regimen. Mucosal cell damage reduces any effective defensive barrier with increased risk of infection, particularly from fungi.[42] Early neutropenic fever is typically assumed to be due to bacterial pathogens, though blood cultures are often negative. The most common fungal infection in this stage is *Candida* followed by *Aspergillus*. Viral reactivation is frequent, especially with HSV, and prophylaxis is commonly given.[43] The early post-graft phase is characterized by impaired cell-mediated and humoral immunity. The development of GVHD and its treatment will further affect immunity, increasing the risk of opportunistic viral and fungal infections. Acute GVHD requiring steroids will enhance the risk of fungal (*Candida* and *Aspergillus*) and viral (CMV and VZV) infections. Bacterial infection is uncommon in this phase.[44] The late phase is from approximately 3 months until normal immunity is regained.[41] Patients with chronic GVHD have a more prolonged period of cell depletion. During this late phase, encapsulated bacterial infections (*Haemophilus influenzae, Neisseria meningitidis,* and *Streptococcus pneumoniae*) predominate along with fungal infections; on the contrary, viral infection (CMV) becomes less frequent. Guidelines exist for the prevention of opportunistic infection following HSCT.[45]

Other noninfective complications of immunosuppression can be divided into vascular disorders and malignancies. They may present with encephalopathic features, frequently associated with pyrexia due to their complications such as aspiration pneumonia.

Several discrete mechanisms may result in stroke in the immunocompromised individual.[46,47] Angioinvasive infections (aspergillosis or mucormycosis) can affect multiple vessels resulting in an encephalopathic presentation. *Aspergillus* destroys the internal elastic lamina of large and medium-size vessels resulting in thrombosis and mycotic aneurysm formation.[48] Mucormycosis, a disorder associated with both immunosuppression and poorly controlled diabetes, invades blood vessels directly from the paranasal sinuses. Extracranial arterial occlusions have been described as a complication of this infection.[49] Vasculitis is associated with both VZV and CMV. Endocarditis from systemic bacterial or fungal infection can result in cardioembolic stroke and some infections may also promote or accelerate atherothrombosis or induce prothrombic states. Intravascular lymphoma may present with "territorial infarction." Finally, drug treatments themselves may induce stroke–like syndromes.

The prevalence of *primary CNS lymphoma (PCNSL)* has increased 3–5-fold in recent years, primarily due to AIDS, but also from immunosuppressive therapy for organ transplantation[50] and autoimmune disorders. Presentation may be with focal signs or with more widespread features. MRI features will be discussed later. CSF can show tumor cells but a stereotactic biopsy is typically necessary (often delayed until the response to anti-toxoplasmosis therapy can be gauged). Treatment with chemotherapy plus radiotherapy significantly prolongs survival. The risk of tumors following transplantation and the role of Epstein-Barr virus in the induction of post-transplant lymphoprolifera-tive disorders have been comprehensively reviewed.[51,52] Recent interest in the possible rela-tionship between gliomas and SOTs[53] requires fur-ther exploration.

In *HIV encephalopathy*, brain CT can show generalized atrophy with low attenuation changes in deep white matter. MRI is more sensitive to these changes, showing them as diffuse, con-fluent, predominately frontal, and reflecting demyelination and gliosis.[54] *Toxoplasmosis* mani-fests as ring-enhancing masses with surrounding edema on contrast CT. On MRI, these lesions are hypo- or isointense on T1, and T2 is more sen-sitive to show multiplicity. MRI is used to monitor treatment with persisting enhancement indicating recurrence.[55] Distinction from lymphoma is diffi-cult. *Lymphoma* is solitary in 70 percent of biopsy-proven cases,[56] and hemorrhage is rare. Thallium SPECT is useful in the differential diagnosis, showing increased uptake in lymphoma but not in toxoplasmosis.[57]

In *progressive multifocal leukoencephalopathy*, brain CT is unhelpful, but MRI shows rounded or oval areas of increased signal on T2. These are con-fluent and involve the basal ganglia and posterior brain regions.[58] However, such appearances may be indistinguishable from HIV encephalopathy or subcortical infarction. In *cryptococcal* infection, MRI reveals multiple areas of increased T2 signal in the basal ganglia that represent gelatinous pseudocysts and dilated Virchow-Robin spaces. The CT is often diagnostic in *tuberculosis*, showing hydrocephalus with meningeal enhancement. Areas of infarction can be seen in the basal ganglia due to occlusion of lenticulostriate vessels by exu-dates.[59] Tuberculomas (granulomas) with solid centers are seen at the gray/white matter junction on MRI with a hypointense core on T1. *Herpes simplex types 1 and 2* show little changes on early CT, though areas of low attenuation with mass effect become obvious after 3–5 days. MRI is more sensitive to early HSV showing gray matter thickening, sulcal effacement, and hyperintense signal on T2; hemorrhagic changes are best seen on

gradient echo sequences.[60] Whilst CT is insensitive to *VZV*, MRI displays multiple lesions on T2 reflecting myelin loss at the gray/white matter junction, often ring-enhancing on T1 with gadolin-ium.[60] MRI best evaluates fungal infections. *Mucormycosis* invades the frontal lobes from con-tiguous sinuses. *Aspergillus* invades along arteries (angioinvasive). *Candida* produces small multiple abscesses.[61]

With this baggage of knowledge, it is illusory to assume that a clinical diagnosis is easily forthcom-ing. The consulting neurologist asked to assess a febrile, confused, immunosuppressed patient has to amass clues from the physical examination and a growing variety of laboratory studies. The follow-ing paragraphs provide succinct guidelines to streamline the initial evaluation of these complex patients.

Neurological Examination

Terms such as confusion or agitation typically fail to convey a description of the patient's mentation. Their vagueness leaves room for erroneous inter-pretation. For example, a focal disorder (e.g., dys-phasia) may be mistaken for a more diffuse encephalopathy. Looking for localizing signs is essential, especially when brain imaging is not immediately available and early CSF examination is indicated. Signs indicative of a mass lesion demand immediate on-site imaging or transfer to where this can best be obtained. The specific clini-cal syndrome (e.g., meningoencephalitis) should be defined when possible. In the absence of focal signs, a drug interaction or side effect, or a meta-bolic derangement, is likely.

General Examination

Full physical examination should be focused on identifying sources of infection and must include detailed inspection of the skin and mucosa.

The drug charts must be studied for possible drug-related side effects, interactions, and increased sensitivity to hypnotics. The results of routine emergent investigations (blood film, liver, renal function, blood glucose, and inflammatory markers such as ESR and CRP) must be reviewed.

Neuroimaging

CT of the brain is rarely sufficient and generally MRI will provide more detail. Use of contrast is generally advisable. Radiological appearances are diverse but may indicate a specific infective process or vascular complication. Additional radiology can be informative in certain situations (chest x-ray for *Aspergillus*, sinus x-ray for mucormycosis).

Cerebrospinal Fluid Examination

Whilst not recommended in patients with intracranial mass lesions and evidence of brain tissue shift, this examination may be of great diagnostic importance especially when applying modern techniques such as polymerase chain reaction (PCR).

■ The Pros and Cons

Many practicing neurologists assess and manage agitated febrile immunosuppressed patients infrequently, and thus it is important to adopt a pragmatic approach to their evaluation. The multiplicity of potential causes, lack of information on sensitivity and specificity of investigations, and absence of outcome data make it impossible to provide an evidence-based approach. One can, however, sensibly construct a "route map" to guide the diagnosis and treatment.[1] The differences in the immunocompromised population are in the range of possible infective agents, the "blunting" of classical presentations, and the catastrophic effect of infection once established. Other compounding differences include the underlying disease causing immunosuppression, the possibility of organ failure or rejection, and the considerations of immunosuppressant-induced encephalopathy and malignancy.

The role of the neurologist is to give additional clarity to the diagnosis where it remains uncertain (Case 1) and also to be aware of the hazards of immunosuppression in neurological patients receiving such treatment regimens (Case 2). The first case illustrates the complexity of the clinical problem of fever and mental changes after bone marrow transplantation. Bone marrow transplantation using matched unrelated donor marrow is performed for an increasing number of conditions such as hematological malignancies and nonmalignant hematological states (e.g., sickle cell anemia), as well as for nonhematological disorders such as solid tumors, genetic disorders, and in certain gene therapy protocols.[62] The latter conditions do not require prior conditioning (or myeloablative therapy) and thus carry a much lesser risk of morbidity and mortality. Neurological complications are common and can be immune-mediated (GVHD), toxic (drug-related), metabolic, cerebrovascular, or infective.[63]

An allogeneic transplant takes 2–4 weeks to function and during this period patients are invariably pancytopenic and have an increased susceptibility to infection. Acute GVHD occurs in up to 60 percent of patients in this acute/subacute phase, manifesting as skin rash, disturbed liver function, and mild gastrointestinal upset.[64,65] The patient had a stormy posttransplant period and was treated empirically for a host of potential infections (bacterial/fungal/viral). Because his donor was CMV positive, his risk of developing this infection was particularly high.

The prime issue is to ensure that potentially treatable infections and PCNSL are not overlooked. The laboratory investigations of these infections are not discussed here. Suffice that the clinicians and laboratory staff confer to ensure that diagnostic studies are comprehensive and that the pitfalls of sensitivity and specificity, where known, are implicitly understood. Mimics of CNS infection in the immunocompromised host have been reviewed.[66] They include organ rejection, GVHD, drug-induced aseptic meningitis, toxic/metabolic abnormalities, primary (PCNSL) or metastatic CNS malignancies, marantic endocarditis, systemic infection, and coagulopathies. Examination of charts and discussion with colleagues will address most of these mimics. Next, when infection is probable, syndromic classification (meningitis, encephalitis, meningoencephalitis, mass lesion) will narrow down diagnostic possibilities and assist the investigative approach (Table 5-2). Also understanding the underlying immune disorder will further help, accepting that there is a considerable overlap (Table 5-3). In transplant patients, the length of time from procedure, nature of procedure (e.g., SOT or HSCT), and treatment regimens used must also be taken into account. Table 5-4 emphasizes these points, showing the specific phases and types of infection in allogeneic HSCT recipients.

Table 5-2. Plan for Investigating CNS Infection in the Immunosuppressed Host

	Diagnostic Procedures	Possible Organisms
Meningitis		
Determine host defense defect	Imaging CT/MRI if available	*Listeria*
Exclude mimics	LP with CSF studies	*Cryptococcus*
Commence empirical treatment	Diff. WBC	Tuberculosis
	Glucose/protein	*Strep. pneumoniae*
	Cytology	*Neisseria meningitidis*
	Bacterial stains/culture	*Hemophilus influenzae*
	AFB/fungal stains and culture	
Encephalitis/Meningoencephalitis or possible mass lesion		
Determine host defense defect	CT/MRI mandatory	*Aspergillus*
Exclude mimics	Review imaging with radiology	CMV/HSV/VZV
	Request (if indicated) further imaging	Toxoplasmosis
		Candida
Commence empirical treatment	Monitor response (MRI)	*Mucormycosis*
In the absence of papilledema	LP with CSF studies	
	Diff. WBC	
	Glucose/protein	
	Cytology	
	AFB/fungal stains and culture	

Ancillary investigation, such as PCR, may be requested after discussion with appropriate laboratories regarding suitability, utility, and availability.

Table 5-3. Disorders of Immunity and CNS Pathogens

Impaired granulocyte function			
Causes:	Hematological malignancies. Chemotherapy and radiation-induced leukopenia. Drug-induced leukopenia. Solid tumors. Lymphomas. Aplastic anaemia. HSCT.		
Pathogens:	Frequent	Infrequent	Rare
	Staphylococcus aureus	*Neisseria meningitidis*	*Candida*
	Streptococcus pneumoniae	*Hemophilus influenzae*	*Aspergillus*
	Pseudomonas aeruginosa		*Enterobacter*
Impaired B-lymphocyte function (humoral immunity)			
Causes:	Multiple myeloma. Splenectomy. B-cell lymphoma. Autoimmune disease (e.g., RA). Hematological malignancy (e.g., CLL). Malnutrition. Hereditary immunoglobulin deficiency.		
Pathogens:	Frequent	Infrequent	Rare
	Hemophilus influenzae	*Neisseria meningitidis*	*Pseudomonas aeruginosa*
	Streptococcus pneumoniae	*Klebsiella pneumoniae*	
Impaired T-lymphocyte function (cellular immunity)			
Causes:	AIDS/HIV. Lymphoreticular malignancies. Chronic immunosuppressive therapy. Organ transplantation (SOT and HSCT). Viral infections (herpes viruses).		
Pathogens:	Frequent	Infrequent	Rare
	Listeria	*Mycobacterium tuberculosis*	PML
	CMV/HSV/VZV	*Aspergillus*	*Pneumocystis carinii*
	Toxoplasma gondii	Mucormycosis	
	Cryptococcus		
	Nocardia		

This table is not intended to be comprehensive but essentially to act as a "rough guide" of what to expect and when.
Adapted from Cunha, BA. Central nervous system infections in the compromised host. *Infect Dis Clin North Am* 2001;15:423–432.)
HSCT, hematopoietic stem cell transplantation; RA, rheumatoid arthritis; CLL, chronic lymphocytic leukemia; SOT, solid organ transplantation.

Table 5-4. The Epochs of Infection after Allogeneic Human Stem Cell Transplantation (HSCT)

	Phase One Pre and early post graft (< 30 days)	Phase Two Post-graft (30 days – 3 months)	Phase Three Late phase (after 3 months)
IMMUNE DEFECT	Neutropenia Acute GVHD Mucosal damage	Impaired cellular immunity Chronic GVHD	Impaired cellular / humoral immunity
CATHETERS CENTRAL LINES	———————————→		
RISK OF SPECIFIC INFECTIONS:			
Bacterial infections	– Staphylococcus ————→	—— encapsulated bacteria —→	
Viral infections	– H. simplex ——→	—— VZV ———→	
	———— Respiratory and enteric viruses ————→		
Fungal infections	– Candida ———→	—— Aspergillus ——→	
	———— Toxoplasma ———→		
Treatment related malignancies (Epstein-Barr related lymphoproliferative)			(late phase)

Adapted from Leather HL, Wingard JR. Infections following hematopoietic stem cell transplantation. *Infect Dis Clin North Am.* 2001;15:483–520.

Bacterial and cryptococcal infections are relatively easily diagnosed by laboratory tests. Other infections are more difficult to confirm (toxoplasmosis) or less rapidly processed (tuberculosis) and empirical treatment may have to be started whilst results are awaited.

■ **The Main Points**

- The diagnostic approach should involve collaboration and consultation with appropriate clinical and laboratory colleagues.
- The initial approach to differential diagnosis should be that considered in the immunocompetent population.
- Mimics of infection must be considered and comprehensively eliminated from the differential diagnosis.
- The nature of the underlying disease must be taken into account, in particular the type of immunodeficiency.
- The time from treatment initiation to the onset of the febrile agitated state will help define possible pathogen or process, as also will the nature of the neurological syndrome.

- MR studies are imperative in most cases.
- Where PCNSL is suspected, stereotactic biopsy is indicated since treatment may result in marked clinical response.
- Empirical treatment of infection is not normally advisable but is sometimes warranted in the critically ill immunosuppressed person.

■ References

1. Cohen JA, Raps EC. Critical neurologic illness in the immunocompromised patient. *Neurol Clin* 1995;13: 659–677.
2. Lee JM, Raps EC. Neurologic complications of transplantation. *Neurol Clin* 1998;16:21–33.
3. Wijdicks EFM. *Neurological Complications of Critical Illness*, 2nd ed. Oxford, Oxford University Press, 2002.
4. Wijdicks EFM, ed. *Neurological Complications in organ transplant recipients.* Boston, Butterworth-Heinemann, 1999.
5. Boerman RH, Kullberg BJ. Opportunistic CNS infections in cancer. In CJ Vecht, ed. *Handbook of Clinical Neurology*, vol. 25(69): *Neuro-oncology*, part 3. Amsterdam, Elsevier, 1997, 431–458.
6. Palella FJ Jr, Delaney KM, Moorman AC, Loveless MO, Fuhrer J, Satten GA, Aschman DJ, Holmberg SD. Declining morbidity and mortality among patients with advanced human immunodeficiency virus infection. HIV Outpatient Study Investigators. *N Engl J Med* 1998;338:853–860.
7. Hofflin JM, Potasman I, Baldwin JC, Oyer PE, Stinson EB, Remington JS. Infectious complications in heart transplant recipients receiving cyclosporine and corticosteroids. *Intern Med* 1987;106:209–216.
8. Ammassari A, Cingolani A, Pezzotti P, De Luca DA, Murri R, Giancola ML, Larocca LM, Antinori A. AIDS-related focal brain lesions in the era of highly active antiretroviral therapy. *Neurology* 2000;55: 1194–1200.
9. Sacktor N, Lyles RH, Skolasky R, Kleeberger C, Selnes OA, Miller EN, Becker JT, Cohen B, McArthur JC. HIV-associated neurologic disease incidence changes: Multicenter AIDS Cohort Study, 1990–1998. *Neurology.* 2001;56:257–260.
10. Antinori A, Murri R, Ammassari A, De Luca A, Linzalone A, Congolani A, Damiano F, Maiuro G, Becchiet J, Scoppettuolo G. Aerosolized pentamidine, cotrimoxazole and dapsone-pyrimethamine for primary prophylaxis of *Pneumocystis carinii* pneumonia and toxoplasmic encephalitis. *AIDS* 1995;9:1343–1350.
11. Ammasssari A, Scoppettuolo G, Murri R, Pezzotti P, Cingolani A, Del Borgo C, De Luca A, Aninori A, Ortona L. Changing disease pattern in focal brain lesion-causing disorders in AIDS. *J Aquir Immune Defic Syndr Hum Retrovirol* 1998;18:365–371.
12. Cote TR, Manns A, Hardy CR, Yellin FJ, Hartge P. Epidemiology of brain lymphoma among people with or without acquired immunodeficiency syndrome. AIDS/Cancer Study Group. *J Natl Cancer Inst* 1996;88:675–679.
13. Deeks S, Grant R, Horton G, et al. *Interscience Conference on Antimicrobial Agents and Chemotherapy.* Toronto, Ontario, 1997:282; abstract I-205.
14. Carne CA, Tedder RS, Smith A, Sutherland S, Elkington SG, Daly HM, Preston FE, Craske J. Acute encephalopathy coincident with seroconversion for anti-HTLV-III. *Lancet* 1985;2:1206–1208.
15. Gray F, Chimelli L, Mohr M, Clavelou P, Scaravilli F, Poirier J. Fulminating multiple sclerosis-like leukoencephalopathy revealing human immunodeficiency virus infection. *Neurology* 1991;41:105–109.
16. Simon DM, Levin S. Infectious complications of solid organ transplantations. *Infect Dis Clin North Am* 2001;15:521–549.
17. Hoggs RS, Heath KV, Yip B, Craib KJ, O'Shaughnessy MV, Schechter MT, Montaner JS. Improved survival among HIV-infected individuals following initiation of antiretroviral therapy. *JAMA* 1998;279:450–454.
18. Rubin AM, Kang H. Cerebral blindness and encephalopathy with cyclosporin A toxicity. *Neurology* 1987;37:1072–1076.
19. Pittock SJ, Rabinstein AA, Edwards BS, Wijdicks EF. OKT3 neurotoxicity presenting as akinetic mutism. *Transplantation* 2003;75:1058–1060.
20. Thomas DM, Nicholls AJ, Feest TG, Riad H. OKT3 and cerebral oedema. *Br Med J (Clin Res Ed)* 1987; 295:1486.
21. Klein NC, Go CH, Cunha BA. Infections associated with steroid use. *Infect Dis Clin North Am* 2001; 15:423–432.
22. Gottesdiener KM. Transplanted infections: donor-to-host transmission with the allograft. *Ann Intern Med* 1989;110:1001–1016.
23. Curtis L. Infections in solid organ transplantation. *Am J Infect Control* 1998;26:364.
24. Fishman JA, Rubin RH. Infection in organ-transplant recipients. *N Engl J Med* 1998;338:1741–1751.
25. Tolkoff-Rubin NE, Cosimi AB, Russell PS, Rubin RH. A controlled study of trimethoprim-sulfamethoxazole prophylaxis of urinary tract infection in renal transplant recipients. *Rev Infect Dis* 1982;4:614–618.
26. Winston DJ, Emmanouilides C, Busuttil RW. Infections in liver transplant recipients. *Clin Infect Dis* 1995;21:1077–1089.
27. Maurer JR, Tullis DE, Grossman RF, Vellend H, Winton TL, Patterson GA. Infectious complications following isolated lung transplantation. *Chest* 1992;101:1056–1059.
28. Tkatch LS, Kusne S, Irish WD, Krystofiak S, Wing E. Epidemiology of legionella pneumonia and factors

associated with legionella-related mortality at a tertiary care center. *Clin Infect Dis* 1998;27:1479–1486.

29. Lorber B. Listeriosis. *Clin Infect Dis* 1997;24:1–9.
30. Paya CV. Fungal infections in solid-organ transplantation. *Clin Infect Dis* 1993;16:677–688.
31. Paterson DL, Singh N. Invasive aspergillosis in transplant recipients. *Medicine* (Baltimore) 1999;78:123–138.
32. Aguado JM, Herrero JA, Gavalda J, Torre-Cisneros J, Blanes M, Rufi G, Moreno A, Gurgui M, Hayek M, Lumbreras C, Cantarell C. Clinical presentation and outcome of tuberculosis in kidney, liver, and heart transplant recipients in Spain. Spanish Transplantation Infection Study Group, GESITRA. *Transplantation.* 1997;63:1278–1286. (Review). Erratum in *Transplantation* 1997;64:942.
33. Singh N, Dummer JS, Kusne S, Breinig MK, Armstrong JA, Makowka L, Starzl TE, Ho M. Infections with cytomegalovirus and other herpesviruses in 121 liver transplant recipients: transmission by donated organ and the effect of OKT3 antibodies. *J Infect Dis* 1988;158:124–131.
34. Gourishankar S, McDermid JC, Jhangri GS, Preiksaitis JK. Herpes zoster infection following solid organ transplantation: incidence, risk factors and outcomes in the current immunosuppressive era. *Am J Transplant* 2004;4:108–115.
35. Sia IG, Patel R. New strategies for prevention and therapy of cytomegalovirus infection and disease in solid-organ transplant recipients. *Clin Microbiol Rev* 2000;13:83–121.
36. Gallino A, Maggiornini M, Kiowski W, Martin X, Wunderli W, Schneider J, Turina M, Follath F. Toxoplasmosis in heart transplant recipients. *Eur J Clin Microbiol Infect Dis* 1996;15:389–393.
37. Fischer SA, Trenholme GM, Levin S. Fever in the solid organ transplant patient. *Infect Dis Clin North Am* 1996;10:197–184.
38. Adams DH, Ponsford S, Gunson B, Boon A, Honigsberger L, Williams A, Buckels J, Elias E, McMaster P. Neurological complications following liver transplantation. *Lancet* 1987;1:949–951.
39. Fraser C. Neurologic manifestations of the uremic state in metabolic brain dysfunction in systemic disorders. *Ann Intern Med* 1992;109:143.
40. Lewis M, Howdle PD. The neurology of liver failure. *Quart J Med* 2003;96:623–633.
41. Bow EJ, Loewen R, Cheang MS, Schacter B. Invasive fungal disease in adults undergoing remission-induction therapy for acute myeloid leukemia: the pathogenic role of antileukemic regimen. *Clin Infect Dis* 1995;21:361–369.
42. Bowden RA. Blood and marrow transplantation. In: Armstrond D, Cohen J, eds. *Infectious Disease: Fungal Infections.* London, Mosby-Wolff, 1999;4:1–18.
43. Saral R, Ambinder RF, Burns WH, Angelopulos CM, Griffin DE, Burke PJ, Lietman PS. Acyclovir prophylaxis against herpes simplex virus infection in patients with leukemia: a randomized, double-blind, placebo-controlled study. *Ann Intern Med* 1983;99:773–776.
44. Leather HL, Wingard JR. Infections following hematopoietic stem cell transplantation. *Infect Dis Clin North Am* 2001;15:483–520.
45. Centers for Disease Control and Prevention; Infectious Disease Society of America; American Society of Blood and Marrow Transplantation. Guidelines for preventing opportunistic infections among hematopoietic stem cell transplant recipients. *MMWR Recomm Rep* 2000;49(RR-10):1–125, CE1–7.
46. Adair JC, Call GK, O'Connel JB, Baringer JR. Cerebrovascular syndromes following cardiac transplantation. *Neurology* 1992;42:819–823.
47. Adams HP Jr, Dawson G, Coffman TJ, Corry RJ. Stroke in renal transplant patients. *Arch Neurol* 1986;3:113–115.
48. Lau AH, Takeshita M, Ishii N. Mycotic (*Aspergillus*) arteritis resulting in fatal subarachnoid hemorrhage: a case report. *Angiology* 1991;42:251–255.
49. Galetta SL, Wulc AE, Goldberg HI, Nichols CW, Glaser JS. Rhinocerebral mucormycosis: management and survival after carotid occlusion. *Ann Neurol* 1990:28:103–107.
50. Patchell RA, White CL III, Clark AW, Beschorner WE, Santos GW. Neurologic complications of bone marrow transplantation. *Neurology* 1985;35:729–750.
51. Gazdar AF. Tumors arising after organ transplantation: sorting out their origins. *JAMA* 1997;277:154–155.
52. Paya CV, Fung JJ, Nalesnik MA, Kieff E, Green M, Gores G, Habermann TM, Wiesner PH, Swinnen JL, Woodle ES, Bromberg JS. Epstein-Barr virus-induced posttransplant lymphoproliferative disorders. ASTS/ASTP EBV-PTLD Task Force and The Mayo Clinic Organized International Consensus Development Meeting. *Transplantation* 1999;68:1517–1525.
53. Schiff D, O'Neill B, Wijdicks E, Antin JH, Wen PY. Gliomas arising in organ transplant recipients: an unrecognized complication of transplantation? *Neurology* 2001;57(8):1486–1488.
54. Barker PB, Lee RR, McArthur JC. AIDS dementia complex: evaluation with proton MR spectroscopic imaging. *Radiology* 1995;195:58–64.
55. Laissy JP, Soyer P, Parlier C, Lariven S, Benmelha Z, Servois V, Casalino E, Bouvet E, Sibert A, Vachon F, et al. Persistent enhancement after treatment for cerebral toxoplasmosis in patients with AIDS: predictive value for subsequent recurrence. *AJNR Am J Neuroradiol* 1994;15:1773–1778.
56. Ciricillo SF, Rosenblum ML. Use of CT and MR imaging to distinguish intracranial lesions and to define the need for biopsy in AIDS patients. *J Neurosurg* 1990;73:720–724.
57. Ruiz A, Ganz WI, Post MJ, Camp A, Landy H, Mallin W, Sfakianakis GN. Use of thallium-201 brain SPECT to differentiate cerebral lymphoma from toxoplasma

encephalitis in AIDS patients. *AJNR Am J Neuroradiol* 1994;15:1885–1894.

58. Davenport C, Dillon WP, Sze G. Neuroradiology of the immunosuppressed state. *Radiol Clin North Am* 1992; 30:611–637.

59. Demaerel P, Wilms G, Robberecht W, Johannik K, Van Hecke P, Carton H, Baert AL. MRI of herpes simplex encephalitis. *Neuroradiology* 1992;34:490–493.

60. Lentz D, Jordan JE, Pike GB, Enzmann DR. MRI in varicella-zoster virus leukoencephalitis in the immuno-compromised host. *J Comput Assist Tomogr* 1993;17: 313–316.

61. Ashdown BC, Tien RD, Felsberg GJ. Aspergillosis of the brain and paranasal sinuses in immuno-compromised patients: CT and MRI findings *AJR Am J Roentgenol* 1994;162:155–159.

62. Krouwer HG, Wijdicks EF. Neurologic complications of bone marrow transplantation. *Neurol Clin* 2003;21: 319–352.

63. Patchell RA. Primary central nervous system lymphoma in the transplant patient. *Neurol Clin* 1988;6: 297–303.

64. Openshaw H, Slatkin NE. Differential diagnosis of the neurological complications in bone marrow transplantation. *Neurologist* 1995;1:191:206.

65. Snider S, Bashir R, Bierman P. Neurologic complications after high-dose chemotherapy and autologous bone marrow transplantation for Hodgkin's disease. *Neurology* 1994;44:681–684.

66. Cunha BA. Central nervous system infections in the compromised host: a diagnostic approach. *Infect Dis Clin North Am* 2001;15:567–590.

Chapter 6
Thunderclap Headache

Christopher J. Boes and Peter J. Goadsby

■ Introduction

The term "thunderclap headache" was introduced into the neurological lexicon by Day and Raskin in 1986.[1] C. Miller Fisher had previously called this headache phenotype "crash migraine" in cases where subsequent lumbar puncture and angiography were found to be normal.[2] His description is classic:

> Crash migraine ... refers to headache that "out of the blue" in 10 or 20 seconds reaches a high intensity, suggesting subarachnoid hemorrhage; yet, both lumbar puncture and angiography are normal. The headache may be situated posteriorly or generalized. Vomiting occurs in about one half of the cases. The patients are usually between 20 and 40 years of age, and males and females are equally represented. There may be a recurrence 2 or 3 days later. ... In some 10 patients, long-term follow-up has revealed no disaster.[2]

Thunderclap headache refers to a sudden, severe, explosive headache with peak intensity at onset, as unexpected as a thunderclap. Patient descriptions have included: "as if the top of my head blew off," "as if hit with a stick from behind," and "as if a grenade went off in my head." This presentation often denotes a neurological or neurosurgical emergency, but its evaluation is complex and controversial, with conflicting views in the literature.

Thunderclap headache is occasionally confused with the "exploding head syndrome." Patients with the exploding head syndrome complain of an explosive noise in the head sometimes associated with a flash of light, but not pain, differentiating

this entity from thunderclap headache.[3] There is a report of SAH presenting with the sudden onset of a brief, loud, painless noise in the head, but that case was associated with protracted nausea and vomiting,[4] thus differentiating it from the typical exploding head syndrome.

■ The Patient

A 65-year-old right-handed female presented to her local emergency department 4 hours after developing a severe headache following sexual intercourse. The headache started immediately after orgasm and had never occurred previously. The pain was maximal at onset and very severe. It lasted 1–2 minutes and then resolved completely. Pain quality was "like a rubber band around her head." There were no other symptoms.

Although the headache had resolved, the quite unusual and frightening experience prompted her to visit the local emergency department. A head CT was obtained and was initially reported to be normal, but closer inspection at a later date revealed a hyperintensity in the left paraclinoid area (Figure 6-1). The instantaneous onset of pain was apparently not appreciated in the local emergency department, or the quick resolution of the pain was considered benign, and thus a spinal fluid examination was not performed.

The following morning after the thunderclap headache, the patient awoke with a mild dull headache. This headache was bifrontal without nausea, vomiting, photophobia, phonophobia,

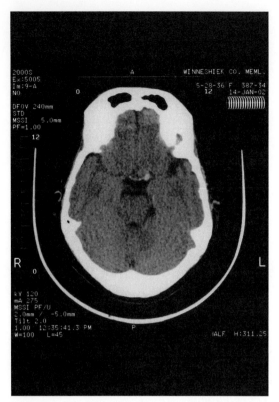

Figure 6-1. CT of the head showing hyperintensity in the left paraclinoid region.

osmophobia, or jaw claudication. It was not associated with a visual, sensory, or motor aura. There was no cough or sneeze effect, and it was not worse with walking up the stairs.

These mild headaches continued on a daily basis, lasting 10–12 hours each day but resolving without treatment. They were not bothersome enough for the patient to take any pain-relievers. She had a history of similar headaches in the past, but those typically occurred once every 6 months.

The patient was seen in outpatient neurological consultation 5 weeks after the thunderclap headache. She had daily mild headaches as described above but had not had any recurrent thunderclap headaches. Her medications included aspirin, cholestyramine, pravastatin, and atenolol. Her past medical history was significant for hypertension, coronary artery disease, and hyperlipidemia. She did not smoke cigarettes or drink alcohol. There was no family history of subarachnoid hemorrhage, cerebral hemorrhage, or intracranial aneurysms. Her brother had migraine without aura. Neurological examination was normal.

MRI of the brain and MRV were normal. MRA revealed an 8 mm saccular aneurysm arising from the left supraclinoid ICA, projecting medially (Figure 6-2). Cerebral angiogram demonstrated an 8 by 7 by 5 mm aneurysm arising from the medial wall of the distal left internal carotid artery proximal to the anterior choroidal artery (Figure 6-3). The aneurysm was somewhat lobulated, and the neck measured 4 mm (see Figure 6-3). Additionally, a 2 mm aneurysm arising from the callosomarginal branch of the right anterior cerebral artery was seen.

Given the fact that no spinal fluid exam had been done shortly after the headache onset, and given the appearance of the left supraclinoid aneurysm, the consulting neurosurgeon recommended repair. The surgery was performed 7 weeks after the patient's thunderclap headache. Since the base of the aneurysm was moderately wide, it was decided that the best treatment was placement of a clip rather than endovascular occlusion with platinum coils. At the time of surgery, the aneurysm was found to arise off the posterior wall of the left internal carotid artery, with the dome projecting medially below the left optic nerve. There was no evidence of old or recent hemorrhage. The base of the aneurysm was estimated at 7 mm in breadth, and one superior hypophyseal branch arose with the aneurysm. The aneurysm was clipped with two right-angled fenestrated clips.

Postoperatively the patient had a short period of drowsiness and confusion. Head CT showed only postoperative changes. Left internal carotid angiogram showed occlusion of the left supraclinoid aneurysm, as well as some narrowing of the left internal carotid artery in the region of the clipped aneurysm (Figure 6-4).

When seen in follow-up 3 months after the aneurysm clipping, the patient continued to have mild headaches consistent with tension-type headaches. They were occurring 5 days per week, lasting 10–12 hours. She had no recurrent thunderclap headaches.

■ The Problem

- Was neurosurgical intervention appropriate in this case?
- Can unruptured intracranial aneurysms present with thunderclap headache?

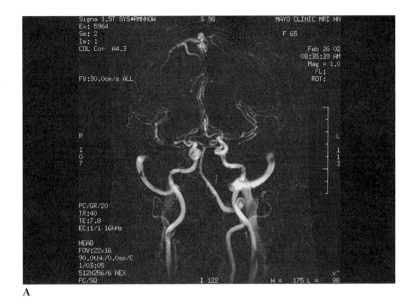

A

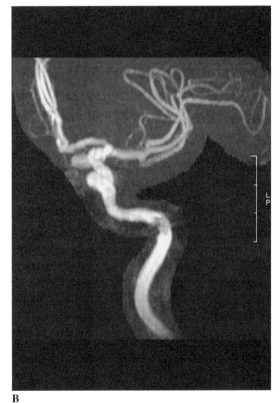

B

Figure 6-2. MRA showing an 8 mm saccular aneurysm arising from the left supraclinoid internal carotid artery, projecting medially.

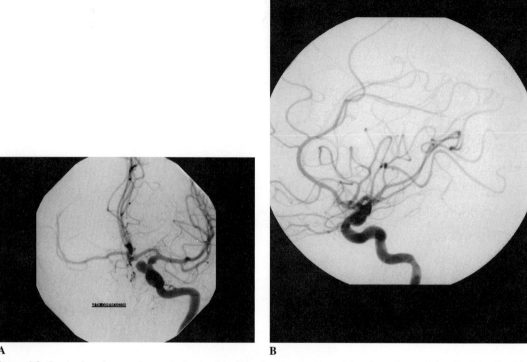

Figure 6-3. Cerebral angiogram demonstrating an 8 by 7 by 5 mm aneurysm arising from the medial wall of the distal left internal carotid artery.

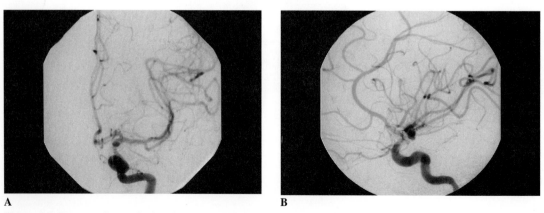

Figure 6-4. Postoperative cerebral angiogram revealing occlusion of the left supraclinoid aneurysm.

- What are the causes of symptomatic thunder-clap headache?
- How should a patient with thunderclap headache be evaluated?

■ The Evidence

Was Neurosurgical Intervention Appropriate in This Case?

Because no spinal fluid examination was done shortly after the patient's thunderclap headache, a subarachnoid hemorrhage had not been excluded. CSF xanthochromia determined by spectropho-tometry is present in over 70 percent of subarach-noid hemorrhage cases 3 weeks after the ictus, and in over 40 percent of cases 4 weeks after the ictus, but there are no data beyond this time period (Table 6-1).[5] Visual inspection for xanthochromia can miss discoloration in up to 50 percent of spec-imens.[6] A negative spinal fluid examination for xanthochromia 5 weeks after the ictus, which is when the neurologist first saw the patient in this case, would have been meaningless. Surgical exploration and intervention was therefore appro-priate and most likely imperative.

Can Unruptured Intracranial Aneurysms Present with Thunderclap Headache?

Day and Raskin were the first to speculate that an unruptured cerebral aneurysm could present with a thunderclap headache.[1] The authors presented a 42-year-old woman who complained of three

stereotyped thunderclap headaches. Neurological exam showed old findings secondary to multiple sclerosis. CT of the head after the first event and CSF examinations after the first and third events were normal. Angiogram after the third event showed diffuse vasospasm in the anterior and pos-terior circulations of both hemispheres, and a 1.0 by 1.5 cm right internal carotid artery aneurysm. The aneurysm was clipped surgically, but no evidence of old or recent hemorrhage was detected by the neurosurgeon. Four-vessel angiography 4 weeks later showed that the vasospasm had resolved. A similar patient was subsequently reported, although in that case repeat angiography was not performed to document resolution of the vasospasm.[7]

Cases of thunderclap headache with normal neurological examinations, unruptured aneurysms, and no evidence of segmental vasospasm have also been reported. Ng and Pulst described a 53-year-old woman who presented to the emergency department with a thunderclap headache.[8] Neurological exami-nation, CT head, and CSF exam were normal. Whether the CSF was checked for xanthochromia by spectrophotometry was not mentioned. She was discharged from the ED after 36 hours as her headache improved on analgesics. Two days later she was readmitted due to recurring headaches, and the following day she was found unresponsive, having suffered a subarachnoid hemorrhage. An angiogram showed a distal right internal carotid aneurysm, and the patient died shortly thereafter. Witham and Kaufmann described a 50-year-old woman who presented with a thunderclap headache and subsequently had a normal neurological exam-ination, CT head, and CSF examination.[9] A 13 mm

Table 6-1. CSF Xanthochromia after SAH[5]

Delay Since Ictus	No. of Patients with Xanthochromia Absent	No. of Patients with Xanthochromia Present	Probability of Detecting Xanthochromia by Spectrophotometry
12–24 hours	0	34	100%
1–2 days	0	37	100%
3–4 days	0	27	100%
5–6 days	0	13	100%
1 week	0	41	100%
2 weeks	0	32	100%
3 weeks	2	20	91% (95% CI 71–99)
4 weeks	4	10	71% (95% CI 42–92)

Data adapted from reference 5 with permission.

left posterior communicating artery aneurysm with a daughter sac was found on angiography. At surgery the aneurysm was thin-walled, but there was no evidence of prior hemorrhage. Hughes presented a 32-year-old man who had a thunderclap headache.[10] He saw a neurologist 12 days after the thunderclap headache, and the neurological exam was normal. CT of the head was normal, and the lumbar puncture revealed 9 red blood cells, 6 white blood cells, protein of 44 mg/dL, and no xanthochromia. A cerebral angiogram demonstrated a 5 mm left middle cerebral artery aneurysm, which was surgically clipped. At the time of surgery there was no evidence of recent hemorrhage.

Furthermore, there have been several other patients with thunderclap headache secondary to unruptured aneurysms reported. In these cases, however, the neurological examination or CT scans were abnormal, and the information concerning spinal fluid examination was incomplete. Raps et al. studied 111 patients with unruptured intracranial aneurysms.[11] Seven of these patients presented with thunderclap headache. CT scan was negative for hemorrhage in these patients, but it is not clear how many had spinal fluid examinations. The unruptured state was confirmed by direct visualization at the time of surgery. Three of the 7 patients had oculomotor palsies. Two of these patients had aneurysmal thrombosis on CT or MRI. Two patients had giant anterior communicating artery aneurysms, one with extensive thrombosis. One headache followed intranasal cocaine use.

A brief case report in the "Images from Headache" section of the journal *Headache* by an anonymous author in January 2002 described a 36-year-old woman who presented with thunderclap headache.[12] Her neurological examination was normal. CT of the head showed a serpiginous lesion in the left frontal region just adjacent to the midline. CSF exam was not performed. Brain MRI showed a partially thrombosed giant aneurysm involving the distal portion of the left anterior cerebral artery. Angiography confirmed a single aneurysm of the left pericallosal artery without vasospasm. At surgery she was found to have a "sausage-shaped, thrombosed aneurysm of the left callosal marginal artery and a large (2.5 cm) aneurysm shaped 'like a bent summer squash' and arising from the left pericallosal artery."[12] The neck of the pericallosal aneurysm was clipped. There was no evidence of

recent bleeding at surgery, but the aneurysm was felt to contain a large amount of clot.

Two non-English-language retrospective studies have presented patients with unruptured aneurysms and thunderclap headache. Takeuchi et al. studied 562 patients presenting with thunderclap headache.[13] All CT scans were normal, and the CSF was colorless. The spinal fluid was not checked by spectrophotometry. Aneurysms were found in 52 patients (9.3 percent). It is unclear what sort of angiography (conventional versus CT angiography) was performed to confirm the presence of an aneurysm, or whether the evaluation involved four-vessel angiography. Forty-six of these patients were taken to surgery and "minor leaks" were found in 8 patients. During surgery hemorrhage was found in the subarachnoid cistern in all 8 cases. Strittmatter et al. retrospectively studied 84 patients presenting with thunderclap headache and negative CT scans and CSF examinations over a period of 1–6 years.[14] One of these patients had an unruptured aneurysm on angiography. None of the patients developed SAH over a 1–6 year period. The authors only recommended cerebral angiography in cases with neurological deficits.

Circumstantial evidence against an association between thunderclap headache and unruptured aneurysms comes from several prospective studies.[15–19] These studies have shown that patients with thunderclap headache who present with bloodless CT scans and CSF exams do not go on to have subarachnoid hemorrhages during follow-up. The authors thus do not recommend conventional angiography routinely in these circumstances.

In the study by Wijdicks et al., 71 patients presented with thunderclap headaches.[15] Neurological examination was normal, except for "doubtful neck stiffness" in 10 and a dilated unreactive pupil in one. All patients had negative CT scans and CSF examinations. Cerebral angiography was normal in 4 patients. Follow-up information was obtained for an average of 3.3 years (range 1–7 years). No evidence of subsequent SAH was found in any patient. Repeat thunderclap headaches occurred in 12 patients. Four of these 12 were readmitted with recurrences, and again brain CT and CSF examination were normal. Two of these 4 had cerebral angiograms performed that were normal.

Harling et al. followed 14 patients for 18–30 months after they presented with thunderclap headaches and negative brain CT/CSF analysis.[16] Eight of these 14 patients had angiograms performed, and all were negative. No patient suffered SAH during follow-up. Markus found the same result after following 16 patients for 14–24 months.[17] Linn et al. followed 93 patients for 1–10 years and no subsequent SAH was diagnosed.[18]

Landtblom et al. studied 137 consecutive patients with thunderclap headache.[19] Brain CT scans were performed acutely and, if no definite cause was found, a CSF exam was done using spectrophotometry to look for xanthochromia. Twenty-three patients were found to have SAH, 5 had cerebral infarcts, 3 had cerebral hematomas, 4 had aseptic meningitis, one had cerebral edema, and one had venous sinus thrombosis. One hundred and three patients were felt to have benign (or primary) thunderclap headache. The non-SAH patients were followed for a year, and none developed subarachnoid hemorrhage. Recurrent attacks of thunderclap headache occurred in 24 percent of the non-SAH patients, who were not re-investigated. Dodick has suggested criteria for primary thunderclap headache (Table 6-2).[20]

Summarizing all of the studies, 297 patients presented with thunderclap headaches and bloodless CT/CSF exams. During a follow-up period of 1–10 years, none developed subarachnoid hemorrhage.

Table 6-2. Diagnostic Criteria for Primary (Idiopathic or Benign) Thunderclap Headache[20]

I.	Very severe pain intensity
II.	Instantaneous or hyperacute onset of pain (<30 seconds)
III.	Appropriate investigations exclude the presence of an underlying cause. These include SAH, cerebral venous sinus thrombosis, pituitary apoplexy, arterial dissection, low CSF volume (pressure) headache, and acute hypertensive crisis.

Comment: Idiopathic thunderclap headache may occur spontaneously or may be precipitated by the Valsalva maneuver, sexual activity, strenuous exercise, or exertion. Headaches may recur over a 7–14-day period. Similar headaches may occur infrequently over subsequent months to years. Investigations are always necessary to rule out secondary causes listed in III. If performed, angiography may demonstrate diffuse segmental cerebral vasospasm, which resolves within weeks to months.

What are the Causes of Symptomatic Thunderclap Headache?

Table 6-3 reviews the reported causes of thunderclap headache.

How Should a Patient with Thunderclap Headache be Evaluated?

In a patient with a normal examination, CT scan, and CSF examination, further neuroimaging studies may be indicated if one of the secondary headache disorders listed in Table 6-3 is suspected clinically. A normal CSF examination should include recording a normal opening pressure. A normal opening pressure can help differentiate a traumatic spinal tap from a SAH, an elevated opening pressure can be a clue to the diagnosis of cerebral venous sinus thrombosis, and a low opening pressure can suggest low CSF volume (pressure) headache.[6] Further testing may include MRI with gadolinium, MR venography (MRV), MRA, CTA, or conventional angiography.

Table 6-3. Differential Diagnosis of Thunderclap Headache[19,21,22]

I.	Primary headache disorders	
	A.	Primary thunderclap headache
		1. Without reversible vasospasm
		2. With reversible vasospasm
	B.	Primary headache associated with sexual activity (explosive type)
	C.	Primary exertional headache
	D.	Primary cough headache
II.	Secondary headache disorders	
	A.	Subarachnoid hemorrhage
	B.	Intracerebral hemorrhage
	C.	Spontaneous retroclival hematoma
	D.	Chronic subdural hematoma
	E.	Pituitary apoplexy
	F.	Cerebral venous sinus thrombosis
	G.	Carotid artery dissection
	H.	Cerebral infarction
	I.	Acute hypertensive crisis
	J.	Low CSF volume (pressure) headache
	K.	Intermittent hydrocephalus
	L.	Meningitis/encephalitis
	M.	Sphenoid sinusitis
	N.	Occipital neuralgia
	O.	Unruptured intracranial aneurysms?

MRI with gadolinium often demonstrates pachymeningeal enhancement in low CSF volume (pressure) headache. In one study, 3 patients with low CSF volume headache presenting as thunderclap headache were reported.[23] All had normal neurological examinations aside from nuchal rigidity. Emergent CT scanning, lumbar puncture, and MRA were performed to rule out aneurysmal SAH. MRI with gadolinium showed pachymeningeal enhancement and brain sagging in all patients. In one patient, the opening pressure was 5 cm H_2O, in one the CSF pressure was "low," and in the remaining patient the pressure was not checked.[23] Details of the CSF studies were not described but were reported to be "typical."[23] The authors noted that xanthochromia could be present in low CSF volume headache patients, possibly secondary to increased subdural vascular permeability.[23]

MRV could be used to look for venous sinus thrombosis. In one study, 10 patients were reported with thunderclap headache as the first symptom of cerebral venous sinus thrombosis.[24] Of these 10 patients, one had a normal exam, CT scan, and CSF analysis, but the opening pressure was not checked. Another patient had a normal exam, CT, and CSF studies. However, the CSF pressure was 50 cm H_2O.[24]

MRA can demonstrate reversible vasospasm in some patients, which is suggestive of primary thunderclap headache even in the presence of an unruptured aneurysm.[25] MRA could also demonstrate evidence of a cervicocephalic arterial dissection. In one study, 6 of 135 carotid dissection patients had thunderclap headache as their first symptom.[26] One thunderclap headache patient with a normal neurological examination aside from carotid artery tenderness, normal CT, and normal CSF studies was reported.[27] Cerebral angiography documented bilateral carotid dissections.

MRA could also show evidence of an unruptured aneurysm. The sensitivity of MRA for the detection of intracranial aneurysms is 69–100 percent, while the specificity is 75–100 percent.[28] For aneurysms >6 mm in diameter, the sensitivity rates are >95 percent.[22] The overall aneurysm detection rate for CTA is 85–98 percent.[22] If an aneurysm is found on MRA or CTA, the International Study of Unruptured Intracranial Aneurysms findings can help guide therapy.[29]

There is no clear compelling evidence to routinely perform an invasive conventional cerebral angiogram in a patient with thunderclap headache and normal examination, CT head, and CSF examination, especially when MRA or CTA are available.

■ The Pros and Cons

It has been estimated that 3.6 to 6.0 percent of individuals over 30 years of age harbor an unruptured aneurysm.[28] The two patients presented by Day, Raskin, and Clarke most likely had incidental aneurysms as well as primary thunderclap headache with reversible vasospasm.[1,7] It is difficult to explain how vasospasm could be caused by an unruptured aneurysm in the absence of subarachnoid blood, and thus the two likely occurred together by chance.

Sudden expansion of an aneurysm independent of bleeding into the wall could lead to thunderclap headache.[1,7,30] After noting that at surgery the unruptured aneurysm had a daughter bleb and a very thin-walled dome, Witham and Kaufmann speculated that the thunderclap headache in their patient was secondary to acute enlargement of the unruptured aneurysm.[9] Hughes likewise favored the notion that aneurysmal expansion might cause thunderclap headache.[10] However, this hypothesis seems difficult to prove without serial neuroimaging documenting the enlargement. Raps et al. speculated that acute headache from an unruptured aneurysm was likely caused by local thrombosis but also mentioned morphological change in the vascular wall, intramural bleeding, or occult hemorrhage as possible contributors.[11] If expansion or morphological change in the wall of an unruptured aneurysm were the cause of thunderclap headache, one would expect several of these patients to develop subarachnoid hemorrhage over the subsequent years, but this does not seem to be the case.[15]

The most convincing evidence that an unruptured aneurysm can cause thunderclap headache and herald a major subarachnoid hemorrhage may be the case reported by Ng and Pulst.[8] Unfortunately, this is only presented in abstract form, and the abstract does not state whether the patient continued to have a normal neurological examination once she was readmitted after discharge from the emergency department. Also, no data are given concerning what studies were used to diagnose subarachnoid hemorrhage as the cause of the patient's unresponsiveness. We are only told that a distal right internal carotid aneurysm was found on angiography and that the patient subsequently died.

In the study by Takeuchi et al., the 8 patients with "minor leaks" at surgery might have been identified preoperatively as having SAH if the CSF had been sent for assessment of xanthochromia by spectrophotometry.[13] That would leave 7.8 percent (44/562) of patients in the study presenting with an unruptured aneurysm and thunderclap headache. Certainly some (and possibly all) of these aneurysms were incidental.

In the study by Raps et al., there were several abnormal examination and neuroimaging findings.[11] These findings would have left little doubt that the thunderclap headache in most of these cases was symptomatic of an underlying cause.[20] Therefore, this study does not help determine whether an unruptured aneurysm can present with thunderclap headache in a patient with a normal exam, brain CT, and CSF examination.

■ The Main Points

- It is unclear if thunderclap headaches may be caused by unruptured aneurysms.
- When evaluating a patient presenting with a thunderclap headache, careful examination of the CT scan and CSF is essential to rule out SAH.
- CT scans must be reviewed closely to ensure that there is no blood before the pons or in the ventricles, and that the basal cisterns are adequately imaged.
- CSF must always be studied with spectrophotometry to exclude xanthochromia. Visual inspection is not sufficient when trying to exclude SAH in a patient presenting with thunderclap headache.
- If an unruptured aneurysm can cause thunderclap headache in a patient with a normal neurological examination, a bloodless CT scan, and a bloodless CSF examination, it would seem to occur rarely. If thunderclap headache were commonly secondary to unruptured

aneurysms, one would expect to find more patients with this combination in the literature.
- In selected clinical circumstances, MRI with gadolinium, MRA or CTA, and MRV may be useful diagnostic tools in patients with thunderclap headaches.
- Conventional cerebral angiography should be reserved for patients with abnormal neurological signs on examination, and for cases with questionable results on less invasive studies (e.g., CSF xanthochromia not excluded by spectrophotometry, noninvasive angiograms of insufficient quality or with equivocal findings).

■ References

1. Day JW, Raskin NH. Thunderclap headache: symptom of unruptured cerebral aneurysm. *Lancet* 1986;2: 1247–1248.
2. Fisher CM. Honored guest presentation: Painful states: a neurological commentary. *Clin Neurosurg* 1984;31: 32–53.
3. Pearce JMS. Clinical features of the exploding head syndrome. *J Neurol Neurosurg Psychiatry* 1989;52: 907–910.
4. Noseworthy JH, Girvin JP. Sentinel tinnitus as symptom of acephalgic subarachnoid haemorrhage. *Lancet* 1987;1:1315.
5. Vermeulen M, Hasan D, Blijenberg BG, Hijdra A, van Gijn J. Xanthochromia after subarachnoid hemorrhage needs no revisitation. *J Neurol Neurosurg Psychiatry* 1989;52:826–828.
6. Edlow JA, Caplan LR. Avoiding pitfalls in the diagnosis of subarachnoid hemorrhage. *N Engl J Med* 2000;342:29–36.
7. Clarke CE, Shepherd DI, Chishti K, Victoratos G. Thunderclap headache. *Lancet* 1988;2:625.
8. Ng PK, Pulst S-M. Not so benign "thunderclap headache." *Neurology* 1992;42(Suppl 3):260.
9. Witham TF, Kaufmann AM. Unruptured cerebral aneurysm producing a thunderclap headache. *Am J Emerg Med* 2000;18:88–90.
10. Hughes RL. Identification and treatment of cerebral aneurysms after sentinel headache. *Neurology* 1992;42:1118–1119.
11. Raps EC, Rogers JD, Galetta SL, Solomon RA, Lennihan L, Klebanoff LM, Fink ME. The clinical spectrum of unruptured intracranial aneurysms. *Arch Neurol* 1993;50:265–268.
12. Anonymous. Aneurysmal "thunderclap" headache without subarachnoid hemorrhage. *Headache* 2002;42:82.

13. Takeuchi T, Kasahara E, Iwasaki M, Kojima S. Necessity for searching for cerebral aneurysm in thunderclap headache patients who show no evidence of subarachnoid hemorrhage: investigation of 8 minor leak cases on operation. *No Shinkei Geka* 1996;24:437–441.
14. Strittmatter M, Zimmermann C, Schimrigk K, Hamann GF. "Thunderclap headache": an independent form of headache? *Wiener Klinische Wochenschrift* 1996;108:326–329.
15. Wijdicks EFM, Kerkhoff H, van Gijn J. Long-term follow-up of 71 patients with thunderclap headache mimicking subarachnoid haemorrhage. *Lancet* 1988;2:68–70.
16. Harling DW, Peatfield RC, Van Hille PT, Abbott RJ. Thunderclap headache: is it migraine? *Cephalalgia* 1989;9:87–90.
17. Markus HS. A prospective follow up of thunderclap headache mimicking subarachnoid haemorrhage. *J Neurol Neurosurg Psychaitry* 1991;54: 1117–1118.
18. Linn FHH, Rinkel GJE, Algra A, van Gijn J. Follow-up of idiopathic thunderclap headache in general practice. *J Neurol* 1999;246:946–948.
19. Landtblom A-M, Fridriksson S, Boivie J, Hillmann J, Johansson G, Johansson I. Sudden onset headache: a prospective study of features, incidence and causes. *Cephalalgia* 2002;22:354–360.
20. Dodick DW. Thunderclap headache. *J Neurol Neurosurg Psychaitry* 2002;72:6–11.
21. Dodick DW. Thunderclap headache. *Headache* 2002;42:309–315.
22. Linn FHH, Wijdicks EFM. Causes and management of thunderclap headache: a comprehensive review. *Neurologist* 2002;8:279–289.
23. Schievink WI, Wijdicks EFM, Meyer FB, Sonntag VKH. Spontaneous intracranial hypotension mimicking aneurysmal subarachnoid hemorrhage. *Neurosurgery* 2001;48:513–517.
24. de Bruijn SFTM, Stam J, Kappelle LJ, for the CVST Study Group. Thunderclap headache as first symptom of cerebral venous sinus thrombosis. *Lancet* 1996;348:1623–1625.
25. Dodick DW, Brown RD, Britton JW, Huston J. Nonaneurysmal thunderclap headache with diffuse, multifocal, segmental, and reversible vasospasm. *Cephalalgia* 1999;19:118–123.
26. Silbert PJ, Mokri B, Schievink WI. Headache and neck pain in spontaneous internal carotid and vertebral artery dissections. *Neurology* 1995;45:1517–1522.
27. Biousse V, Woimant F, Amarenco P, Touboul P-J, Bousser M-G. Pain as the only manifestation of internal carotid artery dissection. *Cephalalgia* 1992;12:314–317.
28. Wardlaw JM, White PM. The detection and management of unruptured intracranial aneurysms. *Brain* 2000;123:205–221.
29. Wiebers DO, Whisnant JP, Huston J III, Meissner I, Brown RD Jr, Piepgras DG, Forbes GS, Thielen K, Nichols D, O'Fallon WM, Peacock J, Jaeger L, Kassell NF, Kongable-Beckman GL, Torner JC; International Study of Unruptured Intracranial Aneurysms Investigators. Unruptured intracranial aneurysms: natural history, clinical outcome, and risks of surgical and endovascular treatment. *Lancet.* 2003;362:103–110.
30. Anonymous Editorial. *Lancet* 1988;2:80–82.

PART II
Tough Calls in Procedures

Chapter 7

When to Intubate Critically Ill Neurological Patients

Cecil O. Borel and David L. McDonagh

Airway assessment and endotracheal intubation remains "terra incognita" for many physicians in hospital practice and more than a few understandably balk at the idea of making this call. The decision to intubate is often based on an assessment of the patient's disease course and the clinical appearance of impending ventilatory collapse.

The most important consequence of compromised ventilation is hypoxemia. Hypoxemia results in a deadly spiral of decreasing oxygen delivery to ischemic neurological tissue, resulting in further end-organ injury and compromised ventilation. Controlling the airway, maintaining ventilation, and supplementing oxygenation can interrupt the process.

Patients with acute life-threatening neurological diseases need endotracheal intubation and mechanical ventilation whenever there is a risk of compromised ventilation. Endotracheal intubation should be performed before compromised ventilation results in secondary neurological injury. Pathophysiological guidelines can help in deciding which patients are at a high risk of ventilatory compromise due to neurological dysfunction. The need for endotracheal intubation may result from the following basic patterns of neurological injury: decreased level of consciousness, injury to brainstem airway reflexes or ventilatory drive, or weak inspiratory effort due to muscle weakness. Neurological illnesses may also affect gas exchange by decreasing lung compliance and increasing intrapulmonary shunting due to neurogenic pulmonary edema. This chapter summarizes the major concerns of practicing physicians (Table 7-1).

■ The Patient

A 45-year-old man presents to the emergency room with an altered level of consciousness following a severe headache. He mutters incomprehensible words, opens his eyes to painful stimulation, and withdraws to pain (Glasgow coma score [GCS] of 8). Pupils are equal and reactive, but there is a decreased corneal response in the right eye, and a right facial droop. The right arm and leg are weak. A CT scan of the head demonstrates a large left thalamic hemorrhage with discernable midline shift, but without compression of the quadrigeminal cistern. His breathing appears satisfactory, and he is able to maintain oxygen saturations of 95 percent with nasal oxygen supplementation at 2 L/min. His chest x-ray is clear.

The patient was intubated in the emergency room.

■ The Problem

- What are the indications for endotracheal intubation in patients with critical neurological disease?
- What are the risks of delaying intubation in these patients?

Table 7-1. Endotracheal Intubation in Patients with Acute Neurological Disorders

Impairment	Physiological Confirmation	Indication	Considerations During Intubation	Technique
Decreased level of consciousness	GCS <10	Prevention of aspiration	Prevent passive regurgitation Minimal sedation necessary	Oral tracheal intubation under direct laryngoscopy
Raised intracranial pressure	GCS <9 CT scan	Prevention of hypoxia or hypercarbia Hyperventilation	Block ↑ in ICP during laryngoscopy Prevent aspiration Avoid cervical or facial injury	Rapid-sequence intubation with cervical stabilization
Posterior fossa injury not affecting consciousness	Positional airway obstruction Decreased gag reflex	Maintain patent airway Prevent aspiration	Exaggerated ↑ or ↓ BP response Minimal sedation necessary	Oral tracheal intubation under direct laryngoscopy
Medullary lesion	↑ Resting PCO_2 No response to inhaled CO_2	Loss of ventilatory drive	Exaggerated response to narcotics and sedatives	Oral tracheal intubation under direct laryngoscopy
High cervical spine injury	↓ Inspiratory muscle effort	Phrenic nerve paralysis	Avoid cervical injury	Best possible cervical stabilization In-line head immobilization Fiber-optic intubation Blind nasal intubation
Lower cervical thoracic injury	↓ Inspiratory and expiratory function ↓ Po_2 from atelectasis, pneumonia	↓ Intercostal, abdominal strength	Avoid cervical injury Rigid stabilization already present ↑K^+ response to succinylcholine	Fiber-optic intubation Oral intubation using laryngeal mask device Blind nasal intubation
Acute polyneuropathy	↓ Po_2 from aspiration, atelectasis, pneumonia ↑ Pco_2 from ↓ ventilation Inspiratory force < 30 mm Hg Vital capacity < 10 mL/kg	↓ Ventilatory muscle strength Airway obstruction	Dysautonomia exaggerates ↓BP with sedation or anesthesia ↑K^+ response to succinylcholine	Topical local anesthesia Oral intubation technique of choice
Neuromuscular junction disease	↓ Po_2 from aspiration, atelectasis, pneumonia ↑ Pco_2 from ↓ ventilation Inspiratory force < 30 mm Hg Vital capacity < 10 mL/kg	↓ Ventilatory muscle strength Airway obstruction	Exaggerated response to nondepolarizing muscle relaxants Unpredictable response to succinylcholine	Topical local anesthesia Light sedation Oral intubation technique of choice
Myopathy	↑ Pco_2 from ↓ ventilation ↓ Po_2 from aspiration, atelectasis, pneumonia Inspiratory force < 30 mm Hg Vital capacity < 10 mL/kg	↓ Ventilatory muscle strength	Risk of malignant hyperthermia with succinylcholine use in some myopathies	Oral intubation technique of choice No succinylcholine (vecuronium, rocuronium, or *cis*-atracurium may be used if necessary)

GCS, Glasgow coma score.

- What are the specific technical adjustments and potential complications to be considered when intubating patients with acute intracranial pathology, spinal cord injury, or neuromuscular respiratory failure?
- What is the value of rapid sequence intubation?

■ The Evidence

Decreased Level of Consciousness

The GCS is the best rapid assessment for patients with acute cortical dysfunction. Generally, a GCS <10 has been used as an indication for intubation. A GSC <10 is found in patients who do not open eyes spontaneously, follow commands, or verbalize. The main purpose of intubation in patients with decreased level of consciousness is to protect airway patency and reduce the risk of aspiration.

Global Cortical Injury and Raised Intracranial Pressure

A reduced level of consciousness, with GCS <10, has been shown to significantly influence mortality in ischemic stroke and intracerebral hemorrhage.[1–4] The requirement for intubation and mechanical ventilation within the first day after the stroke is a valid marker for stroke severity.[5] The GCS at the time of intubation predicts survival at 30 days in patients suffering from both ischemic stroke and spontaneous cerebral hemorrhage.[2] Neurological deterioration resulting in a reduced level of consciousness and the need for airway protection has been shown to be associated with tissue shifts secondary to edema.[6,7] Patients presenting with acutely raised ICP often require control of the airway as the initial therapeutic intervention.[8] Secondary neurological damage from raised ICP can be minimized by preventing hypoxemia, hypercarbia, and acidosis.[9] In patients with decreased level of consciousness (GCS <10) and impaired ability to protect the airway, brief moderate mechanical hyperventilation may be used to control raised ICP.[10] In these patients, early signs of herniation include failure to protect airway or ventilate appropriately (it impairs airway reflexes, coughing, and ventilatory drive).[11,12]

Airway manipulation without adequate pharmacological support can cause precipitous changes in systemic hemodynamic parameters, adversely affecting the injured brain. Laryngoscopy, hypoventilation, struggling, and the use of succinylcholine without defasciculation[13] may increase ICP. Rapid-sequence intubation is the safest approach for the patient with raised ICP.[14] Rapid-sequence intubation proceeds through three phases: (1) preoxygenation, to prevent hypoxemia during intubation; (2) pretreatment with drugs to mitigate the hemodynamic and intracranial pressure effects of intubation (e.g., lidocaine, short-acting barbiturate); and (3) sequential administration of a potent sedative (e.g., propofol) and, when necessary, a rapidly acting nondepolarizing neuromuscular blocking agent (e.g., rocuronium, vecuronium) to induce unconsciousness and paralysis. Succinylcholine may increase intracranial pressure due to widespread muscle fasciculations, increased central venous pressure, and hypercarbia.[15] Thus, the use of succinylcholine in patients with elevated intracranial pressure or pronounced cerebral edema should probably be avoided. Cricoid pressure must be maintained during drug administration to prevent passive regurgitation of stomach contents. In-line cervical stabilization must be maintained to prevent potential cervical vertebral dislocation during laryngoscopy and intubation.[16]

Inability to Protect Airway or Initiate Breathing

Brainstem disease may lead to several well-defined disorders of breathing and require endotracheal intubation. For example, patients with acute basilar artery occlusions may suffer from obstructive or mixed apnea, or impaired airway reflexes which lead to positional airway obstruction or repeated aspiration.

Decreased Gag Reflex

The gag reflex decreases as a general result of decreased level of consciousness or from direct injury to brainstem or cranial nerves IX or X. It is not clear whether the bedside sensory examination can reliably distinguish IX and X nerve lesions, but lack of posterior wall pharyngeal sensation is reported to have practical implications in stroke.[17] A unilateral XII nerve lesion causes the tongue to deviate to the healthy side on retraction due to unopposed action of styloglossus, as well as to the affected side on protrusion from the genioglossus. Volitional cough may be feeble due to depressed level of consciousness or respiratory or laryngeal muscle weakness, whereas a "bovine" cough suggests vocal cord paresis.[18] Patients with corticobulbar lesions may exhibit impaired voluntary control of facial movements, cough, and respiration while retaining emotional or reflex responses. Breathing may be stridorous (laryngeal dystonia), obstructed (laryngeal or pharyngeal occlusion), or abnormal in pattern (respiratory dyskinesia).

Decreased Ventilatory Drive

The dorsolateral medulla is primarily responsible for the integration of effective rhythmic breathing. Central ventilatory control may be relatively normal as long as this area, which includes the nucleus ambiguus and solitarius, is not affected. Thus, even locked-in patients with rostral brainstem infarction may conserve a relatively normal respiratory drive.[19] Disruption of automatic breathing may result from damage to the lateral medulla and pontine tegmentum caudal to trigeminal outflow. Lateral medullary stroke is most commonly due to occlusion of the distal vertebral or posterior inferior cerebellar artery, and large infarcts involving the dorsolateral medulla may be associated with fatal apnea.[20] These patients may suffer from mild hypoventilation while awake, which can be reversed voluntarily. Respirations may cease entirely during sleep. Uncommonly, hemorrhagic or ischemic lesions near the pontomesencephalic junction may result in neurogenic hyperventilation.[21,22] This condition may also be seen after severe global insult from anoxia, hypoglycemia, or metabolic encephalopathy, especially hepatic encephalopathy.[23]

Ventilatory Muscle Weakness

Spinal Cord Injury. Many spinal cord injury patients will require at least temporary endotracheal intubation. Spinal immobilization must be maintained during airway management in any patient with a potential spinal cord injury. The majority of cervical spinal movement occurring during direct laryngoscopy is concentrated in the

upper cervical spine,[24] though the magnitude of movement during airway management rarely exceeds the physiological limits of the spine.[25] Movement is reduced by in-line immobilization but traction forces cause clinically important distraction and should be avoided. Indirect techniques for tracheal intubation cause less cervical movement than direct laryngoscopy.[26] Missed diagnosis is common and associated with a high incidence of severe secondary injury. Failure to immobilize the spine is deemed to be the most relevant factor in secondary injury.[16]

The intubation technique used for patients with suspected cervical cord injuries should avoid further cord injury and prevent aspiration. Blind or fiber-optically guided nasotracheal intubation with local/topical anesthesia are appropriate approaches. Rapid-sequence intubation techniques using a short-acting barbiturate and neuromuscular blocking agent with simultaneous cricoid pressure can also be used.[27] There is no conclusive evidence for or against the use of any particular technique.[28,29] Manual in-line neck traction has fallen out of favor due to concerns about dislocation of an unstable cervical spine.[30] However, in-line head immobilization continues to be recommended.[29]

Patients with spinal cord injury will display hypersensitivity to depolarizing neuromuscular blockers such as succinylcholine. If a depolarizing agent is used to facilitate intubation, it can be used safely within the first 48 hours of the injury. Thereafter, massive release of skeletal muscle potassium can occur after succinylcholine administration, possibly leading to cardiac arrest.[31–33] This may be due to an upregulation of acetylcholine receptors at the motor endplate. The phenomenon is thought to last at least 3–6 months. A rapid-onset nondepolarizing neuromuscular blocker such as rocuronium, vecuronium, or *cis*-atracurium should be used instead of succinylcholine for spinal cord injury patients at risk of hyperkalemia.

Emergent tracheotomy may be needed in the event of severe head and neck injuries. A depressed level of consciousness due to concomitant head injury will necessitate intubation for airway protection. Awake or rapid-sequence intubation techniques can reduce the occurrence of aspiration. High cervical lesions (at or above C3) may result in loss of diaphragmatic function due to inability to activate the phrenic nerves, while lesions below this level will compromise some or all accessory muscles of inspiration. Patients with adequate respiratory movements on admission should be watched carefully for delayed apnea. This has been reported to occur up to a week after a cervical cord injury.[34]

Neuromuscular Ventilatory Failure. The decision to proceed to intubation and ventilatory support should be made as soon as it becomes clear that respiratory failure is imminent or inevitable, so that resources for airway management and mechanical ventilation are readily available. The indications for intubation from neuromuscular failure are complex and often subtle. Patients who manifest diaphragmatic failure invariably have tachycardia and tachypnea.[35,36] Use of accessory muscles is not always appreciated well with the naked eye, and palpation of the sternocleidomastoid muscles may disclose heightened muscle activity during breathing. Contraction of the sternocleidomastoid muscle is present long before florid paradoxical breathing becomes clinically apparent. Patients with diaphragmatic failure manifest with dyspnea at relatively low levels of physical exercise.

Laboratory measurements to detect ventilatory failure are very useful but must be interpreted together with clinical manifestations. Most of these tests are effort-dependent and require clear instruction to the patient. Vital capacity and maximum airway pressures may be spuriously low from inadequate mouth closure, particularly in patients with bilateral facial palsy. Forced vital capacity is defined as the volume of air that can be exhaled by force from the lungs after a full inhalation. Critical values are around 15 mL/kg. The maximum inspiratory pressure (MIP) and maximum expiratory pressure (MEP) are also clinically useful. Another frequent sign of imminent respiratory failure is transient oxygen desaturation during monitoring with a pulse oximeter. These bedside respiratory tests are reliable in patients with Guillain-Barré syndrome[37] but may be of relatively less value in cases of myasthenia gravis due to the fluctuating nature of this disease.[38]

Endotracheal intubation is more difficult in patients with Guillain-Barré syndrome than in other patients requiring emergency airway control because of dysautonomia and the potential for lethal hyperkalemia following succinylcholine administration.

The dysautonomic state in Guillain-Barré syndrome may be severe enough to cause sudden death,[39] and certainly exaggerates the hypotensive response to drugs used to induce anesthesia for intubation.[40] The administration of barbiturates, benzodiazepines, and narcotics must be titrated carefully to prevent hypotensive responses. Cardiac arrhythmias, particularly bradycardia, may also occur during airway manipulation in the dysautonomic patient. Heart rate, heart rhythm, and blood pressure should be monitored during intubation. Anticholinergic drugs (atropine), vasoconstrictors (epinephrine), and antiarrhythmic drugs (lidocaine) should be immediately available to treat sudden cardiovascular compromise. There are numerous case reports of cardiac arrest following succinylcholine administration in patients suffering ventilatory failure from polyneuropathy,[32,41] and Guillain-Barré syndrome.[42] Cardiac arrhythmias and arrest result from hyperkalemia which is due to extrajunctional chemosensitivity of denervated muscles to succinylcholine.

Both orotracheal and nasotracheal intubation can be performed safely. Topical anesthesia of the airway allows orotracheal intubation using a benzodiazepine for short-acting sedation and atropine. Blind nasal endotracheal intubation avoids the need for laryngoscopy and allows preservation of compromised protective airway reflexes and shallow breathing efforts, both of which may improve the safety and success of the procedure. The use of topical, rather than systemic, anesthetics decreases the risk of sudden hypotension and arrhythmias induced by airway manipulation. This approach to airway management is only feasible if the need for intubation has been anticipated and the patient prepared properly. If the patient cannot be adequately prepared or the intubation is emergent, laryngoscopy and endotracheal intubation can be safely performed using rapid-sequence techniques including preoxygenation, cricoid pressure, atropine, lidocaine, and low doses of thiopental intravenously. Short-acting nondepolarizing muscle relaxants can be added to this regimen, but are usually unnecessary.

Failure of Gas Exchange

Hypoxia has been shown to be a major factor in the outcome from acute head injury.[9,43] It is reasonable to assume that hypoxia may worsen other acute brain injuries, such as brain ischemia and intracerebral hemorrhage. Even though lung injuries may not be apparent on presentation, secondary lung injury should be suspected in patients with decreased cerebral function as a result of aspiration pneumonia, neurogenic pulmonary edema, or lung contusion. A widened alveolar-arterial oxygen gradient on an FiO_2 of 1.0, $PaO_2/FiO_2 < 200$, or a PO_2 of less than 60 mmHg on face mask oxygen should be considered indications for prompt ventilatory support. Endotracheal intubation and mechanical ventilation are life-saving in the prevention and treatment of acute hypoxia in neurologically compromised patients. Noninvasive methods of ventilation, such as BiPAP, are only useful when patients are cooperative and have a competent airway.[44]

Aspiration Pneumonia. Aspiration frequently causes impaired gas exchange in patients with neurological injury and is usually not witnessed by caregivers. There is a spectrum of possible lung damage. Patients may have silent, asymptomatic aspiration resulting in arterial desaturation and radiological abnormalities on chest x-ray. Others have mild symptoms such as coughing or wheezing.[45] Some go on to develop a fulminant aspiration pneumonitis (Mendelson's syndrome), with or without concomitant pneumonia. The common radiological findings in adults are right lower lobe infiltrates, atelectasis, and air bronchograms when a segmental infiltrate is present. In supine patients, the infiltrates will be posterior in the upper and lower lobes. Aspiration of large amounts of gastric acid may cause acute hypoxemia, cyanosis, and shock.[46] Occasionally, patients develop the acute respiratory distress syndrome (ARDS), which carries a high mortality.[47]

Neurogenic Pulmonary Edema. Neurogenic pulmonary edema has been often described in the setting of severe acute central nervous system injuries.[48,49] Its clinical presentation is similar to ARDS. Dramatic tachypnea, diaphoresis, hypertension, and frothy sputum are typically present. Diffuse pulmonary infiltrates ("white-out lungs") are seen on chest x-ray. Hypoxic respiratory failure, defined by hypoxemia and markedly increased alveolar-arterial oxygen gradient, occurs despite normal pulmonary artery wedge pressure.

Mechanical ventilation with PEEP (usually 10 to 15 cm H_2O titrated to maximize PO_2) is very effective in reversing the condition and radiographic improvement is achieved within hours. This measure alone is usually sufficient to treat the condition, and weaning is most commonly uneventful.[50,51]

■ The Pros and Cons

Our patient had decreased level of consciousness and he was intubated electively to ensure adequate protection of the airway. In addition, this intervention could prevent worsening cerebral edema from hypercarbia secondary to hypoventilation. Although this particular decision seems rather straightforward, several issues must be considered before intubation of a critically ill neurological patient as detailed above.

There is no question that endotracheal intubation and mechanical ventilation are life-saving procedures in preventing hypoxemia, hypercarbia, and aspiration pneumonia in patients with acute neurological diseases.[52] Patients at risk for sudden onset of ventilatory failure should have the airway controlled and mechanical ventilation initiated before the serious consequences of hypoxia or cardiac arrest indicate a need for emergent intervention.

In modern emergency care, endotracheal intubation is a safe and effective means of controlling the airway and assuring adequate ventilation. Though complications can occur, the risk of complications is decreased when there is time for recruitment of experienced laryngoscopists and procedural planning.

Endotracheal intubation and mechanical ventilation are reversible procedures. If the patient's level of consciousness improves, it is relatively simple to wean ventilation in the absence of lung disease. If the patient is able to maintain a patent airway, a trial of extubation can be scheduled but only if there are providers available to reintubate the patient if the need arises.

The downside of the endotracheal intubation procedure is that it usually requires the use of potent short-acting barbiturates and muscle relaxants. The use of these drugs may make neurological assessment unreliable for a period of several minutes to an hour. Sedation may be necessary to control coughing and struggling during mechanical ventilation, further confusing neurological assessment.

Autonomic hyperactivity with elevation of blood pressure and tachycardia causes additional systemic stress and may lead to secondary cerebral hemorrhage.

Intubated patients are cared for in an intensive care unit, thus increasing the complexity of medical and nursing care, risk of complications, and cost of hospitalization.

■ The Main Points

- Critically ill neurological patients from acute brain lesions often require intubation and mechanical ventilation to protect the airway, and prevent hypoxia and hypercarbia that can result in secondary neurological injury.
- Decreased level of consciousness (GCS <10) compromises airway reflexes.
- Patients with severe head injuries (GCS <8) have better outcomes when endotracheal intubation is performed early.
- Patients with cranial nerve palsies affecting airway control and protection may suffer airway compromise at higher levels of consciousness, because these patients depend on conscious effort to clear their secretions and maintain airway patency.
- In patients with documented or suspected history of trauma, in-line immobilization of the cervical spine must be maintained during intubation.
- Close clinical monitoring, including the use of bedside respiratory tests, is essential in patients with impending neuromuscular respiratory failure from Guillain-Barré syndrome. Emergency intubation in these patients is perilous due to the possible complications of dysautonomia.
- Patients with neurological injuries often have concomitant pulmonary disease due to aspiration pneumonia, neurogenic pulmonary edema, or lung contusion.

■ References

1. Burtin P, Bollaert PE, Feldmann L, Nace L, Lelarge P, Bauer P, Larcan A. Prognosis of stroke patients undergoing mechanical ventilation. *Intensive Care Med* 1994;20:32–36.

2. Bushnell C, Phillips-Bute B, Laskowitz D, Lynch J, Chilukuri V, Borel C. Survival and outcome after endotracheal intubation for acute stroke. *Neurology* 1999;52:1374–1381.

3. Gujjar A, Deibert E, Manno E, Duff S, Diringer M. Mechanical ventilation for ischemic stroke and intracerebral hemorrhage: indications, timing, and outcome. *Neurology* 1998;51:447–451.

4. Steiner T, Mendoza G, De Georgia M, Schellinger P, Holle R, Hacke W. Prognosis of stroke patients requiring mechanical ventilation in a neurological critical care unit. *Stroke* 1997;28:711–715.

5. Horner R, Sloane R, Kahn K. Is use of mechanical ventilation a reasonable proxy indicator for coma among Medicare patients hospitalized for acute stroke? *Health Services Res* 1998;32:841–859.

6. Frank J. Large hemispheric infarction, deterioration, and intracranial pressure. *Neurology* 1995;45:1286–1290.

7. Schwab S, Aschoff A, Spranger M, Albert F, Hacke W. The value of intracranial pressure monitoring in acute hemispheric stroke. *Neurology* 1996;47:393–398.

8. Anonymous. The Brain Trauma Foundation. The American Association of Neurological Surgeons. The Joint Section on Neurotrauma and Critical Care. Initial management. *J Neurotrauma* 2000;17:463–469.

9. Anonymous. The Brain Trauma Foundation. The American Association of Neurological Surgeons. The Joint Section on Neurotrauma and Critical Care. Resuscitation of blood pressure and oxygenation. *J Neurotrauma* 2000;17:471–478.

10. Gildenberg P, Frost E. Respiratory care in head trauma. In Becker D, Povlishock J, eds. *Central Nervous System Trauma*. Bethesda, MD, National Institutes of Health, 1985:161–176.

11. Ampel L, Hott K, Sielaff G, Sloan T. An approach to airway management in the acutely head-injured. *J Emerg Med* 1988;6:1–7.

12. Silvestri S, Aronson S. Severe head injury: prehospital and emergency department management [Review]. *Mount Sinai J Med* 1997;64:329–338.

13. Stirt J, Grosslight K, Bedford R, Vollmer D. Defasciculation with metocurine prevents succinylcholine-induced increases in intracranial pressure. *Anesthesiology* 1987;67:50–53.

14. Walls RM. Rapid-sequence intubation in head trauma. *Ann Emerg Med* 1993;22:1008–1013.

15. Lanier WL Milde JH, Michenfelder JD. Cerebral stimulation following succinylcholine in dogs. *Anesthesiology* 1986;64:551–559.

16. Crosby E. Airway management after upper cervical spine injury: what have we learned? *Can J Anaesthesia* 2002;49:733–744.

17. Kidd D, Lawson J, Nesbitt R, MacMahon J. Aspiration in acute stroke: a clinical study with videofluoroscopy. *Quart J Med* 1993;86:825–829.

18. Hughes TA, Wiles CM. Clinical measurement of swallowing in health and in neurogenic dysphagia. *Quart J Med* 1996;89:109–116.

19. Feldman M. Physiological observations in a chronic case of "locked in" syndrome. *Neurology* 1971;21:459.

20. Devereaux M, Keane J, Davis R. Automatic respiratory failure associated with infarction in the medulla. *Arch Neurol* 1973;29:46.

21. Froman C, Crampton Smith A. Hyperventilation associated with low pH of cerebrospinal fluid after intracranial hemorrhage. *Lancet* 1966;1:780–782.

22. Lane D, Rout M, Williamson D. Mechanism of hyperventilation in acute cerebrovascular accidents. *Br Med J* 1971;3:9–12.

23. Posner J, Plum F. Toxic effects of carbon dioxide and acetazolamide in hepatic encephalopathy. *J Clin Invest* 1980;39:1246.

24. Lennarson PJ, Smith D, Todd MM, Carras D, Sawin PD, Brayton J, Sato Y, Traynelis VC. Segmental cervical spine motion during orotracheal intubation of the intact and injured spine with and without external stabilization. *J Neurosurg* 2000;92(2 Suppl): 201–206.

25. McCrory C, Blunnie WP, Moriarty DC. Elective tracheal intubation in cervical spine injuries. *Irish Med J* 1997;90:234–235.

26. Brimacombe J, Keller C, Kunzel KH, Gaber O, Boehler M, Puhringer F. Cervical spine motion during airway management: a cinefluoroscopic study of the posteriorly destabilized third cervical vertebrae in human cadavers [Comment]. *Anesthesia & Analgesia* 2000;91:1274–1278.

27. Talucci R, Shaikh K, Schwab C. Rapid sequence induction with oral endotracheal intubation in the multiply injured patient. *Am Surg* 1988;54:185–187.

28. Meschino A, Devitt J, Kock J, Schwartz M. The safety of awake tracheal intubation in cervical spine injury. *Can J Anaesthesia* 1992;39:114–117.

29. Suderman V, Crosby E, Lui A. Elective oral tracheal intubation in the cervical spine-injured adult. *Can J Anaesthesia* 1991;38:785–789.

30. Twiner L. Cervical spine immobilization with axial traction: a practice to be discouraged. *J Emerg Med* 1989;7:385–386.

31. Cooperman L, Strobel G, Kennell E. Massive hyperkalemia after administration of succinylcholine. *Anesthesiology* 1970;32:161–164.

32. Cooperman L. Succinylcholine-induced hyperkalemia in neuromuscular disease. *JAMA* 1970;213: 1867–1871.

33. Stone W, Beach T, Hamburg W. Succinylcholine danger in the spinal cord injured patient. *Anesthesiology* 1970;32:168–169.

34. Kang L, et al. Delayed apnea in patients with mid- to lower cervical spinal cord injury. *Spine* 2000;25: 1332–1338.

35. Borel C, Teitlebaum J, Hanley D. Ventilatory drive and CO_2-response in ventilatory failure due to myasthenia gravis and Guillain-Barré. *Critic Care Med* 1993; 21:1717–1726.

36. Borel C, Tilford C, Nichols D, Hanley D, Traystman R. Diaphragmatic performance during recovery from acute ventilatory failure in Guillain-Barré syndrome and myasthenia gravis. *Chest* 1991;99:441–451.

37. Lawn ND, Fletcher DD Henderson RD, Wolter TD, Wijdicks EFM. Anticipating mechanical ventilation in Guillain-Barré syndrome. *Arch Neurol* 2001;58: 893–898.

38. Rabinstein AA, Wijdicks EFM. BiPAP in acute respiratory failure due to myasthenic crisis may prevent intubation. *Neurology* 2002;59:1647–1649.

39. Lichtenfeld P. Autonomic dysfunction in the Guillain-Barré syndrome. *Am J Med* 1971;50:772–780.

40. Dalos N, Borel C, Hanley D. Cardiovascular autonomic dysfunction in Guillain-Barré syndrome: therapeutic implications of Swan-Ganz monitoring. *Arch Neurol* 1988;45:115–117.

41. Fergusson R, Wright D, Willey R, Crompton G, Grant I. Suxamethonium is dangerous in polyneuropathy. *Br J Med* 1981;232:298–299.

42. Sunderrajan EV, Davenport J. The Guillain-Barré syndrome: pulmonary neurologic correlations. *Medicine* 1985;64:333–341.

43. Jiang JY, Gao GY, Li WP, Yu MK, Zhu C. Early indicators of prognosis in 846 cases of severe traumatic brain injury. *J Neurotrauma* 2002;19: 869–874.

44. Evans TW. International Consensus Conferences in Intensive Care Medicine: non-invasive positive pressure ventilation in acute respiratory failure. Organized jointly by the American Thoracic Society, the European Respiratory Society, the European Society of Intensive Care Medicine, and the Société de Réanimation de Langue Française, and approved by the ATS Board of Directors, December 2000. *Intensive Care Med* 2001;27:166–178.

45. Marik P. Aspiration pneumonitis and aspiration pneumonia. *N Engl J Med* 2001;344:665–671.

46. Gibbs C, Modell J. Pulmonary aspiration of gastric contents: pathophysiology, prevention, and management. In Miller R, ed. *Anesthesia,* 4th ed. New York, Churchill Livingstone, 1994:1437–1464.

47. Ware L, Matthay M. The acute respiratory distress syndrome. *N Engl J Med* 2000;342:1334–1349.

48. Chen H, Sun S, Chai C. Pulmonary edema and hemorrhage resulting from cerebral compression. *Am J Physiol* 1973;224:223.

49. Colice G, Matthay M, Bass E, Matthay R. Neurogenic pulmonary edema. *Am Rev Respir Dis* 1984;130: 941–948.

50. Maron M, Holcomb P, Dawson C, Rickaby D, Clough A, Linehan J. Edema development and recovery in

neurogenic pulmonary edema. *J Appl Physiol* 1994;77:1155–1163.

51. Rogers F, Shackford S, Trevisani G, Davis J, Mackersie R, Hoyt D. Neurogenic pulmonary edema in fatal and nonfatal head injuries. *J Trauma, Injury, Infect Dis & Crit Care* 1995;39: 860–868.

52. Rabinstein AA, Wijdicks EF. Warning signs of imminent respiratory failure in neurological patients. *Semin Neurol* 2003;23:97–104.

Chapter 8

When to Use Hyperventilation, Mannitol, or Corticosteroids to Reduce Increased Intracranial Pressure from Cerebral Edema

Edward M. Manno

■ Introduction

Cerebral edema is a consequence of typically severe and irreversible brain injury and includes conditions such as head trauma, stroke, meningitis, encephalitis, hypoxia, and electrolyte imbalance. Treatment will vary according to the neurological clinical condition of the patient, the timing of the intervention, and the proposed mechanism of development of the cerebral edema.

Traditional therapies for cerebral edema are based mostly on anecdotal experience and the extrapolation of data from laboratory models. Evidence from prospective trials is either lacking in some conditions or contradictory in others. As a consequence, treatment of cerebral edema is too often guided by personal or institutional preferences rather than scientific evidence.

Treatment of cerebral edema is one of the most frequently debated controversies in critical care neurology, and thus needs further discussion in this monograph.

■ The Patient

A 22-year-old man was brought to the emergency room after being involved in a high-speed motor vehicle accident. He was ejected from the passenger seat and then found 50 feet from the vehicle. He was intubated at the scene and hyperventilated. His initial blood pressure was 60/30 mmHg, prompting volume resuscitation with albumin and crystalloids. On initial neurological assessment, he was comatose and showed intermittent extensor posturing of all extremities. Pupils were isocoric and large (6 mm) and their direct and consensual response to light was sluggish but symmetric. Corneal, cough, and gag reflexes were present. Oculocephalic reflexes were not examined due to concerns about cervical spine instability. Cold-water caloric responses were not tested. A head CT revealed diffuse cerebral edema with slit-like ventricles. Neurosurgery was unable to place a ventriculostomy, and an ICP parenchymal monitor was used instead. The initial ICP reading was 30 mmHg, which was lowered to 18 mmHg after 75 g of mannitol were infused. A phenylephrine drip was started after the patient was considered euvolemic and then titrated to maintain a cerebral perfusion pressure greater than 70 mmHg.

On the second day of hospitalization, the intracranial pressure increased and became recalcitrant to repeated doses of 1 g/kg of mannitol. A jugular venous catheter was introduced and revealed normal jugular venous oxygen saturation (60 to 70 percent). Due to persistent intracranial hypertension, the patient was started on pentobarbital.

The dose of pentobarbital was titrated to a pattern of burst suppression on continuous bedside EEG monitoring. An aggressive regimen of acetaminophen, ibuprofen, and cooling blankets was initiated to maintain normothermia. Use of hypertonic saline was considered but deemed unnecessary because ICP values remained between 20 and 25 mmHg with CPP greater than 70 mmHg and steadily normal arteriovenous difference in oxygen content. After 3 days of continuous infusion, pentobarbital was slowly tapered over several days. Several months later the patient was transferred to a rehabilitation center with significant but improving cognitive deficits.

■ **The Problem**

- What is the role of intracranial pressure monitors in patients with severe head injury?
- What is the optimal intracranial or cerebral perfusion pressure that needs to be maintained in order to improve patient outcome?
- Is hyperventilation ever indicated? If so, when should it be used?
- What are the available options to treat refractory intracranial hypertension?
- What role do barbiturates play in the treatment of severe head trauma?

■ **The Evidence**

The current Guidelines for the Management of Severe Head Injury supported by the Brain Trauma Foundation and the American Association of Neurological Surgeons recommend ICP monitoring for patients with GCS sum score <8 and abnormal CT scan of the brain. ICP-lowering therapy is typically initiated when sustained measurements greater than 20–25 mmHg are present.[1,2] This threshold is based on evidence that outcome is improved when ICP is steadily maintained below 20 mmHg.[3,4] At present, ventricular catheter connected to an external strain gauge is the most accurate, affordable, and reliable method of monitoring ICP.[5,6] It offers the additional advantage of allowing therapeutic cerebrospinal fluid drainage. ICP transduction via fiber-optic or strain gauge devices placed in ventricular catheters provides similar benefits, but at a higher cost.[1] Parenchymal ICP

monitoring with fiber-optic or strain gauge catheter tip transduction is fairly comparable to ventricular ICP monitoring, but has the potential for measurement drift.[6,7] However, its placement is safer and carries a much lower risk of infection than ventricular catheters (risk of ventriculitis from ventricular catheters reaches 3 to 6 percent despite prophylactic antibiotics and subcutaneous tunneling).[8,9]

ICP monitoring allows calculation of the cerebral perfusion pressure (CPP). CPP results from subtracting the ICP from the mean arterial pressure (MAP). An adequate CPP is not only needed to adequately perfuse the brain but also to avoid a possible increase in ICP secondary to the cerebral vasodilatation that may occur with cerebral hypoperfusion. According to this theory, injured brain is dysautoregulated and cerebral blood flow (CBF) is dependent upon cerebral perfusion pressure. As this pressure drops (due to hypotension, increases in ICP, changes in head position, etc.), the resistance arterioles in the brain will dilate in an attempt to maintain adequate CBF. This arteriolar dilatation will lead to an increase in cerebral blood volume with a subsequent increase in ICP.[10] The threshold CPP needed to avoid this phenomenon has been estimated between 60 and 80 mmHg[1] but likely should be individually tailored.[11]

Hyperventilation

Hyperventilation is very efficacious in reducing elevated ICP. It leads to cerebral vasoconstriction and a decrease in cerebral blood volume. This process is mediated through a decrease in the hydrogen ion concentration in the CSF.[12] Since the blood-brain barrier (BBB) is impermeable to bicarbonate and hydrogen ions but permeable to carbon dioxide, changes in CSF hydrogen ion concentration can be mediated through changes in serum pCO_2.[13,14] The reduction in CBF occurs immediately but can continue for up to 30 minutes. This response requires intact CO_2 autoregulation. Normal CO_2 autoregulation relates a 3 percent change in CBF per torr change in pCO_2. This response lessens with lower levels of pCO_2. Loss of vasomotor reactivity to CO_2 is a grave prognostic indicator after head injury.[1,15,16]

The use of chronic hyperventilation to control intracranial hypertension is generally avoided due to concerns that cerebral vasoconstriction may worsen cerebral ischemia.[11] The choroid plexus equilibrates the induced changes in hydrogen ion concentration approximately 3–4 hours after any acute change, but ICP levels may return to their baseline levels long before this. The addition of weak bases or the buffer agent tromethamine (THAM) can sustain a reduction in intracranial pressure for longer periods of time. However, the only randomized trial evaluating chronic hyperventilation in head trauma found a significantly worse functional outcome at 6 months in hyperventilated patients with initial GCS motor score of 4–5.[17]

A more tailored use of hyperventilation titrated to match arterial-venous oxygen saturation differences has been championed by some authors[18] and may be useful in selected patients.[11,19] Patients who have elevated ICP secondary to cerebral hyperemia will have a decreased arterial-venous difference that can be detected by arterial and jugular venous sampling. Under these circumstances, CBF can best be matched with metabolic demands using

hyperventilation to return the arterial venous difference to normal values. However, the reliability of jugular venous oxygen saturation changes to detect harmful local reductions in cerebral perfusion with moderate hyperventilation has been questioned by the results of a study that also used brain tissue Po_2 measurements to monitor for local hypoperfusion.[20]

Studies of patients with severe brain injury using positron emission tomography (PET) have shown that brief moderate hyperventilation may produce large reductions in CBF but no compromise in oxygen metabolism. This phenomenon has been explained by low baseline metabolic rate and compensatory increase in oxygen extraction fraction.[21–24] However, these areas with "oxygen hunger" represent potentially ischemic brain tissue.[22] In fact, brief moderate hyperventilation has been shown to reduce brain tissue Po_2 below ischemic levels[23] (Figure 8-1) and to increase extracellular concentrations of markers of anaerobic metabolism (pyruvate, lactate) and excitotoxicity (glutamate).[25]

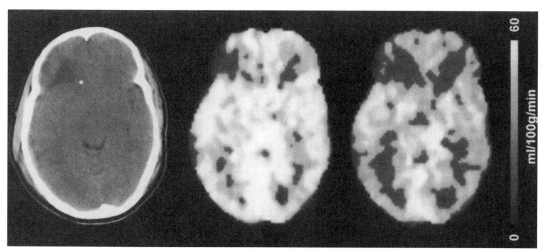

Figure 8-1. Effect of hyperventilation on the burden of hypoperfusion. Radiographic computed tomography (left) and gray scale positron emission tomographic imaging of cerebral blood flow obtained from a 31-year-old man 7 days after injury at relative normocapnia (middle), $Paco_2$ 35 torr (4.7 kPa), and hypocapnia (right) 26 torr (3.5 kPa). Voxels with a cerebral blood flow of <10 mL/100 g/min are shaded in black. Note the right frontal contusion and small parietal subdural hematoma. Baseline ICP was 21 mmHg and baseline CPP was 74 mmHg. Baseline $SjvO_2$ values of 70 percent and $AVDo_2$ of 3.7 mL/dL are consistent with hyperemia and support the use of hyperventilation for ICP control. Hyperventilation did result in a reduction in ICP to 17 mmHg and an increase in CPP to 76 mmHg, with maintenance of $SjvO_2$ and $AVDo_2$ within desirable ranges (58 percent and 5.5 mL/dL respectively). However, despite these $SjvO_2$ and $AVDo_2$ figures, baseline HypoBV was 141 mL and increased to 428 mL with hyperventilation. These increases were observed in both perilesional and normal regions of brain tissue. Reproduced with permission from author. Zornow MH, Prough DS. Does acute hyperventilation cause cerebral ischemia in severely head-injured patients? *Crit Care Med* 2002;30:2774–2775.

Mannitol

Mannitol is the most commonly used osmothera-peutic agent. Osmotherapy can be defined as the use of osmotically active solutes to reduce brain volume.[26] The use of osmotic agents to treat cerebral edema is based primarily on the direct qualitative observations that the administration of water leads to brain swelling while the use of hypertonic solutions results in brain shrinkage.[27] These observations indicated that the brain effectively serves as an osmometer, swelling as osmolality drops and shrinking as osmolality rises.[28]

Urea was historically used as an osmotic agent designed to decrease brain swelling but has been largely abandoned due to problems with electrolyte abnormalities and concerns about rebound intracranial hypertension.[26,28] The ideal osmotic agent is one that establishes a strong osmotic (transendothelial) gradient and can be rapidly cleared or excreted. To that end, mannitol is the preferred agent and the most commonly used in North America and the United Kingdom.[26]

The mechanism of action by which mannitol exerts its effect on brain tissue is a matter of considerable debate. Two competing theories can be broadly categorized into the osmotic and hemodynamic effects of mannitol. The osmotic effect of mannitol increases intravascular tonicity and establishes a concentration gradient across the BBB that allows movement of water from edematous brain tissue into the intravascular space. This is followed by rapid renal excretion of mannitol and water.

This theory has relatively fallen out of favor, due primarily to the observations that the timing and dose of mannitol required to exert a change in brain water content in animal models is not consistent with the changes in ICP that are seen in clinical practice.

Effective changes in ICP clinically occur at much lower doses of mannitol than those used in animal experiments. It has also been difficult to demonstrate that the dosage of mannitol used clinically has any effect on cerebral water.[26]

Paczynski argues, however, that very small changes in diffuse cerebral water content that may have been immeasurable on previous studies could have profound effects on ICP.[26] This is supported by radiological studies using CT[29] and MRI[30] that showed decreases in brain water after mannitol administration. Similarly, reductions in cerebral water content after the use of clinically relevant doses of mannitol have been demonstrated by direct measurements in traumatized human brain[31] and a rat stroke model.[32]

The hemodynamic or rheological effects of mannitol have been emphasized by other authors.[10,33–36] According to this theory, mannitol decreases cerebral blood volume by decreasing blood viscosity and subsequently cerebral blood volume. The osmotic gradient produced by an infusion of mannitol initially causes an influx of extravascular water into the intravascular space. This has two major effects. The first is an increase in blood pressure and cardiac output. The second is a decrease in blood viscosity due to hemodilution of red blood cell mass and fibrinogen.

The subsequent drop in ICP can then be explained through the use of the Hagen–Poiseuille equation. In this equation, flow is directly related to the pressure difference across a vessel (i.e., CPP) and the radius of the vessel to the fourth power. Flow is indirectly related to serum viscosity and a constant, a product of π times the length of the vessel. Assuming constant cerebral blood flow and cerebral vessel reactivity, according to this equation the radius of the vessel must decrease in response to an increase in CPP and a decrease in viscosity. Under these circumstances, cerebral blood flow and cerebral oxygen delivery remain constant due to a reduction in vessel radius. Rosner describes this as a passive vasoconstriction.[10]

This passive vasoconstriction decreases cerebral blood volume and subsequently ICP. Thus, according to this mechanism of action of mannitol, ICP is reduced by a decrease in cerebral blood vessel engorgement and not by an effect on cerebral edema.

The hemodynamic and rheological effects on ICP appear to correlate more closely with the pharmacological profile of mannitol, which exhibits its peak effect 30–60 minutes after infusion.[37] The direct osmotic effect on cerebral edema may occur as a delayed response. Whether this occurs secondary to an osmotic dehydration or secondary to volume depletion remains speculative.

There are other proposed mechanisms of action of mannitol in intracranial hypertension. Suzuki et al. have emphasized the cytoprotective role that mannitol can enact by serving as a free radical scavenger.[38]

This action, however, has been thought to be clinically insignificant by others.[39] Also, mannitol may increase CSF absorption.[40] Regardless of the persisting uncertainties about its precise mechanism of action, mannitol constitutes the mainstay of drug therapy in patients with intracranial hypertension.

There is considerable controversy about dosing and mode of administration of mannitol. A standardized dosing regimen (e.g., 1 g/kg of 20 percent mannitol in a bolus followed by 0.25 to 0.5 g/kg every 4 to 6 hours) may be complicated by volume depletion. There is also concern about possible leakage of mannitol into damaged brain tissue.[41] Mannitol becomes less effective as serum osmolality rises probably secondary to a decrease in the osmolal gradient initially created by bolus dosing of mannitol. This problem has led some authors to suggest maintaining serum osmolality near normal in an attempt to preserve the effectiveness of mannitol.[10] This is usually best achieved by using repeated boluses of mannitol only when required by elevations of the ICP. Still, most experts allow mannitol to produce some dehydration to induce some transient degree of cellular shrinkage.[11] A serum osmolality of 320 mOsm/L is generally quoted as the maximal allowable serum osmolality; however, it is important to understand that this cutoff number is a limitation designed to prevent renal tubular damage.

Corticosteroids

Glucocorticoids are used primarily to treat vasogenic cerebral edema. They are effective in ameliorating the edema encountered with tumors, meningitis, and other cerebral lesions that are believed to have a component of increased BBB permeability. In fact, glucocorticoids have been a mainstay in the treatment of cerebral edema due to primary or secondary brain tumors. The usual initial dose is 10 mg of dexamethasone intravenously or by mouth followed by 4 mg every 6 hours. This is equivalent to 20 times the normal physiological production of cortisol.

Cerebral tumors may have variable amounts of peritumoral edema and response to corticosteroids. This may be due to differences in steroid receptor concentration,[42] variability in the permeability of the tumor vascular endothelium, or differences in the secretion of vascular endothelial growth factors.[43–45]

The reduction in peritumoral edema with corticosteroids may occur because of decreased endothelial cell permeability,[45,46] increased clearance or resolution of cerebral edema,[47] or an inhibition of tumor cell growth.[48] Corticosteroids decrease vascular permeability by stabilizing the endothelial cell membrane. Membrane stabilization occurs secondary to a decrease in lipid peroxidation from the free radical scavenging effect of corticosteroids. This in turn leads to a decrease in the release of arachidonic acid or polyunsaturated fatty acids from the cell membrane.

Glucocorticoids are also useful as adjunctive therapy to antibiotics for the treatment of bacterial meningitis. The rationale for this indication is to decrease the development of cerebral edema induced by the inflammatory reaction initiated after the lysis of bacterial cell walls. The release of bacterial cell wall components is the initial step in the development of an inflammatory cascade that leads to the development of cerebral edema.[49] Inflammation is mediated through the increased production of cytokines and chemokines by microglia, astrocytes, and macrophages. Interleukin-1 (IL-1) and tumor necrosis factor (TNF) increase vascular permeability both directly and indirectly by increasing leukocyte adherence to the endothelium. In addition to the development of vasogenic edema, interstitial edema develops as CSF outflow resistance is increased by the inflammatory exudates that interfere with CSF absorption at the level of the arachnoid granulations.

Glucocorticoids decrease cerebral edema in bacterial meningitis through many of the mechanisms previously discussed. Additionally, glucocorticoids also exert a depressant effect on both the synthesis and translation of IL-1 and TNF mRNA. The timing of glucocorticoid use may be critical as the maximal reduction in the production of these inflammatory cytokines occurs only if therapy is started prior to the release of the bacterial cell wall components.

Glucocorticoid use decreases morbidity and mortality in animal models[50,51] of meningitis and has been shown to be of benefit in reducing hearing loss in pediatric patients with *Haemophilus influenzae* type B meningitis.[52] Other clinical trials have produced conflicting results.[52,53] A meta-analysis of clinical studies, however, supported the use of dexamethasone in children with both *Haemophilus influenzae* type B and *Streptococcus pneumoniae* meningitis.[54] Dexamethasone is currently recommended for children older than 2 months of age with bacterial meningitis. The suggested dose is 0.15 mg/kg given intravenously every 6 hours for the first 4 days of antibiotic treatment. The first dose should be administered before or concurrent with the start of antibiotic treatment.[49]

Corticosteroid use in adults with meningitis has been controversial. The recent development of a *Haemophilus influenzae* type B vaccine has changed the infectious patterns of meningitis in both children and adults. In addition, a global increase in penicillin- and cephalosporin-resistant pneumococci has led to the growing use of vancomycin in the treatment of meningitis in adults.[55] Animal models have shown a decrease of antibiotic penetration into the CSF of animals pretreated with dexamethasone,[55,56] a concern that prematurely stopped an adult trial of dexamethasone in severe meningitis.[57]

Until recently, trials of dexamethasone in adults with meningitis had produced conflicting results.[57,58] The debate, however, appears to have been resolved by the results of a recent prospective, randomized, double-blind trial of adjuvant treatment with dexamethasone versus placebo in adults with bacterial meningitis. In this study, dexamethasone started 15–20 minutes prior to the first dose of antibiotics and given for the first 4 days of treatment (10 mg every 6 hours) was associated with reduced mortality ($p=0.04$) and improved functional outcome ($p=0.03$). Treatment was most effective for the sickest patients as evaluated by an admission Glasgow coma score and in patients with pneumococcal meningitis.[59] Based on the above study, adjunctive therapy with dexamethasone is warranted in adults with suspected meningitis.[60] However, there is lingering concern about the appropriateness of this approach in populations with high incidence of penicillin-resistant pneumococcus or susceptible to infection by *Staphylococcus aureus* (e.g., neurosurgical patients).[61]

In patients with severe head injury, the use of glucocorticoids is not recommended for improving outcome or reducing ICP.[1] Several prospective randomized trials have evaluated different regimens of glucocorticoids in this population and consistently found no evidence of therapeutic benefit.[62–66] At least part of these negative results may be explained by the unfavorable metabolic and nutritional effects exerted by megadoses of glucocorticoids in critically ill patients.[67] Nonetheless, steroids improve functional recovery of brain-injured animals in the laboratory[68] and interest in the early use of steroids after head injury has re-emerged recently, prompting new randomized studies that are currently underway.

Barbiturates

Barbiturates have been shown to be effective in reducing ICP in patients with severe head injury.[3] They are generally reserved for cases of refractory intracranial hypertension in head injury. Barbiturate dosing can be titrated to a predetermined ICP but there is little additional effect on ICP once a burst suppression pattern is present on bedside electroencephalography.

A randomized controlled trial evaluating the prophylactic use of barbiturates in head trauma found no difference in one-year outcomes.[69] However, Eisenberg et al. reported in 1988 a multicenter randomized controlled trial evaluating the use of pentobarbital for intracranial hypertension refractory to conventional treatments. The study had a crossover design to allow treatment failures to be entered into the treatment group at a later point. Six-month outcome was significantly improved for patients whose ICP responded to barbiturate therapy. Mortality was 9.3 percent in the treatment group and 15 percent in the crossover group compared with 88 and 84 percent mortality in the respective groups that did not respond to barbiturate therapy.[3]

Despite the improvement in mortality, barbiturate therapy in head injury remains debatable. Significant side effects including hypotension, and increased infectious complications, limit treatment. In addition, significant questions remain on the quality of life of the survivors after barbiturate therapy.[70]

Other Therapeutic Alternatives

Therapeutic cerebrospinal fluid drainage is an effective means to decrease ICP even in patients without hydrocephalus. Other measures used to control ICP include sedation, paralysis, and head elevation. Sedation is helpful in controlling rises in ICP secondary to agitation but must be balanced against the ability to monitor the neurological exam. Prophylactic neuromuscular paralysis has been associated with an increased length of stay in the intensive care unit and worse clinical outcome.[71] Neuromuscular paralysis is thus reserved to judiciously treat intracranial hypertension. Advocates of cerebral perfusion pressure monitoring claim that head elevation may decrease CPP and eventually result in rising ICP. Others argue that this rarely occurs in patients with adequate volume status. Conversely, elevating the head of the bed in a euvolemic patient may decrease ICP by improving jugular venous drainage. Obviously any obstruction to jugular venous drainage (jugular central lines, endotracheal tube securing ties) should be avoided. Hyperthermia should be avoided and aggressively treated. The result of a multicenter trial evaluating the effects of hypothermia on severe head injury have been disappointing.[72]

Recently, hypertonic saline solutions have been investigated for the treatment of cerebral edema. Initial enthusiasm for this treatment was fueled by small clinical trials using hypertonic saline for volume resuscitation in hemorrhagic shock. In these studies, an improvement in survival seen with hypertonic saline was attributed to a reduction in intracranial pressure and mass effect.[73,74] Since the BBB is relatively impermeable to sodium, osmotherapy with hypertonic saline probably induces similar mechanisms to those invoked in the case of mannitol. There may, however, be some important advantages to the use of hypertonic saline as compared with mannitol. These include an augmentation of intravascular volume without the delayed diuretic effect of mannitol and its potential electrolyte disturbances.[28]

Animal models of focal cryogenic injury have also demonstrated a decrease in cerebral water content with the use of hypertonic solutions.[75,76] Animal models comparing hypertonic solutions with mannitol have shown similar effects on hemodynamics and ICP.[77–79] However, Qureshi et al. were able to demonstrate improved ICP control and CPP values using hypertonic saline in a dog model of intracerebral hemorrhage, thus suggesting that

there may be specific pathologies that respond best to hypertonic solutions.[80]

Various case series have been reported addressing the results of hypertonic saline use for the treatment of intracranial hypertension.[81–85] The most important was one reported by Suarez et al. in which an intravenous bolus of 23.4 percent saline was used as "rescue therapy" for recalcitrant intracranial hypertension in a variety of intracranial pathologies. A greater than 50 percent reduction in ICP was attained in 16 of 20 patients studied.[85] Small randomized trials comparing hypertonic saline with mannitol in head injury have shown better results with hypertonic saline; however, no definite conclusions can be drawn at present due to the fact that equimolar solutions were not used in these studies.[86,87]

Future work evaluating the use of hypertonic saline will require a study of dose escalation and a safety and efficacy profile. The overall impression is that hypertonic saline is at least as effective as mannitol without many of the unwanted side effects. Further studies are needed before hypertonic saline can replace mannitol as the osmotherapeutic agent of choice.[28,88]

In patients with recalcitrant intracranial hypertension who fail to respond to all other therapeutic measures, hemicraniectomy with duraplasty may be a valuable alternative.[89] Good long-term functional outcomes have been reported in more than half of young patients with severe head injury who underwent hemicraniectomy for uncontrollable intracranial hypertension.[90] Table 8-1 summarises the discussed treatment modalities of cerebral edema.

■ The Pros and Cons

Our patient presented refractory intracranial hypertension that required aggressive treatment for its control. All efforts devoted to controlling ICP are justified because there is proof that an aggressive approach to the management of intracranial hypertension by experienced clinicians is associated with a decreased mortality.[91]

The treatment of any patient with recalcitrant intracranial hypertension after head trauma involves the maintenance of adequate intravascular volume and blood flow, the avoidance of hypotension and hyperthermia, limited hyperventilation,

Table 8-1. Treatment of Cerebral Edema

	Proposed Mechanism of Action	Uses	Dosages	Miscellaneous
Corticosteroids	Suppression of phospholipase 2 Decreased endothelial cell permeability Membrane stabilization Decreased lipid peroxidation Free radical scavenging	Meningitis Glioma	10 mg IV/PO every 6 hours for 4 days (adults)	Treat hyperglycemia Provide gastrointestinal prophylaxis
Barbiturates	Decreased cerebral metabolic rate with subsequent decreased CBF and decreased CBV	Severe head trauma Recalcitrant intracranial hypertension	Pentobarbital load 200 mg boluses, max. 1 g, maintenance 60–120 mg/hr	Titrate to ICP control, or burst suppression on EEG, may be limited by decreases in mean arterial pressure. Assuring normovolemia prior to treatment may require vasopressors
Hyperventilation	Active vasoconstriction secondary to decreased CSF hydrogen ion concentration mediated by changes in P_{CO_2}	Acute but transient control of intracranial hypertension	Titrate ventilator respiratory rate to sequentially decrease P_{CO_2} to 25–30 torr	Effect lasts only 90–180 minutes
Mannitol	Osmotic diuresis decrease brain water Rheological effect secondary to changes in viscosity which leads to passive vasoconstriction and subsequent decreased CBV	Sustained control of intracranial hypertension	25–1.0 g/kg used on prn basis Relative limits for serum osmolality 320 mOsm/L Give as rapid bolus over 20–30 minutes	Prevent dehydration
Hypertonic saline	Similar to mannitol	Rescue therapy for recalcitrant ICP	3% normal saline titrate to sodium 144–155 mmol/l[108] 23.4% NaCl 30 ml given over 15–20 minutes[109]	Prevent cardiac failure

IV, intravenous; PO, by mouth; CBF, cerebral blood flow; CBV, cerebral blood volume; ICP, intracranial pressure; prn, as needed; P_{CO_2}, partial pressure of carbon dioxide.

and ICP-guided osmotherapy. This approach has developed over the past several years in contrast to the traditional approach to intracranial hypertension in head trauma that proposed mild volume depletion and sustained hyperventilation. The use of this modern approach has been associated with improved outcomes in several nonrandomized studies.[92,93]

There has been considerable controversy as to the best application of medical measures to treat intracranial hypertension in head trauma. The debate has been centered on whether adequate cerebral perfusion or brain oxygen extraction ratios should be the focus of how therapies designed to lower ICP should be instituted. The answer appears to be best stated by Chesnut, who pointed out that these approaches are not mutually exclusive and that components of each should be applied individually to each patient.[94] For example, the optimal head position for a given patient can be tailored with an ICP monitor by maximizing ICP control while maintaining adequate CPP. Adequate CPP control does not preclude the use of a jugular venous oxygen monitor. In any case it is clear that meticulous ICU care focused on the prevention of secondary injuries after head trauma is crucial to improving patient outcome.

In our patient, the initial priority was achieving appropriate fluid resuscitation. Brief hyperventilation in the field, although it may cause an additional ischemic brain insult, is difficult to criticize when applied to a comatose patient with evidence of posturing. Attempts to place a ventriculostomy catheter were unsuccessful, thus negating the option of therapeutic cerebrospinal fluid drainage. Still, reliable ICP monitoring was accomplished through a parenchymal monitor. Osmotherapy using mannitol was initially effective. Repeated bolus dosing was chosen, as opposed to a scheduled "around-the-clock" regimen, to avoid steady increases in serum osmolality and the possibility that the drug would lose efficacy over time. Nonetheless, mannitol became eventually insufficient and a pentobarbital drip was required. Fortunately, it could be tapered after only 3 days, thus avoiding some of the feared complications commonly encountered with more prolonged use. Jugular oximetry was used as a measure of global (hemispheric) perfusion. If the ICP had not been controlled with mannitol and pentobarbital or CPP had become insufficient, hypertonic saline would have been used. Hemicraniectomy would have been a measure of last resort, but a reasonable alternative in this young and previously healthy patient.

■ The Main Points

- Secondary injury due to the development of delayed intracranial hypertension accounts for significant morbidity and mortality in severe head trauma.
- Treatment focuses on the maintenance of adequate intravascular volume and cerebral perfusion. Hyperthermia and hypotension need to be aggressively treated.
- In some patients the use of brain oxygen extraction ratios obtained through the use of a jugular venous monitor may help tailor therapies to reduce ICP.

- Chronic prophylactic hyperventilation should not be used in patients with severe head injury. Brief moderate hyperventilation is very efficacious in reducing elevated ICP but it must be used with caution to avoid the risk of hypoperfusion and possible ischemia.
- Osmotherapy with mannitol or hypertonic saline is the mainstay of therapy for post-traumatic cerebral edema.
- Pentobarbital infusion and hemicraniectomy should be reserved for patients with intracranial hypertension refractory to more conservative approaches. Yet these aggressive modalities can make good long-term functional outcome possible and should be employed when needed.

■ The Patient

A 76-year-old, right-handed man with previous history of poorly controlled hypertension developed abrupt onset of left-sided weakness. On arrival at the local emergency room he had flaccid hemiplegia and right-sided gaze preference with dense left-sided hemineglect. Head CT scan revealed complete effacement of cortical sulcal marking in the right middle cerebral artery territory and hyperdense MCA sign. The patient was admitted to the neurological intensive care unit for close observation because he was considered to be at risk for potential delayed neurological deterioration secondary to the development of cerebral edema. The following day the patient remained awake and alert with persistent gaze preference, hemineglect, and hemiplegia. Cardiac telemetry monitoring showed intermittent periods of atrial fibrillation. Carotid ultrasound revealed minimal carotid atherosclerosis, and transesophageal echocardiography displayed biatrial enlargement with intact atrial septum. On the second day after the stroke, the patient was noted to be drowsy but aroused easily to command. Repeat head CT revealed complete left middle cerebral infarct with approximately 5 mm midline shift of the pineal gland. No antiedema treatment was initiated. On the third post-stroke day, the patient became progressively more lethargic and developed an ipsilateral 2 mm anisocoria. He was given 75 g of mannitol (approximating 1 g per kg of body weight). One hour later the anisocoria had resolved and the patient had begun to respond to verbal stimuli and to follow simple commands. A new head CT revealed further midline shift of the pineal gland. Another dose of 75 g of mannitol was given approximately 12 hours later because the nurse was concerned that the patient was becoming more lethargic. Mannitol was again successful in improving the patient's level of consciousness. Neurosurgery was consulted and the patient underwent hemicraniectomy before any further neurological deterioration occurred. He remained stable after surgery and was transferred out of the intensive care one week after stroke onset. Six months later the patient remained in a skilled nursing facility with severe functional sequelae.

■ **The Problem**

- What is the mechanism of neurological deterioration in this patient?
- What medical strategies are effective for treating ischemic brain edema?
- What is the optimal timing of the institution of therapies?
- What is the indication of hemicraniectomy after ischemic stroke?

■ **The Evidence**

This case illustrates the development of malignant cerebral edema after a complete infarction of the middle cerebral artery territory. Neurological deterioration is believed to occur due to horizontal displacement of the rostral diencephalon secondary to the development of focal cerebral edema. This displacement was quantified by Ropper through the measurement of the horizontal displacement of the pineal gland.[95] Peak swelling with shift of intracranial contents develops approximately 3–5 days after infarction, although there is an underappreciated range of time when this can occur.[96]

Hyperventilation should only be used in acute stroke as a temporizing measure because it produces vasoconstriction and might exacerbate cerebral ischemia.[97] In selected cases, brief use of moderate hyperventilation may be justified if followed by other safer and more definitive antiedema treatments (such as osmotherapy or hemicraniectomy).

Mannitol is the agent most frequently used to treat ischemic brain edema. The use of mannitol in this situation is not aimed at lowering ICP. Frank demonstrated that only approximately one-third of patients with large MCA infarct have elevated ICP. In fact, ICP monitoring under these circumstances could potentially provide a false sense of security since focal pressure changes can induce brain tissue shifts and herniation even with a normal ICP.[98]

The idea that mannitol can preferentially shrink infarcted tissue has two potential limitations and problems. The first is that mannitol requires an intact BBB to be effective regardless of the believed mechanisms of action. The second is that, after repeated doses, mannitol can leak into the brain area that has a disrupted BBB.[41] Theoretically, then, the use of mannitol could potentially worsen cerebral edema by leaking into infarcted tissue. Manno et al., tested this potential concern by performing sequential MRIs of the brain in patients with large MCA infarcts during mannitol loading. In this study, no worsening of horizontal or vertical displacement of brain tissue could be demonstrated.[99] Videen et al., using MRI volumetric analysis of these same patients, were able to demonstrate a 3 percent decrease in normal but not infarcted brain tissue. In either case, the volumetric changes seem clinically insignificant.[100] These studies did not directly address repeated dosing of mannitol. A recent study with glycerol and serial MRI showed decrease of the volume of cerebral infarction[101] (Figures 8-2 and 8-3).

The effect of mannitol on the outcome of patients with mass effect from hemispheric infarction has never been tested on a randomized clinical trial. Thus a systematic review (Cochrane) on this matter concluded that there was insufficient data to perform an adequate outcome analysis.[102] Current expert guidelines recommend the use of mannitol only when clinical signs of brain tissue shift appear but not before, even if marked edema is present on brain imaging.[97]

Historically, cerebral edema secondary to ischemic stroke was treated with corticosteroids based on early studies suggesting therapeutic benefit.[103,104] Subsequent randomized clinical trials, however, have conclusively proven no value of corticosteroids in the treatment of ischemic stroke,[105–108] and its use has been largely abandoned. A more recent animal study, however, has questioned

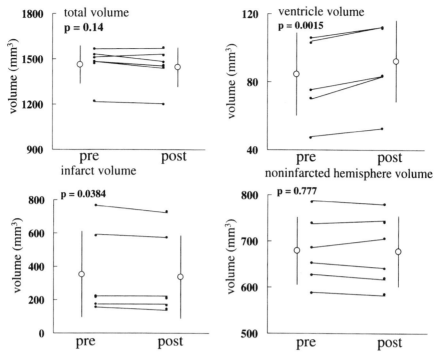

Figure 8-2. Changes in the volume of the total brain, the cerebral infarction, the ventricle, and the noninfarcted hemisphere after administration of glycerol. The volume of the ventricle increased and the volume of the cerebral infarction decreased significantly ($p < 0.05$). Values are means/SD.[101] (Used with permission from author. Sakamaki M, Igarashi H, Nishiyama Y, Hagiwara H, Ando J, Chishiki T, Curran BC, Katayama Y. Effect of glycerol on ischemic cerebral edema assessed by magnetic resonance imaging. *J Neurol Sci* 2003;209:69–74.)

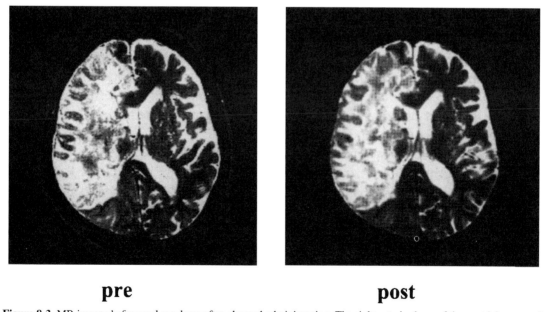

Figure 8-3. MR images before and one hour after glycerol administration. The right arterior horn of the ventricles opened after glycerol administration.[101] (Used with permission from author. Sakamaki M, Igarashi H, Nishiyama Y, Hagiwara H, Ando J, Chishiki T, Curran BC, Katayama Y. Effect of glycerol on ischemic cerebral edema assessed by magnetic resonance imaging. *J Neurol Sci* 2003;209:69–74.)

this dogma by showing a decrease in cerebral edema following temporary but not permanent focal cerebral ischemia. This raises the possibility that corticosteroids may prove useful in patients who receive intravenous or intra-arterial thrombolysis.[109]

Other medical treatment options include alternative osmotic agents, barbiturates, and hypothermia. Glycerol has been tested in randomized trials with conflicting results.[110–112] A systematic review of these studies concluded that a favorable effect is possible but may be minimal and restricted to short-term outcome.[112] Glycerol use is not simple because intravenous infusion can provoke hemolysis. Hypertonic saline has not been studied in randomized clinical trials but it may be effective in patients refractory to mannitol.[113] Barbiturates only seem to offer limited and short-lasting benefits that may be counterbalanced by adverse effects, especially if hypotension occurs.[114] Hypothermia may improve outcome in patients with malignant middle cerebral artery infarction by helping control critically elevated ICP and possibly by exerting neuroprotective actions.[115,116] Hypothermia in acute ischemic stroke is currently being investigated in randomized clinical trials.

Hemicraniectomy is a procedure reserved for patients with medically refractory focal cerebral edema. In this procedure a large portion of the skull is removed and the dura is transected to allow outward expansion of the swollen brain, thus relieving the tissue shifts causing neurological deterioration.

The timing of hemicraniectomy may be critical to its success. Pathological studies in a rat model have shown a decreased size of the initial cerebral infarction if hemicraniectomy is performed prior to the development of cerebral edema. This occurs presumably through increased pial collateral flow to the ischemic penumbra. This finding has led Schwab et al. to recommend hemicraniectomy early in the clinical course after a large cerebral infarct.[117] Hemicraniectomy not only saves lives but also results in good functional recovery and quality of life in a high proportion of young operated patients.[118] However, functional outcome after hemicraniectomy is much less favorable in elderly patients.[119]

A randomized pilot clinical trial of hemicraniectomy versus best medical therapy has recently been completed. The preliminary unpublished results suggest a benefit in survival after hemicraniectomy, although the very small number of patients enrolled limits any definitive conclusion about the efficacy of the intervention. A large European trial is underway.

■ The Pros and Cons

In situations where clinical deterioration secondary to cerebral edema occurs early in the clinical course (within 24 hours), osmotherapy or hyperventilation only provide a temporizing measure until hemicraniectomy can be performed. When neurological deterioration occurs later in the clinical course (e.g., at or near the time of anticipated peak swelling), the edema may often be treated medically.

We try to minimize the use of hyperventilation in patients with ischemic brain edema due to the concern about worsening hypoperfusion from vasoconstriction. Osmotherapy with mannitol remains our pivotal treatment when patients present signs of clinical deterioration from brain tissue shift. Hypothermia may become a helpful adjunct to our presently limited therapeutic options, but its real value and ideal form of implementation remain to be reliably established by appropriate randomized clinical trials.

Some of the staunchest proponents of hemicraniectomy strongly advocate for early surgery in patients at risk of herniation from ischemic brain edema. However, this practice may result in many unnecessary surgeries. Most commonly, hemicraniectomy is only pursued after medical therapy has proven ineffective in treating neurological deterioration secondary to the development of cerebral edema. Patient selection is another controversial issue. Elderly patients often survive but fail to recover meaningful function after hemicraniectomy. The appropriateness of surgery in those patients is debatable.

In our case, mannitol had been successful in reversing the signs of herniation but hemicraniectomy was performed nonetheless. The resulting poor functional outcome was not surprising in an elderly patient with prior comorbidity. Although hemicraniectomy is not considered "standard of care,"[97] withholding a potentially life-saving intervention is always a very difficult decision. More studies addressing the effects of hemicraniectomy on long-term functional outcome are required to define which patients may benefit from this radical treatment.

■ The Main Points

- Neurological deterioration after large cerebral infarcts is due to horizontal shift of brain structures secondary to regional intracranial pressure differences.
- Medical "antiedema" therapy should be reserved for patients with clinical signs of neurological deterioration. Treatment decisions should not be based solely on radiographic findings.
- ICP monitors may provide a false sense of security in cases of focal ischemic brain edema since many patients can deteriorate clinically despite normal intracranial pressure.
- Glucocorticoids have no role in the treatment of cerebral edema after ischemic stroke.
- Hemicraniectomy should be strongly considered in young patients with neurological deterioration due to large cerebral infarcts that are recalcitrant to medical therapy.

■ References

1. Anonymous. Guidelines for the management of severe head injury. Brain Trauma Foundation, American Academy of Neurosurgery, Joint Section of Neurotrauma and Critical Care. *J Neurotrauma* 1996;13:641–734.
2. American College of Surgeons Committee on Trauma. *Advanced Trauma Life Support Course for Physicians: Instructor's Manual*, 2nd ed. Chicago, American College of Surgeons, 1985:1–525.
3. Eisenberg HM, Frankowski RF, Constant CF. High-dose barbiturate control of elevated intracranial pressure in patients with severe head injury. *J Neurosurg* 1988;69:15–23.
4. Marmarou A, Anderson R, Ward J, Choi S, Young H, Eisenberg H, Foulkes M, Marshall L, Jane J. Impact of ICP instability and hypotension on outcome in patients with severe head trauma. *J Neurosurg* 1991;75:59–66.
5. Ostrup RC, Luerssen TG, Marshall LF, Zornow MH. Continuous monitoring of intracranial pressure with a miniaturized fiberoptic device. *J Neurosurg* 1987;67:206–209.
6. Piek J, Bock WJ. Continuous monitoring of cerebral tissue pressure in neurosurgical practice—experiences with 100 patients. *Intensive Care Med* 1990;16:184–188.
7. Schickner DJ, Young RF. Intracranial pressure monitoring: fiberoptic monitor compared with the ventricular catheter. *Surg Neurol* 1992;37:251–254.
8. Lyke KE, Obasanjo OO, Williams MA, O'Brien M, Chotani R, Perl TM. Ventriculitis complicating use of intraventricular catheters in adult neurosurgical patients. *Clin Infect Dis* 2001;33:2028–2033.
9. Poon WS, Ng S, Wai S. CSF antibiotic prophylaxis for neurosurgical patients with ventriculostomy: a randomised study. *Acta Neurochir Suppl (Wien)* 1998;71:146–148.
10. Rosner MJ. Pathophysiology and management of increased intracranial pressure. In Andrews BT, ed. *Neurosurgical Intensive Care*. New York, McGraw-Hill, 1993:57–112.
11. Chesnut RM. Medical management of severe head injury: present and future. *New Horizons* 1995;3:581–593.
12. Traystman RJ. Regulation of cerebral blood flow by carbon dioxide. In Welch KMA, Caplan LR, Reis DJ, Siesjo BK, Weir B, eds. *Primer on Cerebrovascular Disease*. San Diego, Academic Press, 1997:55–57.
13. Kontos HA, Raper AJ, Patterson JL. Analysis of vasoactivity of local pH, P_{CO_2}, and bicarbonate on pial vessels. *Stroke* 1977;8:358–360.
14. Kontos HA, Wei EP, Raper AJ, Patterson JL. Local mechanisms of CO_2 action of cat pial arterioles. *Stroke* 1977;8:226–229.
15. Ropper AH, Rockoff MA. Treatment of intracranial hypertension. In Ropper AH, Kennedy SK, eds. *Neurological and Neurosurgical Intensive Care,* 2nd ed. Rockville, MD, Aspen Publications, 1988:23–42.
16. Schalen W, Messeter K, Nordstrom CH. Cerebral vasoreactivity and the prediction of outcome in severe traumatic brain lesions. *Acta Anaesthesiol Scand* 1991;35:113–122.
17. Muizelaar JP, Marmarou A, Ward JD, Kontos HA, Choi SC, Becker DP, Gruemer H, Young HF. Adverse effects of prolonged hyperventilation in patients with severe head injury. *J Neurosurg* 1991;75:731–735.
18. Cruz J. The first decade of continuous monitoring of jugular bulb oxyhemoglobin saturation: management strategies and clinical outcome. *Crit Care Med* 1998;26:344–351.
19. Oertel M, Kelly DF, Lee JH, McArthur DL, Glenn TC, Vespa P, Boscardin WJ, Hovda DA, Martin NA. Efficacy of hyperventilation, blood pressure elevation, and metabolic suppression therapy in controlling intracranial pressure after head injury. *J Neurosurg* 2002;97:1045–1053.
20. Imberti R, Bellinzona G, Langer M. Cerebral tissue P_{O_2} and $SjvO_2$ changes during moderate hyperventilation in patients with severe traumatic brain injury. *J Neurosurg* 2002;96:97–102.

21. Diringer MN, Videen TO, Yundt K, Zazulia AR, Aiyagari V, Dacey RG Jr, Grubb RL, Powers WJ. Regional cerebrovascular and metabolic effects of hyperventilation after severe traumatic brain injury. *J Neurosurg* 2002;96:103–108.

22. Coles JP, Minhas PS, Fryer TD, Smielewski P, Aigbirihio F, Donovan T, Downey SP, Williams G, Chatfield D, Matthews JC, Gupta AK, Carpenter TA, Clark JC, Pickard JD, Menon DK. Effect of hyperventilation on cerebral blood flow in traumatic head injury: clinical relevance and monitoring correlates. *Crit Care Med* 2002;30:1950–1959.

23. Carmona Suazo JA, Maas AI, van den Brink WA, van Santbrink H, Steyerberg EW, Avezaat CJ. CO_2 reactivity and brain oxygen pressure monitoring in severe head injury. *Crit Care Med* 2000;28:3268–3274.

24. Zornow MH, Prough DS. Does acute hyperventilation cause cerebral ischemia in severely head-injured patients? *Crit Care Med* 2002;30:2774–2775.

25. Marion DW, Puccio A, Wisniewski SR, Kochanek P, Dixon CE, Bullian L, Carlier P. Effect of hyperventilation on extracellular concentrations of glutamate, lactate, pyruvate, and local cerebral blood flow in patients with severe traumatic brain injury. *Crit Care Med* 2002;30:2619–2625.

26. Paczynski RP. Osmotherapy: basic concepts and controversies. *Crit Care Clin* 1997;13:105–129.

27. Weed LH, McKibben PS. Pressure changes in the cerebrospinal fluid following intravenous injection of solutions of various concentrations. *Am J Physiol* 1919;48:512–530.

28. Prough DS, Zornow MH. Mannitol: an old friend on the skids? *Crit Care Med* 1998;26:997–998.

29. Cascino T, Baglivo J, Conti J, Szewczykowski J, Posner JB, Rottenberg DA. Quantitative CT assessment of furosemide and mannitol-induced changes in brain water content. *Neurology* 1983;33:898–903.

30. Bell BA, Kean DM, MacDonald HL, Barnett GH, Douglas RHB, Smith MA, McGhee CNJ, Miller JD, Tocher JL, Best JJK. Brain water measured by magnetic resonance imaging: correlation with direct estimation and changes after mannitol and dexamethasone. *Lancet* 1987;1:66–69.

31. Nath F, Galbraith S. The effect of mannitol on cerebral white matter content. *J Neurosurg* 1986;65:41–43.

32. Paczynski RP, He YY, Diringer MN, Hsu CY. Multiple-dose mannitol reduces brain water content in a rat model of cortical infarction. *Stroke* 1997;28:437–444.

33. Muizelaar JP, Lutz HA, Becker DP. Effect of mannitol on intracranial pressure and cerebral blood flow and correlation with pressure autoregulation in head-injured patients. *J Neurosurg* 1984;61:700–706.

34. Muizelaar JP, Wei EP, Kontos HA, Becker DP. Mannitol causes compensatory cerebral vasoconstriction and vasodilation in response to blood viscosity changes. *J Neurosurg* 1983;59:822–823.

35. Rosner MJ, Coley I. Cerebral perfusion pressure: a hemodynamic mechanism of mannitol and the postmannitol hemogram. *Neurosurgery* 1987;21:147–156.

36. Auer LM, Haselberger K. Effect of intravenous mannitol on cat pial arteries and veins during normal and elevated intracranial pressure. *Neurosurgery* 1987;21:142–146.

37. Cloyd JC, Snyder BD, Cleeremans B, Bundlie SR. Mannitol pharmacokinetics and serum osmolality in dogs and humans. *J Pharmacol Exp Ther* 1986;236:301–306.

38. Suzuki J, Imaizumi I, Kayama T, Yoshimoto T. Chemiluminescence in hypoxic brain: Second report: Cerebral protective effect of mannitol, vitamin E and glucocorticoid. *Stroke* 1985;16:695–700.

39. Gilbe CE, Sage FJ, Gutteridge JM. Commentary: Mannitol: molecule magnifique or a case of radical misinterpretation? *Free Radical Res* 1996;24:1–7.

40. Dimattio J, Hockwald GM, Malhan C, Wald A. Effects of changes in serum osmolality on bulk flow into cerebral ventricles and brain water content. *Pflügers Arch Eur J Physiol* 1975;359:253–264.

41. Kaufman AM, Cardozo E. Aggravation of cerebral edema by multiple dose mannitol. *J Neurosurg* 1992;77:584–589.

42. Yu ZY, Wrange O, Boethius J, Hatam A, Granholm L, Gustafsson JA. A study of the glucocorticoid receptors in intracranial tumors. *J Neurosurg* 1981;55:757–760.

43. Papadopoulos MC, Saadoun S, Davies DC, Bell BA. Emerging molecular mechanisms of brain tumor oedema. *Br J Neurosurg* 2001;15:101–108.

44. Gailicich JH, French LA. Use of dexamethasone in the treatment of cerebral edema resulting from brain tumors and brain surgery. *Am Pract* 1961;12:169–174.

45. Bodsch W, Rommel T, Grosse B, Ophoff BG, Menzel J. Factors responsible for the retention of fluid in human tumor edema and the effect of dexamethasone. *J Neurosurg* 1987;67:250–257.

46. Shapiro WR, Posner JB. Corticosteroid hormones: effects in an experimental brain tumor. *Arch Neurol* 1974;30:217–221.

47. Long DM, Hartmann JF, French LA. The response of human cerebral edema to glucocorticoid administration: an electron microscopic study. *Neurology* 1966;16:521–528.

48. Gurcay O, Wilson C, Barker M, Eliason J. Corticosteroid effect on transplantable rat glioma. *Arch Neurol* 1971;24:266–269.

49. Roos KL. Acute bacterial infections of the central nervous system. In. Aminoff MJ, ed. *Neurology and General Medicine,* 3rd ed. Philadelphia, Churchill Livingstone, 2001:665–682.

50. Tauber MG, Khayam-Bashi H, Sande MA. Effects of ampicillin and corticosteroids on brain water content, cerebrospinal fluid pressure, and cerebrospinal fluid lactate levels in experimental pneumococcal meningitis. *J Infect Dis* 1985;151:528–534.

51. Syrogiannopulos GA, Olsen KD, Reisch JS, McCracken GH Jr. Dexamethasone in the treatment of *Haemophilus influenzae* type b meningitis. *J Infect Dis* 1987;155:213–219.
52. Quagliarello V, Scheld WM. Bacterial meningitis: pathogenesis, pathophysiology, and progress. *N Engl J Med* 1992;327:864–872.
53. Molyneux EM, Walsh AL, Forsyth H, Tembo M, Mwenechanya J, Kayira K, Bwanaisu L, Njobvu A, Rogerson S, Mobenga G. Dexamethasone treatment in childhood bacterial meningitis in Malawi: a randomized controlled trial. *Lancet* 2002;360:211–218.
54. McIntyre PB, Berkey CS, King SM, Schaad UB, Kilpi T, Kanra GY, Perez CM. Dexamethasone as adjunctive therapy in bacterial meningitis: a meta-analysis of randomized clinical trials since 1988. *JAMA* 1997; 278:925–931.
55. Martinez-Lacasa J, Cabellos C, Martos A, Fernandez A, Tubau F, Viladrich PF, Linares J, Gudiol F. Experimental study of the efficacy of vancomycin, rifampin, and dexamethasone in the therapy of pneumococcal meningitis. *J Antimicrob Chemother* 2002; 49:507–513.
56. Cabellos C, Martinez-Lacasa J, Tubau F, Fernandez A, Viladrich PF, Linares J, Gudiol F. Evaluation of combined ceftriaxone and dexamethasone therapy in experimental cephalosporin-resistant pneumococcal meningitis. *J Antimicrob Chemother* 2002;45:315–320.
57. Thomas R, Le Tulzo Y, Bouget J, Camus C, Michelet C, LeCorre P, Bellissant E, Adult Meningitis Steroid Group. Trial of dexamethasone treatment for severe bacterial meningitis in adults. *Intensive Care Med* 1999;25:475–480.
58. Girgis NI, Farid Z, Mikhail IA, Farrag I, Sultan Y, Kilpatrick ME. Dexamethasone treatment for bacterial meningitis in children and adults. *Pediatr Infect Dis J* 1989;8:848–851.
59. de Gans J, van de Beek D. Dexamethasone in adults with bacterial meningitis. *N Engl J Med* 2002;347: 1549–1556.
60. Tunkel AR, Scheld MW. Corticosteroids for everyone with meningitis? *N Engl J Med* 2002;347:1613–1615 (editorial).
61. Abril V, Ortega E. Dexamethasone in adults with bacterial meningitis. *N Engl J Med* 2003;348:954–957 (letter).
62. Braakman R, Schouten HJA, Blaauw-van Dishoeck M, Minderhoud JM. Megadose steroids in severe head injury. *J Neurosurg* 1983;58:326–330.
63. Cooper PR, Moody S, Clark WK, Kirkpatrick J, Maravilla K, Gould AL, Drane W. Dexamethasone and severe head injury: a prospective double-blind study. *J Neurosurg* 1979;51:307–316.
64. Dearden NM, Gibson JS, McDowall DG, Gibson RM, Cameron MM. Effect of high-dose dexamethasone on outcome from severe head injury. *J Neurosurg* 1986;64:81–88.

65. Giannotta SL, Weiss MH, Apuzzo MLJ, Martin E. High dose glucocorticoids in the management of severe head injury. *Neurosurgery* 1984;15:497–501.
66. Saul TG, Ducker TB, Salcman M, Carro E. Steroids in severe head injury: a prospective randomized clinical trial. *J Neurosurg* 1981;54:596–600.
67. Lam AM, Winn HR, Cullen BF, Sundling N. Hyperglycemia and neurologic outcome in patients with head injury. *J Neurosurg* 1991;75:545–551.
68. Malik AS, Narayan RK, Wendling WW, Cole RW, Pashko LL, Schwartz AG, Strauss KI. A novel dehydroepiandrosterone analog improves functional recovery in a rat traumatic brain injury model. *J Neurotrauma* 2003;20:463–476.
69. Ward JD, Becker DP, Miller JD, Miller JD, Choi SC, Marmarou A, Wood C, Newlan PG, Keenan R. Failure of prophylactic barbiturate coma in the treatment of severe head injury. *J Neurosurg* 1985;62:383–388.
70. Schalen W, Sonesson B, Messeter K, Nordstrom G, Nordstrom CH. Clinical outcome and cognitive impairment in patients with severe head injury treated with barbiturate coma. *Acta Neurochir* 1992;17:153–159.
71. Hsiang JK, Chesnut RM, Crisp CB, Klauber MR, Blunt BA, Marshall LF. Early routine paralysis for intracranial pressure control in severe head injury: is it necessary? *Crit Care Med* 1994;22:1471–1476.
72. Clifton GL, Miller ER, Choi SC, Levin HS, McCauley S, Smith KR, Muizelaar JP, Wagner FC, Marion DW, Luerssen TG, Chesnut RM, Schwartz M. Lack of effect of induction of hypothermia after acute brain injury. *N Engl J Med* 2001;344:556–563.
73. Vassar MJ, Perry CA, Gannaway WL, Holcroft JW. 7.5% sodium chloride/dextran for resuscitation of trauma patients undergoing helicopter transport. *Arch Surg* 1991;126:1065–1072.
74. Vassar MJ, Fischer RP, O'Brien P, Bachulis BC, Chambers JA, Hoyt DB, Holcroft JW. A multicenter trial for resuscitation of injured patients with 7.5% sodium chloride: the effect of added dextran 70. The Multicenter Group for the Study of Hypertonic Saline in Trauma Patients. *Arch Surg* 1993;128: 1003–1011.
75. Battistella FD, Wisner DH. Combined hemorrhagic shock and head injury: effects of hypertonic saline (7.5%) resuscitation. *J Trauma* 1991;31:182–188.
76. Sheikh AA, Matsuoka T, Wisner DH. Cerebral effects of hypertonic saline and a new low-sodium hypertonic fluid in hemorrhagic shock and head injury. *Crit Care Med* 1996;24:1226–1232.
77. Zornow MH, Oh YS, Scheller MS. A comparison of the cerebral and hemodynamic effects of mannitol and hypertonic saline in an animal model of brain injury. *Acta Neurochir (Wien)* 1990;51:324–325.
78. Freshman SP, Battistella FD, Matteucci M, Wisner DH. Hypertonic saline (7.5%) versus mannitol: a comparison for treatment of acute head injuries. *J Trauma* 1993;35:344–348.

79. Berger S, Schurer L, Hartl R, Messmer K, Baethmann A. Reduction of post traumatic hypertension by hypertonic/hyperoncotic saline/dextran and hypertonic mannitol. *Neurosurgery* 1995;37:98–107.

80. Qureshi AI, Wilson DA, Traystman RJ. Treatment of elevated intracranial pressure in experimental intracerebral hemorrhage: comparison between mannitol and hypertonic saline. *Neurosurgery* 1999;44:1055–1064.

81. Fisher B, Thomas D, Peterson B. Hypertonic saline lowers raised intracranial pressure in children after head trauma. *J Neurosurg Anesthesiol* 1996;8:137–141.

82. Gemma M, Cozzi S, Piccoli S, Magrin S, De Vitis A, Cenzato M. Hypertonic fluid therapy following brainstem trauma. *J Neurosurg Anesthesiol* 1996;8:137–141.

83. Hartl R, Ghajar J, Hochleuthner H, Mauritz W. Hypertonic/hyperoncotic saline reliably reduces ICP in severely head-injured patients with intracranial hypertension. *Acta Neurochir Suppl* (*Wien*) 1997;70:126–129.

84. Qureshi AI, Suarez JI, Bhardwar A, Mirski M, Schnitzer MS, Hanley DF, Ulatowski JA. Use of hypertonic (3%) saline/acetate infusion in the treatment of cerebral edema: effect on intracranial pressure and lateral displacement of the brain. *Crit Care Med* 1998;26:440–446.

85. Suarez JI, Qureshi AI, Bhardwar A, Williams MA, Schnitzer MS, Mirski M, Hanley DF, Ulatowski JA. Treatment of refractory intracranial hypertension with 23.4% saline. *Crit Care Med* 1998;26:1118–1122.

86. Shackford SR, Bourguignon PR, Wald SL, Rogers FB, Osler TM, Clark DE. Hypertonic saline resuscitation of patients with head injury: a prospective randomized clinical trial. *J Trauma* 1998;44:50–58.

87. Simma B, Burger R, Falk M, Sacher P, Fanconi S. A prospective randomized and controlled study of fluid management in children with severe head injury: lactated Ringer's solution versus hypertonic saline. *Crit Care Med* 1998;26:1265–1270.

88. Qureshi AI, Suarez JI. Use of hypertonic saline solutions in treatment of cerebral edema and intracranial hypertension. *Crit Care Med* 2000;28:3301–3313.

89. Coplin WM. Intracranial pressure and surgical decompression for traumatic brain injury: biological rationale and protocol for a randomized clinical trial. *Neurol Res* 2001;3:277–290.

90. Kunze E, Meixensberger J, Janka M, Sorensen N, Roosen K. Decompressive craniectomy in patients with uncontrollable intracranial hypertension. *Acta Neurochir Suppl* (*Wien*) 1998;71:16–18.

91. Bulger EM, Nathens AB, Rivara FP, Moore M, MacKenzie GJ, Jurkovich GJ. Management of severe head injury: institutional variations in care and effect on outcome. *Crit Care Med* 2002;30:1870–1876.

92. Rosner MJ, Rosner SD, Johnson AH. Cerebral perfusion pressure: management protocol and clinical results. *J Neurosurg* 1995;83:949–962.

93. Cruz J. The first decade of continuous monitoring of jugular bulb oxyhemoglobin saturation: management strategies and clinical outcome. *Crit Care Med* 1998;26:344–351.

94. Chesnut RM. Hyperventilation versus cerebral perfusion pressure management: time to change the question. *Crit Care Med* 1998;26:210–212.

95. Ropper AH. Lateral displacement of the brain and level of consciousness in patients with acute hemispheral mass. *N Engl J Med* 1986;314:953–958.

96. Ng LKY, Nimmannitya J. Massive cerebral infarction with severe brain swelling: a clinicopathological study. *Stroke* 1970;1:158–163.

97. Adams HP Jr, Adams RJ, Brott T, del Zoppo GJ, Furlan A, Goldstein LB, Grubb RL, Higashida R, Kidwell C, Kwiatkowski TG, Marler JR, Hademenos GJ; Stroke Council of the American Stroke Association. Guidelines for the early management of patients with ischemic stroke: a scientific statement from the Stroke Council of the American Stroke Association. *Stroke* 2003;34:1056–1083.

98. Frank JI. Large hemispheric infarction, clinical deterioration, and intracranial pressure. *Neurology* 1995;45:1286–1290.

99. Manno EM, Adams RE, Derdeyn CP, Powers WJ, Diringer MN. The effects of mannitol on cerebral edema after large hemispheric cerebral infarct. *Neurology* 1999;52:583–587.

100. Videen TO, Zazulia AR, Manno EM, Derdeyn CP, Adams RF, Diringer MN, Powers WJ. Mannitol bolus preferentially shrinks non-infarcted brain in patients with ischemic stroke. *Neurology* 2001;57:2120–2122.

101. Sakamaki M, Igarashi H, Nishiyama Y, Hagiwara H, Ando J, Chishiki T, Curran BC, Katayama Y. Effect of glycerol on ischemic cerebral edema assessed by magnetic resonance imaging. *J Neurol Sci* 2003;209:69–74.

102. Bereczki D, Liu M, do Prado GF, Fekete I. Mannitol for acute stroke. *Cochrane Database Syst Rev* 2001;(1):CD001153.

103. Russek HI, Russek AS, Zohman BL. Cortisone in immediate therapy of apoplectic stroke. *JAMA* 1955;159:102–105.

104. Patten BM, Mendell J, Bruun B, Curtin W, Sarter S. Double-blind study of the effects of dexamethasone on acute stroke. *Neurology* 1972;22:377–383.

105. Bauer RB, Tellez H. Dexamethasone as treatment in cerebrovascular disease. 2. A controlled study in acute cerebral infarction. *Stroke* 1973;4:547–555.

106. Norris JW. Steroid treatment in acute cerebral infarction. *Arch Neurol* 1976;33:69–71.

107. Mulley G, Wilcox RG, Mitchell JRA. Dexamethasone in acute stroke. *Br Med J* 1978;2:994–996.

108. Norris JW, Hachinski VC. High-dose steroid treatment in cerebral infarction. *Br Med J* 1986;292:21–23.

109. Slivka AP, Murphy EJ. High-dose methylprednisolone treatment in experimental focal cerebral ischemia. *Exp Neurol* 2001;167:166–172.

110. Bayer AJ, Pathy MS, Newcombe R. Double-blind randomised trial of intravenous glycerol in acute stroke. *Lancet* 1987;1:405–408.

111. Yu YL, Kumana CR, Lauder IJ, Cheung YK, Chan FL, Kou M, Fong KY, Cheung RT, Chang CM. Treatment of acute cortical infarct with intravenous glycerol: a double-blind, placebo-controlled randomized trial. *Stroke* 1993;24:1119–1124.

112. Righetti E, Celani MG, Cantisani T, Sterzi R, Boysen G, Ricci S. Glycerol for acute stroke. *Cochrane Database Syst Rev* 2000;(4):CD000096.

113. Schwarz S, Georgiadis D, Aschoff A, Schwab S. Effects of hypertonic (10%) saline in patients with raised intracranial pressure after stroke. *Stroke* 2002;33:136–140.

114. Schwab S, Spranger M, Schwarz S, Hacke W. Barbiturate coma in severe hemispheric stroke: useful or obsolete? *Neurology* 1997;48:1608–1613.

115. Schwab S, Schwarz S, Spranger M, Keller E, Bertram M, Hacke W. Moderate hypothermia in the treatment of patients with severe middle cerebral artery infarction. *Stroke* 1998;29:2461–2466.

116. Berger C, Schabitz WR, Georgiadis D, Steiner T, Aschoff A, Schwab S. Effects of hypothermia on excitatory amino acids and metabolism in stroke patients: a microdialysis study. *Stroke* 2002;33:519–524.

117. Schwab S, Steiner T, Aschoff A. Early hemicraniectomy in patients with complete middle cerebral artery infarction. *Stroke* 1998;29:1888–1893.

118. Walz B, Zimmermann C, Bottger S, Haberl RL. Prognosis of patients after hemicraniectomy in malignant middle cerebral artery infarction. *J Neurol* 2002;249:1183–1190.

119. Holtkamp M, Buchheim K, Unterberg A, Hoffmann O, Schielke E, Weber JR, Masuhr F. Hemicraniectomy in elderly patients with space occupying media infarction: improved survival but poor functional outcome. *J Neurol Neurosurg Psychiatry* 2001;70:226–228.

Chapter 9

When to Consider Emergency Interventional Procedures

Ricardo A. Hanel, Jawad F. Kirmani, Andrew R. Xavier,
Stanley H. Kim, and Adnan I. Qureshi

Endovascular approaches may potentially offer to patients with an acute stroke or subarachnoid hemorrhage a therapy that is capable of reversing neurological deficits. However, emergency endovascular interventions, such as carotid artery angioplasty and stenting and interventional vasospasm therapy, are in their earlier stages of development, and patient response to such therapies is highly variable. In addition to the nature of the underlying neurological condition, response to endovascular therapy and ultimate outcome depend on various systemic factors including coagulation status, blood pressure, cardiac function, blood glucose levels, and severity of other medical comorbidities. Patient selection and periprocedural care are controversial topics that have captured considerable attention.

In this chapter we illustrate and discuss two urgent procedures, namely the use of stenting for carotid revascularization after carotid endarterectomy and the use of interventional therapy for the treatment of cerebral vasospasm.

■ The Patient

A 43-year-old right-handed man underwent a right carotid endarterectomy (CEA) under general anesthesia for an asymptomatic 80 percent carotid stenosis at an outside institution. The stenosis was diagnosed by an ultrasound duplex study. He had a history of myocardial infarction (MI) followed by a right coronary artery stent placement 6 months prior to the CEA. After clamping of the carotid artery, he developed acute hypotension with systolic blood pressure ranging from 40 to 50 mmHg. The hypotension was treated with vasopressors, and the surgery was continued and completed. While initially neurologically intact after surgery, the patient developed a sudden left hemiplegia in the recovery room. Because of suspicion of possible inferior wall MI based on postoperative electrocardiogram, the patient was transferred to our institution for possible emergent coronary intervention. However, upon evaluation the cardiologist determined that emergent coronary angiogram was not required. The patient was referred to the endovascular neurosurgery service for evaluation of perioperative stroke. A computed tomography (CT) scan of the head revealed no evidence of intracerebral hemorrhage or infarction. The patient remained intubated and sedated with blood pressure of 90/60 mmHg on phenylephrine and norepinephrine.

When evaluated by the neuroendovascular team, 4 hours had elapsed since completion of surgery. Emergent cerebral angiogram was performed for possible endovascular intervention. It revealed occlusion of the right common carotid artery (CCA) at the carotid bifurcation (Figure 9-1). Intravenous bolus of heparin (70 IU/kg) was administered to achieve an activated coagulation

125

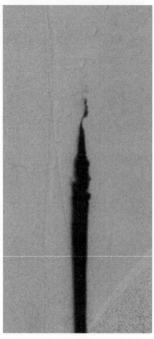

Figure 9-1. Digital subtracting angiography, anteroposterior (AP) view; right CCA injection reveals occlusion of right CCA, compatible with intimal flap dissection.

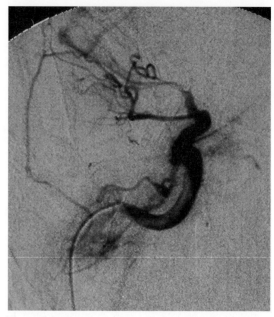

Figure 9-2. Digital subtracting angiography, lateral view. Microcather injection from the distal right ICA reveals the catheter in the true lumen of ICA as well as patency of distal part of the vessel.

time (ACT) greater then 300 seconds. Then a 6F envoy guide catheter (Cordis Neurovascular, Miami Lakes, FL) was advanced over the Glidewire to perform a right and left common carotid angiogram. With the tip of the guide catheter in the proximal right CCA, a prowler plus microcatheter (Cordis Neurovascular) was coaxially advanced over a Transcend EX microwire (Boston Scientific/ Target, Fremont, CA) through the occluded right CCA to the distal cervical internal carotid artery (ICA). Angiography was performed through the microcatheter to ensure the microcatheter was in the true lumen of right ICA (Figure 9-2). The distal normal-appearing ICA measured 4.8 mm and the CCA proximal to bifurcation measured 5.6 mm. Carotid stent placement was performed to revascularize the right ICA and CCA. The microwire was exchanged with a Balance Medium Weight microwire (Guidant, Advanced Cardiovascular Inc., Temecula, CA). A 5.0 × 47 mm Magic Wall stent was deployed from distal to proximal cervical ICA. Then a second Magic Wall stent of the same size was deployed from proximal cervical ICA to CCA below the carotid bifurcation (Figure 9-3).

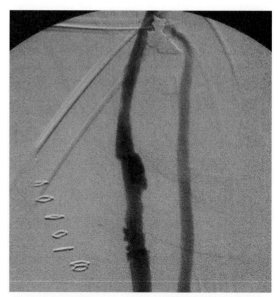

Figure 9-3. Digital subtracting angiography, oblique view demonstrating right common and internal carotid artery recanalization after placement of two overlapping carotid stents.

Recanalization of right CCA and ICA was achieved. Excellent contrast filling of intracranial circulation was observed from right CCA injection (Figure 9-4). The patient was left intubated and he was transferred to an intensive care unit.

In the postoperative period, the patient received 325 mg of aspirin and 75 mg of clopidogrel daily. Postoperative CT of the head revealed infarction involving the distribution of the right middle cerebral artery. He was transferred to a rehabilitation hospital on postoperative day 10. Prior to discharge from the hospital, he was able to ambulate with assistance. Left hemiplegia had improved to mild hemiparesis, and persistent left peripheral visual field loss and mild dysphagia were observed.

■ The Problem

- Should the patient have been submitted to immediate carotid re-exploration just after the discovery of a new profound neurological deficit?
- Is the endovascular approach a reasonable option for the acute treatment of carotid artery occlusion or dissection following CEA?

■ The Evidence

Perioperative stroke following CEA is uncommon and the management of this complication remains controversial. In the North American Symptomatic Carotid Endarterectomy Trial (NASCET), the overall rate of disabling stroke and death was 2.0 percent at 90 days.[1] There were 9 (0.6 percent) stroke-related deaths and 13 (0.9 percent) permanent disabling strokes in the surgical group ($n = 1415$) at 90 days. In the group that died of stroke, 8 of the 9 patients had massive ipsilateral cerebral infarction. Seven of these 9 patients were found to have occlusion at the endarterectomy site with the onset of stroke ranging from immediately after surgery to 3 days after surgery. Four of these patients had returned to surgery for exploration of the endarterectomy site without benefit. In the group that had permanent disabling stroke, 7 of the 13 patients awoke with major deficits due to ischemia in the hemisphere ipsilateral to the CEA. Two of these 7 patients underwent exploration of the endarterectomy site without finding any abnormality. In 4 of the 13 patients, there was a delay in the onset of stroke ranging from 2 to 6 hours. Removal of thrombus at the endarterectomy site resulted in

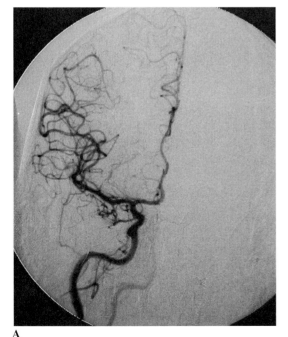
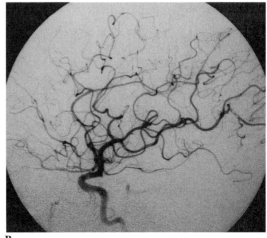

A   B

Figure 9-4. Excellent intracranial circulation is observed in AP (A) and lateral views (B) following carotid stent placement.

no benefit in these 4 patients. It is not clear how many of these patients had diagnostic tests such as cerebral angiography or carotid ultrasound duplex study prior to reoperation. Poor outcome in some of the reoperated patients may have been due to cerebral embolization or delay in reoperation and re-establishment of regional cerebral blood flow.

In contrast to poor results observed in the NASCET, other investigators have emphasized the importance of urgent reoperation. Kwaan et al.[2] reported success of immediate carotid re-exploration in 3 consecutive patients who developed hemiplegia following CEA performed with local anesthesia. In all 3 cases, the authors performed thrombectomy. No diagnostic tests were performed prior to reoperation. The authors concluded that reversal of stroke in such patients could be accomplished if reoperation is carried out within one hour of onset of stroke. Simma et al.[3] described 5 cases of neurological deficits that developed within 18 hours to 10 days after a successful CEA. In 4 of the 5 cases, thrombectomy resulted in complete neurological recovery. Even though cerebral angiogram was performed to diagnose carotid artery occlusion prior to reoperation in 2 cases, they concluded that angiography is neither necessary nor advisable before reoperation in patients who develop sudden neurological deficits after CEA. Treiman et al.[4] investigated the cause of major perioperative stroke after CEA in 19 of 26 patients. In this series, 10 patients had documented carotid thrombosis by angiography, reoperation, or postmortem examination. Oculoplethysmography suggested thrombosis in 3 of these patients. However, in 11 of 26 patients the cause of stroke was unknown. Of 12 patients who were reoperated, the site of carotid endarterectomy was thrombosed in 8 and patent in 4. Only 4 of the patients who had thrombectomy achieved neurological recovery. It is not exactly clear how many patients had diagnostic tests prior to reoperation, but the authors recommended reoperation in such patients provided the stroke occurs within several hours of CEA.

Rosenthal et al. reported a retrospective review of 12 cases of postoperative profound neurological deficits among 818 patients who underwent CEA.[5] Emergent reoperation revealed thrombus at the endarterectomy site in 7 and patent carotid artery in 5 patients. Angiography showed cerebral emboli in 3 of the 5 patients in the distribution of a patent carotid artery. Of the 7 patients with a thrombosed endarterectomy site, reoperation showed thrombus in 4, carotid dissection in 2, and a lateral tear at the repair site in one case. The authors recommended urgent reoperation if a profound neurological deficit was found immediately after CEA. If a pulsatile vessel is found in surgery, the authors recommended an intraoperative angiogram. If the vessel is pulseless, the endarterectomy site should be reopened and thrombectomy and revascularization should be performed. These studies emphasized the importance of urgent reoperation in the management of perioperative stroke but did not demonstrate a consistent reliable diagnostic tool to evaluate the mechanisms leading to cerebral ischemia.

Recently, several reports have incorporated routine diagnostic evaluation of perioperative stroke. Aburahma et al. made a retrospective review of the etiology and management of perioperative stroke following CEA in a series of 32 patients.[6] One or more of the following methods determined the cause of stroke: oculopneumoplethysmography (OPG), carotid duplex ultrasound, CT scan of the head, cerebral angiogram, or carotid exploration. These tests were done immediately after the stroke in the operating room, recovery room, or intensive care unit. The OPG had an overall accuracy of 95 percent in detecting postoperative thrombosis at the endarterectomy site. They recommended that if noninvasive testing such as duplex study or OPG is negative, cerebral angiography should be performed to evaluate cerebral embolization and avoid unnecessary reoperation. Anzuini et al. reported emergent carotid angioplasty and stent (CAS) placement in a series of 13 cases who developed perioperative stroke just after CEA.[7] Diagnostic angiography revealed dissection in 5 (39 percent) and definite or possible thrombus in 8 cases (61 percent). Pre-stent stenosis ranged from 75 to 95 percent. The authors attempted to use a distal protection device called the PercuSurge GuardWire system (PercuSurge Inc., Santa Rosa, CA), but none of the patients tolerated temporary balloon occlusion of the parent carotid artery. Self-expanding Wall stents (Boston Scientific) were used in all patients. Complete remission of neurological symptoms occurred in 11 of 13 patients treated by CAS and in 1 of 5 patients treated by surgical re-exploration. These 5 patients were explored surgically because angiography equipment was not available. The authors emphasized the importance of early investigation and potential benefit of CAS in the treatment of perioperative stroke.

The technique of CAS to treat acute carotid dissection and occlusion has been previously reported. Melissano et al. reported 2 cases of CAS to treat acute carotid dissection after eversion carotid endarterectomy.[8] In one of his cases, an introducer sheath was placed in the common carotid artery and CAS was completed in the operating room. In the other case, a transfemoral approach was used to perform CAS in a symptomatic patient in the angiography suite with neurological recovery.

■ The Pros and Cons

Review of the above studies underscores the importance of a careful but prompt investigation of differential diagnoses in the management of acute perioperative stroke following CEA. Emergent reoperation will not benefit patients with clamping ischemia, intracranial embolization, or intracerebral hemorrhage. Therefore, an emergent noncontrast CT of the head to rule out an intracerebral hemorrhage and a carotid duplex may be performed to evaluate an obstructive carotid lesion. However, these noninvasive tests do not provide information about the extent of thrombosis in the carotid artery or possible intracranial embolization. Diagnostic angiography performed in a timely fashion may provide information about not only the endarterectomy site but also intracranial embolization and collateral circulation. Recent advances in the endovascular treatment of acute stroke such as mechanical thrombolysis have allowed treatment of intracranial embolizations with low-dose thrombolytics.

In our case report, carotid duplex ultrasound study could have been used but we chose to perform an urgent diagnostic angiography to investigate the cause of the neurological deficit. The diagnostic angiogram via the microcatheter in the distal ICA revealed a possible dissection at the endarterectomy site. As a result, we proceeded to treat the dissection with two self-expanding Magic Wall stents (Boston Scientific) after crossing the lesion with a microwire and a microcatheter. The fact that the stents were able to reopen the carotid artery suggested that an intimal flap could have been the cause of near-carotid occlusion as opposed to a thrombus at the endarterectomy site, especially since no thrombolytic agent was administered. Using a distal protection device to capture any particles that may embolize distally during CAS would have been advisable if a device had been available at the time of the procedure. No gross evidence of intracranial vessel occlusion was seen following CAS. We avoided using thrombolytic agents during the procedure because of risk of intracerebral hemorrhage and wound hematoma.

Surely, an urgent carotid endarterectomy site exploration would not be appropriate in this particular case, since the dissection was extending intracranially and therefore not amenable to surgery. Cases like this illustrate the need for preoperative imaging before surgical re-exposure.

■ The Main Points

- The use of rapid noninvasive imaging methods such as carotid duplex and CT angiography are highly recommended before surgical site exploration.
- Emergent carotid artery stenting should be considered as an alternative method of treatment for symptomatic carotid artery dissection or occlusion following CEA. More experience and long-term evaluation are needed to evaluate the validity and durability of this treatment modality.

■ The Patient

A 48-year-old woman was admitted to an outside institution with acute subarachnoid hemorrhage (SAH). She was initially in poor clinical condition but spontaneously improved to a Hunt and Hess grade 1. Subsequently, she became more lethargic due to hydrocephalus, requiring ventriculostomy. Digital subtracted angiography (DSA) showed a basilar tip aneurysm and she was referred to our institution for endovascular treatment of the aneurysm on post-SAH day 1. At admission, she was confused and had a Hunt-Hess grade of 2. Computed tomography showed a diffuse subarachnoid hemorrhage (Figure 9-5), classified as Fisher grade 3.

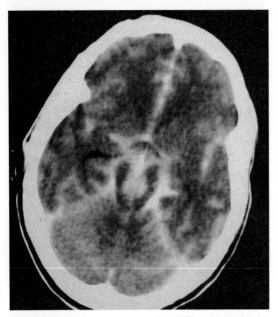

Figure 9-5. CT scan, axial, revealing diffuse subarachnoid hemorrhage.

A four-vessel angiogram confirmed the presence of a basilar tip aneurysm which measured 4.7 × 5.3 mm in the anteroposterior view and 7.4 mm in length on the lateral view (Figure 9-6). Intravenous bolus of heparin (2000 U) was administered to achieve an activated coagulation time (ACT) of 300 seconds. Then a 6F angled guide catheter (Cordis Neurovascular, Miami Lakes, FL) was advanced over the Glidewire, into the left vertebral artery (VA). The guide catheter was placed in the low cervical segment of the VA. An Excel 14, two-tip microcatheter (Boston Scientific/Target, Fremont, CA) was advanced under roadmap guidance over a Transcend 0.014-inch microwire (Boston Scientific/Target, Fremont, CA) into the basilar artery and the aneurysm. The microcatheter tip was left in a mid-position inside the aneurysm. Three coils were deployed: Micrus 10, 5 mm spherical; Micrus 10, 4 mm spherical; and GDC 10, 3 × 8 mm soft. After the deployment of the third coil, an acute elevation of the patient's intracranial pressure was noted. An angiogram demonstrated some contrast extravasation, representing intraoperative rupture of the aneurysm.

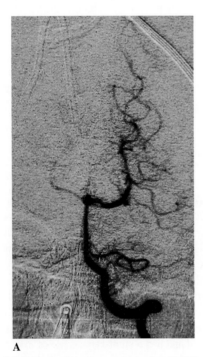
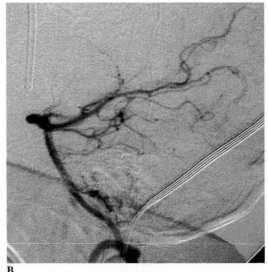

A   B

Figure 9-6. Digital subtracting angiography, AP (A) and lateral (B), demonstrating a basilar tip aneurysm projecting anteriorly.

After rapid reversal of heparin using protamine, we decided to proceed with a rapid packing of the residual aneurysm. Another GDC 10, 3 × 8 mm soft coil was deployed, with cessation of contrast extravasation. Another two GDC 10, 2 × 8 mm soft coils were deployed, resulting in a near-complete occlusion of the aneurysm (Figure 9-7). She had a stable immediate postoperative course. Four days after coiling, she presented with confusion, mild pronator drift, and right facial weakness. Transcranial Doppler revealed increased velocities in both anterior and posterior circulations suggesting diffuse vasospasm. Despite maximal medical therapy with hypervolemia and hypertension for 2 hours, the patient did not improve. The patient was referred for a diagnostic angiogram and possible intervention. Angiography revealed severe vasospasm in the basilar artery, both posterior cerebral arteries (Figure 9-8), and moderate vasospasm on both supraclinoid carotid arteries and middle cerebral arteries (MCAs). Balloon angioplasty was contemplated for the basilar artery and a 1.5 mm (diameter) by 20 mm (length) Ninja balloon was selected. Once the balloon was placed in the mid-basilar artery, the

table was repositioned to acquire a new roadmap to further navigate the balloon. Under fluoroscopy, just before contrast injection, we noticed that the position of the balloon had changed. It represented a rupture of the basilar apex with the balloon, probably due to further advancement of the guide catheter at the vertebral artery, as verified by fluoroscopy. An angiogram showed contrast extravasation superiorly to the tip of the ventriculostomy catheter. At this time, it was decided to abort the procedure. The heparin anticoagulation effect was reversed with intravenous protamine injection. CT scan performed just after this procedure demonstrated intraventricular hemorrhage but no intraparenchymal blood. Two days later, the patient underwent repeat angiography which revealed persistent vasospasm, most severe on the right MCA (Figure 9-9A). Angioplasty of the M1 segment of the right MCA was performed (Figure 9-9B) with good angiographic result. Papaverine was infused into the left internal carotid and left MCA with good angiographic response (Figure 9-10). No angioplasty or papaverine infusion was attempted in the vertebrobasilar system due to the recent hemorrhagic event.

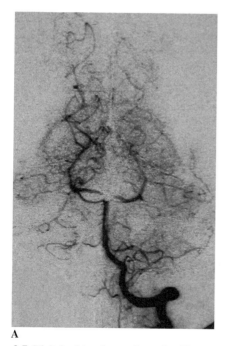
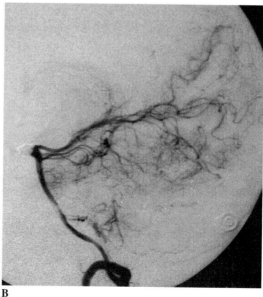

A   B

Figure 9-7. Digital subtracting angiography, AP (A) and lateral (B), showing a near-complete occlusion of the aneurysm after coiling.

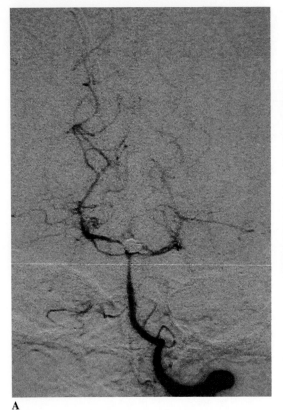
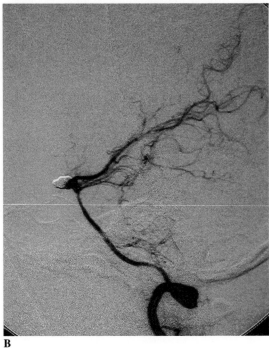

A   **B**

Figure 9-8. Digital subtracting angiography, AP (A) and lateral (B), 4 days after initial aneurysm rupture, revealing severe vasospasm on the basilar artery and its branches.

Three days after the procedure, the patient presented with another episode of neurological deterioration progressing to coma and left hemiplegia. A new angiogram demonstrated severe vasospasm in the vertebrobasilar system, right supraclinoid carotid artery, A1 segment of left anterior cerebral artery and M2 segments of the left MCA. We performed angioplasty on the supraclinoid segment of the right internal carotid artery (Figure 9-11), and infused papaverine into both right and left MCAs and anterior cerebral arteries (Figure 9-12). Both interventions achieved good angiographic results.

One day later she underwent angioplasty of the left supraclinoid internal carotid artery and M1 segment of the left MCA, due to recurrence of the spasm.

On day 11 after aneurysm embolization with coils, transcranial Doppler revealed persistently increased velocities in the vertebrobasilar system. Since CT scan showed no evidence of infarction, we proceeded with cerebral angiogram. Papaverine was infused in the basilar artery after angiography demonstrated severe basilar artery spasm. Considerable improvement was observed in the filling of the basilar artery.

Thirty-four days after admission, she underwent a ventriculoperitoneal shunt placement due to symptomatic persistent hydrocephalus. Upon discharge to a rehabilitation unit, the patient was oriented, had no focal deficits, and was walking without assistance. A 6-month follow-up angiography revealed some residual filling of the aneurysm neck (Figure 9-13) but no growth of the remnant when compared to the previous angiogram. Nineteen months after bleeding, she had no neurological deficit and was completely independent in all her activities of daily living.

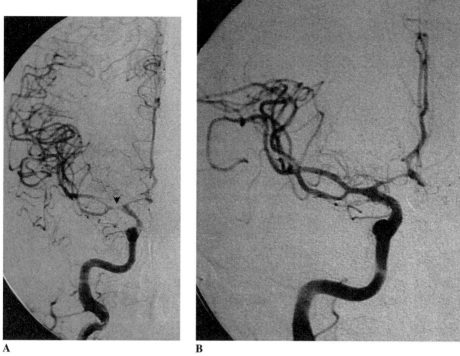

A   B

Figure 9-9. Digital subtracting angiography demonstrating severe vasospasm, more marked on the M1 segment of the right middle cerebral artery (arrow) (A). Resolution of vasospasm after a balloon angioplasty (B).

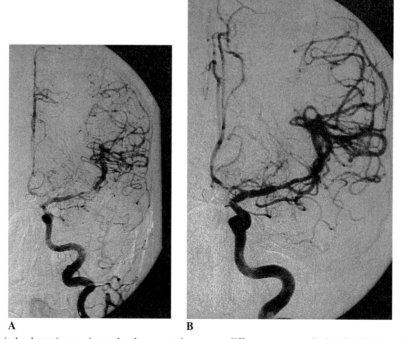

A   B

Figure 9-10. Digital subtracting angiography demonstrating severe diffuse vasospasm in the distribution of the left middle cerebral and anterior cerebral arteries (A). Improvement after intra-arterial papaverine infusion (B).

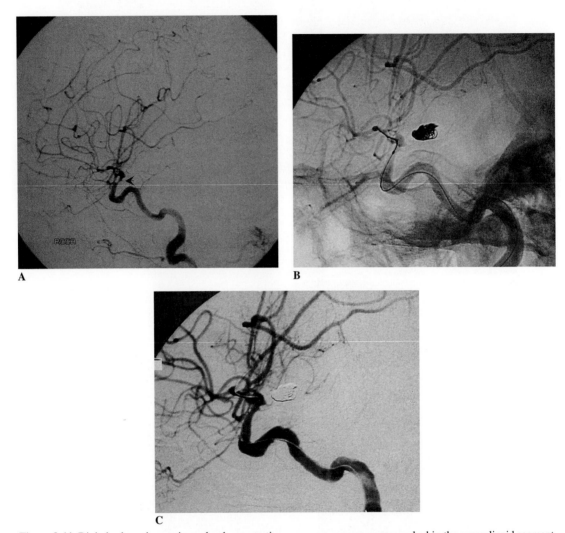

Figure 9-11. Digital subtracting angiography demonstrating severe vasospasm, more marked in the supraclinoid segment of the internal carotid cerebral artery (arrow) (A). Note the position of the angioplasty balloon over the wire on this unsubtracted image (B). The vasospasm resolved after angioplasty (C).

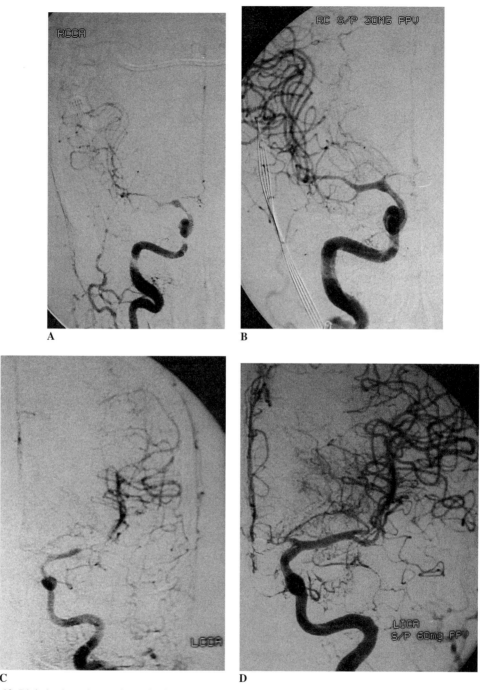

Figure 9-12. Digital subtracting angiography demonstrating severe diffuse vasospasm bilaterally in the distribution of middle cerebral and anterior cerebral arteries (A, right, C, left). Note the improvement after intra-arterial papaverine infusion (B, right, D, left).

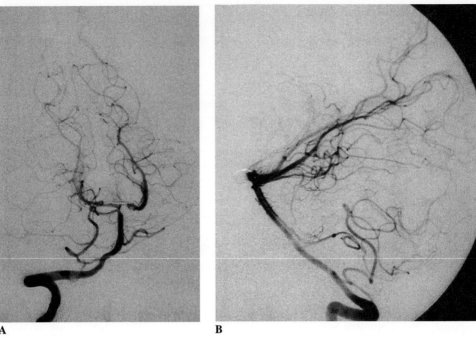

A   B

Figure 9-13. Six-month follow-up angiograms, AP (A) and lateral (B), showing near-complete occlusion of the aneurysm, with some residual filling at the neck area.

■ The Problem

- When should we consider endovascular treatment of vasospasm?
- Which endovascular options are available and how safe are the techniques?
- When should one select each endovascular procedure?
- Does this aggressive approach improve patient outcomes?

■ The Evidence

Cerebral vasospasm after SAH is the delayed narrowing of large capacitance arteries at the base of the brain after SAH, often associated with radiographic and/or clinical evidence of diminished cerebral perfusion in the distal territory of the affected artery. After the benefits of early aneurysm treatment[9] for the prevention of rebleeding became widely accepted, vasospasm turned into the major cause of delayed morbidity and death in patients with subarachnoid hemorrhage.[10]

In 1987, the Cooperative Aneurysm Study reported an incidence of angiographic vasospasm of more than 50 percent, with symptomatic vasospasm in 32 percent of patients.[11] These values have remained consistent in contemporary retrospective reviews.[12–15]

Clinical examination, transcranial Doppler ultrasound, and cerebral angiography are helpful in diagnosing and monitoring cerebral vasospasm. Recently, CT perfusion,[16] brain tissue oxygen content monitoring,[17] microdialysis,[18–21] and diffusion/perfusion MR techniques[22,23] have been shown to be useful modalities for the early diagnosis and follow-up of these cases.

Angiographic vasospasm has a typical temporal course, with onset between 3 and 5 days after the hemorrhage, maximal narrowing at 5 to 14 days, and gradual resolution over 2 to 4 weeks.[24] In about one-half of cases, vasospasm is manifested by the occurrence of a delayed ischemic neurological deficit (DIND), which can lead to stroke with disability and even death. In contemporary series, 15 to 20 percent of DIND patients suffer permanent neurological deficits or die from vasospasm despite maximal therapy.[25,26] The DIND associated with symptomatic vasospasm usually appears shortly after the onset of angiographic vasospasm with the acute or subacute development of focal or generalized symptoms and signs.[24,27] Progression to cerebral infarction occurs in approximately 50 percent of symptomatic cases; recovery without deficit in the remaining individuals may occur despite the persistence of angiographic vasospasm.[24,28]

Early aneurysm clipping or embolization followed by hypervolemic, hypertensive therapy has been advocated as the treatment of choice for this clinical and radiological entity. However, Lennihan et al.[29] showed that patients maintained in a normovolemic state (CVP >5 mmHg, PADP >7 mmHg) did not have a higher risk of symptomatic vasospasm, compared with those treated with prophylactic hypervolemic therapy (CVP >8 mmHg, PADP >14 mmHg). Thus, avoiding hypovolemic states, sometimes a difficult task on these patients due to cerebral salt wasting syndrome and inappropriate antidiuretic hormone secretion, may be effective in preventing DIND.

Pharmacological treatment with calcium channel blockers has been shown to improve the outcome after SAH.[30] Nimodipine is the agent of choice in patients with aneurysmal SAH. It has been shown to improve the overall outcome in SAH cases, in spite of not changing the absolute incidence of radiographic vasospasm.[31] The mechanisms by which nimodipine exerts its beneficial effect after aneurysmal subarachnoid hemorrhage remain uncertain, but possible neuroprotective actions have been implicated.[31] There is no evidence that nicardipine improves overall outcome.[31]

Recently, therapy with intravenous magnesium sulfate infusion has been proposed.[32,33] This agent seems to be neuroprotective, reducing the incidence of clinical vasospasm and improving outcome in patients with symptomatic vasospasm. The exact mechanisms of action of magnesium remain uncertain. This agent may prevent vasospasm by acting as a calcium antagonist, because calcium and magnesium have opposing effects on vascular tone.[34] Thus, magnesium sulfate may have a similar action to calcium channel blockers in blocking the activation of smooth-muscle contraction. Also, magnesium may produce beneficial effects by antagonizing the detrimental effects of increased intracellular calcium concentration induced by cerebral ischemia.[33] Magnesium may compete with calcium for intracellular sites or limit the influx of calcium from damaged cellular membranes.[34]

Even with the use of maximal medical therapy, some patients continue to show neurological deterioration with progression of vasospasm. In such patients, early endovascular intervention could play a very important role.

In recent years, endovascular treatment of vasospasm using balloon angioplasty has been performed in selected patients by mechanical dilatation of the stenotic arteries through a microballoon catheter under fluoroscopic guidance. Balloon dilatation of arteries leads to a transient alteration in myocyte structure,[35] resulting in a degree of functional impairment of vascular smooth muscle that persists for at least 7 days.[36] However, balloon dilatation may cause permanent disruption of the normal architecture of the collagen matrix in the arterial wall.[37] The results from initial clinical trials using angioplasty showed no recurrence of vasospasm within 7 days of treatment, with some rare cases of vessel dissection or rupture.[26,38–41] Angioplasty is effective in reversing vessel constriction and may lead to significant and sustained neurological improvement in many cases. Recurrent vasospasm at the angioplasty site is very rare, although it may occur in the segments of the vessel just proximal and distal to the dilated segment.

Table 9-1 summarizes some case series using balloon angioplasty to treat cerebral vasospasm. One of the potential limitations of angioplasty is that despite successful dilatation of vasospastic arteries in all cases, the clinical improvement is not seen in one-third of the patients. Zubkov et al.[42] found that improvement was most prominent in patients who presented with Hunt-Hess grade 1 or 2 and subsequently deteriorated (all 13 patients improved). Among SAH patients in Hunt-Hess grade 3 at presentation, 85 percent improved with angioplasty compared with 40 percent improvement in grades 4 and 5. Eskridge et al.[40] found that angioplasty was most successful if done within 12 hours of onset of symptoms (presumably before irreversible ischemic damage has occurred). Most studies excluded patients who had CT evidence of cerebral infarction. Coyne et al.[38] included patients with cerebral infarction on the CT scan and found no cases of hemorrhagic transformation after angioplasty treatment; however, limited clinical

Table 9-1. Summary of Case Series on Balloon Angioplasty on the Treatment of Cerebral Vasospasm

Series and No. of Patients	Patients' Characteristics	Timing of Angioplasty	Rate of Angiographic Success	Rate of Clinical Success	Recurrence	Complications
Zubkov et al.[42] (N = 89)	All grades, (+) vasospasm	51 pts pre-op 16 pts post-op	100%	72%	0% at 5–7 days	3 pts arterial rupture 1 pt TIA 1 pt worsened
Eskridge et al.[40] (N = 48)	Refractory to HV and HTN	Within 18 hr of DIND	100%	66%	0%	2 pts arterial rupture 2 rebleeds from unclipped aneurysm 1 thrombosis after 6 weeks
Higashida et al.[26] (N = 13)	Refractory to HV and HTN	No evidence of infarction on CT	100%	69%	0%	1 pt hemorrhagic infarct
Coyne et al.[38] (N = 13)	Refractory to HV and HTN	<48 hr of DIND	100%	31%	Not reported	None
Takahashi et al.[43] (N = 20)	Refractory to HV and HTN	No evidence of infarct on CT	100%	70%	0%	1 pt ruptured aneurysm
Firlik et al.[44] (N = 14)	Refractory to HV and HTN	Day 6 to day 12	100%	92% (12/13) improved 58% complete resolution	0%	Not reported
Nemoto[45] (N = 10)	Refractory to HV and HTN	Not available	60%	40%	Not reported	Not reported
Elliot et al.[46] (N = 52)	Comparison between angioplasty and IA papaverine Refractory to HV and HTN	Not reported	100% initially Sustained 45% mean decrease in TCD velocities after angioplasty	GOS favorable in 67% of angioplasty cases	1%	1 death, cause not specified
Polin et al.[47] (N = 38)	Comparison between 38 patients treated by balloon angioplasty and matched controls (North American Tirilazad Trial)	Not reported	Not reported 39% improved by TCD	No difference in outcome between groups by logistic regression	Not reported	Not reported

Abbreviations: HV, hypervolemia; HTN, hypertension; IA, intra-arterial; TIA, transient ischemic attack; DIND, delayed ischemic neurological deficit; TCD, transcranial Doppler; pt, patient.
Modified from Newell DW et al. Endovascular treatment of intracranial aneurysms and cerebral vasospasm. *Clin Neurosurg* 1992;39:348–360.[48]

benefit was observed. These findings suggest that the maximum benefits with angioplasty may be seen in patients with a good clinical status at admission who experience subsequent acute deterioration due to vasospasm that is unresponsive to intensive medical therapy. Although there may be a time window for intervention extending for up to 12 hours, earlier intervention may increase the chances of successful treatment with good clinical outcomes.

In animal models of subarachnoid hemorrhage, early angioplasty was shown to prevent vasospasm development.[36] Based on these findings, Muizelaar et al.[20] conducted a phase I study where 13 patients with a Fischer grade 3 SAH were submitted to a multivessel angioplasty within 3 days of bleeding. None of these patients developed clinical vasospasm, but one of them had a vessel rupture during the procedure. Their results led to a current ongoing trial for prophylactic use of angioplasty.

Despite continuous advances in catheter industry technology, vessel rupture and dissection remain the main complications of angioplasty, as illustrated in our case.[39,40,49] Patients with angioplasty proximal to an unsecured aneurysm may be at risk for rupture of the aneurysm.[40] Therefore, treatment of the aneurysm prior to angioplasty has been recommended for patients with unsecured ruptured aneurysms.[39,50] Murayama et al. reported their experience with combined endovascular treatment for cerebral aneurysm occlusion and vasospasm in a single session.[51] They concluded that this combination is both feasible and safe. This has been also our approach to these cases.

Papaverine is an opium alkaloid that causes vasodilatation of cerebral vessels via its action on smooth muscle. It also prevents the constriction of smooth muscle secondary to a wide variety of stimuli.[52] It is essential that papaverine be infused just proximal to the spastic arterial segments in order to maximize the therapeutic effect of the drug. Intrathecal administration of papaverine in animal models has shown to be ineffective.[21] Larger doses of papaverine are required for intravenous administration, which can lead to systemic hypotension. Theoretically, the timing of papaverine infusion is also important because papaverine may be ineffective for dilating narrowed arteries in the chronic phase of vasospasm (starting after 3 to 5 days), since this period is characterized by collagen remodeling of the arterial wall.[53]

Several case series have been reported on the use of intra-arterial injection of papaverine for the treatment of cerebral vasospasm (Table 9-2). These studies suggest that the vasodilating effect of intra-arterial papaverine is long-lasting and can be seen even after 10 days of SAH onset. The benefit was most prominent in patients who underwent angioplasty along with intra-arterial papaverine administration for symptomatic vasospasm in vascular territories not accessible to angioplasty.[55] The doses of papaverine in these patients were selected empirically and ranged from 60 to 600 mg administered as boluses or infusion. Kassell et al.,[54] after evaluating various doses, concluded that using 300 mg of papaverine in 100 ml saline was adequate and safe in most cases.

Recurrence rates of up to 20 percent were seen in patients who received only intra-arterial papaverine. In the series published by Kassell et al.,[54] vasospasm recurred in 2 patients 5 days after the first infusion. Both of these patients improved markedly after a second infusion of papaverine. Delay in initiation of papaverine treatment, insufficient doses, and inadequate duration of treatment have been suggested as possible mechanisms for vasospasm recurrence.[54,61] Adverse effects reported after administration of papaverine include transient mental status changes, ophthalmic complications, seizures, and increases in heart rate and in intracranial pressure.

Thus, intra-arterial papaverine may be a valuable therapeutic modality for the treatment of vasospasm in vessels not accessible to angioplasty. The hypothesis of a papaverine-resistant phase of vasospasm does not seem consistent with the data, as a number of patients continue to improve with infusion as long as 19 days after SAH. The procedure appears to have minimal permanent complications. However, recurrence of vasospasm, probably due to the short duration of action of the drug,[53] appears to be a major limitation of this treatment.

■ The Pros and Cons

If the patient presents with SAH, ruptured cerebral aneurysm and severe vasospasm, we tend to treat both situations in a single session, attempting to secure the aneurysm first and act on the vasospasm later. In some case this is not possible because the

Table 9-2. Summary of Case Series on Intra-arterial Injection of Papaverine on the Treatment of Cerebral Vasospasm

Series (No. of Patients)	Study Characteristics	Dosage and Timing of Papaverine	Rate of Angiographic Success	Rate of Clinical Success	Recurrence	Comments
Kassell et al.[54] (N = 12)	Not candidates for balloon angioplasty	100–300 mg by infusion	66%	33%	17%	1 pt transient mental status and hemiparesis
Kaku et al.[55] (N = 14)	No response to HV and HTN; No evidence of infarct on CT	6–20 mg in repeated doses with angioplasty and IA nicardipine	92%	80%	0%	Tachycardia
Clouston et al.[56] (N = 10)	No response to HV and HTN	150–600 mg by manual injection <48 hr after DIND	93%	50%	21%	1 pt permanent monocular blindness; 1 pt arterial rupture without neurological decline
Numaguchi et al.[57] (N = 24)	Analysis of repeat IA papaverine; 12 with no improvement	Not specified	100%	50% improved after 2nd infusion; 33% after 3rd infusion	100%	Not reported
Milburn et al.[58] (N = 34)	81 arterial territories	300 mg infusion over 15 to 60 min Day 3 to day 19 post-SAH	100%	Not reported	100%	Not reported
Fandino et al.[59] (N = 10)	23 vascular territories; No response to HV and HTN	360 mg/120 ml, infusion rate of 0.1 ml/sec Day 4 to day 16 post-SAH	100%	Good recovery (n = 7); Moderate disability (n = 3)	Not reported	Improvement of cerebral oxygenation
Firlik et al.[44] (N = 15)	32 arteries	Not reported	78%	26%	6 of 15 patients	4 complications; 1 brainstem signs; 1 systemic hypotension; 1 seizure; 1 aggravation of spasm
Polin et al.[60] (N = 31)	Comparison between patients treated by balloon angioplasty and matched controls (North American Tirilazad Trial)	Not reported	13% immediate improvement	Logistic regression, no difference in outcome between groups	Not reported	Not reported

Abbreviations: HV, hypervolemia; HTN, hypertension; TIA, transient ischemic attack; DIND, delayed ischemic neurological deficit; TCD, transcranial Doppler; pt, patient. Modified from Qureshi et al.[10] Recent advances in the management of vasospasm in patients with subarachnoid hemorrhage. *Neurologist* 1996;2:53–65.

Table 9-3. Summary of Pros and Cons of Balloon Angioplasty and Intra-arterial Injection of Papaverine on the Treatment of Cerebral Vasospasm

Modality	Pros	Cons
Papaverine injection	Low risk of vessel injury Possibility of treating branches distal to A1, M2, and P1	High incidence of recurrence Can cause increase in intracranial pressure Can cause seizures
Balloon angioplasty	Very low incidence of recurrence Re-establishes vessel lumen diameter May be useful as prophylactic maneuver (to be determined)	Risky to treat branches distal to A1, M2, and P1 Risk of vessel dissection Risk of vessel rupture during balloon inflation May be limited by tortuous anatomy and severe spasm distal to the target vessel

severity of spasm precludes aneurysm catheterization. In these cases we try to dilate the vessel injecting a 30 mg dose of papaverine. This injection is repeated until a reasonable vessel diameter for microcatheter and wire manipulation is obtained. We use angioplasty to treat vasospasm resistant to medical therapy in the major intracranial branches that are amenable to catheter manipulation and balloon dilatation. We reserve intra-arterial papaverine to treat diffuse vasospasm and vasospasm involving more distal arteries that are inaccessible to the balloon catheter.

Since the timing of these endovascular treatments may have an impact on its chances of success, we try to intervene as soon as the patient fails to improve with a reasonable trial of hemodynamic augmentation therapy. When the patient develops recurrent or worsening neurological symptoms secondary to refractory vasospasm, the endovascular treatments are repeated. Cerebral vasospasm is a self-limited phenomenon; every effort should be made to prevent irreversible brain ischemia during its course. As illustrated by our case, repeated aggressive endovascular treatments carry some risks but also have the potential to avert major neurological morbidity.

The pros and cons for both interventional therapeutic modalities, namely balloon angioplasty and papaverine infusion, are further summarized in Table 9-3.

■ The Main Points

- Endovascular intervention to treat vasospasm is recommended if aggressive hypervolemic,

hypertensive therapy does not result in rapid patient improvement.

- The safety and efficacy of prophylactic angioplasty remains to be established. Therefore, this intervention cannot be recommended at present in asymptomatic patients with vasospasm.

- Since balloon angioplasty gives a more durable result, we perform it as first choice, whenever the vessel characteristics (size, accessibility) are permissive. We use papaverine infusion as a second choice modality, predominantly as adjunct therapy to angioplasty.

- Prospective, randomized trials comparing angioplasty and intra-arterial papaverine with standard medical therapy are needed to determine the optimal management strategy for vasospasm secondary to SAH.

■ References

1. Ferguson GG, Eliasziw M, Barr HW, Clagett GP, Barnes RW, Wallace MC, Taylor DW, Haynes RB, Finan JW, Hachinski VC, Barnett HJ. The North American Symptomatic Carotid Endarterectomy Trial: surgical results in 1415 patients. *Stroke* 1999;30:1751–1758.
2. Kwaan JH, Connolly JE, Sharefkin JB. Successful management of early stroke after carotid endarterectomy. *Ann Surg* 1979;190:676–678.
3. Simma W, Hesse H, Gilhofer G, Menner C, Muck G. Management of immediate occlusion after carotid reconstruction. *J Cardiovasc Surg (Torino)* 1987;28:176–179.
4. Treiman RL, Cossman DV, Cohen JL, Foran RF, Levin PM. Management of postoperative stroke after carotid endarterectomy. *Am J Surg* 1981;142:236–238.

5. Rosenthal D, Zeichner WD, Lamis PA, Stanton PE Jr. Neurologic deficit after carotid endarterectomy: pathogenesis and management. *Surgery* 1983;94:776–780.

6. Aburahma AF, Robinson PA, Short YS. Management options for post carotid endarterectomy stroke. *J Cardiovasc Surg (Torino)* 1996;37:331–336.

7. Anzuini A, Briguori C, Roubin GS, Pagnotta P, Rosanio S, Airoldi F, Carlino M, Pagnotta P, Dmario C, Sheiban I, Magnani G, Jannello A, Melissano G, Chiesa R, Colombo A. Emergency stenting to treat neurological complications occurring after carotid endarterectomy. *J Am Coll Cardiol* 2001;37:2074–2079.

8. Melissano G, Chiesa R, Sheiban I, Colombo A, Astore D. Intraoperative stenting of the internal carotid artery after unsuccessful eversion endarterectomy. *J Vasc Surg* 1999;30:355–356.

9. Haley EC Jr, Kassell NF, Torner JC. The International Cooperative Study on the Timing of Aneurysm Surgery: the North American experience. *Stroke* 1992;23:205–214.

10. Qureshi AI, Dawson R, Frankel MR, et al. Recent advances in the management of vasospasm in patients with subarachnoid hemorrhage. *Neurologist* 1996;2: 53–65.

11. Adams HP Jr, Kassell NF, Torner JC, Haley EC Jr. Predicting cerebral ischemia after aneurysmal subarachnoid hemorrhage: influences of clinical condition, CT results, and antifibrinolytic therapy. A report of the Cooperative Aneurysm Study. *Neurology* 1987; 37:1586–1591.

12. Auer LM. Acute operation and preventive nimodipine improve outcome in patients with ruptured cerebral aneurysms. *Neurosurgery* 1984;15:57–66.

13. Awad IA, Carter LP, Spetzler RF, Medina M, Williams FC Jr. Clinical vasospasm after subarachnoid hemorrhage: response to hypervolemic hemodilution and arterial hypertension. *Stroke* 1987;18:365–372.

14. Megyesi JF, Vollrath B, Cook DA, Findlay JM. In vivo animal models of cerebral vasospasm: a review. *Neurosurgery* 2000;46:448–460.

15. Treggiari-Venzi MM, Suter PM, Romand JA. Review of medical prevention of vasospasm after aneurysmal subarachnoid hemorrhage: a problem of neurointensive care. *Neurosurgery* 2001;48:249–261.

16. Nabavi DG, LeBlanc LM, Baxter B, Lee DH, Fox AJ, Lownie SP, Ferguson GG, Craen RA, Gelb AW, Lee TY. Monitoring cerebral perfusion after subarachnoid hemorrhage using CT. *Neuroradiology* 2001;43:7–16.

17. Vath A, Kunze E, Roosen K, Meixensberger J. Therapeutic aspects of brain tissue pO_2 monitoring after subarachnoid hemorrhage. *Acta Neurochir Suppl* 2002;81:307–309.

18. Sarrafzadeh AS, Sakowitz OW, Kiening KL, Benndorf G, Lanksch WR, Unterberg AW. Bedside microdialysis: a tool to monitor cerebral metabolism in subarachnoid hemorrhage patients? *Crit Care Med.* 2002;30:1062–1070.

19. Unterberg AW, Sakowitz OW, Sarrafzadeh AS, Benndorf G, Lanksch WR. Role of bedside microdialysis in the diagnosis of cerebral vasospasm following aneurysmal subarachnoid hemorrhage. *J Neurosurg* 2001;94:740–749.

20. Muizelaar JP, Zwienenberg M, Rudisill NA, Hecht ST. The prophylactic use of transluminal balloon angioplasty in patients with Fisher Grade 3 subarachnoid hemorrhage: a pilot study. *J Neurosurg* 1999;91: 51–58.

21. Ogata M, Marshall BM, Lougheed WM. Observations on the effects of intrathecal papaverine in experimental vasospasm. *J Neurosurg* 1973;38:20–25.

22. Condette-Auliac S, Bracard S, Anxionnat R, Schmitt E, Lacour JC, Braun M, Meloneto J, Cordebar A, Yin L, Picard L. Vasospasm after subarachnoid hemorrhage: interest in diffusion-weighted MR imaging. *Stroke* 2001;32:1818–1824.

23. Phan T, Huston J, Campeau N, Wijdicks EF, Atkinson JL, Fulgham JR. Value of diffusion-weighted imaging in patients with a non-localizing examination and vasospasm from subarachnoid hemorrhage. *Cerebrovasc Dis* 2003;15:177–181

24. Sundt TM Jr, Kobayashi S, Fode NC, Whisnant JP. Results and complications of surgical management of 809 intracranial aneurysms in 722 cases: related and unrelated to grade of patient, type of aneurysm, and timing of surgery. *J Neurosurg* 1982;56:753–765.

25. Heros RC, Zervas NT, Varsos V. Cerebral vasospasm after subarachnoid hemorrhage: an update. *Ann Neurol* 1983;14:599–608.

26. Higashida RT, Halbach VV, Cahan LD, Brant-Zawadzki M, Barnwell S, Dowd C, Hieshima GB. Transluminal angioplasty for treatment of intracranial arterial vasospasm. *J Neurosurg* 1989;71:648–653.

27. Longstreth WT Jr, Nelson LM, Koepsell TD, van Belle G. Clinical course of spontaneous subarachnoid hemorrhage: a population-based study in King County, Washington. *Neurology* 1993;43:712–718.

28. Kassell NF, Sasaki T, Colohan AR, Nazar G. Cerebral vasospasm following aneurysmal subarachnoid hemorrhage. *Stroke* 1985;16:562–572.

29. Lennihan L, Mayer SA, Fink ME, Beckford A, Paik MC, Zhang H, Wu YC, Klebanoff LM, Raps EC, Solomon RA. Effect of hypervolemic therapy on cerebral blood flow after subarachnoid hemorrhage: a randomized controlled trial. *Stroke* 2000;31:383–391.

30. Allen GS, Ahn HS, Preziosi TJ, Battye R, Boone SC, Chou SN, Kelly DL, Weir BK, Crabbe RA, Lavik PJ, Rosenbloom SB, Dorsey FC, Ingram CR, Mellits DE, Bertsch LA, Boisvert DP, Hundley MB, Johnson RK, Strom JA, Transou CR. Cerebral arterial spasm— a controlled trial of nimodipine in patients with subarachnoid hemorrhage. *N Engl J Med* 1983; 308:619–624.

31. Feigin VL, Rinkel GJ, Algra A, Vermeulen M, van Gijn J. Calcium antagonists in patients with

aneurysmal subarachnoid hemorrhage: a systematic review. *Neurology* 1998;50:876–883.

32. Boet R, Mee E. Magnesium sulfate in the management of patients with Fisher Grade 3 subarachnoid hemorrhage: a pilot study. *Neurosurgery* 2000;47:602–606.

33. Veyna RS, Seyfried D, Burke DG, Zimmerman C, Mlynarek M, Nichols V, Marrocco A, Thomas AJ, Mitsias PD, Malik GM. Magnesium sulfate therapy after aneurysmal subarachnoid hemorrhage. *J Neurosurg* 2002;96:510–514.

34. Ram Z, Sadeh M, Shacked I, Sahar A, Hadani M. Magnesium sulfate reverses experimental delayed cerebral vasospasm after subarachnoid hemorrhage in rats. *Stroke* 1991;22:922–927.

35. Chavez L, Takahashi A, Yoshimoto T, Su CC, Sugawara T, Fujii Y. Morphological changes in normal canine basilar arteries after transluminal angioplasty. *Neurol Res* 1990;12:12–16.

36. Megyesi JF, Findlay JM, Vollrath B, Cook DA, Chen MH. In vivo angioplasty prevents the development of vasospasm in canine carotid arteries: pharmacological and morphological analyses. *Stroke* 1997;28:1216–1224.

37. Yamamoto Y, Smith RR, Bernanke DH. Mechanism of action of balloon angioplasty in cerebral vasospasm. *Neurosurgery* 1992;30:1–5.

38. Coyne TJ, Montanera WJ, Macdonald RL, Wallace MC. Percutaneous transluminal angioplasty for cerebral vasospasm after subarachnoid hemorrhage. *Can J Surg* 1994;37:391–396.

39. Eskridge JM, McAuliffe W, Song JK, Deliganis AV, Newell DW, Lewis DH, Mayberg MR, Winn HR. Balloon angioplasty for the treatment of vasospasm: results of first 50 cases. *Neurosurgery* 1998;42:510–517.

40. Eskridge JM, Newell DW, Pendleton GA. Transluminal angioplasty for treatment of vasospasm. *Neurosurg Clin N Am* 1990;1:387–399.

41. Zubkov AY, Lewis AI, Scalzo D, Bernanke DH, Harkey HL. Morphological changes after percutaneous transluminal angioplasty. *Surg Neurol* 1999;51:399–403.

42. Zubkov YN, Alexander LF, Smith RR, Benashvili GM, Semenyutin V, Bernanke D. Angioplasty of vasospasm: is it reasonable? *Neurol Res* 1994;16:9–11.

43. Takahashi A, Yoshimoto T, Mizoi K, et al. Transluminal balloon angioplasty for vasospasm after subarachnoid hemorrhage. In Sano K, Takakura K, Kassell NF, et al., eds. *Cerebral Vasospasm.* Tokyo, University of Tokyo Press, 1990:429–432.

44. Firlik KS, Kaufmann AM, Firlik AD, Jungreis CA, Yonas H. Intra-arterial papaverine for the treatment of cerebral vasospasm following aneurysmal subarachnoid hemorrhage. *Surg Neurol* 1999;51:66–74.

45. Nemoto S. [Percutaneous transluminal angioplasty.] *No To Shinkei* 2000;52:571–579.

46. Elliott JP, Newell DW, Lam DJ, Eskridge JM, Douville CM, LeRoux PD, Lewis DH, Mayberg MR, Grady MS, Winn HR. Comparison of balloon angioplasty and papaverine infusion for the treatment of vasospasm following aneurysmal subarachnoid hemorrhage. *J Neurosurg* 1998;88:277–284.

47. Polin RS, Coenen VA, Hansen CA, Shin P, Baskaya MK, Nanda A, Kassell NF. Efficacy of transluminal angioplasty for the management of symptomatic cerebral vasospasm following aneurysmal subarachnoid hemorrhage. *J Neurosurg* 2000;92:284–290.

48. Newell DW, Eskridge J, Mayberg M, Grady MS, Lewis D, Winn HR. Endovascular treatment of intracranial aneurysms and cerebral vasospasm. *Clin Neurosurg* 1992;39:348–360.

49. Linskey ME, Horton JA, Rao GR, Yonas H. Fatal rupture of the intracranial carotid artery during transluminal angioplasty for vasospasm induced by subarachnoid hemorrhage: case report. *J Neurosurg* 1991;74:985–990.

50. Le Roux PD, Newell DW, Eskridge J, Mayberg MR, Winn HR. Severe symptomatic vasospasm: the role of immediate postoperative angioplasty. *J Neurosurg* 1994;80:224–229.

51. Murayama Y, Song JK, Uda K, Gobin YP, Duckwiler GR, Tateshima S, Patel AB, Martin NA, Vinuela F. Combined endovascular treatment for both intracranial aneurysm and symptomatic vasospasm. *AJNR Am J Neuroradiol* 2003;24:133–139.

52. Bolton TB. Mechanisms of action of transmitters and other substances on smooth muscle. *Physiol Rev* 1979;59:606–718.

53. Vorkapic P, Bevan RD, Bevan JA. Longitudinal time course of reversible and irreversible components of chronic cerebrovasospasm of the rabbit basilar artery. *J Neurosurg* 1991;74:951–955.

54. Kassell NF, Helm G, Simmons N, Phillips CD, Cail WS. Treatment of cerebral vasospasm with intra-arterial papaverine. *J Neurosurg* 1992;77:848–852.

55. Kaku Y, Yonekawa Y, Tsukahara T, Kazekawa K. Superselective intra-arterial infusion of papaverine for the treatment of cerebral vasospasm after subarachnoid hemorrhage. *J Neurosurg* 1992;77:842–847.

56. Clouston JE, Numaguchi Y, Zoarski GH, Aldrich EF, Simard JM, Zitnay KM. Intraarterial papaverine infusion for cerebral vasospasm after subarachnoid hemorrhage. *AJNR Am J Neuroradiol* 1995;16:27–38.

57. Numaguchi Y, Zoarski GH, Clouston JE, Zagardo MT, Simard JM, Aldrich EF, Sloan MA, Maurer PK, Okawara SH. Repeat intra-arterial papaverine for recurrent cerebral vasospasm after subarachnoid haemorrhage. *Neuroradiology* 1997;39:751–759.

58. Milburn JM, Moran CJ, Cross DT III, Diringer MN, Pilgram TK, Dacey RG Jr. Increase in diameters of vasospastic intracranial arteries by intraarterial papaverine administration. *J Neurosurg* 1998;88:38–42.

59. Fandino J, Kaku Y, Schuknecht B, Valavanis A, Yonekawa Y. Improvement of cerebral oxygenation

patterns and metabolic validation of superselective intraarterial infusion of papaverine for the treatment of cerebral vasospasm. *J Neurosurg* 1998;89:93–100.

60. Polin RS, Hansen CA, German P, Chadduck JB, Kassell NF. Intra-arterially administered papaverine for the treatment of symptomatic cerebral vasospasm. *Neurosurgery* 1998;42:1256–1257.

61. Marks MP, Steinberg GK, Lane B. Intraarterial papaverine for the treatment of vasospasm. *AJNR Am J Neuroradiol* 1993;14:822–826.

Chapter 10
When and How to Monitor Acute Brain Injury

Marek Czosnyka

Detailed neurological examination has been traditionally used to monitor brain function. However, physical signs are often poorly sensitive and may be obscured by pharmacological interventions in the intensive care setting. It is in those cases that the advances in technology have come to aid cliniciensist. Therefore, one could argue that the first part of the question included in the title is relatively easy to answer. Brain function should be monitored in all acute cases when a patient is unconscious or requires anesthesia, paralysis and ventilation in intensive care, or during major neurological or cardiac surgery.

The choice of appropriate candidates and variables to monitor is essential. First, the majority of sensors used for monitoring are invasive. Limiting brain monitoring only to those patients who are most likely to benefit from its use is necessary to reduce the risk of complications. Several questions must be answered when considering the use of brain monitoring. Are all monitoring techniques sensitive and specific to detect the pathological states that are most likely to happen? For example, can we monitor local ischemia of cerebral tissue with transcranial Doppler ultrasonography or with an intracranial pressure (ICP) probe located in the contralateral frontal lobe? Some sensors reflect global measurements (such as intracranial pressure or regional cerebral blood flow), whilst others study local changes (e.g., brain tissue oxygenation, microdialysis). Are they all accurate and is their accuracy likely to decline over time? Examples of decreased accuracy over time include zero drift of intraparenchymal pressure transducers, and the notorious technical problems observed with prolonged use of jugular bulb oxygen saturation fiberoptic transducers. Do they provide early warning about fatal complications that are going to happen in the near future, or when we see something wrong in their readings it is usually too late?

Most clinical knowledge of cerebral pathophysiology has been derived from studying patients with traumatic or vascular injuries in the neurointensive care unit. It is becoming increasingly clear that although these patients are highly heterogeneous, basic pathophysiological responses to injury of the brain share considerable common ground. For instance, the modern treatment of patients with brain trauma shares the same concepts applied to patients with subarachnoid hemorrhage, intracerebral hematomas, and brain swelling due to infection or inflammation.

Secondary ischemic brain damage arises from insults to the brain generally due to episodes of intracranial hypertension, arterial hypotension, and hypoxemia.[1] In addition, physiological brain-protective mechanisms, such as cerebral pressure autoregulation[2,3] or intracranial pressure-volume compensation, can be impaired following head injury.[4] With impaired intrinsic protection, the brain may be more vulnerable to the effects of secondary insults, and less capable of optimally distributing cerebral blood flow, stabilizing blood volume, and maintaining the correct metabolic balance.[5]

Following brain trauma, a complex multiloop control system of cerebrovascular circulation works without feedback information. The aim of intensive brain monitoring is to provide missing feedback data and close the disrupted control loop by appropriate therapy. An ideal monitoring system should not only detect the secondary insults but also identify states of cerebral dysfunction that render the brain more susceptible to such insults and provide this information in a clear form.

Monitoring of cerebral pressure autoregulation, cerebrovascular reactivity, and cerebrospinal compensation have a very special place among the techniques used in the intensive care treatment of head trauma. Most of the methods are based on the observation of the specific response of cerebral blood flow to a provoked increase or decrease in arterial blood pressure,[6] therefore they can be repeated with limited frequency. More recently, methods suitable for continuous assessment of autoregulatory and compensatory reserves, utilizing endogenous variations in cerebral perfusion pressure, have been described.[7–11]

Since secondary insults to the brain may be frequent and of short duration (a few minutes), continuous observation is an essential component with one-minute epochs being generally accepted as a basic period for averaging.[12,13] User-dependent selection of the modalities for monitoring and their online interpretation is a complex task in neuromonitoring.

In terms of directing and optimizing treatment, the monitoring of only one component may be misleading. The inability to reliably distinguish hyperemia from vasospasm using transcranial Doppler ultrasonography is an example where an inappropriate interpretation of the data could lead to potentially dangerous therapeutic interventions.[14] In both cases, blood flow velocity is elevated, hence a second modality (such as jugular vein oxygen saturation [SjO_2] monitoring) is necessary for differentiating these two very different states.

In contrast to experimental studies on cerebral ischemia and different head injury models, the scientific basis of clinical management of head-injured patients is still poorly elucidated. The aim of this chapter, in some respects complementary to Chapter 8, is to present different brain monitoring techniques, and methods of testing of cerebral autoregulation, which show promise in the provision of clinically relevant information, and could improve our understanding of the injured brain.

It remains an important dilemma to subject patients to costly and largely untested technology. The topic, however, is included in this monograph to introduce the reader to the fascinating possibilities that may become standards in the near future. In this chapter, these monitoring devices are only briefly presented with pictorial explanations and references for more detailed readings for those interested in pursuing these techniques.

■ The Patient

A 23-year-old male was hit by a slow-moving car, at an approximate speed of 25 miles/hour, while crossing the road outside language college. He lost consciousness immediately at the scene for 12 minutes but then awakened while awaiting the ambulance, opened his eyes spontaneously, and was obeying commands—although still unable to talk. On arrival at the emergency department of the local hospital, his Glasgow coma scale sum score was 13 but 4 hours later deteriorated to 6. At that time, he was sedated and intubated. Head CT scan showed generalized brain swelling without apparent contusions and small left-to-right middle line shift. He was admitted to a neurointensive care unit (NICU) where, after checking the coagulation profile, a triple-lumen bolt was inserted to introduce a parenchymal ICP transducer that revealed an ICP of 18 mmHg. A right jugular bulb fiber-optic catheter to measure venous oxygen saturation (SjO_2) was inserted. Initial cerebral perfusion pressure (CPP) was 58 mmHg. An intraparenchymal tissue oxygen probe was placed using the second lumen of the bolt. The second day after the injury, CPP increased to 73 mmHg with infusion of noradrenaline but ICP also increased to 27 mmHg. Transcranial Doppler recording demonstrated that the blood flow velocity on the left side was much greater than on the right side, with a diminished pressure autoregulation on the left. Later that day, the ICP increased further to 35 mmHg, causing some instability in CPP, with frequent readings below 65 mmHg. SjO_2 tended to decrease below 55 percent and tissue oxygen partial pressure fell below 17 mmHg. A new CT scan showed more brain swelling with effacement of basal cisterns and increasing midline shift. Emergency bifrontal decompressive craniectomy was performed. Subsequently, the ICP decreased to 10 mmHg and, with some fluctuations, it normalized over the next 4 days. Continuously monitored brain compensatory reserve recovered following surgery and cerebral autoregulation, at first disturbed after surgery, recovered 4 days later. Tissue oxygenation and SjO_2 normalized. Sedation and paralysis were withdrawn successfully, and the patient started breathing spontaneously. Two weeks after discharge from the NICU with a GCS of 14, the patient was transported to his home country, reporting good recovery 6 months after injury.

■ The Problem

- Does sophisticated monitoring influence patient management?
- Which modalities can be chosen for monitoring?
- How should one weigh precision versus risk of complications when deciding whether to use invasive versus noninvasive forms of monitoring?
- Which variables should be measured?

■ The Evidence

Modalities

Generally, there is no "class I" evidence that any of the available brain monitoring methods improve quality of management and outcome following head injury. Most of the methods have been investigated using prospective or retrospective clinical studies (usually of good quality), and a vast number of references support their usefulness in clinical practice. For some newer methods, clinical research is in progress. Table 10-1 attempts to summarize the methods, their use, and essential attributes.

Intracranial Pressure and Cerebral Perfusion Pressure

As discussed in Chapter 8, the brain is a lump in a box. Its environmental pressure, called intracranial pressure (ICP), is an essential parameter that

reflects many of the brain regulating mechanisms.[16] ICP is determined by the circulation of cerebral blood and of cerebrospinal fluid (CSF). Change in the volumes or rates of circulation of CBF or CSF can cause abrupt change in ICP. Factors that influence ICP include physiological variables (head position, arterial carbon dioxide tension, blood pressure) as well as pathological factors (brain swelling, space-occupying lesions, obstruction of CSF circulatory pathways, active vasodilation, or vasoconstriction, obstruction of cerebral venous drainage). Because such changes can occur rapidly (see Figure 10-1), continuous ICP measurement is currently considered a core modality in any brain monitoring system. Most contemporary methods of monitoring relay on intraparenchymal microtransducers.[17]

CPP represents the pressure gradient acting across the cerebrovascular bed, and is therefore an important factor in determining cerebral blood flow. It can be estimated using the simple formula:

$$CPP = MAP - ICP$$

where MAP is mean arterial pressure. CPP is therefore clearly pulsatile. In head injury patients, CPP-oriented therapy[18] to keep CPP above 60–70 mmHg has been introduced as part of management protocols in many neurocritical care centers. (For additional discussion see Chapter 22.)

Monitoring of CBF and Brain Metabolism

Direct Methods. Contemporary techniques for quantitative determination of global CBF include *continuous jugular thermodilution,*[19] or a double-indicator method based on injections of dye and iced water providing noncontinuous measurements.[20] Both methods are novel.

Thermal diffusion (TD) monitors focal cortical blood flow. A probe is inserted through a burr hole and placed in a cortical region of interest. Recently, an improved version of this technique using an intraparenchymal probe with thermistors has been evaluated in brain-injured patients.[21]

More recently, a method based on two angled probes to measure both *Doppler flow* velocity and the diameter of the internal carotid artery has been introduced for direct blood flow measurement.[22]

Brain imaging methods such as xenon CT, SPECT, PET, CT perfusion, and perfusion MRI

Table 10-1. Methods for Brain Monitoring

Method	Continuous	Resolution	Invasive	Quantitative	Remarks
Intracranial pressure	Yes	Global	Yes	Yes	Intraparenchymal probes; intraventricular catheter, subdural drain, epidural sensors are available
Cerebral perfusion pressure	Yes	Global	Yes	Yes	Requires simultaneous ICP and direct arterial pressure monitoring
Brain temperature	Yes	Regional	No	Yes	
CBF jugular thermodilution	Yes	Global	Yes	Yes	
CBF double indicator dilution	No	Global	Yes	Yes	
CBF laser Doppler flowmetry	Yes	Local (1–2 mm^3)	Yes	No	Unknown physiological zero
CBF thermal diffusion	Yes	Local	Yes	Yes	Cortical probe; with parenchymal probe bigger region can be monitored (5 cm^2)
CBF velocity: transcranial Doppler ultrasonography	Yes	MCA (ACA/PCA)	No	No	Problems with probe holders. It may provide information on autoregulation and asymmetry of CBF
NIRS	Yes	Regional	No	No	Technology yet to be refined; some machines prone to extracranial contamination; % tissue oxygen saturation debatable
SjvO$_2$	Yes	Global	Yes	No	Requires frequent (every 2 hours?) co-oximetry
Brain tissue pO$_2$	Yes	Local	Yes	No	
Microdialysis	No	Regional	Yes	No	Various compounds can be monitored

NIRS, near infra-red spectroscopy; SjvO$_2$, jugular bulb venous oxygen saturation; MCA, middle cerebral artery; ACA, anterior cerebral artery; PCA, posterior cerebral artery.

Modified from Steiner LA, Czosnyka M. Should we measure cerebral blood flow in head-injured patients? *Br J Neurosurg* 2002;16:429–439.[19]

cannot be used for monitoring. Rather than dynamic information, they provide precision "snapshot pictures" of the distribution of CBF, brain metabolism, or cerebral blood volume.

Indirect Methods. *Jugular bulb oximetry* provides information about the adequacy of global CBF in relation to metabolic demands. The clinical usefulness of SjO$_2$ monitoring is debatable; while a recent publication found that SjO$_2$ monitoring does not substantially influence the management of head-injured patients,[23] other studies indicate a clear and practical benefit.[24]

Transcranial Doppler (TCD) ultrasonography is easy to use, noninvasive, does not involve ionizing radiation, and can therefore be used repeatedly and also over a longer time period.[25] However, it measures blood flow velocity (BFV) instead of CBF and the linear relationship between CBF and BFV (CBF = BFV × area of the insonated vessel × cosine of angle of insonation) is only present if neither the diameter of the insonated vessel nor the angle of insonation change during the examination. This assumption is probably fulfilled in most situations where examinations of the basal cerebral arteries are performed, with the

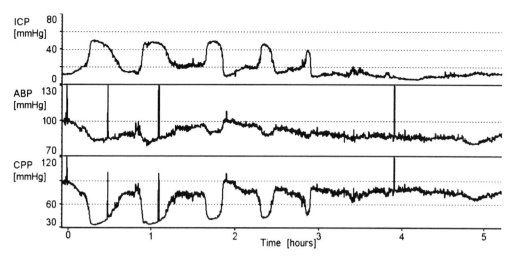

Figure 10-1. Recording of intracranial pressure (ICP), arterial blood pressure (ABP), and cerebral perfusion pressure (CPP) after head injury. ICP and CPP may be highly variable (here we can see repetitive plateau waves of ICP of the magnitude of 10–50 mmHg). Therefore continuous minute-to-minute monitoring is essential.

exception of cases of subarachnoid hemorrhage with vasospasm.

Near-infrared spectroscopy (NIRS) measures the chromophore level of oxygenated and deoxygenated hemoglobin (i.e., "cerebral hemoglobin saturation") via photon scattering, albeit in a target volume that cannot be clearly defined.[26] Changes in these parameters have been used to estimate relative changes in CBF or brain tissue oxygen saturation, with variably enthusiastic reports.

Laser Doppler flowmetry (LDF) allows continuous real-time measurements of local perfusion (red cell flux) with excellent dynamic resolution[27] (Figure 10-2). It has two major disadvantages: the sample volume is small (1–2 mm^3) and only relative changes can be assessed.

Brain tissue pO_2 ($PtiO_2$) has been used as an estimator of local adequacy of perfusion. The method is promising because of its good temporal resolution. In some centers, clear clinical benefit has been reported.[28]

Multiparameter *intraparenchymal brain probes* to measure simultaneously such parameters as $PtiO_2$, CO_2 partial pressure, pH, and temperature are becoming increasingly more available.[29] They also provide local measurements.

Finally, there have been attempts to use *microdialysis* to assess adequacy of CBF. Lactate/pyruvate ratio is widely used as a marker of ischemia.

The temporal resolution of microdialysis is limited and the position of the probe will influence results. The method may be used to monitor energy-related metabolites, markers of brain tissue damage, or neurotransmitters.[30]

Brain temperature probes may be used alone or in combination with other intraparenchymal sensors (e.g., Camino ICP monitor or Neurotrend).[31] They are important in controlling brain hypothermia (although use of hypothermia protocols is still controversial) and avoiding pyrexia.

Monitoring Cerebral Function: EEG and Evoked Potentials

Indications for EEG monitoring in head injury include diagnosis and management of seizures, and assessment of drug effects (dose control for EEG burst suppression). A *standard EEG* consists of an 8–32-channel trace printed on paper at 30 mm/sec (or 300 pages/hour) and provides an enormous amount of raw data. The technique that is most commonly used calculates a spectral array.

Bispectral analysis provides a new approach to computerized EEG analysis. It takes into account not only the frequency and phase angles of the components of a signal but also the interactions of some waves with others, with the calculation of new summary measures of EEG activity. The BIS is

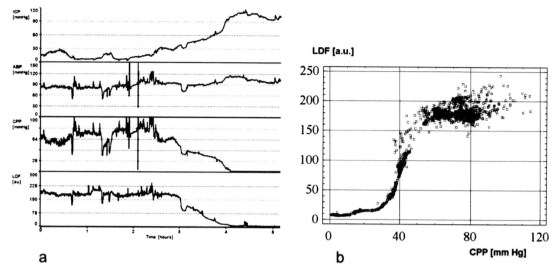

a   b

Figure 10-2. Tracing physiology: example of brain monitoring during terminal rise in ICP followed by decrease in CPP and decrease in cortical CBF (laser Doppler flux [LDF] in arbitrary units). LDF plotted against CPP replicates an almost ideal "autoregulation curve."[2] Horizontal extension of the curve for low CPP (below 40 mmHg) expresses that zero blood flow is represented by certain nonzero flux (so-called "biological zero"). Testing autoregulation in clinical practice should be done using much more limited changes in cerebral perfusion pressure!

a dimensionless number ranging from 0 to 100 and gives information on depth of anesthesia or coma.[32]

Evoked potentials are a measurement of potentials that are produced in response to a stimulus. They allow assessment of defined neural tracts including peripheral nerves and subcortical regions. The most frequently used evoked potentials in anesthesia are somatosensory evoked potentials (SSEPs).[33] Evoked potentials can be used for the assessment of head-injured patients. Certain patterns of SSEPs from stimulation of the median nerve (absent scalp potentials with preserved cervical spine responses) can predict unfavorable outcome with a reasonable degree of accuracy.

Invasive Versus Noninvasive

The choice of purely noninvasive methodology for brain monitoring may lead to a substantial error of judgment. The exception is when the readings are interpreted as a response to known medication and therapeutic or diagnostic maneuvers (for example, change in transcranial Doppler blood flow velocity, SjO_2, or NIRS in response to change in $PaCO_2$, change in laser Doppler flux or tissue oxygenation

after bolus of mannitol, etc.). In continuous monitoring following head injury, the core of brain monitoring variables—ICP and CPP—should always be used and other modalities should be interpreted against their changes. Attempts to monitor CPP and ICP noninvasively should at present be interpreted as research tools. The following paragraphs briefly mention some of these noninvasive methods. For more precise technical details, the reader should consult the references provided.

Compliant branches of the middle cerebral artery (MCA) can be compared to two "physiological" pressure transducers. The pattern of blood flow inside these elastic tubes is certainly modulated by transmural pressure (approximated by cerebral perfusion pressure) and the proximal vascular resistance (also modulated by CPP). But what is the calibration factor, and how should we compensate for unknown nonlinear distortion? While there is a reasonable correlation between the pulsatility index of the MCA velocity and ICP,[34] the absolute measurements are far from being accurate. Other authors have suggested that the "critical closing pressure" derived from BFV and arterial pressure waveforms approximates the ICP.[35] The accuracy of this method has, however, never been satisfactory.

Aaslid et al.[36] suggested that an index of cerebral perfusion pressure could be derived from the ratio of the amplitudes of the first harmonics of the arterial blood pressure and the MCA flow velocity multiplied by mean flow velocity.

Recently a new method for the noninvasive assessment of CPP has been reported, derived from MAP multiplied by the ratio of diastolic to mean BFV.[37] This estimator can predict real CPP with an error of less than 10 mmHg for more than 74 percent of the time. This is of potential benefit for continuous monitoring of changes in real CPP over time in situations where the direct measurement of CPP is not readily available.

Another method aimed at the noninvasive assessment of ICP has been introduced by Schmidt et al.[38] The method is based on the presumed linear transformation between arterial pressure and ICP waveforms. The method is complex and relies on a database of previously recorded ICP, MAP, and BFV of patients sharing the same pathology, but it appears amazingly promising.

Recent studies have described good relationship between the flow velocity of venous blood in straight sinus and ICP. Increasing ICP is supposed to squeeze the sinus and produce proportional increase in blood flow velocity. A calibration coefficient was reported to be convergent in a group of patients, making this method possibly quantitative.[39]

Other methods are based on ultrasonography but do not use the Doppler principle. The most promising of them evaluates the time of flight of ultrasound through the skull, which theoretically depends on ICP.[40]

Monitoring of Physiological Reserves of the Brain

Two essential brain-protecting reserves may be listed:

1. Compensatory reserve can be understood as the hypothetical maximal cerebral volume load below which we do not notice any substantial (exponential) increase in ICP.
2. Autoregulatory reserve represents how far the CPP can be reduced without substantial decrease in CBF.

Waveform Analysis of ICP Used to Monitor Brain Compensatory Reserve

The shape of the ICP waveform theoretically includes information about the transmission of arterial pulse pressure through the arterial walls to the compliant CSF pool. This information is not always clear and demands highly specific analysis and careful interpretation. As CPP falls and the tension in the vascular walls relaxes, the transmission of the arterial pulse wave to the intracranial contents increases. Additionally, as ICP increases, the compliance of the brain diminishes and the pressure-wave transmission becomes heightened, which also forces the amplitude of the ICP waveform to increase. Therefore, as long as cerebral vessels are reactive, a decrease in CPP will provoke an increase in the pulsatility of ICP. However, in advanced stages of intracranial hypertension the cerebral vessels may cease to be pressure-reactive as the reserve in cerebral vasodilatation becomes exhausted. Under these circumstances, the relationship is reversed and ICP pulse amplitude flattens or starts to decrease.

Computer-supported data analysis is required to demonstrate the relationships between ICP, MAP, and CPP. By way of example, data is collected online over 5 minutes. Mean ICP and the average pulse amplitude (AMP) of the ICP waveform are calculated for 60 consecutive 5-second periods. These 60 paired variables are correlated and this action is repeated with a moving time window. The coefficient of this correlation is named the RAP (from R = symbol of correlation, A = amplitude, P = pressure). A low RAP (close to zero or negative) associated with low ICP (below 20 mmHg) indicates good cerebrospinal compensatory reserve. A high RAP (close to +1) indicates an exhausted compensatory reserve. The most obvious clinical example is an increasing compensatory reserve (i.e., decrease in RAP) following decompressive craniectomy (Figure 10-3). However, a low RAP with high ICP (above 25 mmHg) indicates a decrease in ICP pulse amplitude and terminal vasoplegia. This has proven to be highly predictive of fatal outcome following head injury.[41]

Pressure Reactivity

The correlation between MAP and ICP is dependent on the autoregulatory reserve of cerebral vasculature.

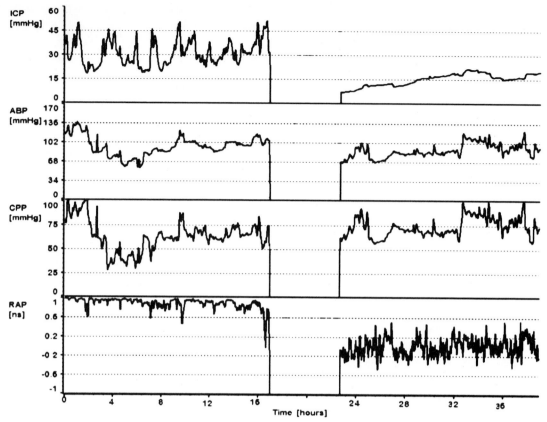

Figure 10-3. Example of monitoring of ICP, ABP, and CPP together with index of cerebrospinal compensatory reserve (RAP) before and after decompressive craniectomy. After craniectomy, although ICP may increase in time, pressure-volume compensatory reserve persists much better than before (RAP close to +1 before and fluctuating around 0 after surgery).

If autoregulation is intact, a rise in MAP produces vasoconstriction, a decrease in cerebral blood volume, and a fall in ICP. The correlation coefficient between MAP and ICP is named the pressure-reactivity index (PRx) and is near to zero, or negative, when cerebral vessels are reactive to perfusion pressure changes. However, when autoregulation is disturbed, the vessels can no longer respond actively to changes in MAP, which are transmitted passively to the intracranial compartment resulting in similar changes in ICP. A positive correlation coefficient (PRx) therefore indicates disturbed autoregulation. This index can fluctuate with time, but its average (over a minimum of 2–3 hours) is predictive of outcome, i.e., the greater the disturbance in autoregulation, the poorer the outcome[42] (Figure 10-4).

Cerebral Autoregulation

Transcranial Doppler ultrasonography can be used to assess the brain autoregulatory reserve. Although cerebral autoregulation is frequently disturbed following head injury, the extent of this disturbance may fluctuate with time. Regular assessment is therefore an essential component of this type of evaluation. Several methods are available.

(i) *Static test of autoregulation* relies on recording MCA flow velocity during changes in MAP induced by an infusion of vasopressors. The static rate of autoregulation (SRoR) is calculated as the percentage increase in vascular resistance (CPP/BFV) divided by the percentage rise in CPP. The common error here is considering only

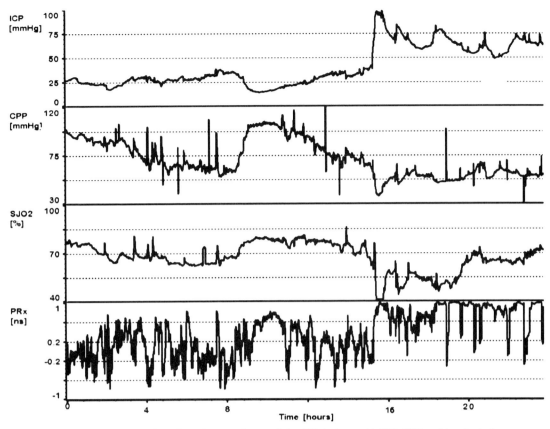

Figure 10-4. Continuous monitoring of cerebrovascular reactivity (PRx) along with ICP, CPP, and jugular bulb oxygen saturation (SjO$_2$) in a patient who died because of refractory intracranial hypertension. Increase in ICP and decrease in CPP and SjO$_2$ were followed or even anticipated (episode around 10th hour of monitoring and another past 15th hour) by a deterioration in vascular reactivity (PRx >0.3).

changes in MAP instead of CPP—this may lead to an error when ICP changes proportionally to the testing step increase in MAP. A SRoR of 100 percent indicates fully intact autoregulation, whereas a SRoR of 0 percent indicates that autoregulation is fully exhausted.[6]

(ii) Testing for *CO$_2$ cerebrovascular reactivity* has been shown to have an important application in the assessment of severely head-injured patients as well as other cerebrovascular diseases. Although cerebral vessels are reactive to changes in PaCO$_2$ even when cerebral pressure autoregulation has been impaired, disturbed CO$_2$ reactivity correlates significantly with worse outcome following head injury.[43]

(iii) Aaslid et al.[44] described a method in which a step decrease in arterial blood pressure was achieved by the deflation of compressed leg cuffs whilst simultaneously measuring TCD flow velocity in the MCA. An index, called the *dynamic rate of autoregulation* (RoR), describes how quickly cerebral vessels react to the sudden fall in blood pressure.

(iv) Short-term compression of the common carotid artery produces a marked decrease in the ipsilateral MCA flow velocity. If autoregulation is intact, the distal cerebrovascular bed dilates during compression. Upon release of the compression, a transient hyperemia lasting for a few seconds occurs until the distal cerebrovascular bed constricts to its former diameter. This sequence of events, which underlies the *transient hyperemic response test* (THRT), indicates a positive autoregulatory response (Figure 10-5). A positive correlation

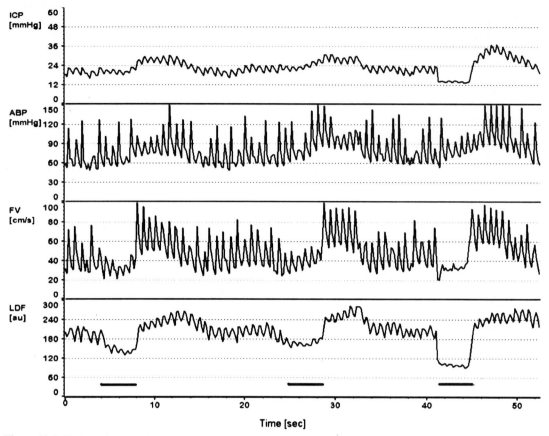

Figure 10-5. Testing of autoregulation using the transient hyperemic response test. Blood flow velocity (FV) and cortical laser Doppler flux (LDF) recorded along with ICP and ABP after three 4-second compressions of the carotid artery (marked with horizontal lines) showed postcompression hyperemia, indicating intact autoregulation. Changes in ABP and ICP may be encountered (although rarely) during compression and complicate interpretation of the test.

between the presence of a hyperemic response and better outcome following head injury has been demonstrated.[45]

(v) An interesting noninvasive method of deriving autoregulatory status from natural fluctuations in MCA flow velocity involves the assessment of *phase shift between the superimposed respiratory and arterial blood pressure waves* during slow and deep breathing. A 0° phase shift indicates absent autoregulation, whereas a phase shift of 90° indicates intact autoregulation.[9]

(vi) By *continuous monitoring* over 60 consecutive 5–10-second periods, a correlation coefficient between mean CPP and mean BFV can be calculated. This coefficient has been termed the mean index (Mx). A positive coefficient signifies a positive association between BFV and CPP, i.e., disturbed autoregulation. A zero or negative correlation

coefficient signifies an absent or negative association, implying intact autoregulation. This index seems to be ideal to monitor transient changes in autoregulation in response to a cerebral intrinsic phenomenon, such as ventilation, drugs, etc. (Figure 10-6). Group analysis has demonstrated that the autoregulation index averaged daily was related to clinical outcome following head injury; a positive Mx (disturbed autoregulation) was associated with worse outcome.[10] Similar methods are becoming popular in multiple clinical applications.[7,8,11]

■ The Pros and Cons

It is obvious that CPP-oriented therapy requires continuous monitoring of CPP, just as various ICP protocols also require direct ICP measurements.

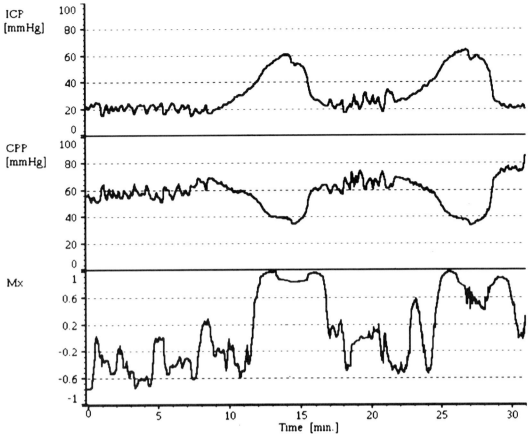

Figure 10-6. Monitoring of pressure autoregulation (Mx index). Example shows temporary loss of autoregulation during ICP plateau waves, when the vascular bed is maximally dilated. This example shows that autoregulation may be intact (before the wave) and become disturbed in a matter of minutes! This illustrates why continuous monitoring of autoregulation is important in clinical practice.

Continuously derived pressure reactivity (PRx index—see the previous section) plotted against CPP shows a "U-shaped" curve.[46] This indicates that in a majority of patients there is a value of the CPP for which pressure reactivity is the best. This pressure has been named "optimal" pressure and a simple protocol, by plotting and analysing the PRx vs. CPP curve in a moving 6-hour-long time window, can be applied to evaluate it online. It has been demonstrated that greater distance between current and "optimal" CPP is associated with worse outcome in a group of retrospectively evaluated patients. This useful methodology attempts to refine CPP-oriented therapy. Both too low (ischemia) and too high CPP (hyperemia leading to secondary increase in ICP) are detrimental; therefore,

CPP should be optimized to maintain global cerebral perfusion in the most favorable state.

There are many controversies and unanswered questions regarding the above-mentioned methods of brain monitoring. Even such a well-established modality as ICP monitoring is not free from frequently raised criticisms. With contemporary intraparenchymal probes we cannot control zero drift of the pressure sensor, which in some cases may be substantial.[47] In some cases, many compartmentalized ICPs may be present but they are difficult to define and monitor. These pressure gradients between CSF compartments may appear when free circulation of CSF is disrupted (brain swelling, mass lesions). They can be recorded with direct two-sensor monitoring[48] or evidenced by noninvasive methods based on transcranial Doppler ultrasonography.[37,38] Moreover, when there are no normal CSF pools, can ICP be considered as ruled by the Pascal law or rather by the stress in the heterogeneous environment? In the second case, intraparenchymal ICP readings may vary from point to point, and a bedside ICP monitor may express highly local values that are not representative for the whole brain. There are also quite a few controversies about new methods based on measurement of brain compliance. Is this new modality useful in intensive care or simply a derivative of ICP that adds no additional value to the traditional set of brain monitoring variables?[49]

The value of TCD in brain monitoring as a noninvasive method giving real-time quantification of BFV, which can be used for optimizing management, is well established. However, an unsolved problem is the fixation of the probes for prolonged monitoring. TCD holds great promise as an alternative noninvasive technique to monitor cerebral autoregulation, noninvasive estimates for ICP and CPP, and the asymmetry of cerebral hemodynamic parameters. However, its value in optimizing management needs to be further validated by prospective studies. TCD technology is progressing very rapidly, as noted by the recent introduction of the volume flowmeter, based on the Doppler principle and currently only applicable to carotid blood inflow.[22]

Jugular bulb oxygenation is widely used in many neurointensive care units, but the reliability of contemporary oximeters remains questionable. The frequency of faulty measurements because of low light intensity recorded by the receiving optic fiber and other technical difficulties (e.g., apposition of the tip of the catheter against the jugular vein wall) is still considerable. Frequent direct blood gasometry should be performed (the common knowledge says once every couple of hours!) to confirm the fidelity of interim continuous monitoring. It has also been documented that cerebral blood may be drained asymmetrically, therefore it is not clear on which side the jugular vein should be monitored. Bilateral catheterization may impede cerebral blood outflow and cause substantial rise in ICP. Nevertheless, a well-working SjO_2 catheter in experienced hands is a key modality to measure adequacy of brain oxygenation. Arteriovenous oxygen difference with known value of CBF allows the measurement of $CMRO_2$.[50] An alternative to SjO_2

may be the use of brain tissue oxygenation. This direct method requires the introduction of an invasive intraparenchymal probe. It is reliable and gives absolute values but the reading is local. Injured brain is extremely heterogeneous, therefore a one-point measurement may not be representative of the situation in other areas of the brain. Good time response with a possibility of keeping the probe over a longer time period partially compensates for this disadvantage. Recently described $PtiO_2$-based management protocols rely on the reactivity of $PtiO_2$ to changes in ventilation and CPP.[51] In fact, it may be argued that monitoring of SjO_2 and $PtiO_2$ should ideally be used every time hyperventilation is induced in order to prevent the risk of brain ischemia from vasoconstriction.

Near-infrared spectroscopy can measure proportions between oxygenated and deoxygenated hemoglobin, but continuous noninvasive tissue oxygen saturation is still debatable. Thanks to new technologies, contamination of readings by extracranial circulation can be minimized.

Thermal diffusion or laser Doppler probes are used in a few centers to measure cortical cerebral blood flow. The clinical impact of these monitoring modalities is rather limited to assessment of rCBF reactivity to changes in $PaCO_2$ or CPP. Similarly, brain microdialysis is criticized as being a research rather than a clinical tool. On the other hand, as with almost all brain monitoring modalities, monitoring never helps by itself, unless the information is used by experienced clinicians to optimize patients' management.[52]

Secondary ischemic insults can be very short-lived and may be missed because of the limited temporal and spatial resolution as well as the limited sensitivity of our monitoring devices. This has led to the concept of continuous multimodality monitoring. The combination of several monitors and integration of the complex information using dedicated software can improve our understanding of the injured brain and also increases the likelihood of recording relevant insults[12,13,53] (Figure 10-7).

Recent studies involving brain imaging are rapidly extending our understanding of the pathophysiology of injured brain. The tools used in those studies are highly specialized, requiring dedicated and expensive technology. Complex data processing extends the time gap between scanning and obtaining clinically useful information. Snapshot images

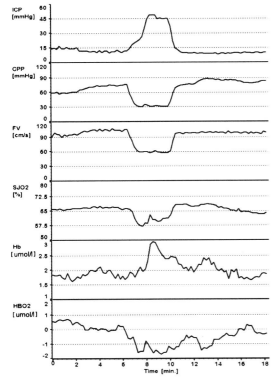

Figure 10-7. Monitoring of short-term brain insults requires computer support. Decrease in transcranial Doppler blood flow velocity (FV), jugular bulb oxygenation (SjO₂), deoxygenated (Hb) and oxygenated (HbO₂) hemoglobin using near-infrared spectroscopy during a short-term ICP plateau wave (duration of 4 minutes).

like PET or perfusion MRI can be performed only from time to time (because of limitations of patient transport and radiation exposure), and highly dynamic information about what happens to the brain between scans can only be derived from the sensors and transducers used for continuous brain monitoring. Recent validation studies have improved our understanding of the relationship between the information provided by PET imaging and brain monitoring. Dysautoregulation monitored continuously using the pressure-reactivity index correlates with a state of high oxygen extraction fraction and diminished oxygen metabolism documented by PET.[54] Poor stability of PET-CBF during test change in CPP, indicating faulty autoregulation, may be assessed continuously using the same PRx index.[55]

Finally, there is (mainly class II) evidence showing a correlation between different modalities

and outcome following head injury. Too low or too high CPP, low brain oxygenation, low CBF, poor autoregulation, and reduced compensatory reserve have been shown to correlate with poor outcome following brain trauma. This, again, seems to support the usefulness of continuous brain monitoring.

The case presented at the beginning of this chapter is a good example of how continuous multimodality brain monitoring may allow for the rapid and reliable recognition of secondary insults. In this case, different modalities concurred in the diagnosis of those secondary insults, thus justifying a radical intervention such as decompressive craniectomy. Thanks to this decision, the patient achieved a remarkable functional recovery.

■ The Main Points

- In appropriately selected cases, the information provided by brain monitoring can lead to dramatic changes in management with a favorable impact on outcome.
- Different brain monitoring modalities should be used in combination and integrated to optimize the recognition of erroneous abnormal measurements.
- Core variables in brain monitoring following head injury are intracranial pressure, cerebral perfusion pressure, and tissue oxygenation.
- Intrinsic mechanisms of brain protection such as autoregulation or sufficient compensatory reserve are probably more important than "high CPP," "low ICP," or "adequate tissue oxygenation." Continuous monitoring of these parameters is available.
- Contemporary brain imaging is very informative. But in contrast to brain monitoring, it cannot be performed continuously over time. Direct brain monitoring allows interpolation of changes in evolving brain pathology between "snapshot" images and can facilitate timely decisions about necessary interventions.

Acknowledgments

Many thanks to my colleagues who participated in the head injury program in Cambridge, UK, between

1991 and 2002: Dr. M. Hiler, Mrs. P. Al-Rawi, Miss M. Balestreri, Dr. L.A. Steiner, Mr. R. Kett-White, Mr. P. Hutchinson, Dr. E.A. Schmidt, Dr. P. Smielewski, Dr. S.K. Piechnik, Mr. P.J. Kirkpatrick, Dr. F.K. Matta, Dr. A. Gupta, Professor D.K. Menon, and Professor J.D. Pickard.

■ References

1. Miller JD, Becker DP. Secondary insults to the injured brain. *J Roy Coll Surg Ed* 1982;27:292–298.
2. Lassen NA. Control of cerebral circulation in health and disease. *Circ Res* 1974;34:749–760.
3. Overgaard J, Tweed WA. Cerebral circulation after head injury. 1. Cerebral blood flow and its regulation after closed head injury with emphasis on clinical correlations. *J Neurosurg* 1974;41:531–541.
4. Avezaat CJJ, von Eijndhoven JHM, Wyper DJ. Cerebrospinal fluid pulse pressure and intracranial volume-pressure relationships. *J Neurol Neurosurg Psychiatry* 1979;42:687–700.
5. Obrist WD, Langfitt TW, Jaggi JL, Cruz J, Gennarelli TA. Cerebral blood flow and metabolism in comatose patients with acute head injury: relationship to intracranial hypertension. *J Neurosurg* 1984;61:241–255.
6. Strebel S, Lam AM, Matta B, Mayberg TS, Aaslid R, Newell DW. Dynamic and static cerebral autoregulation during isoflurane, desflurane, and propofol anesthesia. *Anesthesiology* 1995;83:66–76.
7. Panerai RB, White RP, Markus HS, Evans DH. Grading of cerebral dynamic autoregulation from spontaneous fluctuations in arterial blood pressure. *Stroke* 1998;29:2341–2346.
8. Hu HH, Kuo TB, Wong WJ, Luk YO, Chern CM, Hsu LC, Sheng WY. Transfer function analysis of cerebral hemodynamics in patients with carotid artery stenosis. *J Cereb Blood Flow Metab* 1999;19:460–465.
9. Diehl RR, Linden D, Lucke D, Berlit P. Spontaneous blood pressure oscillations and cerebral autoregulation. *Clin Auton Res* 1998;8:7–12.
10. Czosnyka M, Smielewski P, Kirkpatrick P, Menon DK, Pickard JD. Monitoring of cerebral autoregulation in head-injured patients. *Stroke* 1996;27:829–834.
11. Steinmeier R, Bauhuf C, Hubner U, Bauer RD, Fahlbusch R, Laumer R, Bondar I. Slow rhythmic oscillations of blood pressure, intracranial pressure, microcirculation, and cerebral oxygenation: dynamic interrelation and time course in humans. *Stroke* 1996;27:2236–2243.
12. Miller JD, Piper IR, Jones PA. Integrated multimodality monitoring in the neurosurgical intensive care unit. *Neurosurg Clin N Am* 1994;5:661–670.
13. Czosnyka M, Whitehouse H, Smielewski P, Kirkpatrick P, Pickard JD. Computer supported multimodal monitoring bed-side in neurointensive care. *Int J Clin Monit Comput* 1994;11:223–232.
14. Chan KH, Dearden NM, Miller JD, Midgley S, Piper IR. Transcranial Doppler waveform differences in hyperemic and nonhyperemic patients after severe head injury. *Surg Neurol* 1992;38:433–436.
15. Steiner LA, Czosnyka M. Should we measure cerebral blood flow in head-injured patients? *Br J Neurosurg* 2002;16:429–439.
16. Pickard JD, Czosnyka M. Management of raised intracranial pressure. *J Neurol Neurosurg Psychiatry* 1993;56:845–858.
17. Zhong J, Dujovny M, Park HK, Perez E, Perlin AR, Diaz FG. Advances in ICP monitoring techniques. *Neurol Res* 2003;25:339–350.
18. Rosner MJ, Rosner SD, Johnson AH. Cerebral perfusion pressure: management protocol and clinical results. *J Neurosurg* 1995;83:949–962.
19. Melot C, Berre J, Moraine JJ, Kahn RJ. Estimation of cerebral blood flow at bedside by continuous jugular thermodilution. *J Cereb Blood Flow Metab* 1996;16:1263–1270.
20. Wietasch GJ, Mielck F, Scholz M, von Spiegel T, Stephan H, Hoeft A. Bedside assessment of cerebral blood flow by double-indicator dilution technique. *Anesthesiology* 2000;92:367–375.
21. Sioutos PJ, Orozco JA, Carter LP, Weinand ME, Hamilton AJ, Williams FC. Continuous regional cerebral cortical blood flow monitoring in head-injured patients. *Neurosurgery* 1995;36:943–949.
22. Soustiel JF, Glenn TC, Vespa P, Rinsky B, Hanuscin C, Martin NA. Assessment of cerebral blood flow by means of blood-flow-volume measurement in the internal carotid artery: comparative study with a 133-xenon clearance technique. *Stroke* 2003;34:1876–1880.
23. Latronico N, Beindorf AE, Rasulo FA, Febbrari P, Stefini R, Cornali C, Candiani A. Limits of intermittent jugular bulb oxygen saturation monitoring in the management of severe head trauma patients. *Neurosurgery* 2000;46:1131–1138.
24. Gopinath SP, Robertson CS, Contant CF, Hayes C, Feldman Z, Narayan RK, Grossman RG. Jugular venous desaturation and outcome after head injury. *J Neurol Neurosurg Psychiatry* 1994;57:717–723.
25. Manno EM. Transcranial Doppler ultrasonography in the neurocritical care unit. *Crit Care Clin* 1997;13:79–104.
26. Kirkpatrick PJ, Smielewski P, Czosnyka M, Menon DK, Pickard JD. Near-infrared spectroscopy use in patients with head injury. *J Neurosurg* 1995;83:963–970.
27. Lam JM, Hsiang JN, Poon WS. Monitoring of autoregulation using laser Doppler flowmetry in patients with head injury. *J Neurosurg* 1997;86:438–445.
28. van den Brink WA, van Santbrink H, Steyerberg EW, Avezaat CJ, Suazo JA, Hogesteeger C, Jansen WJ,

Kloos LM, Vermeulen J, Maas AI. Brain oxygen tension in severe head injury. *Neurosurgery* 2000; 46:868–876.

29. Charbel FT, Du X, Hoffman WE, Ausman JI. Brain tissue Po_2, Pco_2, and pH during cerebral vasospasm. *Surg Neurol* 2000;54:432–437.

30. Ungerstedt U. Microdialysis—principles and applications for studies in animals and man. *J Intern Med* 1991;230:365–373.

31. Dietrich WD. The importance of brain temperature in cerebral injury. *J Neurotrauma* 1992;9(Suppl 2): S475–485.

32. Vivien B, Paqueron X, Le Cosquer P, Langeron O, Coriat P, Riou B. Detection of brain death onset using the bispectral index in severely comatose patients. *Intensive Care Med* 2002;28:419–425.

33. Brown JI, Moulton RJ, Konasiewicz SJ, Baker AJ. Cerebral oxidative metabolism and evoked potential deterioration after severe brain injury: new evidence of early posttraumatic ischemia. *Neurosurgery* 1998; 42:1057–1063.

34. Klingelhofer J, Conrad B, Benecke R, Sander D, Markakis E. Evaluation of intracranial pressure from transcranial Doppler studies in cerebral disease. *J Neurol* 1988;235:159–162.

35. Dewey RC, Pieper HP, Hunt WE. Experimental cerebral hemodynamics: vasomotor tone, critical closing pressure, and vascular bed resistance. *Neurosurgery* 1974;41:597–606.

36. Aaslid R, Lundar T, Lindegaard K-F, et al. Estimation of cerebral perfusion pressure from arterial blood pressure and transcranial Doppler recordings. In Miller JD, Teasdale GM, Rowan JO, Galbraith SL, Mendelow AD, eds. *Intracranial Pressure*, vol. VI. Berlin, Springer Verlag, 1986:229–231.

37. Schmidt EA, Czosnyka M, Gooskens I, Piechnik SK, Matta BF, Whitfield PC, Pickard JD. Preliminary experience of the estimation of cerebral perfusion pressure using transcranial Doppler ultrasonography. *J Neurol Neurosurg Psychiatry* 2001;70:198–204.

38. Schmidt B, Klingelhofer J, Schwarze JJ, Sander D, Wittich I. Noninvasive prediction of intracranial pressure curves using transcranial Doppler ultrasonography and blood pressure curves. *Stroke* 1997;28: 2465–2472.

39. Schoser BG, Riemenschneider N, Hansen HC. The impact of raised intracranial pressure on cerebral venous hemodynamics: a prospective venous transcranial Doppler ultrasonography study. *J Neurosurg* 1999;91:744–749.

40. Petkus V, Ragauskas A, Jurkonis R. Investigation of intracranial media ultrasonic monitoring model. *Ultrasonics* 2002;40:829–833.

41. Czosnyka M, Guazzo E, Whitehouse H, Smielewski P, Czosnyka Z, Kirkpatrick P, Piechnik S, Pickard JD. Significance of intracranial pressure waveform analysis after head injury. *Acta Neurochir (Wien)* 1996;138: 531–542.

42. Czosnyka M, Smielewski P, Kirkpatrick P, Laing RJ, Menon D, Pickard JD. Continuous assessment of the cerebral vasomotor reactivity in head injury. *Neurosurgery* 1997;41:11–19.

43. Lee JH, Kelly DF, Oertel M, McArthur DL, Glenn TC, Vespa P, Boscardin WJ, Martin NA. Carbon dioxide reactivity, pressure autoregulation, and metabolic suppression reactivity after head injury: a transcranial Doppler study. *J Neurosurg* 2001;95: 222–232.

44. Aaslid R, Lindegaard KF, Sorteberg W, Nornes H. Cerebral autoregulation dynamics in humans. *Stroke* 1989;20:45–52.

45. Smielewski P, Czosnyka P, Kirkpatrick P, McEroy H, Rutkowska H, Pickard JD. Assessment of cerebral autoregulation using carotid artery compression. *Stroke* 1996;27:2197–2203.

46. Steiner LA, Czosnyka M, Piechnik SK, Smielewski P, Chatfield D, Menon DK, Pickard JD. Continuous monitoring of cerebrovascular pressure reactivity allows determination of optimal cerebral perfusion pressure in patients with traumatic brain injury. *Crit Care Med* 2002;30:733–738.

47. Piper I, Barnes A, Smith D, Dunn L. The Camino intracranial pressure sensor: is it optimal technology? An internal audit with a review of current intracranial pressure monitoring technologies. *Neurosurgery* 2001;49:1158–1164.

48. Wolfla CE, Luerssen TG, Bowman RM, Putty TK. Brain tissue pressure gradients created by expanding frontal epidural mass lesion. *J Neurosurg* 1996;84: 642–647.

49. Kiening K, Schoening W, Stover J, Unterberg AW. Continuous monitoring of intracranial compliance after severe head injury: relation to data quality, intracranial pressure and brain tissue Po_2. *Br J Neurosurg* 2003;17:311–318.

50. Robertson CS, Contant CF, Narayan RK, Grossman RG. Cerebral blood flow, $AVDo_2$, and neurologic outcome in head-injured patients. *J Neurotrauma* 1992;9 (Suppl 1):S349–358.

51. Unterberg AW, Kiening KL, Hartl R, Bardt T, Sarrafzadeh AS, Lanksch WR. Multimodal monitoring in patients with head injury: evaluation of the effects of treatment on cerebral oxygenation. *J Trauma* 1997; 42(5 Suppl):S32–37.

52. Nordstrom CH, Reinstrup P, Xu W, Gardenfors A, Ungerstedt U. Assessment of the lower limit for cerebral perfusion pressure in severe head injuries by bedside monitoring of regional energy metabolism. *Anesthesiology* 2003;98:809–814.

53. Smielewski P, Czosnyka M, Zabolotny W, Kirkpatrick P, Richards HK, Pickard JD. A computing system for the clinical and experimental investigation of

cerebrovascular reactivity. *Int J Clin Monit Comput* 1997;14:185–198.

54. Steiner LA, Coles JP, Czosnyka M, Minhas PS, Fryer TD, Aigbirhio FI, Clark JC, Smielewski P, Chatfield DA, Donovan T, Pickard JD, Menon DK. Cerebrovascular pressure reactivity is related to global cerebral oxygen metabolism after head injury. *J Neurol Neurosurg Psychiatry* 2003;74:765–770.

55. Steiner LA, Coles JP, Johnston AJ, Chatfield DA, Smielewski P, Fryer TD, Aigbirhio FI, Clark JC, Pickard JD, Menon DK, Czosnyka M. Assessment of cerebrovascular autoregulation in head-injured patients: a validation study. *Stroke* 2003;34:2404–2409.

PART III
Tough Calls in Major Disease Categories

Chapter 11

Asymptomatic Carotid Stenosis Before General or Vascular Surgical Procedures

Magdy Selim and Louis R. Caplan

The incidence of perioperative stroke varies with the timing and type of surgery. More postoperative strokes occur after emergent rather than elective procedures.[1] Stroke after general, noncardiac, surgical procedures is uncommon; its incidence ranges from 0.08 to 0.7 percent.[1–3] This rises to 0.8–3 percent in peripheral vascular surgery;[4,5] 4.8 percent in resection of head and neck tumors;[6] and 2–6 percent in cardiac procedures.[5,7–9]

Although surgery and anesthesia, in general, increase the risk of stroke,[10] patients' comorbid conditions have a dominant role. Risk factors for stroke in patients undergoing surgery are similar to those in the general population. These include history of previous stroke or transient ischemic attacks (TIAs), hypertension, atherosclerosis, diabetes, cardiovascular and peripheral vascular disease, and advancing age.[11–15] Most studies have shown that the most consistent predictor of perioperative stroke is the occurrence of preoperative symptoms of brain ischemia, i.e., TIAs or stroke. Patients with previous stroke or TIAs are at increased risk of recurrent brain ischemia after surgery.[11–14] A number of studies have shown that the presence of a carotid bruit[16–18] or asymptomatic carotid stenosis[19–22] increases the risk for perioperative stroke.

Special attention has been given to the significance of the presence of an asymptomatic carotid bruit or stenosis before elective surgery and its potential impact on the incidence of perioperative stroke. Patients with coronary or peripheral vascular disease often also have coexisting carotid occlusive disease and vice versa. Indeed, studies have shown that up to 22 percent of patients undergoing coronary artery bypass graft (CABG)[21] and 28 percent of patients undergoing lower extremity revascularization[23] have concomitant asymptomatic carotid stenosis of 50 percent in at least one artery.

The Asymptomatic Carotid Atherosclerosis Study (ACAS) showed that carotid endarterectomy (CEA) and medical therapy are more effective than medical therapy alone in reducing the long-term risk of ipsilateral stroke in patients with asymptomatic carotid stenosis ≥60 percent.[24] Although reservations have been expressed about the general applicability and cost-effectiveness of the ACAS data, its results have led some clinicians to advocate diagnosing and treating asymptomatic carotid stenosis in patients presenting for cardiac and noncardiac vascular surgery.

Most of the data presented will apply to cardiac surgery, CABG in particular.

■ The Patient

A 68-year-old, right-handed musician with carotid bruits is referred for evaluation for carotid endarterectomy (CEA). His risk factors for atherosclerosis are hyperlipidemia, coronary artery disease, and a history of smoking cigarettes 15 years ago. He developed progressive angina 2 months before, and cardiac catheterization revealed three-vessel coronary artery disease. His symptoms progressed despite medical therapy.

On examination, carotid bruits were noted bilaterally. Peripheral arterial pulses were palpable. There were no focal neurological findings. A cardiovascular surgeon considered that CABG was indicated. Given the presence of the carotid bruits, he questioned the patient about any history of neurological symptoms, but the patient denied any visual, sensory, speech, or motor disturbances. The surgeon obtained a carotid ultrasound examination, which revealed a calcified plaque in the right internal carotid artery (ICA) that was occluded and a 70 percent stenosis of the left ICA. The surgeon advised the patient to undergo elective left CEA prior to CABG to "minimize the risk of perioperative stroke."

■ The Problem

- What are the predictors of carotid occlusive disease in patients undergoing surgery?
- What is the validity of preoperative screening for carotid disease?
- What is the effect of asymptomatic carotid disease on the perioperative stroke risk?
- If stroke occurs, what is its pathogenesis?
- What, if any, is the risk of carotid endarterectomy?

■ The Evidence

Predictors of Carotid Occlusive Disease

Several studies designed to determine the prevalence and preoperative predictors of carotid occlusive disease in patients undergoing cardiac and vascular surgical procedures have shown that peripheral vascular disease, smoking history, female sex, left main stem coronary artery stenosis, and presence of a carotid bruit are associated with a higher incidence of carotid stenosis.[25–27]

Significance of Asymptomatic Carotid Bruit

Clinically, carotid stenosis is often suspected through the detection of a cervical bruit during preoperative evaluation. Asymptomatic cervical bruit can be detected in 10–14 percent of all surgical patients and up to 20 percent of patients evaluated for CABG and peripheral vascular surgery.[28–30]

Studies evaluating the relationship between asymptomatic bruits and the risk for perioperative stroke have produced inconsistent results.[17,18,28,30,31] In a recent retrospective analysis of 10,860 patients undergoing coronary artery bypass, carotid bruits emerged as one of three independent variables for predicting perioperative stroke (odds ratio 1.9); other variables included advancing age and previous stroke or TIAs.[16] Similar results were reported by McKhann et al.[17] in a prospective cohort of 456 patients undergoing isolated CABG, where five factors were correlated with the risk of peri-CABG stroke: previous stroke, presence of carotid bruit, increasing age, hypertension, and diabetes. Ropper et al.[28] prospectively studied 735 patients having all types of elective surgery including CABG; the authors reported only one stroke among 104 patients with carotid bruits and none in any of 72 patients with asymptomatic bruits during the study's 3-day postoperative follow-up period. Other studies have shown no correlation between asymptomatic carotid bruits and increased risk of stroke after abdominal aortic operations.[32,33]

There is more persuasive evidence that the presence of a carotid bruit may be associated with increased risk for delayed versus perioperative stroke. In a study of 256 patients who had undergone operations for arterial occlusive disease of the lower extremities, Cooperman et al.[34] found that 35 percent of patients with carotid bruits, versus 16 percent of patients without bruits, had stroke/ TIAs during the 2–7-year postoperative follow-up study period. There was no difference in perioperative stroke or TIAs between the two groups.

A number of studies suggest that the risk for stroke correlates with the severity of the underlying carotid stenosis and not the mere presence of a bruit. Table 11-1 shows the frequency of carotid strokes or TIAs in patients with asymptomatic cervical bruits according to the severity of the underlying carotid stenosis in three different series.[35–37] Gutierrez et al.[38] used oculoplethysmography to assess the hemodynamic significance of asymptomatic carotid bruits in patients undergoing elective peripheral vascular procedures. They also reported that the incidence of perioperative stroke in patients

Table 11-1. The Frequency of Carotid Ischemic Events (Strokes and TIAs), According to Severity of the Underlying Carotid Stenosis, in Patients with Asymptomatic Bruits

Study	No. of Patients/ (Bruits)	Mean Duration of Follow-up Period	Diagnostic Modality	Frequency of Carotid Ischemic Events According to Severity of Carotid Stenosis		
				<75%	75–90%	90–100%
Norris and Zhu[35]	500/(n/a)	52 months	Carotid duplex	21.9%	43.5%*	25%
Endean et al.[36]	273/(374)	29.6 months	Carotid duplex	5.5%	13.6%*	
Mackey et al.[37]	715/(n/a)	43.2 months	Carotid duplex	11.5%†	13.2%†	
					(9.9%* with stenosis >80%)	

n/a = not available.
*Statistically significant difference.
†Annual rate.

with hemodynamically significant bruits was 16 percent versus 0 percent in patients without bruits or with nonhemodynamically significant bruits.

Patients with asymptomatic bruit often present with TIAs prior to stroke onset. Ellis and Greenhalgh[39] reported that TIAs were four times more likely to occur in patients with asymptomatic bruits (26 percent) than in control subjects (6 percent), while the incidence of stroke without warning was not different between the two groups (8–9 percent). The Asymptomatic Cervical Bruit Study Group[37] showed that the severity of carotid stenosis was the main risk factor predicting the occurrence of stroke and that progression from 50 percent to 80 percent stenosis is associated with a 3 percent increase in annual rate of stroke without warning.

The incidence of late-onset (up to 8-year follow-up) stroke, myocardial infarction, and death were significantly higher in the Framingham study cohort with asymptomatic carotid bruits.[40] However, more often than not, strokes occurred in a vascular territory different from that of the carotid bruit.[40] Barnes et al.[41] reported similar findings in patients undergoing coronary or peripheral revascularization, where the presence of asymptomatic bruit correlated poorly with perioperative stroke and patients with asymptomatic carotid disease/bruit had a higher incidence of late death and myocardial infarction. In a small study of 37 Japanese patients with asymptomatic carotid bruits using brain computed tomography (CT) scan and carotid Doppler, Iwamoto et al.[42] showed that the incidence of stroke was high in this population, where 35 percent of

patients had silent infarction on CT; most were basal ganglia lacunes. Interestingly, the CT findings did not correlate with the side of the bruit or the degree of carotid stenosis, and occurred significantly more frequently in patients with hypertension and ischemic heart disease. Taken together, these data indicate that an asymptomatic carotid bruit is an indicator of increased stroke risk, chiefly as a sign of generalized atherosclerotic disease. However, its presence per se correlates poorly with perioperative stroke risk.

Correlation Between the Presence of Bruit and Carotid Occlusive Disease

The question arises, in the presence of asymptomatic bruit or preoperative evidence of left main stem coronary stenosis, as to whether further evaluation of the carotid arteries is required. In order to arrive at an answer, one must first answer the following questions: Is there a correlation between the presence of an audible bruit and the degree of carotid stenosis? Is the degree of carotid stenosis predictive of perioperative stroke risk? And if so, would the finding of a significant asymptomatic stenosis change patient management?

The sensitivity and specificity of a cervical bruit as a sign of carotid disease is poor, since it may be caused by other conditions such as transmitted murmurs, hyperdynamic circulation, or improper auscultation. Also, an audible bruit may be absent in the presence of a hemodynamically significant carotid artery stenosis.

Cervical bruits, when they are of carotid origin, do not reflect the degree of carotid stenosis. Studies using carotid duplex ultrasound, conventional angiography, and oculoplethysmography found that the overall correlation between demonstrable carotid stenosis of 50 percent and bruits is 20–60 percent.[40,42] Thus, an audible cervical bruit is not necessarily an indicator of underlying carotid disease or local arterial stenosis.

Asymptomatic Carotid Stenosis and Risk for Perioperative Stroke

Studies have shown that the risk of stroke during CABG is high in patients with carotid stenosis and a history of previous stroke/TIAs, i.e., symptomatic carotid disease.[43,44] However, the role of existing occlusive carotid disease as an independent cause of perioperative stroke remains uncertain, especially when it is asymptomatic. Some studies suggest that patients with asymptomatic carotid disease who undergo CABG are not at increased risk for perioperative stroke.[44–46] Others have shown that the risk of perioperative stroke is increased in patients with asymptomatic carotid stenosis who undergo cardiac[19,22,47–49] and intraabdominal vascular surgery.[20] In a recent study, Evans and Wijdicks found a higher than expected risk of 3.6 percent of stroke in 284 patients undergoing general surgical procedures. One-half of the patients had strokes ipsilateral to a severe carotid stenosis.[50] Table 11-2 summarizes the risk of perioperative stroke in the territory of a diseased carotid artery in patients undergoing surgery.

Evidence suggests that the risk of perioperative stroke in patients with asymptomatic carotid disease may increase with increasing severity of the arterial stenosis.[21,48,49,51–54] In a recent case-control study using preoperative carotid ultrasound in 3069 patients undergoing isolated cardiac surgery, Hill et al.[53] showed that the presence of an asymptomatic carotid stenosis of 80–90 percent at the time of surgery increases the risk of postoperative ipsilateral hemispheric stroke by 24.3-fold. Kartchner and McRae[54] reported that preoperative oculoplethysmography indicative of 30 percent flow reduction in patients undergoing cardiac and vascular surgery was associated with increased risk for perioperative stroke. Das et al.[55] calculated the 30-day accrued mean rate, from four published series, of perioperative stroke following isolated CABG in patients with asymptomatic carotid stenosis; the mean stroke rate for patients with >80 percent carotid stenosis was 14 percent versus 3.8 percent in those with 50–80 percent stenosis. Mickleborough et al.[49] showed that the risk of stroke in patients undergoing first-time CABG increased with ultrasound-documented severity of carotid disease and ranged from 0 percent in patients without stenosis to 3.2 percent in those with >70 percent stenosis and 27.3 percent in those with carotid occlusion. The authors concluded that patients with carotid occlusion are at high risk for perioperative stroke on the occluded side. Brener et al.[48] reported a stroke rate of 16 percent after CABG in 32 patients with carotid occlusion. Furlan and Craciun[51] studied the risk of stroke associated with CABG in patients with angiographically documented carotid stenosis of 50 percent. Ipsilateral stroke occurred in 1 percent of patients with 50–90 percent stenosis, 6 percent of patients with 90–99 percent stenosis, and 2 percent with carotid occlusion. In contrast to Mickleborough et al.,[49] they

Table 11-2. Incidence of Perioperative Stroke in the Territory of Carotid Disease

Study	Surgery	% Stroke or TIA
Schwartz et al.[21]	Cardiopulmonary bypass	3.8
Gutierrez et al.[38]	Peripheral vascular	16
Barnes et al.[41]	Peripheral vascular	0
Cartier et al.[44]	Coronary revascularization	0
Dashe et al.[47]	CABG	6.25
Brener et al.[48]	CABG	9.2
Turnipseed et al.[5]	CABG and valve replacement	5
Evans and Wijdicks[50]	General surgery	3.6

concluded that asymptomatic unilateral carotid stenosis less than 90 percent or occlusion does not increase the risk of peri-CABG stroke. Schwartz et al.[21] found that 5 percent of patients undergoing cardiopulmonary bypass with unilateral 80–99 percent carotid stenosis, bilateral 50–99 percent stenosis, or unilateral occlusion with contralateral stenosis of 50 percent had perioperative hemispheric stroke. Subgroup analysis showed that no strokes occurred in patients with unilateral 50–79 percent stenosis; stroke rate for patients with bilateral carotid stenosis >80 percent was 8 percent versus 7 percent in those with bilateral stenosis >50 percent. The authors concluded that patients with bilateral asymptomatic carotid stenosis >50 percent are at greater risk for peri-CABG stroke than those with unilateral 50–79 percent stenosis.

Overall the foregoing data suggest that (1) there is minimal, if any, increase in the risk of perioperative stroke in patients with asymptomatic carotid stenosis <70 percent; (2) the risk of perioperative stroke becomes greater with increasing severity of carotid stenosis; (3) some patients with asymptomatic stenosis >75 percent are at slightly increased risk for perioperative stroke; and (4) patients with bilateral carotid stenosis, especially if high-grade, are at increased risk for stroke. There is insufficient data to accurately assess the significance of carotid occlusions in perioperative strokes. It is important to recognize that most of the above studies evaluating the risk of perioperative stroke in patients with asymptomatic carotid disease are not comparable because of confounding variables, such as differences in design (retrospective versus prospective, institutional versus multicenter), sample size, duration of follow-up, age and composition of patient population, surgical techniques, availability of imaging data, definition of the neurological deficit, and the specialty of the diagnosing physician. These variations make it difficult to reach concordant conclusions.

Mechanisms of Perioperative Stroke

Establishing a direct cause-effect relationship between carotid stenosis and perioperative stroke can be difficult. Knowledge of the pathophysiological mechanisms, timing, and subtypes of perioperative stroke provides insight to better understand the relationship between carotid disease and risk for stroke.

Atherosclerotic carotid occlusive disease is characterized by intimal thickening and plaque formation at the carotid artery. These pathological changes may be asymptomatic. However, if collateral perfusion becomes inadequate, the atheromatous plaque may give rise to symptoms either by reducing blood flow or by producing emboli. Predisposition to either of these mechanisms is believed to be facilitated by intraoperative hypotension,[48] neck manipulation during induction of anesthesia, or improper head positioning during surgery.[6,14] A hypercoagulable state, attributed to dehydration, bed rest and stasis, general anesthesia, decreased fibrinolytic activity, enhanced platelet aggregation, and increased generation of thrombin, is well known in the postoperative period.[56–58] This prothrombic state, when combined with an atheromatous plaque, may initiate thrombosis in a previously asymptomatic lesion.

Perioperative stroke can be attributed to thromboembolism, arterial stenosis, hemodynamic insufficiency, coagulopathy, or hemorrhage associated with the use of perioperative anticoagulation and hypertension.[3,11,57] There is substantial evidence that the vast majority of perioperative strokes occur in patients without carotid disease and are embolic. Emboli can originate from the heart, aorta, carotid or vertebral arteries, particulate matter, or air from the bypass pump. Hart and Hindman[57] retrospectively studied the mechanism of perioperative stroke among 24,500 patients undergoing general surgical procedures. They found that 83 percent of strokes occurred in the first 10 days of the postoperative period and were not related to intraoperative hypotension; myocardial infarction antedated stroke in 17 percent of patients; and cardiogenic embolism was the cause in 42 percent of perioperative strokes. Their study and others[1,2] indicated that perioperative atrial fibrillation is a significant cause of a large number of perioperative strokes.

Results from radiological and pathological studies also suggest that most strokes after surgery are cardioembolic.[14,59–62] Libman et al.[62] showed that up to 70 percent of strokes after cardiac surgery are hemispheric and most are bilateral or multiple, implicating proximal embolic sources such as the heart or the aortic arch. A prospective multicenter study of 2417 cardiac surgery patients from 24 U.S.

medical institutions[13] identified three principal predictors of perioperative stroke, all related to the presence or manipulation of intracardiac thrombus or aortic atheromatous plaque. The significance of aortic atherosclerosis as an important cause of CABG-associated stroke is highlighted by results from postmortem studies showing that nearly half of the patients with significant carotid stenosis have severe aortic disease as well,[63] and studies in which transesophageal echocardiography (TEE),[64] epiaortic ultrasound,[65] and transcranial Doppler[66] have shown that most microemboli are produced during surgical manipulation of the aortic arch in the presence of severe atheroma, i.e., during aortic cannulation and cross-clamping. In a recent study, Birincioglu et al.[52] prospectively investigated the effect of ultrasound-documented asymptomatic carotid stenosis of 60 percent on perioperative stroke risk in patients undergoing CABG with the off-pump technique. All patients with irregular plaques or marked calcification of the ascending aorta, detected by intraoperative epiaortic ultrasound, and those undergoing combined intracardiac procedures were excluded to minimize potential cardiac and aortic embolic sources. The authors found that carotid stenosis of 60 percent independently increased the incidence of perioperative stroke by 5.7 percent. However, they failed to report the rate of hemispheric strokes ipsilateral to the arterial stenosis and did not designate a presumed stroke mechanism.

Brain hypoperfusion is a potential threat during hypothermic cardiopulmonary bypass. Hypoperfusion and microembolization could theoretically interact to cause stroke during cardiopulmonary bypass. Reduced brain perfusion associated with low mean arterial pressure may be compounded in the presence of hemodynamically significant carotid stenosis, with resultant reduction in the clearance (washout) of microemboli.[67] The border zone regions, where blood flow is tenuous, are the most frequently affected in these low flow states.[68] Wijdicks and Jack[59] studied the radiological topography of CABG-associated strokes in 25 patients. Nineteen patients had single-territory infarcts, 6 had multiple subcortical and cortical infarcts, and no watershed infarcts were found in any patient. Libman et al.[62] reported that only 14 percent of strokes after heart surgery were in border zone regions. Limburg et al.[14] studied the

arterial territory of perioperative stroke in 122 patients undergoing general, noncardiac, surgical procedures. They found that 61 percent of strokes were middle cerebral artery territory infarcts, 18 percent posterior circulation, 10 percent multiple vascular territories, and 11 percent border zone, and that hypotension rarely accounted for postoperative strokes. Dashe et al.[47] retrospectively evaluated the topography and presumed mechanism of perioperative stroke in 1022 patients undergoing CABG and reported a higher incidence of border zone infarcts (8/22). Among 224 patients with carotid stenosis of 50 percent, 7/14 strokes were border zone, 4 of which were attributed to low perfusion. Inzitari et al.[68] recently examined the causes of stroke in the territory of a carotid artery with asymptomatic stenosis in 1820 patients participating in the North American Symptomatic Carotid Endarterectomy Trial (NASCET). They found that 45 percent of strokes in patients with asymptomatic 60–99 percent lesions are attributable to lacunes or cardioembolism. It is important to recognize that patients with cardiac diseases were excluded from this trial, which implies that the reported number of cardioembolic strokes is likely to be higher in patients with concomitant cardiac and carotid disease. Furthermore, studies using xenon CT to measure cerebral blood flow during CABG found no evidence of low flow during bypass in patients with carotid stenosis.[69]

The above data clearly indicate that (1) most perioperative strokes occur during the postoperative period and not during surgery; (2) although causes of perioperative stroke in patients with carotid stenosis are multifactorial, embolism appears to be the most important mechanism; and (3) stroke risk may be related to associated cardiac pathology, prothrombotic milieu, and surgical manipulation of the atheromatous aorta rather than the degree of carotid stenosis and its related limitation of flow.

Benefit versus Risk of Carotid Endarterectomy in CABG Patients

The risk reduction of perioperative stroke gained by prophylactic CEA in asymptomatic patients depends on several factors including the perioperative morbidity and mortality of the procedure itself.

For CEA to be beneficial it must be of low risk and the long-term probability of postoperative ipsilateral stroke must be minimal.

According to a consensus of the American Heart Association, the acceptable risk for operative morbidity or mortality on asymptomatic disease should be <3 percent.[70] The 2.7-year combined morbidity and mortality in the ACAS was 2.7 percent and the estimated 5-year risk of post-CEA stroke is 5 percent, compared to 11 percent for medically treated patients.[24] The 5-year risk of a first stroke was 8 percent (1.6 percent annually) in patients with asymptomatic carotid stenosis <60 percent, and 16.2 percent (3.2 percent annually) with 60–99 percent stenosis in the NASCET cohort.[71] Patients with severe coronary artery disease were excluded from both the ACAS and NASCET; the actual figures for morbidity and mortality of CEA are probably higher in patients with peripheral and coronary artery disease.

History of diabetes, hyperlipidemia, poor cardiac function, and high-grade stenosis or occlusions of the contralateral carotid artery are associated with increased risk for stroke following CEA.[72] These comorbidities are common in patients undergoing cardiac and peripheral vascular surgery. Myocardial infarction is the major cause of mortality following CEA.[73] Studies have shown that the actuarial rates of myocardial infarction, angina, and cardiac death are much higher in patients with pre-existing coronary artery disease who undergo CEA than in those without it.[73,74] The experience of the surgical team also influences the outcome of CEA.[75] Collectively, the above data indicate that the postoperative morbidity and mortality of CEA is likely to be higher in patients with severe coronary artery disease requiring CABG. A recent tabulation of 13 published series reported a total 30-day stroke/death risk of 7.4 percent, after CEA in patients scheduled for CABG,[55] almost twice the acceptable risk adopted by the consensus of the American Heart Association.[70] Hertzer et al.[71] reported a 5-year survival rate of 92 percent for patients who had isolated CABG without CEA versus 81 percent for patients who had both operations, suggesting that CEA does not seem to improve the long-term survival in cardiac patients with carotid disease.

There is no consensus regarding the potential benefit of CEA for asymptomatic disease prior to general and cardiac surgical procedures. Bechtel et al.[76] safely performed CEA in 41 patients, with angiographically confirmed high-grade carotid stenosis, prior to major abdominal aortic surgery. They reported a total perioperative mortality related to aortic reconstruction of 3.5 percent; no mortality or morbidity related to CEA, and only one perioperative stroke. Hines et al.[77] retrospectively analyzed the benefit of CEA in 68 patients with high-grade (80–99 percent) carotid stenosis, of which 15 underwent CABG without carotid surgery, 9 underwent CEA prior to CABG, and 44 underwent simultaneous CEA and CABG. None of the patients undergoing CEA developed postoperative stroke/TIA versus 4/15 in patients undergoing isolated CABG. The authors concluded that patients with 80–99 percent carotid stenosis undergoing CEA prior to or in conjunction with CABG have a decreased incidence of postoperative stroke. In a prospective nonrandomized study by Bilfinger et al.,[78] the risk of postoperative stroke in patients undergoing combined CABG/CEA was higher than in patients undergoing CABG alone (4.7 percent vs. 1.7 percent). However, CEA was not a significant risk factor by either univariate or multivariate analysis. The authors suggested that patients with carotid disease fall into a higher surgical risk group than those without it. Brener et al.[48] also reported that the operative mortality rate after cardiac surgery was three times higher in patients with carotid disease. However, they indicated that patients with asymptomatic carotid disease could undergo CABG safely with or without prior CEA. Palerme et al.[79] analyzed pooled data from 58 papers for 1109 patients with asymptomatic carotid disease >50 percent undergoing CABG with (554 patients) and without CEA (555 patients). The combined stroke and death rate was not statistically different for the two groups, although the trend was toward a higher stroke/death rate in patients with stenosis >70 percent who underwent combined CABG and CEA (5.5 percent vs. 5.3 percent). Goldstein et al.[80] analyzed the frequency of postoperative complications in 463 patients undergoing CEA for asymptomatic disease in 12 academic medical centers. The rate of postoperative stroke or death was 1.8 percent, rising to 8.6 percent in patients with congestive heart failure and 18.7 percent in 16 patients who had CEA performed in combination with CABG.

It is our impression after reviewing these conflicting data that (1) combined CABG and CEA is associated with higher rates of morbidity and mortality than either surgery alone; and (2) although CEA, by itself, does not appear to increase the risk for postoperative complications, it has not been shown to confer a significant reduction in short-term risk of post-CABG stroke. There are no data regarding long-term follow-up of patients with concomitant coronary and asymptomatic carotid disease who underwent CABG with or without CEA. Therefore, a long-term benefit from CEA in CABG patients can only be speculative at this time.

Bilateral Carotid Stenosis

Some physicians advocate treatment of at least one carotid artery before CABG in patients known to have bilateral hemodynamically significant lesions. Safa et al.[81] retrospectively examined the perioperative course in 94 patients with asymptomatic high-grade carotid stenosis undergoing CABG ± valve replacement. The authors reported only one perioperative stroke and no death in this group of patients, which included 17 patients with bilateral high-grade lesions and 6 with unilateral high-grade stenosis and contralateral occlusion. They concluded that asymptomatic high-grade carotid stenosis could be safely ignored during cardiac surgical procedures. Ali et al.[82] prospectively examined the perioperative course of 46 patients with asymptomatic carotid stenosis >60 percent undergoing various open-heart procedures without CEA. Twenty-seven of 46 patients had bilateral carotid occlusive disease in this series; no patient had postoperative stroke or death during a mean follow-up of 7 days. The authors concluded that cardiac procedures, without prior CEA, can be done in patients with asymptomatic carotid disease with no added risk of stroke. They recommended that blood pressure be kept stable intra-operatively, at slightly higher than normal pressure.

Timing of Carotid Endarterectomy

Among those advocating prophylactic CEA for asymptomatic occlusive disease in patients undergoing cardiac surgery, the optimal timing of CEA

in relationship to CABG is debatable. While some endorse combined procedures (CEA + CABG) under the same anesthesia, others recommend reverse-staged, where CEA is performed a short time after CABG, or prior-staged CEA, i.e., CEA before CABG. Brow et al.[83] retrospectively examined the perioperative outcome of 35 patients with carotid stenosis >70 percent undergoing CABG. The 30-day perioperative mortality rate was 4.3 percent and the stroke rate was 8.6 percent among 23 patients who had simultaneous CABG and CEA. No perioperative strokes occurred in 12 patients who had staged CEA (9 reverse and 3 prior staged); the mortality was 2.7 percent. The authors concluded that staged management of concomitant coronary and carotid disease achieves better results. Other investigators[71,84–89] have reported that simultaneous CEA and CABG can be performed with low morbidity and mortality, and that staging of these procedures may not be necessary in most patients. A meta-analysis of 16 studies revealed a trend toward increased risk for stroke and death (9.5 percent vs. 5.7 percent) during combined procedures when compared to staged procedures.[89] A more comprehensive meta-analysis of 56 studies showed that the perioperative risk for stroke was 5 percent for prior-staged CEA, 6 percent for combined CEA and CABG, and 10 percent for reversed-staged CEA.[79]

Das et al.[55] recently compiled data from several published reports from 1966 to 1999 and calculated the 30-day outcome of the following surgical strategies: isolated CABG in the presence of carotid stenosis, combined CEA and CABG, and reverse- and prior-staged procedures. Their analysis revealed that the mean stroke rate was 3.8 percent and the mortality rate was 4 percent among patients who underwent isolated CABG in the presence of carotid stenosis >50 percent. The mean stroke and mortality rates in the combined CABG + CEA series were 3.9 percent and 4.5 percent, respectively, versus 2.4 percent and 4.8 percent in the reverse-staged and 1.5 percent and 6 percent in the prior-staged series. Subsequent subgroup analysis, limited to patients with asymptomatic carotid stenosis, revealed no significant differences in stroke or mortality rate between all treatment groups. Palerme et al.[79] recently surveyed 108 Canadian surgeons concerning their beliefs and management of asymptomatic carotid disease at the time of CABG; only 1 in 5 surgeons endorsed CEA at the time of CABG.

Considering all the data, it appears that patients may do slightly better, when carefully selected, by staging the operations. The lack of significant improvement in outcome and higher rate of complications with combined CABG + CEA cast doubt on its role in patients with asymptomatic carotid disease. It has often been reserved for the sickest urgent patients with bilateral or symptomatic carotid disease and poor cardiac function. The reverse-staged approach is recommended when cardiac morbidity and mortality outweigh the risks of neurological complications, and prior staging may be suitable for patients with minimal cardiac disease.

In summary, the incidence of stroke after general, noncardiac, surgical procedures is too low to justify any routine preoperative prophylactic regimen. It is difficult to ascertain the degree of risk for perioperative stroke due to asymptomatic carotid stenosis, per se, in patients undergoing cardiac surgery. The currently available data do not substantiate an increased risk for perioperative stroke in patients with asymptomatic carotid stenosis <75 percent. Therefore, there is little evidence to support the contention that CEA before major surgery is indicated in these patients. There is some evidence to suggest that stroke risk increases with increasing severity of the arterial stenosis. A subgroup of patients with asymptomatic carotid stenosis >80 percent or bilateral high-grade stenosis may be at a slightly increased risk for perioperative stroke. Current data do not persuasively support routine prophylactic CEA prior to cardiac surgery in this subgroup. A plethora of evidence indicates that the vast majority of perioperative strokes are secondary to thromboembolism of cardiac and aortic origin. Only a minority of perioperative strokes are caused by low perfusion, attributed to carotid stenosis. This latter group, with hemodynamically significant carotid lesion, might derive benefit from early recognition and CEA. It is not certain from our review of the literature which management strategy would best minimize the risk of perioperative stroke in this subset of patients. The decision whether to do staged or combined CEA and CABG, or CABG alone, should be based on the individual patient and the surgical and anesthetic team. However, there appear to be little sound data

to support combined simultaneous CEA + CABG in patients with asymptomatic carotid disease. The available literature has not demonstrated a significant reduction in short-term risk from CABG and CEA; a long-term benefit from CEA for asymptomatic carotid stenosis to decrease the risk of post-CABG stroke is yet to be verified. The advent of carotid angioplasty/stenting adds further complexity to this problem since little data exist concerning the role of endovascular therapy in the treatment of carotid disease.

■ The Pros and Cons

Clarification of the optimal management strategy for concomitant carotid and coronary artery disease still awaits adequately powered, multicenter, randomized trials. In the absence of such trials, we advise the following approach. Routine screening for carotid occlusive disease among asymptomatic patients prior to cardiac surgery is probably unnecessary and cost-ineffective. Screening should be considered on a patient-by-patient basis. Those with TIAs and strokes with cervical bruits, and risk factors that may increase their susceptibility to stroke, should be carefully evaluated to assess the severity of their coronary and carotid disease. Noninvasive Doppler ultrasound is the most appropriate screening method. Magnetic resonance angiography (MRA) and CT angiography (CTA) provide alternative noninvasive techniques. We do not advise invasive catheter-based angiography because of its risk of complications. Although screening for asymptomatic carotid stenosis does not appear to be helpful in predicting a patient's perioperative risk of stroke, knowledge of the status of the carotid circulation is important in guiding individualized treatment plans. When significant carotid stenosis is detected, further examination should be done to clarify the carotid hemodynamics and brain protection during the operation should be employed. Transcranial Doppler,[90] perfusion MRI,[91] PET or SPECT,[91,92] or xenon CT[93] can be used to assess cerebral hemodynamic compromise from significant carotid stenosis. These techniques are likely to be increasingly utilized in the future in preoperative assessment of the cerebral reserve capacity and status of the collateral circulation.

If a patient has asymptomatic carotid disease and severe coronary artery disease, CABG or coronary angioplasty is warranted. There is a tendency among many vascular surgeons to perform both (CABG and CEA) procedures when both abnormalities are found (coronary artery disease and high-grade carotid stenosis).[94–96] We believe the carotid arteries are often given too much attention and the aorta and heart too little attention in the preoperative assessment of patients undergoing CABG. We strongly recommend that TEE should be done before cardiac surgery to identify possible cardiac and aortic lesions predisposing to perioperative clot formation. This could potentially lead to modification of the operative technique, such as changing the site of aortic cannulation and clamping, to avoid the sequelae of atheromatous arch disease. We emphasize the importance of postoperative care, including adequate hydration, and rapid treatment of cardiac arrhythmias and hypotension. The patient could be subsequently evaluated for possible CEA, if still appropriate.

In the vast majority of patients, it is safe to wait for the onset of symptoms, i.e., TIAs, before considering CEA. It is appropriate to manage such patients conservatively, by controlling comorbid risk factors, treating the concomitant cardiac disease, and using antiplatelet agents, HMG-CoA reductase inhibitors (statins) or warfarin, if indicated. However, frequent outpatient evaluation and careful review of symptoms is necessary to determine when the stenosis has become symptomatic. Carotid endarterectomy is indicated when TIAs occur during the follow-up period, since the risk of stroke rises sharply thereafter. The greatest risk for stroke is among patients with the highest degree of stenosis, history of diabetes, presence of silent brain infarction ipsilateral to the stenosis, or a combination of these factors.[68]

In patients with coronary artery disease requiring surgery and concomitant hemodynamically significant bilateral carotid stenoses or occlusions in whom surgical correction of the carotid lesion(s) is contemplated before the cardiac surgery, we recommend angioplasty with or without stenting of the carotid or coronary arteries or both.[97,98] Angioplasty and stenting should be considered when there is an experienced operator with documented low operative complication rate available. These interventional treatments for arterial stenosis are not available at all medical institutions and their value is yet to be widely confirmed by randomized trials.

Therefore, in our case, we recommend a trial of lovastatin, more vigorous dietary restrictions, and regular exercise. We also suggest repeating duplex ultrasound of the neck and TCD of the intracranial arteries. If the degree of ICA stenosis remains unchanged and the TCD does not show decreased blood flow velocities in the intracranial left ICA and its branches, we would not pursue the evaluation further at this time. If the stenosis is rapidly progressing or flow is diminished intracranially, and the patient would consider surgery, then we would order a cranial MRI/MRA of the head and neck to determine if an unsuspected infarct is present, which might shift the balance toward a decision for surgery, and to further clarify the anatomy of the left ICA lesion.

In summary, management decision-making in patients with carotid stenosis before cardiac surgery should be individualized on a patient-by-patient basis. Screening for carotid occlusive disease should be performed in those with history of stroke or TIA, and carotid revascularization is advisable if a hemodynamically significant, symptomatic stenosis is detected. Routine screening in patients without prior history of stroke or TIA is unnecessary. Although the risk of stroke or TIA may be slightly higher in patients with asymptomatic carotid bruits, this risk does not justify prophylactic carotid endarterectomy. The vast majority of perioperative strokes are embolic. The best strategy to prevent perioperative stroke is by maximizing medical management of patients' comorbidities, risk factors, and postoperative care.

■ The Main Points

- The incidence of stroke after noncardiac surgery is too low to justify any routine preoperative prophylactic regimen.
- Routine screening for carotid occlusive disease among asymptomatic patients prior to general surgical procedures is unnecessary. It should be considered on a patient-by-patient basis.
- The vast majority of perioperative strokes are thromboembolic. Only a minority of such strokes are caused by low perfusion, associated with carotid stenosis.

- Available data do not substantiate an increased risk for perioperative stroke in patients with asymptomatic carotid stenosis, per se.
- There is little evidence to persuasively support routine prophylactic carotid revascularization procedures prior to major surgery in these patients.
- Surgical patients with high-grade carotid stenosis may derive benefit from early recognition and additional evaluation, with TCD, MRA, or CTA, to assess the status of cerebral hemodynamics and vascular reserve capacity.
- Patients in whom carotid stenosis results in hemodynamically significant low cerebral perfusion, might benefit from preoperative carotid revascularization.
- It is not certain which management strategy would best minimize the risk of perioperative stroke in this subset of patients. However, there appear to be little sound data to support combined simultaneous CEA and CABG. Staged procedures are preferable.

■ References

1. Larsen SF, Zaric D, Boysen G. Postoperative cerebrovascular accidents in general surgery. *Acta Anaesthesiol Scand* 1988;32:698–701.
2. Parikh S, Cohen JR. Perioperative stroke after general surgical procedures. *NY State J Med* 1993;93:162–165.
3. Kam PC, Calcroft RM. Perioperative stroke in general surgical patients. *Anaesthesia* 1997;52:879–883.
4. Gutierrez R, Barone DL, Makula PA, Currier C. The risk of perioperative stroke in patients with asymptomatic carotid bruits undergoing peripheral vascular surgery. *Am J Surg* 1987;153:487–489.
5. Turnipseed WD, Berkoff HA, Belzer FO. Postoperative stroke in cardiac and peripheral vascular disease. *Ann Surg* 1980;192:365–368.
6. Nosan DK, Gomez CR, Maves MD. Perioperative stroke in patients undergoing head and neck surgery. *Ann Otol Rhinol Laryngol* 1993;102:717–723.
7. Mills MD. Cerebral injury and cardiac operations. *Ann Thorac Surg* 1993;5(Suppl):S86–91.
8. Breuer AC, Furlan AJ, Hanson MR, Lederman RJ, Loop FD, Cosgove DM, Greenstreet RL, Estafanous FG. Central nervous complications of coronary artery bypass graft surgery: prospective analysis of 421 patients. *Stroke* 1983;14:682–687.
9. Roach G, Kanchuger M, Mangano C, Newman M, Nussmeier M, Wolman R, Aggarwal A, Marschall K, Graham SH, Ley C. Adverse cerebral outcomes after coronary bypass surgery: multicenter study of Perioperative Ischemia Research Group and the Ischemia Research and Education Foundation Investigators. *N Engl J Med* 1996;335:1857–1863.
10. Wong GY, Warner DO, Schroeder DR, Offord KP, Warner MA, Maxson PM, Whisnant JP. Risk of surgery and anesthesia for ischemic stroke. *Anesthesiology* 2000;92:425–432.
11. Kim J, Adrian WG. Predicting perioperative stroke. *J Neurosurg Anesthesiol* 1995;7:211–215.
12. Hogue CW, Murphy SF, Schechtman KB, Davila-Roman VG. Risk factors for early or delayed stroke after cardiac surgery. *Circulation* 1999;100:642–647.
13. Wolman RL, Nussmeier NA, Aggarwal A, Kanchuger MS, Roach GW, Newman MF, Mangano CM, Marschall KE, Ley C, Boisvert DM, Ozanne GM, Herskowitz A, Graham SH, Mangano DT. Cerebral injury after cardiac surgery: identification of a group at extraordinary risk. *Stroke* 1999;30:514–522.
14. Limburg M, Wijdicks EF, Li H. Ischemic stroke after surgical procedures: clinical features, neuroimaging and risk factors. *Neurology* 1998;50:895–901.
15. Goto T, Baba T, Yoshitake A, Shibata Y, Ura M, Sakata R. Craniocervical and aortic atherosclerosis as neurologic risk factors in coronary surgery. *Ann Thorac Surg* 2000;69:834–840.
16. Puskas JD, Winston AD, Wright CE, Gott JP, Brown WM III, Craver JM, Jones EL, Guyton RA, Weintraub WS. Stroke after coronary operation: incidence, correlates, outcome, and cost. *Ann Thorac Surg* 2000;69:1053–1056.
17. McKhann GM, Goldsborough MA, Borowicz LM Jr, Mellits ED, Brookmeyer R, Quaskey SA, Baumgartner WA, Cameron DE, Stuart RS, Gardner TJ. Predictors of stroke in coronary bypass patients. *Ann Thorac Surg* 1997;63:516–521.
18. Reed GL III, Singer DE, Picard EH, DeSanctis RW. Stroke following coronary artery bypass surgery: a case-control estimate of the risk from carotid bruits. *N Engl J Med* 1988;319:1246–1250.
19. Ricotta JJ, Faggioli GL, Castilone A, Hassett JM. Risk factors for stroke after cardiac surgery. Buffalo Cardiac Cerebral Study Group. *J Vasc Surg* 21:359–363.
20. Harris EJ Jr, Moneta GL, Yeager RA, Taylor LM Jr, Porter JM. Neurologic deficits following non-carotid vascular surgery. *Am J Surg* 1992;163:537–540.
21. Schwartz LB, Bridgman AH, Kieffer RW, Wilcox RA, McCann RL, Tawil MP, Scott SM. Asymptomatic carotid artery stenosis and stroke in patients undergoing cardiopulmonary bypass. *J Vasc Surg* 1995; 21:146–153.
22. Brener BJ, Brief DK, Alpert J, Goldenkranz RJ, Parsonnet V, Feldman S, Gielchinsky I, Abel RM, Hochberg M, Hussain M. A four-year experience with preoperative noninvasive carotid evaluation of two thousand twenty-six patients undergoing cardiac surgery. *J Vasc Surg* 1984;1:326–338.

23. Gentile AT, Taylor LM Jr, Moneta GL, Porter JM. Prevalence of asymptomatic carotid stenosis in patients undergoing infrainguinal bypass surgery. *Arch Surg* 1995;130:900–904.

24. Executive Committee for the Asymptomatic Carotid Atherosclerosis Study. Endarterectomy for asymptomatic carotid artery stenosis. *JAMA* 1995;273:1421–1428.

25. D'Agostino RS, Svensson LG, Neumann DJ, Balkhy HH, Williamson WA, Shahian DM. Screening carotid ultrasonography and risk factors for stroke in coronary surgery patients. *Ann Thorac Surg* 1996;62:1714–1723.

26. Fujitani RM, Kafie F. Screening and preoperative imaging of candidates for carotid endarterectomy. *Semin Vasc Surg* 1999;12:261–274.

27. Vigneswaran WT, Sapsford RN, Stanbridge RD. Disease of the left main coronary artery: early surgical results and their association with carotid artery stenosis. *Br Heart J* 1993;70:342–345.

28. Ropper AH, Wechsler LR, Wilson LS. Carotid bruit and the risk of stroke in elective surgery. *N Engl J Med* 1982;307:1388–1390.

29. Evans WE, Cooperman M. The significance of asymptomatic unilateral carotid bruits in preoperative patients. *Surgery* 1978;83:521–522.

30. Hertzer NR, Beven EG, Young JR, O'Hara PJ, Graor RA, Ruschhaupt WF. Incidental asymptomatic carotid bruits in patients scheduled for peripheral vascular reconstruction: results of cerebral and coronary angiography. *Surgery* 1984;96:535–544.

31. Skotnicki SH, Schulte BP, Leyten QH, Tacke TJ, Arntz IE. Asymptomatic carotid bruit in patients who undergo coronary artery surgery. *Eur J Cardiothorac Surg* 1987;1:11–15.

32. Carney WI Jr, Stewart WB, DePinto DJ, Mucha SJ, Roberts B. Carotid bruit as a risk factor in aortoiliac reconstruction. *Surgery* 1977;81:567–570.

33. Treiman RL, Foran RF, Cohen JL, Levin PM, Cossman DV. Carotid bruit: a follow-up report on its significance in patients undergoing an abdominal aortic operation. *Arch Surg* 1979;114:1138–1140.

34. Cooperman M, Martin EW Jr, Evans WE. Significance of asymptomatic carotid bruits. *Arch Surg* 1978;113:1339–1340.

35. Norris JW, Zhu CZ. Stroke risk and critical carotid stenosis. *J Neurol Neurosurg Psychiatry* 1990;53:235–237.

36. Endean ED, Steffen G, Chmura C, Gupta SR, Littooy FN. Outcome of asymptomatic cervical bruits in a veteran population. *J Cardiothorac Surg (Torino)* 1991;32:620–626.

37. Mackey AE, Abrahamowicz M, Langlois Y, Battista R, Simard D, Bourque F, Leclerc J, Cote R. Outcome of asymptomatic patients with carotid disease. Asymptomatic Cervical Bruit Study Group. *Neurology* 1997;48:896–903.

38. Gutierrez IZ, Barone DL, Makula PA, Currier C. The risk of perioperative stroke in patients with asymptomatic carotid bruits undergoing peripheral vascular surgery. *Am Surg* 1987;53:487–489.

39. Ellis MR, Greenhalgh RM. Management of asymptomatic carotid bruit. *J Vasc Surg* 1987;5:869–873.

40. Wolf PA, Kannel WB, Sorlie P, McNamara P. Asymptomatic carotid bruit and risk of stroke: the Framingham study. *JAMA* 1981;245:1442–1445.

41. Barnes RW, Liebman PR, Marszalek PB, Kirk CL, Goldman MH. The natural history of asymptomatic carotid disease in patients undergoing cardiovascular surgery. *Surgery* 1981;90:1075–1083.

42. Iwamoto T, Ami M, Kubo H, Shimizu T, Tanaka Y, Umahara T, Takasaki M. Brain computerized tomographic and ultrasonographic findings in patients with asymptomatic carotid bruits. *Nippon Ronen Igakkai Zasshi* 1999;36:803–810.

43. Gerraty RP, Gates PC, Doyle JC. Carotid stenosis and perioperative stroke risk in symptomatic and asymptomatic patients undergoing vascular or coronary surgery. *Stroke* 1993;24:1115–1118.

44. Cartier R, Hamani I, Leclerc Y, Herbert Y. Influence of carotid atheroma on the neurologic status after myocardial revascularization. *Ann Chir* 1997;51:894–898.

45. Schultz RD, Sterpetti AV, Feldhaus RJ. Early and late results in patients with carotid disease undergoing myocardial revascularization. *Ann Thorac Surg* 1988;45:603–609.

46. Attum AA, Girarde R, Barbie R, Yared S, Raleigh D, Mathew T, Hymes W, Lansing A. Risk of cerebrovascular events related to open heart surgery. *J Ky Med Assoc* 1998;96:290–295.

47. Dashe JF, Pressin MS, Murphy RE, Payne DD. Carotid occlusive disease and stroke risk in coronary artery bypass graft surgery. *Neurology* 1997;49:678–686.

48. Brener BJ, Brief DK, Alpert J, Goldenkranz RJ, Parsonnet V. The risk of stroke in patients with asymptomatic carotid stenosis undergoing cardiac surgery: a follow-up study. *J Vasc Surg* 1987;5:269–279.

49. Mickleborough LL, Walker PM, Takagi Y, Ohashi M, Ivanov J, Tamariz M. Risk factors for stroke in patients undergoing coronary artery bypass grafting. *J Thorac Cardiovasc Surg* 1996;112:1250–1258.

50. Evans BA, Wijdicks EF. High-grade carotid stenosis detected before general surgery: is endarterectomy indicated? *Neurology* 2001;57:1328–1330.

51. Furlan AJ, Craciun AR. Risk of stroke during coronary artery bypass graft surgery in patients with internal carotid artery disease documented by angiography. *Stroke* 1985;16:797–799.

52. Birincioglu CL, Bayazit M, Ulus AT, Bardakci H, Kucuker SA, Tasdemir O. Carotid disease is a risk factor for stroke in coronary bypass operations. *J Card Surg* 2000;14:417–423.

53. Hill AB, Obrand D, O'Rourke K, Steinmetz OK, Miller N. Hemispheric stroke following cardiac surgery: a case-control estimate of the risk resulting from ipsilateral asymptomatic carotid artery stenosis. *Ann Vasc Surg* 2000;14:200–209.

54. Kartchner MM, McRae LP. Carotid occlusive disease as a risk factor in major cardiovascular surgery. *Arch Surg* 1982;117:1086–1088.

55. Das SK, Brow TD, Pepper J. Continuing controversy in the management of concomitant coronary and carotid disease: an overview. *Int J Cardiol* 2000;74:47–65.

56. Modig J, Borg T, Bagge L, Saldeen T. Role of extradural and of general anaesthesia in fibrinolysis and coagulation after total hip replacement. *Br J Anaesthesiol* 1983; 55:625–629.

57. Hart R, Hindman B. Mechanisms of perioperative cerebral infarction. *Stroke* 1982;13:766–773.

58. Ygge J. Changes in blood coagulation and fibrinolysis during the postoperative period. *Am J Surg* 1970; 119:225–232.

59. Wijdicks EF, Jack CR. Coronary artery bypass grafting-associated ischemic stroke: a clinical and neuroradiological study. *J Neuroimaging* 1996;6:20–22.

60. Moody DM, Bell MA, Challa VR, Johnston WE, Prough DS. Brain microemboli during cardiac surgery or aortography. *Ann Neurol* 1990;28:477–486.

61. Masuda J, Yutani C, Ogata J, Kuriyama Y, Yamaguchi T. Atheromatous embolism in the brain: a clinicopathological analysis of 15 autopsy cases. *Neurology* 1994;44:1231–1237.

62. Libman RB, Wirkowski E, Neystat M, Barr W, Gelb S, Graver M. Stroke associated with cardiac surgery: determinants, timing, and stroke subtypes. *Arch Neurol* 1997;54:83–87.

63. Myers SI, Valentine RJ, Estrera A, Clagett GP. The intra-aortic balloon pump, a novel addition to staged repair of combined symptomatic cerebrovascular and coronary artery disease. *Ann Vasc Surg* 1993;7:239–242.

64. Hartman G, Yao F, Bruefach M, Barbu D, Peterson J, Prucell M, et al. Severity of aortic atheromatous disease diagnosed by transesophageal echocardiography predicts stroke and other outcomes associated with coronary artery surgery: a prospective study. *Anesth Analg* 1996;83:701–708.

65. Davila-Roman V, Barzilai B, Wareing T, Murphy S, Kouchoukos N. Intraoperative ultrasonographic evaluation of the ascending aorta in 100 consecutive patients undergoing cardiac surgery. *Circulation* 1991;84: III47–53.

66. Barbut D, Hinton R, Szatrowski T, Hartman G, Bruefach M, Williams-Russo P, Charlson ME, Gold JP. Cerebral emboli detected during bypass surgery are associated with clamp removal. *Stroke* 1994;25: 2398–2402.

67. Caplan LR, Hennerici M. Impaired clearance of emboli is an important link between hypoperfusion, embolism, and ischemic stroke. *Arch Neurol* 1998;55:1475–1482.

68. Inzitari D, Eliasziw M, Gates P, Sharpe B, Chan R, Meldrum H, Barnett HJ. The causes and risk of stroke in patients with asymptomatic internal carotid artery stenosis. *N Engl J Med* 2000;342:1693–1700.

69. Johnsson P, Algotsson L, Ryding E, Stahl E, Messeter K. Cardiopulmonary perfusion and cerebral blood flow in bilateral carotid artery disease. *Ann Thorac Surg* 1991;51:579–584.

70. Moore W, Barnett H, Beebe H, Bernstein E, Brener B, Brott T, Caplan L, Day A, Goldstone J, Hobson R. Guidelines for carotid endarterectomy: a multidisciplinary consensus statement from the Ad Hoc Committee, American Heart Association. *Stroke* 1995;26:188–201.

71. Hertzer NR, Loop FD, Beven EG, O'Hara PJ, Krajewski LP. Surgical staging for simultaneous coronary and carotid disease: a study including prospective randomization. *J Vasc Surg* 1989;9:455–463.

72. Barnett HJM, Taylor DW, Eliasziw M, Fox AJ, Ferguson GG, Haynes RB, Rankin RN, Clagett GP, Hachinski VC, Sackett DL, Thorpe KE, Meldrum HE. Benefit of carotid endarterectomy in patients with symptomatic moderate or severe stenosis. The North American Symptomatic Carotid Endarterectomy Trial Collaborators. *N Engl J Med* 1998;339:1415–1425.

73. Salenius JP, Harju E, Rickkinen H. Early cerebral complications in carotid endarterectomy: risk factors. *J Cardiovasc Surg* 1990;31:162–167.

74. Hertzer NR, Lees CD. Fatal myocardial infarction following carotid endarterectomy. *Ann Surg* 1981;194: 212–218.

75. Riles TS, Kopelman I, Imparato AM. Myocardial infarction following carotid endarterectomy: a review of 683 operations. *Surgery* 1979;85:249–252.

76. Bechtel JF, Bartels C, Hopstein S, Horsch S. Carotid endarterectomy prior to major abdominal aortic surgery. *J Cardiovasc Surg (Torino)* 2000;41:269–273.

77. Hines GL, Scott WC, Schubach SL, Kofsky E, Wehbe U, Cabasino E. Prophylactic carotid endarterectomy in patients with high-grade carotid stenosis undergoing coronary bypass: does it decrease the incidence of perioperative stroke? *Ann Vasc Surg* 1998;12:23–27.

78. Bilfinger TV, Reda H, Giron F, Seifert FC, Ricotta JJ. Coronary and carotid operations under prospective standardized conditions: incidence and outcome. *Ann Thorac Surg* 2000;69:1792–1798.

79. Palerme LP, Hill AB, Obrand D, Steinmetz OK. Is Canadian cardiac surgeons' management of asymptomatic carotid artery stenosis at coronary artery bypass supported by the literature? A survey and a critical appraisal of the literature. *Can J Surg* 2000;43:93–103.

80. Goldstein LB, Samsa GP, Matchar DB, Oddone EZ. Multicenter review of prospective risk factors for endarterectomy of asymptomatic carotid artery stenosis. *Stroke* 1998;29:750–753.

81. Safa TK, Friedman S, Mehta M, Rahmani O, Scher L, Pogo G, Hall M. Management of coexisting coronary artery and asymptomatic carotid artery disease: report of a series of patients treated with coronary bypass alone. *Eur J Endovasc Surg* 1999;17:249–252.

82. Ali M, Cummings B, Sullivan J, Francis S. The risk of cerebrovascular accident in patients with asymptomatic critical carotid artery stenosis who undergo open-heart surgery. *Can J Surg* 1998;41:374–378.

83. Brow TD, Kakkar VV, Pepper JR, Das SK. Toward a rational management of concomitant carotid and coronary artery disease. *J Cardiovasc Surg (Torino)* 1999;40:837–844.

84. Donatelli F, Pelenghi S, Pocar M, Moneta A, Grossi A. Combined carotid and cardiac procedures: improved results and surgical approach. *Cardiovasc Surg* 1998;6:506–510.

85. Carrel T, Stillhard G, Turina M. Combined carotid and coronary artery surgery: early and late results. *Cardiology* 1992;80:118–125.

86. Minami K, Fukahara K, Boethig D, Bairaktairs A, Fritzsche D, Koerfer R. Long-term results of simultaneous carotid endarterectomy and myocardial revascularization with cardiopulmonary bypass used for both procedures. *J Thorac Cardiovasc Surg* 2000;119: 764–773.

87. Busch T, Sirbu H, Aleksic I, Kazmaier S, Friedrich M, Buhre W, Dalichau H. Combined approach for internal carotid artery stenosis and cardiovascular disease in septuagenarians—a comparative study. *Eur J Cardiothorac Surg* 1999;16:602–606.

88. Terramani TT, Rowe VL, Hood DB, Eton D, Nuno IN, Yu H, Yellin AE, Starnes VA, Weaver FA. Combined carotid endarterectomy and coronary artery bypass grafting in asymptomatic carotid artery stenosis. *Am Surg* 1998;64:993–997.

89. Borger MA, Fremes SE, Weisel RD, Cohen G, Rao V, Lindsay TF, Naylor CD. Coronary bypass and carotid endarterectomy: does a combined approach increase risk? A meta-analysis. *Ann Thorac Surg* 1999;68:14–20.

90. Fulesdi B, Valikovics A, Orosz L, Olah L, Limburg M, Dink L, Kaposzta Z, Csiba L. Assessment of cerebrovascular reactivity in patients with symptomatic and asymptomatic atherosclerotic carotid artery lesions. *Orv Hetil* 1998;139:623–628.

91. Kim JH, Lee SJ, Shin T, Kang KH, Choi PY, Gong JC, Lim BH. Correlative assessment of hemodynamic parameters obtained with T2*-weighted perfusion MR imaging and SPECT in symptomatic carotid artery occlusion. *AJNR Am J Neuroradiol* 2000;21: 1450–1456.

92. Kuwabara Y, Ichiya Y, Sasaki M, Yoshida T, Fukumura T, Masuda K, Fujii K, Fukui M. PET evaluation of cerebral hemodynamics in occlusive cerebrovascular disease pre- and post-surgery. *J Nucl Med* 1998;39: 760–765.

93. Shumann MU, Mirzai S, Samii M, Vorkapic P. Xenon CT CBF measurements as valuable diagnostic tool in a case of bilateral occlusive cerebrovascular disease associated with intracranial aneurysm. *Acta Neurol Scand Suppl* 1996;166:104–109.

94. Char D, Cuadra S, Ricotta J, Bilfinger T, Giron F, McLarty A, Krukenkamp I, Saltman A, Seifert F. Combined coronary artery bypass and carotid endarterectomy: long-term results. *Cardiovasc Surg* 2002;10:111–115.

95. Zacharias A, Schwann TA, Riordan CJ, Clark PM, Martinez B, Durham SJ, Engoren M, Habib RH, Operative and 5-year outcomes of combined carotid and coronary revascularization: review of a large contemporary experience. *Ann Thorac Surg* 2002;73: 491–497.

96. Vitali E, Lanfranconi M, Bruschi G, Colombo T, Russo C. Combined surgical approach to coexistent carotid and coronary artery disease: early and late results. *Cardiovasc Surg* 2003;11:113–119.

97. Babatasi G, Massetti M, Theron J, Khayat A. Asymptomatic carotid stenosis in patients undergoing major cardiac surgery: can percutaneous carotid angioplasty be an alternative? *Eur J Cardiothorac Surg* 1997;11:547–553.

98. Leisch F, Kerschner K, Hofmann R. Percutaneous interventions combined with carotid artery stenting. *Dtsch Med Wochenschr* 2000;125:273–279.

Chapter 12

Management of Incidental Aneurysms and Vascular Malformations

Mustafa K. Baskaya, Andrew Jea, and Roberto C. Heros

Aneurysms, arteriovenous malformations (AVMs), and cavernous angiomas are a diverse group of disease entities. The debate and controversy as to when to treat incidental, asymptomatic, and unruptured aneurysm, AVMs, and cavernous malformations continues. Therefore, we only hope to familiarize the reader with the treatment dilemmas in dealing with incidental aneurysms, AVMs, and cavernous angiomas. For each disease, we shall present what we know of the natural history, trying to justify conservative or more aggressive treatment. We then explore the risks and outcome of each accepted treatment modality for the particular lesion. Finally, we shall summarize our approach to these controversies, based on existing data and our experience.

■ Incidental Intracranial Aneurysm

The Patient

A 48-year-old woman was involved in a motor vehicle accident and experienced brief loss of consciousness. The patient was brought to the local trauma center for further evaluation. On admission, she was awake, alert, and oriented but was amnestic for the events that brought her to the hospital. She had a deep frontal scalp laceration from striking her windshield but was neurologically intact.

A plain CT scan of the brain showed a small hyperdense lesion in the right sylvian fissure along the course of the middle cerebral artery (MCA). The neurosurgical service was consulted, and the patient was admitted for further studies. MRA of the brain was suggestive of a small aneurysm originating from the MCA. A cerebral angiogram confirmed the existence of a 6 mm MCA aneurysm (Figure 12-1).

Delving deeper into the history the following morning, the attending physician finds that the patient has a previous history of polycystic kidney disease and never had sudden onset of new headaches, neck stiffness, or photophobia. The passenger in the vehicle gives a clear account that the patient was fully conscious before striking her head on the windshield; the patient had not experienced syncope or seizures just prior to the accident.

Based on the patient's history, examination, and imaging studies, a diagnosis of an unruptured asymptomatic 6 mm MCA aneurysm was made. Despite the relatively small aneurysm size, the neurosurgical team decided to proceed with surgical clipping given the accessible location of the aneurysm and the low surgical risk of the patient. The aneurysm was secured without complications and the patient remained asymptomatic.

The Problem

- When is it appropriate to secure an unruptured intracranial aneurysm?
- What is the risk of rupture if the aneurysm is not treated?

177

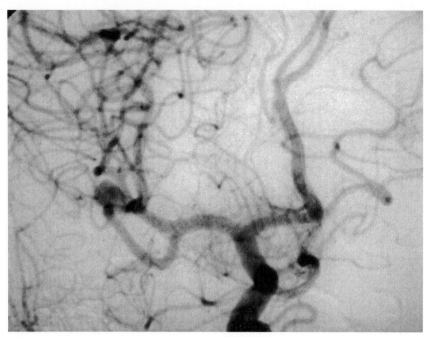

Figure 12-1. Angiogram of the patient described in case 1 with history of autosomal dominant polycystic kidney disease. A 6 mm aneurysm of the right distal middle cerebral artery is seen. This patient underwent surgery for clipping of her aneurysm because of relatively superficial location of this aneurysm and her young age. She had uneventful postoperative course and remained asymptomatic on distant follow-up.

- What treatment modality should be used if treatment is pursued?
- How should the patient be followed if the aneurysm remains unsecured?

The Evidence

The majority of aneurysms are saccular in shape and result from a combination of factors including degeneration and weakening of the internal elastic lamina and collagen fibers of the arterial wall, as well as hemodynamic effects of fluid pulsations. Certain inherited factors can increase the likelihood of aneurysm formation. Autosomal dominant polycystic kidney disease (ADPKD) is one of the most common medical conditions associated with saccular aneurysms, followed by coarctation of the aorta and a number of collagen vascular diseases. Hypertension, cigarette smoking, and cocaine use increase risk of aneurysm development and rupture.[1] Hypertension may also predict fatal outcome after aneurysm rupture.[2]

Histopathology of ruptured and unruptured aneurysms shows different features. One pathological report[3] studied walls of 45 ruptured and 27 unruptured aneurysms with immunohistochemistry. They found more significant endothelial damage, inflammatory cell invasion, and structural changes in the ruptured aneurysms. The walls of ruptured aneurysms were also more fragile. The activity of the elastase and collagenase in the vascular wall was found to be higher in cases of ruptured aneurysms than in those of unruptured aneurysms. Histopathological signs of impending rupture include unusually thin areas in the wall, sac-like pouches extending outward, patchy fibrin infiltration, layers of thrombus in the sac, inflammatory cells in the wall, and blood pigment containing macrophages and erythrocytes within the wall.[4]

Natural History

The prevalence of saccular aneurysms in the general population is estimated at 0.2–6.8 percent.[5] Because of advances in neuroimaging, the rate of detection of aneurysms has increased from 0.3 to 2 per 100,000 person-years between 1965 and 1995.[6] Annual hemorrhage risk of an unruptured intracranial aneurysm had been estimated at 1–2 percent in previous studies until the results of the International Study of Unruptured Intracranial Aneurysms (ISUIA)[7] were first published in 1998. In this study, 1400 patients with 1937 unruptured aneurysms were divided into two groups in the retrospectively studied arm: patients with no history of SAH (group 1) and those with previous SAH (group 2). Patients in group 1 ($n = 727$) had a mean age of 56 years and 25 percent harbored multiple aneurysms. Mean aneurysm diameter was 10.9 mm, and 58 percent were smaller than 10 mm. Only 10 percent were located along the anterior communicating artery (AComA) or anterior cerebral artery, and 16.9 percent were located in the cavernous sinus. In group 2 ($n = 722$), the mean age was 49.4 years and 25.2 percent still harbored multiple lesions. Annual risk of SAH from an aneurysm less than 10 mm in group 1 patients was 0.05 percent per year, far less than previously estimated. In this group, aneurysm size was the best predictor of future rupture. Also, aneurysm location independently predicted a higher risk of future SAH (aneurysms located at the basilar tip, vertebrobasilar system, posterior communicating arteries, and posterior cerebral arteries had a relatively higher risk of rupture). In group 2 patients, the annual risk of SAH from an aneurysm less than 10 mm was 0.5 percent per year, 10 times higher than that in group 1. In this group, size alone did not predict risk of future rupture and basilar tip location was the only factor associated with a higher risk of future SAH.

A recent study[8] has reported data on the long-term natural history of unruptured intracranial aneurysms (UIAs) in 142 patients with 181 UIAs. Median follow-up was 19.7 years (range 0.8–38.9 years), which is longer than in the initial report of the ISUIA. They estimated the overall annual incidence of SAH to be 1.3 percent (2.6 percent in symptomatic patients, 1.3 percent in patients with prior SAH, and 1 percent in incidental aneurysms). Smoking, aneurysm size, and age were independent predictors for aneurysm rupture.

In a recent single-institution Japanese study, the authors showed that the risk of rupture in incidental aneurysms with no history of SAH was much higher than in previous reports.[9] In particular, the risk with aneurysms larger than 10 mm was extremely high: 33.5 percent in 5 years and 55.9 percent in 10 years. The risk of bleeding in aneurysms smaller than 10 mm was similar to the results reported in many other studies, 13.9 percent risk in 10 years, which is substantially higher than reported in the ISUIA study.[9]

Results of the initial report of the ISUIA have created much controversy, and the study has been criticized based on the select nature of the retrospective cohort and the comparison between the prospectively gained morbidity data and the very low rupture rate for patients in the historical cohort who had been selected for the nonoperative intervention. It was suggested that the retrospective group had excluded patients with the highest risk of rupture and introduced data-collection bias, artificially lowering the estimated annual hemorrhage rate. This combined retrospective/prospective ISUIA report did not make a clear distinction between the risks of symptomatic and truly incidental unruptured aneurysms and did not determine the influence of genetic factors, smoking history, or concurrent diseases such as ADPKD. It is likely that the patients enrolled in the retrospective cohort between 1970 and 1991 might represent only a small portion of the total group of patients harboring unruptured aneurysms seen at the 53 participating centers. Patients may have been selectively included who were considered to harbor calcified, partly extrasubarachnoid aneurysms, who were elderly and had other medical problems, or who harbored tiny and laterally located aneurysms with low risk of rupture.

There is considerable documentation in the literature that the majority of ruptured aneurysms are smaller than 10 mm. In the analysis by Kassell and Torner[10] of 1092 patients admitted to the Cooperative Aneurysm Study between 1970 and 1977, angiographic studies revealed a mean maximal diameter of 8.2 ± 3.9 mm and a median diameter of 7 mm. 71 percent of the sacs were smaller than 10 mm and 13 percent were less than 5 mm in diameter. The MCA aneurysms were the largest and anterior communicating artery lesions were the smallest.[10]

Members of the Stroke Council[11] recommended that incidental aneurysms smaller than 10 mm in

Table 12-1. Five-Year Cumulative Rupture Rates of Intracranial Aneurysms According to Size and Location in 4060 Patients Prospectively Studied in the ISUIA

	<7 mm		7–12 mm	13–24 mm	>24 mm
	No Prior SAH	Prior SAH*			
Cavernous carotid (*n* = 210)	0	0	0	3%	6.4%
ACA/MCA/ICA (*n* = 1037)	0	1.5%	2.6%	14.5%	40%
PCom/PCA/VB (*n* = 445)	2.5%	3.4%	14.5%	18.4%	50%

SAH, subarachnoid hemorrhage; ACA, anterior communicating artery or anterior cerebral artery; MCA, middle cerebral artery; ICA, internal carotid artery; PCom, posterior communicating artery; PCA, posterior cerebral artery; VB, vertebrobasilar system.
*From a different aneurysm.

patients without a previous SAH should be observed rather than treated. Exceptions to this are aneurysms approaching the 10 mm diameter size and those with daughter sac formations and other unique hemodynamic features. Patients with a family history of aneurysmal SAH also deserve special consideration for treatment. In a study conducted in Finland, the relative risk for intracranial aneurysms among first-degree relatives in families with familial intracranial aneurysms was 4.2 (95 percent confidence interval, 2.2 to 8.0) and among first-degree relatives in families with only one affected family member it was 1.8 (95 percent confidence interval, 0.7 to 4.8) compared with the general population.[12] Surgery is favored in young patients with a previous aneurysm rupture, a family history of lesion rupture, larger aneurysms, symptoms, observed aneurysm growth, and a predictably low treatment risk. Factors favoring conservative treatment include advanced age, decreased life expectancy, comorbid medical conditions, and asymptomatic small aneurysms. A Japanese report[13] offered similar guidelines for treatment of patients with incidental aneurysms: (1) if the patient is in good medical and neurological condition, surgical intervention should be recommended when the aneurysm can easily be approached surgically and when the aneurysm size is larger than 5 mm in diameter; and (2) repeat follow-up studies using noninvasive angiogram are recommended for conservatively managed patients.

Results of a continuation of the prospective arm of ISUIA have recently been presented.[14] In a study population of 4060 patients, 1692 had no aneurysm treatment, 1917 had open neurosurgery, and 451 had endovascular treatment. The 5-year cumulative rupture rates according to aneurysm size and location are shown in Table 12-1. Compared with rupture rates in the retrospective cohort, rupture rates were higher in patients from group 1 (no prior SAH) of the prospective cohort who had unruptured aneurysms at least 7 mm in diameter, and this difference was most pronounced for aneurysms 7–9 mm in diameter. Size had little predictive value in patients with history of SAH from a different aneurysm (group 2). Aneurysms located in the posterior circulation had greater risk of rupture regardless of lesion size. On multivariate analysis, age >50 years (relative risk [RR] 2.4, 95 percent CI 1.7–3.3), aneurysm size >12 mm (RR 2.6, 95 percent CI 1.8–3.8), posterior circulation location (RR 1.6, 95 percent CI 1.1–2.4), previous ischemic cerebrovascular disease (RR 1.9, 95 percent CI 1.1–3.0), and aneurysm symptoms other than rupture (RR 1.59, 95 percent CI 1.2–2.4) were predictive of poor outcome after craniotomy. In patients treated endovascularly, only size >12 mm (RR 2.4, 95 percent CI 1.0–5.9) and posterior circulation location (RR 2.25, 95 percent CI 1.1–4.4) were associated with poor outcome. Comparison between the surgical and endovascular cohorts is not possible because of the unbalanced distribution of patients in the treatment groups of this nonrandomized study. Although the overall treatment-related morbidity and mortality at one year was lower in patients who underwent endovascular therapy, there was a high rate of incomplete aneurysm obliteration in the endovascular cohort (obliteration was judged to be complete in only 51 percent of these patients).

Surgical Indications

The presence of severe progressive symptoms from an aneurysm within the subarachnoid space is considered to be a good indication for treatment, regardless of the size of the unruptured aneurysm. In a series of 111 patients with 132 UIAs,[15] 17 percent of patients presented with acute symptoms, 32 percent with chronic symptoms, and 51 percent were asymptomatic. In patients who presented acutely, ischemia was the presenting symptom in 37 percent, headache in 37 percent, seizure in 18 percent, and cranial nerve deficits in 12 percent of cases. In patients presenting with chronic signs or symptoms, these included headache in 51 percent, decreased visual acuity in 29 percent, pyramidal signs in 11 percent, and facial pain in 9 percent. Risk of hemorrhage was not studied in this series.

An increase in aneurysm size may make treatment of UIA necessary. In a study reported from Finland, the authors followed 111 UIAs, which were mostly multiple, for almost 19 years.[16] Subsequent rupture of these aneurysms was significantly associated with lesion growth during the follow-up period. Lesions that ruptured had grown significantly more than the largest aneurysms harbored in patients who had not experienced lesion rupture. The mean diameter of intact aneurysms at the time of rupture was 11.2 mm compared with 6 mm for the remaining lesions. The mean diameter of fatal ruptured aneurysms was 13.2 mm compared with 10 mm for nonfatal ruptured lesions.[16]

Several lines of evidence suggest that AComA aneurysms, pericallosal aneurysms, and basilar artery aneurysms should be treated earlier than more laterally situated lesions. In 88 percent of 90 cases in which there were multiple aneurysms, the one with the greatest maximum external diameter ruptured.[17] Of 36 cases in which two or more aneurysms were located on the same side or on the same artery or its branch, the proximal lesion ruptured in 70 percent. The increased tendency of AComA aneurysms to rupture was supported by the fact that, of 11 cases in which the distal aneurysm ruptured, 7 cases were a combination of ruptured AComA and unruptured ICA lesions.[17,18]

The mortality rate from rupture of previously unruptured aneurysms is high and reaches up to 80 percent in some series. In the ISUIA, 1449 patients with intact aneurysms, there were 32 lesions that subsequently ruptured.[7] The mortality rate was 83 percent in the group of patients who had not experienced previous SAH from different aneurysms, and the rate was 55 percent in those who had a history of SAH. A 1993 study[19] reported a 52 percent mortality rate for patients with 27 ruptures of previously intact aneurysms. A similar mortality rate was reported in their follow-up study published in 2000.[8]

Surgical Clipping Versus Endovascular Coiling

The difficulties of evaluating coil embolization technology come from the fact that the procedure is constantly being refined and additional experience is being gained. In general, patients selected for coil embolization have had aneurysms in difficult locations for surgical approaches and, in some series, were in poorer clinical condition than those undergoing surgery. It is possible that coil embolization will be refined or replaced by new technologies.[20] In a recent review, the authors reported that elective clipping of asymptomatic unruptured aneurysms is associated with a morbidity rate of 10.9 percent and a mortality rate of 3.8 percent.[21] A meta-analysis that analyzed 28 articles published between 1966 and 1992, containing data on 733 patients with UIAs, found that morbidity and mortality rates were 4.1 percent and 1 percent, respectively. There was no statistically significant association between morbidity or mortality rates and factors such as year of publication, gender, age, aneurysm size, and location.[22] Another study[23] demonstrated that size, and not location of the aneurysm, is the main variable predicting the incidence of complications during surgery for UIAs. In properly selected patients, aneurysms less than 10 mm in size can be surgically repaired with a risk of major morbidity of about 1 percent. Surgical treatment of intermediate-sized aneurysms, between 10 and 25 mm in diameter, carries an approximately 5 percent risk of major morbidity. Conversely, aneurysms greater than 25 mm in diameter imply a 20 percent risk of significant surgical morbidity or poor outcome after surgery.

A meta-analysis that included 61 studies and involved 2460 patients and 2568 unruptured aneurysms (27 percent >25 mm and 30 percent located in the posterior circulation) reported

Table 12-2. Comparison of Surgical Morbidity and Mortality Rates for Clipped Unruptured Intracranial Aneurysms

Author	Morbidity (%)	Mortality (%)
Wardlaw and White[21]	10.9	3.8
King et al.[22]	4.1	1.0
Solomon et al.[23]	1.0 (for UIA size <10 mm)	
	5.0 (for UIA size 10–25 mm)	
	20.0 (for UIA size >25 mm)	
Raaymakers et al.[24]	10.9*	2.6*
Orz et al.[25]		0.3

*27 percent of UIAs >25 mm and 30% of UIAs in posterior circulation.

a 2.6 percent mortality rate. Permanent morbidity occurred in 10.9 percent of patients.[24]

A large study reported the experience with 1558 patients with intracranial aneurysms that were treated by surgical clipping.[25] 20 percent of these patients harbored UIAs. Of these patients with UIAs, 95 percent had a favorable outcome. Mortality rate in this group was 0.3 percent. Excellent outcome was more common in patients with aneurysms of the anterior circulation than in those with aneurysms of the posterior circulation. Table 12-2 summarizes the major morbidity and mortality results of the previous five surgical series after microsurgical clipping of UIAs.

A comparative study[26] looked at the outcome between coil embolization and surgical clipping in 216 patients who were retrospectively judged in a blinded fashion to have been eligible for either surgical or endovascular treatment. Of these 216, 118 were treated with open surgery and 98 by coil embolization. In this study, surgery was found to be associated with greater rates of early and persistent disability and more procedure-related complications.[26]

Another study[27] reported the aneurysmal regrowth in 102 patients with 160 aneurysms that were treated with direct surgical clipping at Barrow Neurological Institute. Mean angiographic follow-up was 4.4 years after clipping. Of 135 aneurysms clipped surgically that showed no residual aneurysm, 1.5 percent exhibited recurrence on later follow-up angiograms. Of 12 aneurysms with known remnant, 25 percent showed enlargement on follow-up. Rehemorrhage rate after surgery was 1.9 percent.

An outcome study[23] reported no postoperative hemorrhage from 202 aneurysms surgically treated during a mean follow-up period of 33 months. In a series of 100 patients who underwent coil embolization of 104 aneurysms, clinical outcomes were evaluated at an average of 3.5 years. None of the small aneurysms rebled, but 4 percent of large aneurysms and 33 percent of giants rebled after coil embolization.[28]

In another series containing 200 patients who underwent coil embolization, recanalization occurred in 17 percent of patients with small aneurysms with small necks, 42 percent of patients with small aneurysms with wide necks, and 87 percent of patients with large aneurysms.[29] 90 percent of giant aneurysms recanalized.

In short, in unruptured aneurysms less than 25 mm in diameter, essentially 90 percent of patients can expect a satisfactory outcome when operated by an experienced aneurysm surgeon.[23] Coil embolization treatment, for which there is less long-term follow-up data, has been found to be associated with a 4 percent morbidity rate and a 1 percent mortality rate; however, aneurysm occlusion has only been achieved in 52–78 percent of cases.[21]

The Pros and Cons

First of all, we are very careful to differentiate unruptured symptomatic aneurysms from those that are truly incidental. With rare exceptions, we recommend treatment of unruptured symptomatic aneurysms. Unruptured aneurysms become symptomatic most frequently as a result of mass effect in the brain or on cranial nerves. Much less commonly, they present with ischemic symptoms from arterial branch occlusion or emboli from clot within the aneurysm. In the first instance, the mass effect and compression of neural structures occurs usually because the aneurysm is very large or giant; when this is the case, we know that the prognosis is very poor and therefore treatment is indicated. A third nerve palsy is a special situation because the third nerve can be compressed by a relatively small aneurysm in the posterior communicating region or in the basilar artery at the origin of the superior cerebellar artery. However, even though these aneurysms may be small, the development of a new oculomotor palsy is taken by most to indicate sudden expansion or perhaps an intramural hemorrhage in the aneurysm, which could indicate that a major rupture is imminent. In these cases, treatment of the aneurysm is considered urgent by most neurosurgeons. In addition to exerting mass effect on neural structures, unruptured aneurysms may become symptomatic and present with a sudden significant headache even though there is no evidence of a subarachnoid hemorrhage on CT scan. We believe these aneurysms should also be treated urgently. Finally, aneurysms may become symptomatic through ischemic symptoms caused by unstable clot within a partially thrombosed sac. We consider this occurrence as an indication for relatively urgent treatment of the aneurysm. The possible exceptions to recommending treatment for symptomatic aneurysms include older patients with mild symptoms from an intracavernous aneurysm and elderly patients with serious comorbidities. There are also situations in which the symptomatology is relatively minor and the risk of treating the aneurysm appears to be excessive because of the location or configuration of the aneurysm. A conservative course of action in these instances may be preferable, particularly in older patients.

Whether or not to treat a truly incidental (asymptomatic) aneurysm remains controversial. There is no question that the results of the ISUIA study have influenced our practice, and we have become more conservative since learning of these results. It is clear that size of the aneurysm is important; however, it is also clear that there is no cutoff size below which rupture is not possible. Small aneurysms have a risk of hemorrhage even though this risk may be less than that of larger aneurysms. Although we have no definitive protocol or guidelines in our institution and we consider each case individually, in general, we would recommend treatment of incidental aneurysms that are more than 7 mm in diameter if the patient is relatively young and without major comorbidities (see Figure 12-1). If the patient is very young or has a family history of aneurysms or has had a subarachnoid hemorrhage from another aneurysm, we will most often recommend treatment even for aneurysms of a significantly smaller size. With larger aneurysms, we "stretch" the indications for treatment, and we treat patients who are older but still in relatively good medical health or younger patients with some comorbidities who are still likely to tolerate general anesthesia. The decision becomes more problematic with very large or even giant aneurysms that are truly incidental, but where the risk of treatment, because of location or configuration of the aneurysm, is very high. In these cases, age is important and we may tend to take the risk in a younger patient, but observe an older patient with periodic imaging. If we find prominent growth of the aneurysm on follow-up imaging, we take this as an indication for a more aggressive approach and generally pursue treatment.

The issue of treating the aneurysm with open microsurgery or endovascular occlusion remains very contentious. It may suffice to affirm that the situation is very different with unruptured aneurysms than with aneurysms that have resulted in acute subarachnoid hemorrhage. In the latter case, we pay attention to the neurological status of the patient and, under equal circumstances, prefer endovascular treatment for patients with poor clinical grade and surgery for those in good condition (grades I and II and some grade III). The size, location, and configuration of the aneurysm must be taken into consideration each time in terms of determining what is the best treatment. With unruptured aneurysms, we do not have the problem of a swollen, hyperemic, and friable brain that may be injured by retraction at surgery, and we do not have the problem of vasospasm that may be exacerbated by surgery. Therefore, we tend to lean more toward open microsurgery under equal circumstances in patients with unruptured aneurysms. The reason for this is the uncertainty about the long-term durability of aneurysm coiling as opposed to our long experience with microsurgical clipping, which clearly indicates that once an aneurysm is clipped it is extremely unlikely, though clearly not impossible, that is aneurysm will bleed in the future. However, we still pay considerable attention to the configuration and location of the aneurysm. In general, we recommend open microsurgical clipping for most aneurysms of the anterior circulation, as well as for aneurysms of the vertebral artery including those in the origin of the PICA or distal PICA or AICA aneurysms. We also tend to recommend open surgical treatment rather than endovascular treatment for aneurysms at the origin of the superior cerebellar artery and for aneurysms of the posterior cerebral artery. However, our own surgical experience with aneurysms of the basilar artery, with the exception of those at the origin of the superior cerebellar artery, has not been as satisfactory as the results we are currently seeing with endovascular treatment of these aneurysms. Therefore, for most basilar aneurysms, we currently recommend endovascular treatment.

A point that we wish to emphasize is that the evaluation of "risk versus benefit" is an ongoing process that continues until the aneurysm is secured either by clipping or coiling. It must be clearly kept in mind knowing that the risk of hemorrhage of incidental aneurysms is likely to be 1 percent or less per year. Therefore, when we undertake treatment of these aneurysms, whether by open microsurgery or by endovascular surgery, we do so under the presumption that the risk of the treatment will be very low. If we find during surgery unexpected circumstances that clearly increase the risk of treatment, we do not hesitate to "back off." This may be the case in open surgery when, for example, we find that the neck of the aneurysm is calcified or that there are vital perforators that cannot be saved and still achieve a satisfactory clipping; in these cases, we feel comfortable "backing off" and either treating the patient conservatively or recommending endovascular therapy. We take the same attitude with endovascular therapy and expect our endovascular colleagues to "back off" whenever they encounter particular difficulties at attempted coiling that would significantly increase the risk of the procedure. Similarly, these patients may then be treated conservatively or by open microsurgery depending on the circumstances.

The Main Points

- The presence of symptoms attributed to the aneurysm is essential in evaluating patients with a UIA.

- Size of the aneurysm is the most important but not the only factor to consider when deciding whether to treat a UIA.
- Individual variables such as age, comorbid conditions, aneurysm location, and presence of compressive symptoms should be weighed when considering treatment of a UIA.
- The choice of treatment modality must be flexibly adjusted to each case. However, open microsurgery offers the advantage of proven durability and higher rates of total aneurysm obliteration.
- The risk-benefit ratio should be constantly reassessed until the aneurysm is secured. If unexpected circumstances that may increase the risk of treatment are encountered during open surgery or endovascular embolization, the right decision is often to "back off" and reconsider the therapeutic approach.

■ Incidental Arteriovenous Malformation

The Patient

A 23-year-old healthy medical student volunteered for the control arm of a study on functional MRIs and mapping of speech centers in the normal population. The MRI showed findings suggestive of an AVM in the left frontal cortex (Figure 12-2A). The student was referred to the university's neurosurgery department for further evaluation.

Upon questioning and examination in a neurosurgeon's clinic, the student was found to be asymptomatic and neurologically intact. A cerebral angiogram confirmed a 3 cm nidus in the left frontal lobe with feeders from the anterior and middle cerebral arteries and with superficial venous drainage (Figure 12-2B,C). The diagnosis of an incidental Spetzler-Martin grade I AVM was made (see Table 12-3 for Spetzler-Martin AVM grading). The patient underwent uneventful surgical excision of the lesion.

The Problem

- When is it appropriate to consider treatment of an asymptomatic AVM?

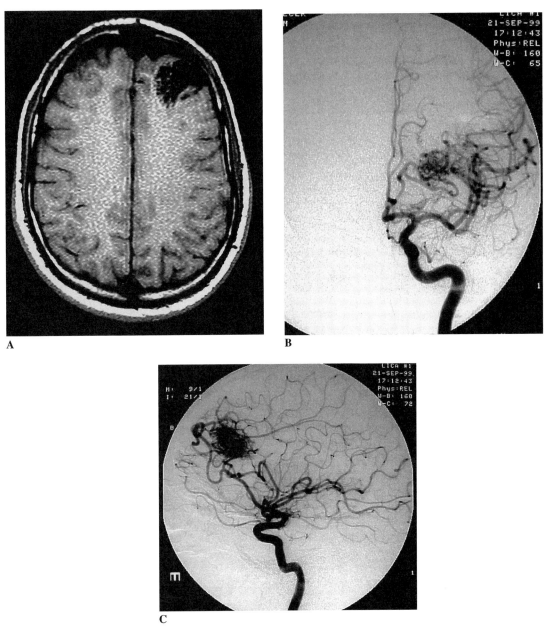

Figure 12-2. (A) T1-weighted MRI scan shows hypointense lesion in the left frontal lobe. (B, C) Angiogram shows a 3 cm AVM supplied by feeders from the left anterior and middle cerebral arteries. This patient underwent surgical removal of this AVM and made an excellent recovery without any neurological morbidity.

- What are the risks of these lesions if left untreated?
- How should the patient be followed if no intervention if pursued?
- What is the best treatment modality for these lesions?

The Evidence

AVMs are vascular abnormalities leading to a fistulous connection of arteries and veins without a normal intervening capillary bed. In the cerebral hemispheres, they frequently occur as cone-shaped

Table 12-3. Spetzler-Martin Grading of Arteriovenous Malformations

Feature	Characteristic	Points
Size[†]	<3 cm	1
	3–6 cm	2
	>6 cm	3
Venous drainage	Superficial	0
	Deep	1
Location	Noneloquent cortex	0
	Eloquent cortex	1

[†]Largest diameter on cerebral angiogram, brain MRI, or head CT scan.

lesions with the apex of the cone reaching toward the ventricles. Nearly all AVMs are thought to be congenital. Supratentorial location is the most frequent (90 percent). The most common presentation of an AVM is intracerebral hemorrhage (ICH). After ICH, seizure is the second most common presentation. Other presentations of AVMs include headache and focal neurological deficits that may be related to steal phenomenon or other alteration in perfusion in the tissue adjacent to the AVM, such as venous hypertension from arterialization of normal draining veins.

In managing unruptured AVMs, it is important to understand the natural history of these vascular malformations. The decision against treatment or to pursue a single- or multi-modality treatment paradigm also involves being familiar with the outcomes and risks of each treatment modality—microvascular resection, endovascular embolization, and stereotactic radiosurgery. Patient-related factors, such as age, general medical condition, neurological condition, and occupation, must also be taken into consideration before reaching a conclusion. The treatment of AVMs is highly individualized and opinions often conflict. There is no established algorithm or protocol to be followed when dealing with these unique problems. Recommendations are most often based on personal experience.

Natural History

A number of series have evaluated the natural history of AVMs with regard to the risk of hemorrhage. In a series of 168 patients without a history of

previous hemorrhage, 18 percent of patients had subsequent hemorrhage over a mean follow-up of 8.2 years.[30] Annualized hemorrhage rate was 2.2 percent. In another study,[31] hemorrhage risk at 1 year was 2 percent, at 5 years 14 percent, and at 10 years 31 percent. An important prospective study[32] outlined the natural history of AVMs among 160 patients who presented with symptomatic AVMs and were followed for a mean follow-up of 23.7 years. The mean age at presentation was 33 years. The rehemorrhage rate was 4 percent per year with an average interval of 7.7 years between hemorrhagic episodes. The yearly morbidity rate was 1.7 percent, and the mortality rate was 1 percent. This study demonstrated the high morbidity and mortality associated with AVMs regardless of initial mode of presentation including hemorrhage, headache, or seizure.

In a retrospective study of 96 patients with AVMs located in the basal ganglia and thalamus, the effect of deep location on natural history was emphasized.[33] The authors found a higher annual hemorrhage rate (9.8 percent per year) in AVMs located in the basal ganglia and thalamus than that of AVMs in other locations (2–4 percent per year).[33]

Several angioarchitectural factors influence the risk of hemorrhage for AVMs.

Size of AVM. In a series of 168 patients without a prior hemorrhage, the size of the AVM was not found to be predictive of future hemorrhage, utilizing a multivariate statistical analysis.[34] However, other studies have found AVMs of small size to carry higher risk of hemorrhage. One study compared the feeding artery pressures in small and large AVMs.[35] It found higher feeding artery pressures in the small AVMs and suggested that small AVMs bleed more often than large ones. However, the relationship between size of AVM and risk of hemorrhage continues to be controversial at present.

Draining Veins. Deep drainage has been thought to be an important risk factor for hemorrhage from an AVM. One correlative report[36] commented on a strong relationship between frequency of hemorrhages and presence of deep drainage in AVMs. AVMs with a single draining vein were found to have a higher risk in some studies.[37,38] This can be explained by the fact that impaired drainage through a single vein leads to a high risk of hemodynamic overload and eventual rupture. Impairment in venous drainage caused by stenosis or kinking increases the risk of bleeding.[38]

AVMs and Aneurysms.   Prevalence of the association of AVMs with aneurysms varies from 2.7 to 22.7 percent. This association seems to be correlated with a high risk of hemorrhage. A report[39] studied 91 patients with unruptured AVMs. Among these, 16 patients had 26 saccular intracranial aneurysms. They found the risk of ICH in patients with coexisting AVM and aneurysm to be 7 percent at 1 year compared with 3 percent among those with AVM alone. At 5 years, the risk persisted at 7 percent per year, while it decreased to 1.7 percent per year in those with an AVM unassociated with aneurysms. 96 percent of 26 aneurysms were located on an AVM arterial feeder.

Microsurgical Resection.   The size, location, and drainage pattern of an AVM are responsible for much of the technical difficulty encountered in surgical resection. Of the several grading systems proposed, the Spetzler-Martin grading system took these factors into consideration. It showed the best correlation for all outcome parameters and offered the best predictive value for operative difficulty and postoperative neurological condition. In assigning a grade to an AVM, the size, pattern of venous drainage, and eloquence of adjacent brain are determined based on neuroradiological studies, such as MRI and angiogram. Adding the points incurred in each category gives the grade I–V of the lesion.[40]

AVMs are considered to be small (see Table 12-3) if they are less than 3 cm in diameter (1 point on the Spetzler-Martin grading scale); medium, if between 3 and 6 cm in diameter (2 points); and large, if more than 6 cm in diameter (3 points). Venous drainage is considered superficial if all draining veins are cortical (0 points); deep if all or part of the drainage is through the deep venous system (1 point). Lesions are considered noneloquent (0 points) or eloquent (1 point) if they involve or are immediately adjacent to the sensorimotor, language, and visual cortex, the hypothalamus and thalamus, the internal capsule, the brainstem, the cerebellar peduncles, and deep cerebellar nuclei.

Total microsurgical excision of an AVM is the ideal method of treatment because it eliminates the risk of hemorrhage immediately and permanently. It may also produce improvement in neurological function and a decrease in the incidence of seizures.[41,42] There are considerable data on immediate and long-term outcome after microsurgical excision of AVMs. The morbidity and mortality is minimal for patients with Spetzler-Martin grades I and II AVMs and acceptably low for patients with grade III AVMs. However, with higher grades (IV and V), morbidity and mortality rates with surgical excision increase significantly.

In a series of 176 patients who underwent microsurgical excision of their AVMs, the authors[43] reported 0 percent serious morbidity or mortality in grade I AVMs and 100 percent of patients had excellent or good outcome while 95 percent of patients with grade II AVMs had excellent or good outcome without mortality. In grade III patients, they achieved excellent or good outcome in 88.2 percent of patients with 2 percent poor outcome and 2 percent mortality. Morbidity and mortality rates were 12.2 percent in grade IV and 38.4 percent in grade V patients. In the study[44] in which the Spetzler-Martin grading was applied prospectively to 120 patients, permanent serious neurological morbidity was reported as 0 percent in grades I to III, and 21.9 percent and 16.7 percent in grades IV and V, respectively.

Radiosurgery.   Stereotactic radiosurgery is an accepted alternative to surgical excision for the treatment of selected AVMs, particularly small lesions located in deep eloquent brain regions such as the brainstem, basal ganglia, thalamus, and internal capsule, or more superficial lesions located in the motor, speech, or visual areas. Surgical removal of these lesions is likely to result in neurological morbidity. Radiosurgery is also a valuable option in patients who are poor surgical candidates.

Stereotactic radiosurgery leads to complete angiographic obliteration in about 80 percent of lesions with a diameter of less than 3 cm at 2–3 years after radiation.[45–47] The main drawback of radiosurgery is that patients remain at risk for hemorrhage until the AVM is completely obliterated, and this risk appears to be the same as the risk of hemorrhage in untreated AVMs.[48,49] Some studies reported a hemorrhage rate after radiosurgery before complete obliteration that is even higher than in untreated patients.[50–52] One possible explanation is that radiosurgical treatment induces inhomogeneous obliteration of an AVM, leading to hemodynamic changes, such as disproportional occlusion of venous outflow in relation to arterial inflow, which could increase the risk of hemorrhage.[53]

Endovascular Embolization. Embolization serves as a useful adjunct to surgery but is rarely successful as the sole mode of therapy. Only small AVMs with one or a few easily accessible feeders can be occluded totally and permanently; these are usually the AVMs that could be removed surgically with a very high rate of efficacy and a low rate of permanent morbidity. Occlusion rates after embolization alone have been reported to be between 5 and 18 percent in the majority of series.[54] The highest rate of complete obliteration reported for AVMs selected for embolization has been 40.8 percent.[55] It should be emphasized that the reported obliteration rate refers only to AVMs selected for embolization as primary treatment, frequently because it was presumed that they could be completely obliterated endovascularly; it does not reflect the percentage of all AVMs that could be obliterated completely by embolization alone.

Even in experienced hands, embolization of AVMs carries significant morbidity and mortality. One study[56] reported 25 percent overall morbidity and 8 percent mortality rates. In another outcome study,[57] embolization resulted in severe complications in 6.6 percent, moderate complications in 15.3 percent, and mild complications in 17.3 percent of 150 patients.

There is no question about the value of embolization as a preoperative adjunct in selected patients. It significantly reduces the chance of intraoperative normal perfusion pressure breakthrough in large AVMs with very high flow[58] and decreases operative time and blood loss.[59] It is also accepted that palliative embolization (incomplete obliteration) has a role in the treatment of some patients with significant headache related to dural feeders,[57] patients with associated intracranial aneurysms,[60] and patients with a progressive neurological deficit due to steal.[61] However, the important question of whether partial embolization alone alters the natural history of AVMs remains unsettled. One study[62] compared patients with inoperable AVMs treated conservatively (seizure and headache control with medications) with patients treated palliatively with

embolization alone and found that 25 percent of patients in the conservatively treated group and 45.5 percent of patients in the palliative embolization group suffered an episode of intracranial hemorrhage during follow-up. Even though this series contained a small number of patients, their results do not support the hypothesis that partial embolization decreases the risk of hemorrhage.

In conclusion, careful consideration of the size, location, and unique angioarchitecture of each AVM is essential in evaluating the treatment risks. The final recommendation should also take into account the patient's age, medical condition, neurological status, profession, and lifestyle, with the goal of treatment being total AVM elimination with the least risk to the patient. In addition, the skill and experience of the treating team should also be carefully considered.

The Pros and Cons

With cerebral AVMs, it is important to keep in mind that the treatment is most frequently aimed at preventing hemorrhage in the future. Rarely, we treat a cerebral AVM to improve symptomatology such as intractable seizures or a progressive neurological deficit from "steal" or venous hypertension. In this context, it must be kept in mind that the risk of hemorrhage is essentially the same in a patient with an arteriovenous malformation that has never bled than that presented by a patient with arteriovenous malformations that have bled in the past (more than 6 months before).[63] In other words, in general, the risk of hemorrhage of an AVM whether it has bled or not is about 3 to 4 percent per year. After hemorrhage, the risk is about 6 percent during the first 6 months, but then it settles down to about the same 3 to 4 percent per year. This risk of hemorrhage from an unruptured AVM is considerably greater than from incidental aneurysms, a fact that is not widely recognized. Granted, the morbidity of aneurysmal subarachnoid hemorrhage is significantly higher than the morbidity of hemorrhage from an AVM, but still the latter is significant (about a 10 percent risk of death and about a 30 percent risk of serious neurological morbidity from each hemorrhage due to AVM). With these considerations in mind, we choose to treat patients harboring cerebral AVMs, regardless of whether they have bled or not in the past, whenever treatment is possible with acceptable risks.[63]

Each patient with an AVM must be approached considering a myriad of factors including the size, configuration, and location of the AVM, the age, health, and occupation of the patient, and the skill and experience of the treating team.

The ideal treatment for cerebral AVMs is microsurgical excision because it eliminates immediately the risk of future hemorrhage. Therefore, in general, we recommend surgical excision of the AVM in patients who are relatively young and in good health provided that the treatment can be accomplished with relatively low risk. As stated above, this is the case with practically all patients with Spetzler-Martin grades I and II AVMs and with most patients with grade III AVMs. As a result of an analysis of our own series,[42] as well as others from the literature, we have concluded that the treatment of grade V AVMs carries an unacceptable risk, and therefore we rarely recommend treatment of these lesions. The same is the case with the majority of grade IV AVMs, although by careful selection we have kept the risk of surgery in patients with grade IV AVMs to an acceptable level (serious morbidity and mortality of 12.2 percent).[42] When we use embolization, we use it specifically for the purpose of making the overall treatment plan of preoperative embolization and surgical excision safer. Thus, when we consider the risk of embolization, we must be convinced that the combined risk of preoperative embolization and surgery is smaller than the risk of surgical excision without embolization.

Additionally, we carefully discuss the aim of preoperative embolization with our endovascular colleagues which is simply to make the surgery safer. Generally, this entails occluding deep feeding pedicles that are inaccessible during the early surgical stages. There is no point in taking the risk of occluding endovascularly feeding pedicles to which the surgeon has immediate access upon exposure of the AVM, such as cortical middle cerebral branches in a superficial AVM. Another aim of preoperative embolization is to significantly decrease flow in AVMs that are adjacent to critical areas of the brain. This allows the surgeon to work at the very margin of the AVM with a considerably reduced risk of hemorrhage and damage to critical areas of the brain. Embolization is also useful in cases of high-flow AVMs where there is a risk of "perfusion breakthrough" from sudden occlusion of the shunt by removal of the AVM.[58] We do not feel that embolization is justified under most circumstances simply for the sake of reducing flow and making the surgery quicker and easier. We believe that there are few indications for primary treatment of an AVM by embolization without subsequent surgical excision. Simply reducing the flow to an AVM without obliterating it completely by embolization does not appear to reduce the risk of future hemorrhage, and it may even increase it. Clearly, there are AVMs that can be occluded completely with embolization, but these are usually AVMs that can be readily excised with minimal risk. Most often, when facing this choice, we prefer the latter approach because the risk is generally lower than the risk of embolization. Of course, there are patients who, because of their age or comorbidities, may be best treated by embolization to completely occlude their AVM if this is possible. There are other indications for embolization simply to reduce the flow of the AVM, such as in patients that present with symptoms from steal, with intractable headaches due to dilated dural feeders, or in patients who have particular features such as aneurysms or direct fistulae that make us presume a higher risk of hemorrhage if left untreated. We have also used "palliative" embolization in patients with large, unresectable AVMs that present with accumulating deficits from multiple hemorrhages, but we do not know if this favorably alters the natural history in these patients.

Radiosurgery is a most welcome addition to our armamentarium for treating cerebral AVMs. We recommend radiosurgery to patients who have a relatively small AVM (generally less than 3 cm, although we may stretch that limit size to 3.5 or 4 cm in some circumstances) located in critical areas of the brain where the surgical morbidity would be unacceptable. For patients with small AVMs in accessible areas of the brain, we recommend microsurgical excision given its very low operative risk and immediate elimination of the risk of hemorrhage. However, in elderly patients or in patients with significant comorbidities, radiosurgery may be considered. One treatment paradigm that we have not been enthusiastic about is that of using preoperative embolization to "reduce the size of the AVM" so that it then becomes amenable to radiosurgery.

We remain unconvinced that those parts of the AVM that appear to be completely obliterated by embolization in the immediate postembolization angiogram remain in fact occluded and without risk of hemorrhage; therefore, when we recommend radiosurgery, we recommend including all of the AVM, whether embolized or not, in the radiation field.

The Main Points

- The average hemorrhage risk of unruptured AVMs is 3–4 percent per year.
- Lesion size, location, and angioarchitecture must be considered when deciding whether to treat an AVM.
- Surgical excision remains the ideal form of treatment because it achieves immediate and total elimination of the risk of hemorrhage.
- Presurgical embolization is useful in selected instances to make surgery safer. Its objective should be to occlude deep feeding pedicles that are inaccessible during early surgical stages.
- Radiosurgery is the modality of choice for small lesions (usually less than 3 cm) located in critical areas of the brain where surgical excision is expected to result in high morbidity.

■ Incidental Cavernous Angioma

The Patient

A well-informed, well-educated, 30-year-old woman passed a billboard next to a local highway on the way to work. The billboard advertized for "whole-body MRIs" at a nearby MRI center. Having not seen a doctor for the past couple of years, the woman thought that it would be a good idea to get a whole-body MRI for screening.

A couple of days after undergoing whole-body MRI, the woman received a call from the radiologist who read her MRI. The radiologist asked her to pick up a copy of her MRI and then go to the nearest emergency room. She checked in the ER with her brain MRI. The patient denied any history of headaches, seizures, or family history of vascular malformations of the brain. Neurological examination was normal. The consultant neurosurgeon

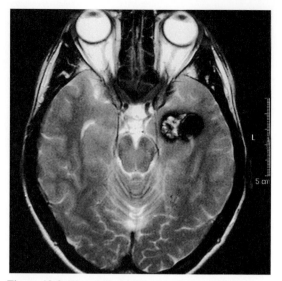

Figure 12-3. T2-weighted MRI scan shows a cavernous malformation with hemosiderin ring and a hematoma resulting from clinically silent hemorrhage. Because of the patient's young age and radiologically documented hemorrhagic event, although clinically asymptomatic, we elected to remove this lesion. The patient remained asymptomatic upon follow-up.

reviewed the MRI with the patient and explained that she had a cavernous malformation (CM) of the temporal lobe (Figure 12-3). Despite the absence of symptoms, the MRI showed signs of previous hemorrhage. Given the young age and good health of the patient, surgery was proposed. Total excision of the lesion was successfully achieved and the patient recovered without any symptoms.

The Problems

- When is treatment indicated in patients with asymptomatic CMs?
- What is the natural history of CMs according to lesion location?
- What is the role of different treatment modalities—microsurgical excision and stereotactic radiosurgery?

The Evidence

Cavernous malformations, also known as cavernous angiomas or cavernomas, are compact lesions comprised of sinusoidal vascular channels lined by a single layer of endothelium and lacking the full complement of mature vessel wall components. Between the vascular channels in the core of the lesion, there is loose connective tissue stroma without intervening brain parenchyma. Varying degrees of gliotic neural tissue may be found in the periphery of the lesion. The channels are often filled with stagnated blood in varying degrees of thrombosis and degradation.[64]

The spectrum of cerebrovascular malformations includes arteriovenous malformations, cavernous malformations, venous angiomas, and capillary telangiectasias. In a representative autopsy series, almost 5 percent of the general population harbored one of these malformations.[64,65] Although there is no reliable study that reflects the true incidence and prevalence of CMs in the population at present, the prevalence of CMs has been estimated to be between 0.4 and 0.9 percent of the population, with CMs representing 8–15 percent of all vascular malformations.[64–66]

The majority of CMs are located supratentorially, and most supratentorial CMs are located in the white matter of the cerebral hemispheres. Infratentorial CMs are located in the pons, cerebellum, midbrain, and medulla. Less frequent locations of CMs are the lateral and third ventricles, cranial nerves, and optic chiasm. Among extracerebral locations, the cavernous sinus, the orbits, and the spinal cord are the most common.

Because CMs are low-flow lesions without arterialized veins or large feeding arteries, they are poorly visualized by angiography. Computerized tomography is more sensitive at detecting CMs, but its specificity is low since most appear simply as high-density lesions with little or no contrast enhancement. This is in contrast to the high sensitivity and specificity of MRI for CMs. The MRI appearance of cavernomas has been divided into four types: a hyper-intense core representing subacute hemorrhage; a "classic" picture of mixed-signal, reticulated core surrounded by a low-signal rim; a markedly hypo-intense lesion corresponding to chronic hemorrhage; and punctate, poorly visualized hypointense foci.[67]

Conservative management with close follow-up is the right management strategy for most patients with asymptomatic CMs. In contrast to a bleeding episode from an AVM, a bleeding episode from a CM is rarely life-threatening.[68] There is more controversy with symptomatic cavernous malformations from hemorrhage in deep locations that are difficult to access. In these cases there are arguments for and against treatment and the best type of treatment—open surgery versus stereotactic radiosurgery—is the subject of debate. The key to making a proper recommendation to the patient is an understanding of the natural history of CMs; unfortunately, however, available evidence is not as solid as with cerebral AVMs.

Natural History

The rate of hemorrhage for CMs is not as well defined as for AVMs. There are several reasons for this problem. First of all, some of the published studies dealing with natural history of CMs calculated the retrospective hemorrhage rate, whereas others calculated the prospective hemorrhage rate by using new databases. The latter studies seem to be more likely to reflect the true risk of hemorrhage from a CM but their period of follow-up is shorter. Secondly, there is variability of the definition of hemorrhage in published series. Hemorrhage from a CM may not always be identifiable clinically or radiologically in contrast to hemorrhage from an AVM. This is because there is no uniform pattern of bleeding from CMs, nor is there homogenous terminology to define hemorrhagic episodes. One study[69] suggested that radiologically defined hemorrhage might miss clinically significant events. It therefore proposed to use "event rates," defined as neurological deterioration experienced by the patient as subjective worsening and associated with objective worsening of clinical status, independently of the radiological findings. Another study[70] described three patterns of hemorrhage from CMs: "slow ooze" producing the hemosiderin ring seen with MRI; "intralesional hemorrhage" producing an expansion of the lesion in MRI with or without subtle increase in symptomatology; and "gross hemorrhage" producing acute severe symptoms and intra- or extralesional acute hemorrhage in MRI. Thirdly, the clinical importance of hemorrhage from a CM is not only dependent on the degree of hemorrhage but also on the location of CM in the brain. For example, a moderate-sized intracerebral hemorrhage in the non-dominant anterior frontal lobe may not cause any neurological symptoms warranting radiological workup, while even a small intralesional hemorrhage from a CM in the brainstem or optic chiasm may produce significant neurological symptoms.

Retrospective studies have reported annual hemorrhage rates ranging between 0.25 and 2.3 percent per patient-year.[71–73] A prospective study reported a 0.7 percent hemorrhage rate per lesion-year. Another prospective study of 162 patients with CMs[71] reported an overall hemorrhage rate of 2.6 percent per patient-year. Rebleeding rate in patients with previous hemorrhage from their CMs was 4.5 percent per year in contrast to a bleeding rate of 0.6 percent in patients without prior evidence of hemorrhage. Other researchers observed a 3.1 percent symptomatic hemorrhage rate per patient per year in a series of 69 patients including 30 percent of familial cases.[65]

A study restricted to familial cavernomas[67] reported a prospective hemorrhage rate of 1.1 percent per lesion-year (6.5 percent per patient-year). The disparity in this familial series between lesional and patient hemorrhage rates underscores the high frequency of multiple lesions in familial cases. Table 12-4 summarizes the hemorrhage rates found in the previous seven retrospective and prospective case series.

Actual hemorrhage rates likely lie between the lowest retrospective rates and the highest prospective rates. Series of patients with asymptomatic lesions have traditionally included those presenting with mild headache and nonspecific symptoms. Although there are insufficient data to precisely identify which patients progress to develop symptoms or the risk factors associated with symptomatic transformation,[68] several authors have reported different factors that may influence natural history. Hemorrhage risk from a CM may be higher in females and in CMs located in the brainstem.[74] In one study, estrogen receptors were demonstrated in a few CMs in females.[75]

Immunohistochemical studies demonstrated the presence of proliferating cell nuclear antigen and angiogenic growth factors (vascular endothelial factor, basic fibroblast growth factor, and transforming growth factor alpha) in the endothelium of CMs.[66,76,77] These findings led some authors to hypothesize that CMs should be classified as slowly growing vascular neoplasms rather than true developmental vascular malformations.[66,76,77]

Familial Cavernous Malformations. Familial cases of cavernous malformations constitute 30 to 50 percent of all cases, although a referral bias may be responsible for exaggerating this frequency.[78] Familial cavernomas are believed to be transmitted as an autosomal dominant trait. The gene responsible for familial cavernomas has been localized to the long arm of chromosome 7.[79–81] They were initially characterized in patients of Hispanic descent.[78] Compared with sporadic cases, familial patients harbor multiple lesions more often. In a series of familial cases only, 84 percent of patients had multiple lesions versus roughly 20 percent of patients in nonfamilial series.[67] Sporadic and familial forms of these lesions either behave similarly or there are insufficient data to conclusively show a difference.[65]

Cavernous Malformations of the Brainstem. CMs of the brainstem constitute a special entity and pose a challenge to neurosurgeons dealing with these lesions for different reasons. CMs of the

Table 12-4. Annual Hemorrhage Rates of Cavernous Malformations

Author	Series Type	Annual Hemorrhage Rate
Kondziolka et al.[71]	Retrospective	1.3%/patient-year
Del Curling et al.[72]	Retrospective	0.25%/patient-year
Kim et al.[73]	Retrospective	2.3%/patient-year
Robinson and Awad[70]	Prospective	0.7%/lesion-year
Kondziolka et al.[71]	Prospective	2.6%/patient-year (4.5%/patient-year in rebleeding; 0.6%/patient-year without prior bleed)
Moriarty et al.[65]	Retrospective	3.1%/patient-year (including 30% familial cases)
Zabramski et al.[67]	Prospective	6.5%/patient-year and 1.1%/lesion-year (in familial cases)

brainstem rarely present incidentally. They produce more severe symptoms and neurological deficits than CMs in other locations. Clinically these patients generally present with sudden symptoms, most commonly headache, vertigo, nausea, and diplopia. The most common focal deficits are palsies of cranial nerves III to VII. In a series of 41 patients and a review of another 98 cases from the literature, none of the brainstem cavernomas presented as an incidental finding.[82]

Secondly, there is evidence in the literature that the hemorrhage rate of brainstem CMs is greater than in other locations. A series of 100 patients with CMs of the brainstem found a 5 percent per person annual risk of hemorrhage. Of 12 patients who were followed up without surgical intervention for an average of 35 months, 7 were in the same condition or better (58 percent), 4 were worse (42 percent), and one died. Another study[82] reported a 2.7 percent annual rate of hemorrhage in patients without previous hemorrhagic event and 21 percent in those with previous hemorrhage. However, it is possible that this higher rate of hemorrhages in the brainstem may be due to the fact that hemorrhages in this location are usually symptomatic and therefore easier to identify than hemorrhages from lesions in less eloquent locations.

Particularly in the brainstem, multiple bleeding episodes may increase the likelihood of a persistent neurological deficit. In the series of Porter et al., rebleeding caused debilitating and persistent deficits in 50 percent of patients with CMs of the brainstem and thalamus.[75]

Because of their critical location, brainstem CMs represent a formidable challenge to neurosurgeons. The consensus among most neurosurgeons is that patients presenting with significant neurological deficits should be treated surgically if the lesion comes to an "accessible" pial surface, such as the floor of the fourth ventricle or the lateral aspect of the brainstem. Patients with deeper lesions are generally monitored and surgically treated only if they exhibit severe progressive symptoms or if they develop permanent neurological deficits such as those that would be expected to result from surgery.

Outcomes for patients treated surgically and conservatively have been compared retrospectively. Of the patients treated surgically, approximately 84 percent had no or only slight deficit during the follow-up period. This compared favorably with the 66 percent of patients with a similar outcome among those managed conservatively.[65] Careful selection plays an essential role in obtaining acceptable surgical results.

Cavernous Malformations of the Third Ventricle. Patients with lesions in the region of the third ventricle present with a more insidious onset of symptoms related to their mass effect rather than an acute hemorrhagic episode. These lesions are typically not identified incidentally.[83,84]

Outcome is related to premorbid status, and preoperative cognitive difficulties are unlikely to resolve after surgery. Given the location of these lesions—suprachiasmatic region, the region of the foramen of Monro, the wall of the third ventricle, and the floor of the third ventricle—surgery carries a significant risk of at least transient endocrinological or neurological dysfunction.[65]

Cavernous Malformations of the Spinal Cord. A descriptive study[85] found four modes of clinical presentation in patients with CMs of the spinal cord. These presentations relate directly to the degree of extralesional hemorrhage. Patients may present with an acute onset followed by a rapid decline, an acute onset followed by a gradual decline, a slow progressive decline, or discrete episodes of decline with intervening remission. The latter clinical picture of exacerbations and partial or complete remissions is seen also with CMs of the brainstem and accounts for the fact that CMs of the spinal cord or brainstem are often initially misdiagnosed as multiple sclerosis. The symptoms of spinal cord CMs generally consist of a painful myelopathy progressing to paraparesis or paraplegia.[86] As with cavernous malformations in the region of the third ventricle, there is little information on the hemorrhage rate of these lesions.

Outcome in most recent series is good, with almost all patients showing improvement in their symptoms following surgery.[85,86] Most authors advocate surgery for symptomatic patients and believe that postoperative outcome is related to preoperative status. [85,86] These authors also advocate following lesions found incidentally in asymptomatic patients.

Extra-axial Cavernous Malformations. The majority of these lesions grow within the cavernous sinus and expand the sinus, stretching the third, fourth, and fifth cranial nerves over the pseudocapsule of the CM. The sixth cranial nerve is contained within the substance of the malformation.[87] Patients present with acute or subacute onset of visual symptoms such as diplopia, ptosis, exophthalmos, and visual acuity disturbances.

In contrast to cerebral CMs, these lesions do not have a characteristic MRI appearance. However, a radiological study[88] reported MRI features of CMs of the cavernous sinus that may help in differentiating them from meningiomas, such as dumbbell shape with a small part in the suprasellar region and a large part in the cavernous sinus, and higher signal intensity on T2-weighted images.

Surgery of CMs of the cavernous sinus carries a 36 percent mortality rate as a result of excessive bleeding. In fact, although histologically these cavernous sinus lesions look like typical CMs, at surgery they behave more like hemangioblastomas with a potential for catastrophic bleeding. This may occur if the lesion itself is entered without previous maneuvers aimed at decreasing their vascularity, such as direct intralesional embolization. In 27 of the 53 cases reviewed, outcomes for cranial neuropathies were analyzed. Twelve patients showed worsening after surgery, 11 patients showed improvement, and 4 patients showed no change.[87] Considering the benign nature of these lesions and the disability associated with an irreversible cranial neuropathy, less aggressive management may be advisable.

Stereotactic Radiosurgery. Most neurosurgeons do not currently recommend stereotactic radiosurgical treatment for cavernous malformations. The long-term efficacy and safety of radiosurgery in obliterating these lesions have not been demonstrated, and there are no series reporting even a 5-year follow-up in such patients. Evaluation of the significance of post-treatment MRI has been problematic, without clear evidence that residual lesions no longer have a hemorrhagic potential. Cavernous malformations seem to react idiosyncratically to stereotactic radiosurgery. Edema and mass effect may occur after treatment rather than obliteration of the malformation.[89] Although some centers claim that stereotactic radiosurgery for small CMs in deep locations might be superior to microsurgical excision, recent studies of stereotactic radiosurgery have revealed that, in general, radiosurgery is not a useful treatment modality for prevention of hemorrhage from a CM.[90–92]

The Pros and Cons

With increasing frequency, incidental (completely asymptomatic) CMs are being discovered during workup of a number of unrelated neurological symptoms. This is particularly true since the advent of MRI, which is very sensitive and specific for detecting CMs. However, it should be kept in mind that in spite of the great specificity of MRI for the diagnosis of these lesions, there are still occasions in which a small tumor that has bled has an identical MRI appearance to that of a CM. For this reason and to prevent future hemorrhage, we will generally recommend surgical excision of lesions that have the typical appearance of a CM and are located in an area of the brain where excision is very unlikely to lead to morbidity. We are particularly aggressive in this respect with very young, healthy patients. In a few occasions, we have been unpleasantly surprised by having found a hemorrhagic tumor in a lesion that we, as well as the neuroradiologists, thought to be a CM in the preoperative MRI.

It should be pointed out that in determining surgical morbidity for CMs, the important factor is the eloquence of the brain that has to be traversed to get to the lesion. Once the surgeon gets to the CM, excising the lesion itself is not problematic because these are very low flow lesions that can be removed essentially like a tumor without the risk of hemorrhage encountered with true cerebral AVMs. Most deep lesions, if they are not located in critical areas of the brain, can be reached through a safe trajectory with the help of intraoperative ultrasound or frame-based or frameless stereotactic guidance. The exceptions are lesions in the brainstem, basal ganglia, internal capsule, thalamus, and, of course, lesions of the primary motor or sensory regions and the visual cortex. Malformations in these locations should be managed conservatively with clinical and MRI follow-up if they are truly incidental. Another group of patients in whom surgery is not indicated are patients with incidental CMs and a clear familial history (in these cases, the diagnosis is practically certain, and there is no need to obtain pathological confirmation) or patients with multiple incidental CMs, whether familial or sporadic.

The Main Points

- Asymptomatic supratentorial CMs have a relatively low risk of hemorrhage and hemorrhage-related morbidity.
- Lesion location is the most important factor when deciding surgical treatment. Supratentorial lesions may be safely treated if no eloquent brain tissue needs to be transversed to access the lesion or if a safe trajectory can be followed with stereotactic aid to reach deeper lesions.
- Asymptomatic brainstem CMs are best managed conservatively.
- Stereotactic radiosurgery has a very limited role in the treatment of CMs.

■ References

1. Broderick JP, Viscoli CM, Brott T, Kernan WN, Brass LM, Feldmann E, Morgenstern LB, Wilterdink JL, Horwitz RI; Hemorrhagic Stroke Project Investigators. Major risk factors for aneurysmal subarachnoid hemorrhage in the young are modifiable. *Stroke* 2003;3: 1375–1381.
2. Juvela S. Prehemorrhage risk factors for fatal intracranial aneurysm rupture. *Stroke* 2003;34:1852–1857.
3. Kataoka K, Taneda M, Asai T, Yamada Y. Difference in nature of ruptured and unruptured cerebral aneurysms. *Lancet* 2000;355:203.
4. Stehbens WE. *Pathology of the Cerebral Blood Vessels*. St. Louis, Mosby, 1972:351–470.
5. Connoly PJ, Biller J, Pritz MB. Aneurysm observation versus intervention: a literature review. *Neurol Res* 2002;24:S84–95.
6. Menghini VV, Brown RD Jr, Sicks JD, O'Fallon WM, Wiebers DO. Incidence and prevalence of intracranial aneurysms and hemorrhage in Olmsted county, Minnesota, 1965 to 1995. *Neurology* 1998;51:405–411.
7. The International Study of Unruptured Intracranial Aneurysms Investigators. Unruptured intracranial aneurysms—risk of rupture and risks of surgical intervention. *N Engl J Med* 1998;339:1725–1733.
8. Juvela S, Porras M, Poussa K. Natural history of unruptured aneurysms: probability of and risk factors for aneurysm rupture. *J Neurosurg* 2000;93:379–387.

9. Tsutsumi K, Ueki K, Morita A, Kirino T. Risk of rupture from incidental cerebral aneurysms. *J Neurosurg* 2000;93:550–553.
10. Kassell NF, Torner JC. Size of intracranial aneurysms. *Neurosurgery* 1983;12:291–297.
11. Bederson JB, Awad IA, Wiebers DO, Piepgras D, Haley EC Jr, Brott T, Hademenos G, Chyatte D, Rosenwasser R, Caroselli C. Recommendations for the management of patients with unruptured intracranial aneurysms: a statement for healthcare professionals from the Stroke Council of the American Heart Association. *Stroke* 2000;31:2742–2750.
12. Ronkainen A, Miettinen H, Karkola K, Papinaho S, Vanninen R, Puranen M, Hernesniemi J. Risk of harboring an unruptured intracranial aneurysm. *Stroke* 1998;29:359–362.
13. Mizoi K, Yoshimoto T, Nagamine Y, Kayama T, Koshu K. How to treat incidental cerebral aneurysms: a review of 139 consecutive cases. *Surg Neurol* 1995;44: 114–121.
14. Wiebers DO, Whisnant JP, Huston J III, Meissner I, Brown RD Jr, Piepgras DG, Forbes GS, Thielen K, Nichols D, O'Fallon WM, Peacock J, Jaeger L, Kassell NF, Kongable-Beckman GL, Torner JC. International Study of Unruptured Intracranial Aneurysms Investigators. Unruptured intracranial aneurysms: natural history, clinical outcome, and risks of surgical and endovascular treatment. *Lancet* 2003;362:103–110.
15. Raps EC, Rogers JD, Galetta SL, Solomon RA, Lennihan L, Klebanoff LM, Fink ME. The clinical spectrum of unruptured intracranial aneurysms. *Arch Neurol* 1993;50:265–268.
16. Juvela S, Poussa K, Porras M. Factors affecting formation and growth of intracranial aneurysms: a long term follow-up study. *Stroke* 2001;32:485–491.
17. Crompton MR. Mechanism of growth and rupture in cerebral berry aneurysms. *Br Med J* 1966;1:1138–1142.
18. Weir B, Disney L, Karrison T. Sizes of ruptured and unruptured aneurysms in relation to their sites and ages of patients. *J Neurosurg* 2002;96:64–70.
19. Juvela S, Porras M, Heiskanen O. Natural history of unruptured intracranial aneurysms: a long-term follow-up study. *J Neurosurg* 1993;79:174–182.
20. Marshall LF. Effect of Guglielmi detachable coils on aneurysm management. *J Neurosurg* 2000;93:719–721 (letter).
21. Wardlaw JM, White PM. The detection and management of unruptured intracranial aneurysms. *Brain* 2000; 123:205–221.
22. King JT Jr, Berlin JA, Flamm ES. Morbidity and mortality from elective surgery for asymptomatic, unruptured, intracranial aneurysms: a meta-analysis. *J Neurosurg* 1994;81:837–842.
23. Solomon RA, Fink ME, Pile-Spellman J. Surgical management of unruptured intracranial aneurysms. *J Neurosurg* 1994;80:440–446.

24. Raaymakers TWM, Rinkel GJE, Limburg M, Algra A. Mortality and morbidity of surgery for unruptured intracranial aneurysms: a meta-analysis. *Stroke* 1998; 29:1531–1538.

25. Orz YI, Hongo K, Tanaka Y, Nagashima H, Osawa M, Kyoshima K, Kobayashi S. Risks of surgery for patients with unruptured intracranial aneurysms. *Surg Neurol* 2000;53:21–29.

26. Johnston JC, Wilson CB, Halbach VV, Higashida RT, Dowd CF, McDermott MW, Applebury CB, Farley TL, Gress DR. Endovascular and surgical treatment of unruptured cerebral aneurysms: comparison of risks. *Ann Neurol* 2000;48:11–19.

27. David CA, Vishteh AG, Spetzler RF, Lemole M, Lawton MT, Partovi S. Late angiographic follow-up review of surgically treated aneurysms. *J Neurosurg* 1999;91:396–401.

28. Malisch TW, Guglielmi G, Vinuela F, Duckwiler G, Gobin YP, Martin NA, Frazee JG. Intracranial aneurysms treated with the Guglielmi detachable coil: midterm clinical results in a consecutive series of 100 patients. *J Neurosurg* 1997;87:176–183.

29. Wong JH, Berenstein A, Setton A, et al. Safety of endovascular coil placement in unruptured cerebral aneurysms: a 10-year experience. *J Neurosurg* 2001; 94:187A (abstract).

30. Brown RD Jr, Wiebers DO, Torner JC, O'Fallon WM. Incidence and prevalence of intracranial vascular malformations in Olmsted county, Minnesota, 1965 to 1992. *Neurology* 1996;46:949–952.

31. Graf CJ, Perret GE, Torner JC. Bleeding from cerebral arteriovenous malformations as part of their natural history. *J Neurosurg* 1983;58:331–337.

32. Ondra SL, Troupp H, George ED, Schwab K. The natural history of symptomatic arteriovenous malformations of the brain: a 24 year follow-up assessment. *J Neurosurg* 1990;73:387.

33. Fleetwood IG, Marcellus ML, Levy RP, Marks MP, Steinberg GK. Deep arteriovenous malformations of the basal ganglia and thalamus: natural history. *J Neurosurg* 2003;98:747–750.

34. Lunsford LD, Kondziolka D, Flickinger JC, Bissonette DJ, Jungreis CA, Maitz AH, Horton JA, Coffey RJ. Stereotactic radiosurgery for arteriovenous malformations. *J Neurosurg* 1991;75:512–524.

35. Spetzler RF, Hargraves RW, McCormick PW, Zabramski JM, Flom RA, Zimmerman RS. Relationship of perfusion pressure and size to risk of hemorrhage from arteriovenous malformations. *J Neurosurg* 1992; 76:918–923.

36. Nataf F, Meder JF, Roux FX. Angioarchitecture associated with haemorrhage in cerebral arteriovenous malformations: a prognostic statistical model. *Neuroradiology* 1997;39:52–58.

37. Albert P, Salgado H, Polaoina M, Trujillo F, Ponce de Leon A, Durand F. A study on the venous drainage of 150 cerebral arteriovenous malformations as related to haemorrhagic risks and size of the lesion. *Acta Neurochir* 1990;103:30–34.

38. Miyasaka Y, Yada K, Ohwada T, Kitahara T, Kurata A, Irikura K. An analysis of the venous drainage system as a factor in hemorrhage from arteriovenous malformations. *J Neurosurg* 1992;76:239–243.

39. Brown RD, Wiebers DO, Forbes GS. Unruptured intracranial aneurysms and arteriovenous malformations: frequency of intracranial hemorrhage and relationship of lesions. *J Neurosurg* 1990;73:859–863.

40. Spetzler RF, Martin NA. A proposed grading system for arteriovenous malformations of the brain stem. *J Neurosurg* 1986;65:476.

41. Drake CG. Cerebral arteriovenous malformations: considerations for and experience with surgical treatment in 166 cases. *Clin Neurosurg* 1979;26:145–208.

42. Heros RC, Korosue K, Diebold PM. Surgical excision of cerebral arteriovenous malformations: late results. *Neurosurgery* 1990;26:570–578.

43. Heros RC, Korosue K. Radiation treatment of cerebral arteriovenous malformations. *N Engl J Med* 1990;323: 127–129.

44. Hamilton MG, Spetzler RF. The prospective application of a grading system for arteriovenous malformations. *Neurosurgery* 1994;34:2–7.

45. Flickinger JC, Kondziolka D, Maitz AH, Lunsford LD. Analysis of neurological sequela from radiosurgery of arteriovenous malformations: how location effects outcome. *Int J Radiat Oncol Biol Phys* 1998;40: 273–278.

46. Friedman WA, Bova FJ, Mendenhall WM. Linear accelerator radiosurgery for arteriovenous malformations: the relationship of size to outcome. *J Neurosurg* 1995;82:180–189.

47. Yamamoto M, Jimbo M, Kobayashi M. Long term results of radiosurgery for arteriovenous malformations: neurodiagnostic imaging and histological studies of angiographically confirmed nidus obliteration. *Surg Neurol* 1992;37:219–230.

48. Friedman WA, Blatt DL, Bova FJ. The risk of hemorrhage after radiosurgery for arteriovenous malformations. *J Neurosurg* 1996;84:912–919.

49. Steinberg GK, Chang SD, Levy RP, Marks MP, Frankel K, Marcellus M. Surgical resection of large incompletely treated intracranial arteriovenous malformations following stereotactic radiosurgery. *J Neurosurg* 1996;84:920–928.

50. Colombo F, Pozza F, Chierego G, Casentini L, De Luca G, Francescon P. Linear accelerator radiosurgery of cerebral arteriovenous malformations: an update. *Neurosurgery* 1994;34:14–21.

51. Pollock BE, Flickinger JC, Lunsford LD. Hemorrhage risk after stereotactic radiosurgery of cerebral arteriovenous malformations. *Neurosurgery* 1996;38: 652–659.

52. Yamamoto M, Jimbo M, Hara M. Gamma knife radiosurgery for arteriovenous malformations: long term

follow up results focusing on complications occurring more than 5 years after irradiation. *Neurosurgery* 1996; 38:906–914.

53. Lo EH, Fabrikant JI, Levy RP, Phillips MH, Frankel KA, Alpen EL. An experimental compartmental flow model for assessing the hemodynamic response of intracranial arteriovenous malformations to stereotactic radiosurgery. *Neurosurgery* 1991;28:251–259.

54. Frizzel RT, Fisher WS III. Cure, morbidity, and mortality associated with embolization of brain arteriovenous malformations: a review of 1246 patients in 32 series over a 35-year period. *Neurosurgery* 1995;37: 1031–1039.

55. Valavanis A, Yasargil MG. The endovascular treatment of brain arteriovenous malformations. *Adv Tech Stand Neurosurg* 1998;24:131–214.

56. Deruty R, Pelissou-Guyotat I, Amat D, Mottolese C, Bascoulergue Y, Turjman F, Gerard JP. Complications after multidisciplinary treatment of cerebral arteriovenous malformations. *Acta Neurochir* 1996;138: 119–131.

57. Wickholm G, Lundqvist C, Svendsen P. Embolization of cerebral arteriovenous malformations: Part I. Technique, morphology, and complications. *Neurosurgery* 1996;39:448–457.

58. Spetzler RF, Wilson CB, Weinstein P, Mehdorn M, Townsend J, Telles D. Normal perfusion pressure breakthrough theory. *Clin Neurosurg* 1978;25: 651–672.

59. Jafar JJ, Davis A, Berenstein A, Choi I, Kupersmith M. The effect of embolization with *N*-butyl cyanoacrylate prior to surgical resection of cerebral arteriovenous malformation. *J Neurosurg* 1993;78:60–69.

60. Marks MP, Lane B, Steinberg GK, Snipes GJ. Intranidal aneurysms in cerebral arteriovenous malformations: evaluation and endovascular treatment. *Radiology* 1992;183:355–360.

61. Heros RC. Prevention and management of therapeutic complications. In Jafar JJ, Awad IA, Rossenwasser RH, eds. *Vascular Malformations of the Central Nervous System*. Philadelphia, Lippincott, Williams & Wilkins, 1999:363–373.

62. Kwon OK, Han DH, Han MH, Chung YS. Palliatively treated cerebral arteriovenous malformations: follow-up results. *J Clin Neurosci* 2000;7(Suppl):69–72.

63. Heros RC, Tu Y-K. Is surgical therapy needed for unruptured arteriovenous malformations? *Neurology* 1987;37:279–286.

64. Jafar JJ, Awad IA, Huang PP. Intracranial vascular malformations: clinical decisions and multimodality management strategies. In Jafar JJ, Awad IA, Rosenwasser RH, eds. *Vascular Malformations of the Central Nervous System.* Philadelphia: Lippincott Williams & Wilkins, 1999:219–232.

65. Moriarity JL, Clatterbuck RE, Rigamonti D. The natural history of cavernous malformations. *Neurosurg Clin North Am* 1999;10:411–417.

66. Bertalanffy H, Benes L, Miyazawa T, Alberti O, Siegel AM, Sure U. Cerebral cavernomas in the adult: review of the literature and analysis of 72 surgically treated patients. *Neurosurg Rev* 2002;25:1–53.

67. Zabramski JM, Wascher TM, Spetzler RF, Johnson B, Golfinos J, Drayer BP, Brown B, Rigamonti D, Brown G. The natural history of familial cavernous malformations: results of an ongoing study. *J Neurosurg* 1994;80:422.

68. Maraire JN, Awad IA. Intracranial cavernous malformations: lesion behavior and management strategies topic review. *Neurosurgery* 1995;37:591–605.

69. Porter PJ, Willinsky RA, Harper W, Wallace MC. Cerebral cavernous malformations: natural history and prognosis after clinical deterioration with or without hemorrhage. *J Neurosurg* 1997;87:190–197.

70. Robinson JR, Awad IA. Clinical spectrum and natural course. In Awad IA, Barrow DL, eds. *Cavernous Malformations*. Park Ridge, IL, AANS, 1993:25–36.

71. Kondziolka D, Lunsford LD, Kestle JRW. The natural history of cerebral cavernous malformation. *J Neurosurg* 1995;83:820.

72. Del Curling OD Jr, Kelly DL Jr, Elster AD, Craven TE. An analysis of the natural history of cavernous angiomas. *J Neurosurg* 1991;75:702–708.

73. Kim DS, Park YG, Choi JU, Chung SS, Lee KC. An analysis of the natural history of cavernous malformations. *Surg Neurol* 1997;48:9–17.

74. Robinson JR, Awad IA, Little JR. Natural history of cavernous angioma. *J Neurosurg* 1991;75:709.

75. Porter RW, Detwiler PW, Spetzler RF, Lawton MT, Baskin JJ, Derksen PT, Zabramski JM. Cavernous malformations of the brainstem: experiences with 100 patients. *J Neurosurg* 1999;90:50–58.

76. Sonstein WF, Kader A, Hirano A. Expression of vascular endothelial growth factor in pediatric and adult cerebral arteriovenous malformations: an immunohistochemical study. *J Neurosurg* 1996;85: 838–845.

77. Sure U, Butz N, Schlegel J, Siegel A, Mennel HD, Bien S, Bertalanffy H. Endothelial proliferation, neoangiogenesis and potential de novo generation of cerebral vascular malformations. *J Neurosurg* 2001;94: 972–977.

78. Rigamonti D, Hadley MN, Drayer BP, Johnson PC, Hoenig-Rigamonti K, Knight JT, Spetzler RF. Cerebral cavernous malformations: incidence and familial occurrence. *N Engl J Med* 1988;319:343.

79. Hayman LA, Evans RA, Ferrell RE, Fahr LM, Ostrow P, Riccardi VM. Familial cavernous angiomas: natural history and genetic study over a 5-year period. *Am J Med Genet* 1982;11:147–160.

80. Dubovsky J, Zabramski JM, Kurth J, Spetzler RF, Rich SS, Orr HT, Weber JL. A gene responsible for cavernous malformations of the brain maps to chromosome 7q. *Hum Mol Genet* 1995;4:453–458.

81. Gunel M, Awad IA, Finberg K, Anson JA, Steinberg GK, Batjer HH, Kopitnik TA, Morrison L, Giannotta SL,

Nelson-Williams C, Lifton RP. A founder mutation as a cause of cerebral cavernous malformation in Hispanic Americans. *N Engl J Med* 1996;334: 946–951.

82. Fritschi JA, Reulen HJ, Spetzler RF, Zabramski JM. Cavernous malformations of the brain stem: a review of 139 cases. *Acta Neurochir (Wien)* 1994; 130:35–46.

83. Katayama Y, Tsubokawa T, Maeda R, Yamamoto T. Surgical intervention of cavernous malformations of the third ventricle. *J Neurosurg* 1994;80:64–72.

84. Sinson G, Zager EL, Grossman RI, Gennarelli TA, Flamm ES. Cavernous malformations of the third ventricle. *Neurosurgery* 1995;37:37–42.

85. Ogilvy CS, Louis DN, Ojemann RG. Intramedullary cavernous angiomas of the spinal cord: clinical presentation, pathological features, and surgical management. *Neurosurgery* 1992;31:219–229.

86. Anson JA, Spetzler RF. Surgical resection of intramedullary spinal cord cavernous malformations. *J Neurosurg* 1993;78:446–451.

87. Linskey ME, Sekhar LN. Cavernous sinus hemangiomas: a series, a review, and a hypothesis. *Neurosurgery* 1992;30:101–108.

88. Suzuki Y, Shibuya M, Baskaya MK, Takakura S, Yamamoto M, Saito K, Glazier SS, Sugita K. Extracerebral cavernous angiomas of the cavernous sinus in the middle fossa. *Surg Neurol* 1996;45:123–132.

89. Frim DM, Scott RM. Management of cavernous malformations in the pediatric population. *Neurosurg Clin North Am* 1999;10:513–518.

90. Karlsson B, Kihlstrom L, Lindquist C, Ericson K, Steiner L. Radiosurgery for cavernous malformations. *J Neurosurg* 1998;88:293–297.

91. Mitchell P, Hodgson TJ, Seaman S, Kemeny AA, Forster DMC. Stereotactic radiosurgery and the risk of hemorrhage from cavernous malformations. *Br J Neurosurg* 2000;14:96–100.

92. Pollock BE, Garces YI, Stafford SL, Foote RL, Schomberg PJ, Link MJ. Stereotactic radiosurgery for cavernous malformations. *J Neurosurg* 2000;93: 987–991.

Chapter 13
Recurrent Cerebral Infarcts in Antiphospholipid Antibody Syndrome

Osvaldo Fustinoni and José Biller

Multiple recurrent strokes are a complex clinical problem that demands extensive diagnostic evaluation to establish the underlying mechanism. Conditions as dissimilar as coagulopathies, cerebral vasculitis, endocarditis, cardiac arrhythmias, and large-artery atherothrombosis must be considered in the differential diagnosis. Thus, possible causes are numerous and secondary prevention can only be successful if the responsible cause is identified in each patient.

The antiphospholipid antibody syndrome (APAS) is increasingly recognized as an important risk factor for recurrent ischemic strokes, especially in young patients. Long and continuous high-intensity oral anticoagulation is required to prevent them, but patients are subsequently at risk of hemorrhage. The most feared hemorrhagic complication is intracranial bleeding. A patient suffering a cerebral hemorrhage under high-intensity oral anticoagulation for APAS-related strokes becomes a difficult therapeutic challenge. The physician must reconsider whether to discontinue anticoagulation altogether (at the risk of further cerebral infarcts), reduce its intensity, or switch to other anticoagulation schemes (heparin, low molecular weight heparins), antiplatelet therapy, or both. If, in addition, the patient becomes pregnant, the management becomes even more complex.

■ The Patient

A 44-year-old right-handed woman was admitted with a sudden onset of slurred speech and weakness of her right arm and leg that had been preceded by vomiting. She had a previous history of stroke, pregnancy-induced hypertension, preeclampsia, and a stillbirth at 9 months of gestation. Her first ischemic stroke had occurred 9 years before, resulting in left hemiparesis. At that time, a mitral valve thickening had been noticed on 2-D echocardiography and she had been placed on warfarin. Nearly 3 years later, she had an abrupt episode of transient loss of consciousness. An acute hemorrhage in the pineal region was found on MRI (Figures 13-1, 13-2, and 13-3). As a result, she developed acute obstructive hydrocephalus. A ventriculoperitoneal (VP) shunt was placed (Figure 13-4), and warfarin discontinued. No underlying pineal structural lesion was observed on follow-up MRI (Figure 13-5). She then suffered two recurrent ischemic strokes in the following 2 months, with worsening right-sided hemibody deficit. An antiphospholipid antibody syndrome (APAS) was eventually diagnosed. Aspirin 1300 mg/day was prescribed after her second stroke. Subsequently, after her third ischemic insult, she was switched to aspirin plus extended-release dipyridamole.

When examined, her blood pressure was 110/70 mmHg and her pulse 64 per minute and regular. There was a grade III/VI apical systolic murmur on cardiac auscultation. Skin examination showed extensive livedo reticularis. Her speech was hesitant and her verbal output had decreased fluency and frequent word-finding difficulties. She had right homonymous hemianopia, some right-left disorientation, spastic right hemiparesis, bilateral Babinski signs, and hemiparetic gait.

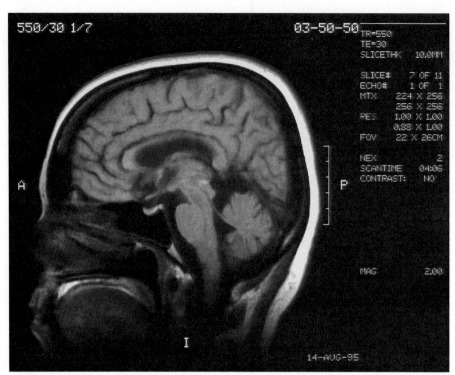

Figure 13-1. Three years after the first ischemic stroke, under high-intensity warfarin. Nonenhanced T1-weighted brain MRI (sagittal view) shows a hyperintense lesion in the pineal region extending to the upper aspect of the midbrain and obstructing the aqueduct of Sylvius.

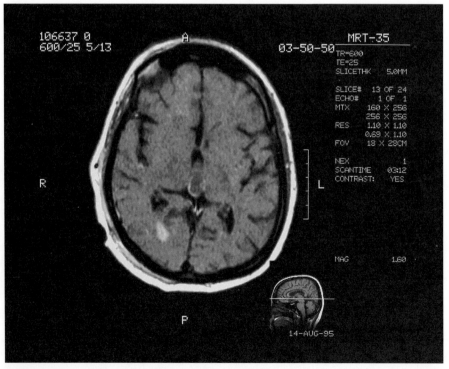

Figure 13-2. Enhanced T1-weighted brain MRI (axial view) shows slight ring enhancement of the pineal lesion. There is also evidence of blood in the right posterior lateral ventricle.

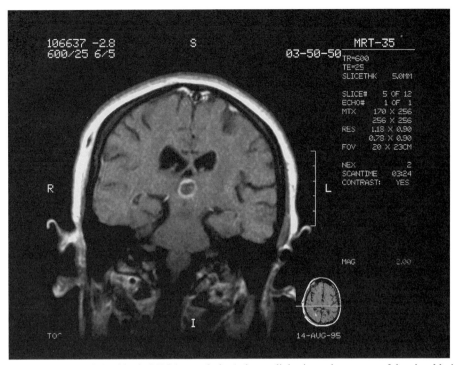

Figure 13-3. Enhanced T1-weighted brain MRI (coronal view) shows slight ring enhancement of the pineal lesion.

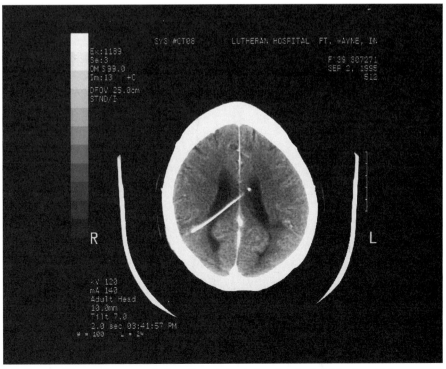

Figure 13-4. Follow-up CT scan shows ventriculoperitoneal shunt placed on the left lateral ventricle.

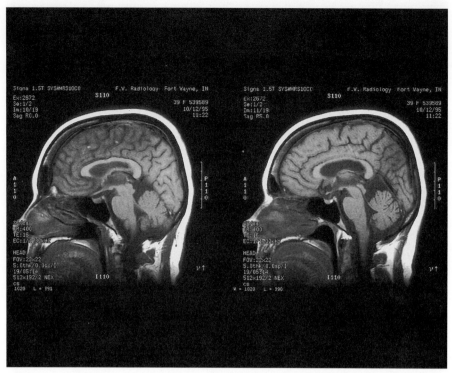

Figure 13-5. Follow-up nonenhanced T1-weighted brain MRI (sagittal view) shows no underlying structural pineal lesion.

Brain MRI showed an old right cortical frontal infarct, bilateral occipital infarcts, and white matter cerebral and cerebellar gliosis ascribed to end vessel infarcts (Figures 13-6 and 13-7). A recent left cortical parietal infarct was seen on diffusion-weighted MRI (Figure 13-8). Brain MRA revealed truncation of left mid-posterior cerebral artery, hypoplastic right posterior communicating artery, and no occlusive disease of the extracranial carotid arteries or their proximal intracranial branches.

On transthoracic echocardiogram the left ventricular function was normal, and there was minimal mitral and aortic regurgitation with no evidence of aortic atherosclerosis or patent foramen ovale.

The aPTT was 70.1 seconds and the Dilute Russell Venom Viper Time (DRVVT) was 71.9 seconds. Lupus anticoagulant was positive. Serum for testing antiphospholipid antibodies was obtained following the cerebrovascular event; it was separated from the clot by centrifugation (3000g) within 24 hours of collection, aliquoted, and stored at −70°C until tested for the presence of IgG, IgA, and IgM to phosphatidylserine (PS), cardiolipin (CL), phosphatidylethanolamine (PE), and phosphatidylcholine

(PC) by an in-house solid-phase enzyme-linked immunosorbent assay (ELISA) as previously reported.[1,2] High titers of IgG aPS, aCL, and aPE were found. These results did not vary substantially on repeated examinations. The antiphospholipid antibody ELISA results are displayed in Table 13-1.

Crithidia (native deoxyribonucleic acid) NDNA antibodies were positive. Anti-DNA antibodies were 25.2 IU/mL. Luetic serology, antiribosomal P and antineuronal antibodies, rheumatoid factor, and C-reactive protein were all negative. Plasma homocysteine was normal. Total cholesterol was 212, LDL 141, HDL 35, and triglycerides 180 mg/dL. A skin biopsy was negative.

The diagnoses at that point were multiple bilateral hemispheric infarcts due to antiphospholipid antibody syndrome (APAS), prior pineal gland hemorrhage with obstructive hydrocephalus requiring a VP shunt, and history of pregnancy-induced hypertension. Because of the presence of positive *Crithidia* NDNA and elevated anti-DNA antibodies, secondary APAS due to systemic lupus erythematosus (SLE) could not be excluded.

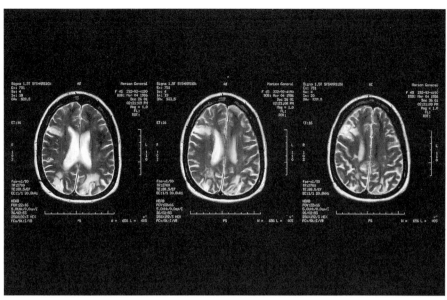

Figure 13-6. Nine years after the first ischemic stroke, under aspirin plus extended-release dipyridamole. Nonenhanced T2-weighted brain MRI shows a right cortical frontal and bilateral cortical occipital infarcts.

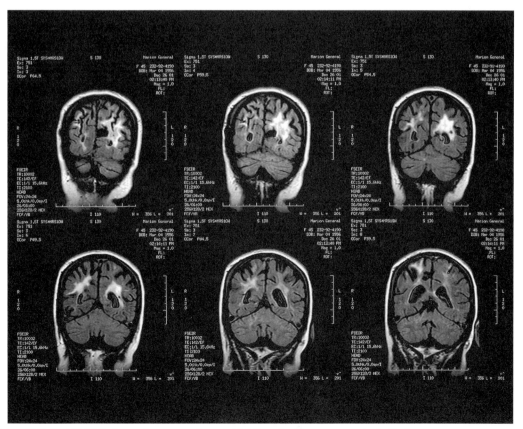

Figure 13-7. FLAIR MRI shows changes consistent with bilateral white matter cerebral gliosis.

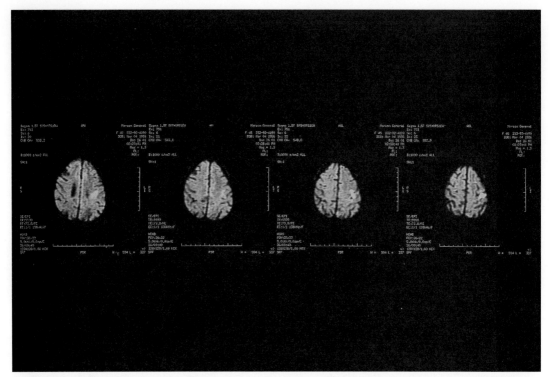

Figure 13-8. Diffusion-weighted brain MRI shows a focal area of restricted diffusion consistent with a recent evolving left cortical parietal infarct.

The patient's motor deficit improved partially with comprehensive rehabilitation. The combination of aspirin plus extended-release dipyridamole was discontinued. She was then placed on aspirin and hydroxychloroquine, and had no further ischemic strokes over one year of follow-up.

■ The Problem

- What are the possible causes of multiple recurrent cerebral infarcts?
- What is the optimal therapy in APAS (heparin, warfarin, ASA, dipyridamole, clopidogrel, or a combination of these agents)?

Table 13-1. Antiphospholipid Antibody (aPA) ELISA Results

		Patient β_2GP1 PL Binding Protein		
Antibody	**Isotype**	**Dependent**	**Independent**	**Normal Range**
Antiphosphatidylserine (aPS)	IgG	40	15	≤ 4
	IgA	3	2	≤ 3
	IgM	2	1	≤ 5
Anticardiolipin (aCL)	IgG	14	3	≤ 4
	IgA	2	1	≤ 4
	IgM	3	1	≤ 6
Antiphosphatidylethanolamine (aPE)	IgG	3	17	≤ 4
	IgA	1	2	≤ 3
	IgM	3	3	≤ 5
Antiphosphatidylcholine (aPC)	IgG	1	1	≤ 4
	IgA	1	1	≤ 3
	IgM	3	≤ 4	≤ 4

- What is the role of long term unfractionated heparin or long term low molecular weight heparin in preventing further strokes?
- The patient has not had any children and would like to get pregnant. What is the best advice and prenatal management?
- After discontinuing warfarin the patient suffered recurrent ischemic strokes under antiplatelet therapy. Would you consider reinitiating oral anticoagulation in spite of her prior pineal gland hemorrhage?
- Under aspirin the patient had further cerebral infarcts. If you decided not to switch to warfarin, what other antiplatelet therapy or agent would you choose: increase the dose of aspirin; switch to aspirin in combination with extended-release dipyridamole; switch to clopidogrel; or switch to aspirin in combination with clopidogrel?
- Can rt-PA be administered in case of a new life-threatening acute ischemic stroke?

■ The Evidence

Ischemic stroke recurrence is not uncommon. Population-based studies have reported recurrence rates of approximately 15 percent in the first 2 years.[3,4] Risk is highest early after the first stroke. Diabetes mellitus and atrial fibrillation might increase the risk of recurrence during the first year after a first stroke, but most recurrences cannot be explained by traditional cerebrovascular risk factors.[4] The situation is very complex and the subtypes of the first and subsequent strokes may often differ (that was the case in 45 percent of patients in a population-based study from London).[4] Large-artery atherothrombosis was associated with higher risk of early recurrence in one study,[5] but other researchers have not found any association between stroke subtype and risk of recurrence.[3,4]

The list of conditions associated with the occurrence of multiple recurrent ischemic strokes is extensive and heterogeneous. These conditions are summarized in Table 13-2.

This patient's history is consistent with APAS. Antiphospholipid antibodies are a recognized cause of recurrent arterial and venous thromboembolism. Ischemic stroke is the most common arterial thrombotic event in APAS.[6–17] Antibodies binding

Table 13-2. Differential Diagnosis of Multiple Recurrent Ischemic Stroke

Most frequent mechanisms
  Large-artery atherothrombosis
  Cardioembolism
    Atrial fibrillation
    Dilated cardiomyopathy
    Valvular disease
    Endocarditis (marantic or infectious)
  Small-vessel occlusion
Less frequent mechanisms
  Patent foramen ovale
  Thrombotic diathesis
    Coagulation disorders*
      APAS (anticardiolipin antibodies, lupus anticoagulant)
      Prothrombin gene mutation
      Activated protein C resistance
      Factor V Leiden mutation
      Protein C deficiency
      Protein S deficiency
      Antithrombin III deficiency
      Fibrinogen disorders
      Elevated factor VIII level
      Malignancies
    Hemoglobinopathies
      Sickle-cell disease
    Platelet disorders
      Essential thrombocythemia
      Thrombotic thrombocytopenic purpura
    Other hematopoietic disorders
      Polycythemia vera
      Paroxysmal nocturnal hemoglobinuria
  Cerebral angiitis
    Isolated CNS angiitis
    Giant cell arteritis
    Takayasu's arteritis
    Cogan syndrome
    Associated with systemic diseases
      Behçet's disease
      Polyarteritis nodosa
      Systemic lupus erythematosus
      Wegener's granulomatosis
      Ulcerative colitis
      Scleroderma
      Sjögren's syndrome
      Sarcoidosis
    Infectious vasculitides
      Viral (HZV, CMV, others)
      Bacterial
      Spirochetal (Lyme, syphilis)
      Fungal (aspergillosis, mucormycosis)
      Parasitic

Continued

Table 13-2. (continued)

Drug-induced vasculitides
  Amphetamines
  Heroin
  Cocaine
Genetic disorders
  CADASIL
  Mitochondrial disorders (MELAS, MERRF,
    Kearns-Sayre, Leigh's disease)
  Homocystinuria
  Hereditary dyslipoproteinemias
  Organic acidemias
  Fabry's disease
  Heritable connective tissue disorders
Miscellaneous
  Moyamoya disease
  Fibromuscular dysplasia
  Migrainous infarction
  Intravascular lymphomatosis
  Radiation-induced vasculopathy
  Thromboangiitis obliterans with cerebral involvement
  Susac syndrome

*Association is strongest for venous thrombosis.
CADASIL, Cerebral autosomal dominant arteriopathy
  with subcortical infarcts and leukoencephalopathy.
MELAS, Mitochondrial myopathy encephalopathy lactic
  acidosis and stroke-like episodes.
MERRF, Myoclonus epilepsy and ragged red fibers.

phospholipids have been often found in SLE and referred to as lupus anticoagulants (LA)[18–21] and in sera from patients with syphilis binding to cardiolipin extracts of beef hearts. However, they are not specific to these diseases.[22–25] Antiphospholipid antibodies act as coagulation inhibitors that prolong in vitro clotting time tests. In vivo, however, they are not associated with bleeding but with venous and arterial thrombosis and spontaneous early pregnancy loss.[26] The presence of antiphospholipid antibodies (APAS) in high titers is associated with recurrent arterial or venous thromboses, fetal loss, and livedo reticularis.[27] Several antiphospholipid antibodies have been described, in IgG, IgA, or IgM isotypes: anticardiolipin (aCL), antiphosphatidylethanolamine (aPE), antiphosphatidylserine (aPS), and antiphosphatidylcholine (aPC). Affinity-purified aCLs do not bind to cardiolipin in the absence of serum or plasma. The component required for aCL binding is β_2-glycoprotein 1 (β_2GP1).[27–30] It is the β_2GP1-dependent aCLs of the IgG isotype that have been significantly associated with stroke and myocardial infarction.[31]

Other stroke studies have reported a significant association with aPE.[29]

APAS can be primary, or secondary to underlying diseases such as SLE, rheumatoid arthritis, Sjögren's syndrome, malignancies, syphilis, AIDS, and others. High rates of recurrence for APAS have been found in retrospective and prospective studies.[32–43] Patients may have arterial occlusions, venous occlusions, or both.[31,36] Antithrombotic treatment, especially for the secondary prevention of arterial thromboembolism, is therefore considered appropriate.

Anticoagulation

Intensity

In retrospective studies, high-intensity (International Normalized Ratio [INR] 3.0–3.5) as compared to low- or standard-intensity (INR 2.0–3.0) oral anticoagulation has been shown to reduce recurrence of thrombotic events in APAS. In 70 cases, recurrence was lower in patients treated with an INR ≥ 3.0 than in those treated with a lower INR or aspirin.[39] A study assessing the efficacy of warfarin, low-dose aspirin (75 mg daily), or both in 147 patients with APAS indicated that treatment with high-intensity warfarin, with or without low-dose aspirin, was significantly more effective than treatment with low-intensity warfarin, with or without low-dose aspirin, or aspirin alone, in preventing further thrombotic events. The rate of recurrence was highest (1.3 per patient-year) during the first 6 months after the cessation of warfarin.[34] In 61 patients, warfarin reduced the recurrent yearly arterial event rate by about 70% (relative risk [RR] 0.25; 95% CI, 0.08–0.75; $p = 0.01$).[35] Both venous and arterial events were included in these studies, which are summarized in Table 13-3. Guidelines published in the United Kingdom have recommended an INR target of either 3.5[44] or 2.5[45] for the secondary prevention of thrombotic events in APAS.

Two prospective studies including only venous events reported absence of recurrences with an INR range of <3.0.[41,46] These studies did not address the issue of intensity of anticoagulation or compare between groups treated with different target INRs, and only a small number of their patients were aPL-positive.[47]

The Warfarin and Aspirin Recurrent Stroke Study (WARSS) assessed the possible benefit of oral

Table 13-3. APAS: Comparison of Antithrombotic Treatments in Retrospective Studies

Study	No. of Patients	Treatment	Events per Year of Follow-up	Patient-Years of Follow-up	P Values
Rosove and Brewer[39]	70	None	0.19	161.2	NS
		Aspirin alone	0.36	27.5	NS
		Warfarin			
		INR ≤ 1.9	0.57	11.3	NS
		INR 2.0–2.9	0.07	40.9	0.12 (NS)
		With aspirin	0.38	5.3	Short follow-up
		INR ≤ 3.0	0	110.2	<0.001
		With aspirin	0	5.0	Short follow-up
Khamashta et al.[34]	147	None	0.29	280.6	
		Aspirin	0.18	240.3	0.013
		Warfarin			
		INR < 3	0.23	141.3	0.270
		With aspirin	0.22	31.4	0.531
		INR ≥ 3	0.015	197.3	<0.001
		With aspirin	0	39.8	<0.001
Krnic-Barrie et al.[35]	61	None	0.192	124.9	
		Aspirin	0.082	36.6	0.15
		Any warfarin	0.051	99.0	0.003
		Warfarin	0.048	63.0	0.01
		With aspirin	0	30.6	0.03
		Any prednisone	0.204	34.3	0.89

anticoagulation (INR 1.4–2.8) over aspirin in the secondary prevention of noncardioembolic stroke, and showed no difference between both treatments in that setting.[48] The Antiphospholipid Antibodies and Stroke Study (APASS) group carried out a collaborative study with WARSS to clarify the role of aPA in predicting recurrent vascular events and to compare the effect of positivity for aPA (LA and aCL) on recurrent thrombotic events in each of the two WARSS treatment groups. Positivity for aPA at the time of an ischemic stroke did not confer increased risk for thrombotic events and did not predict a differential treatment response to aspirin or warfarin (median INR for APASS 1.9). The authors concluded that routine screening for aPA in ischemic stroke patients meeting eligibility criteria for WARSS does not appear warranted, and that future analyses would address titers, isotypes, serial data, and significance of positivity on more than one aPA assay.[49]

There have been no prospective studies comparing different intensities of anticoagulation in the secondary prevention of APAS, but such trials are in progress. The Warfarin in the Antiphospholipid Syndrome study randomizes patients to high-intensity (INR 3.0–4.5) or standard-intensity (INR < 3) treatment.[50] The PAPRE trial in Canada will compare high-intensity (INR 3.1–4.0) with moderate-intensity (INR 2.0–3.0) anticoagulation in APAS patients with one previous thrombotic event.[51]

Duration

It is generally accepted that patients should be anticoagulated for at least 6 months after deep-vein thrombosis or pulmonary embolism.[52] In patients with APAS, some authors assume that anticoagulation is required "as long as antiphospholipid antibodies are present." This implies retesting of patients regularly to determine whether to maintain or to discontinue anticoagulation.[53] However, patients have developed thrombotic episodes after becoming negative for antiphospholipid antibodies.[54] These patients may have had still unidentified antibodies at the time of their report. In a series of 19 patients with APAS, venous thromboembolism, and long-term follow-up, those treated with oral anticoagulation had a 100 percent probability of survival without recurrence at 8 years. In contrast, patients in whom anticoagulants were discontinued had a 50 percent probability of recurrent thromboembolism at 2 years and a 78 percent probability of recurrence at 8 years.[32] In a recent study, 66 patients had a high rate of thrombotic recurrence (9.1 cases per 100 patient-years) despite oral anticoagulation for one year to a target INR of 3.5 (3.0–4.0).[40] To date, no prospective trials have addressed this issue, but the evidence so far seems to favor long-term oral anticoagulation in APAS patients.

Choice of Anticoagulant

Although it is accepted that oral anticoagulation with warfarin is the preferred treatment for the prevention of thromboembolic events in patients with APAS, other anticoagulants should be chosen in pregnancy due to the potential teratogenicity of warfarin. The risk of warfarin embryopathy is about 5 percent. Provided that warfarin is replaced within 2 weeks of the first missed menstrual period, conception under warfarin therapy should be safe, because the period of greatest teratogenic risk is between the sixth and twelfth weeks of gestation. Also, warfarin used in the second trimester may be associated with microcephaly.[55]

There are certain instances of "warfarin resistance" in which patients cannot be maintained in an adequate INR range and should be switched to other drug regimens. It is still unclear whether this "warfarin resistance" is not really inadequate patient compliance or pharmacological interaction with other medications.[51]

To our knowledge, there have been no prospective trials evaluating long-term prevention with heparin in APAS. In one retrospective study, heparin was given to 12/70 patients for 7.5 patient-years. There were 4 thrombotic recurrences in 4 patients (0.53 recurrences per patient-year), 2 during "low-intensity" (PTT ratio ≤ 1.4) and 2 during "high-intensity" (PTT ratio 2.1–2.5) heparin therapy. During high-intensity treatment, one patient had multiple pulmonary emboli in the third trimester of pregnancy, and another had complete thrombotic occlusion of the left common iliac vein that extended during treatment in the postpartum period; in both cases there were no bleeding complications. The authors concluded that follow-up for heparin therapy was "too short to draw conclusions" but that the thrombotic events in the two patients on high-intensity heparin therapy indicated that the APAS "can constitute an intense state of hypercoagulability."[39]

Heparin can cause thrombocytopenia and paradoxical thromboembolism.[56,57] Long-term heparin treatment carries the risk of heparin-induced osteoporosis[58–61] and aldosterone deficiency.[62–65] Low molecular weight heparins (LMWH) may be preferred in patients in whom warfarin is to be avoided. LMWH have a longer half-life and increased bioavailability, which enables administration once or twice a day. They also have a lower risk of thrombocytopenia. Although instances of aldosterone deficiency[63,66,67] and, especially, osteoporotic vertebral collapse[68] with LWMH have been reported, the risk of osteoporosis seems substantially lower.[69] LMWH do not have antithrombin effect and their activity must be determined by anti-factor Xa levels. However, only in very few cases have doses of LMWH had to be changed during pregnancy as a result of these measurements.[70] Some authors, therefore, do not advocate routine measurement of anti-factor Xa to monitor treatment.[71]

In a study involving 42 women with 57 pregnancies and APAS (fetal loss or thrombotic events), 11 were treated with warfarin and 31 with LMWH (subcutaneous enoxaparin 0.7 mg/kg/day) plus aspirin 100 mg/day. There was no significant difference in the incidence of thrombosis, week of delivery, or birth weight between both groups. However, in the enoxaparin group there were episodes of recurrent amaurosis fugax in one pregnancy and "black dots in the visual fields" in three. These disappeared after substitution by warfarin, but recurred when warfarin was replaced by enoxaparin toward the end of the pregnancy.[72]

Complications During Oral Anticoagulation

Recurrence. Lupus anticoagulants may also prolong the prothrombin time and interfere with the measurement of INR. Recurrence might be due in some cases to overestimation of the intensity of anticoagulation caused by prolongation of the prothrombin time by LA.[73,74] Measurement of chromogenic factor Xa levels or application of an instrument-specific International Sensitivity Index (ISI) may be required in such cases.[74,75] However, it has also been shown that LA prolongation of prothrombin time depends on the reagent used to obtain INR values, and that the INR system is valid for monitoring patients with antiphospholipid antibodies provided the reagents that display the interference are identified and excluded.[76] These authors also found that the reliability of measuring the INR was increased when patients' plasma was calibrated against plasma standards that had three different levels of INR.

Bleeding. There is always a risk of bleeding with long-term oral anticoagulation. However, in retrospective studies,[34,35,39] hemorrhagic events in patients on warfarin are clearly lower than recurrences in untreated patients, and comparable to recurrences in patients on warfarin. In all three studies, severe hemorrhages occurred in patients receiving high-intensity or supratherapeutic anticoagulation treatments (Table 13-4). In a recent study of 15 patients with major hemorrhages while on oral anticoagulation for APAS, no relationship could be established with age or duration of treatment, though concomitant drugs, mainly aspirin, and high blood pressure were present at the time of bleeding in many patients.[77]

Antiplatelet Therapy

Aspirin has so far only been studied prospectively in women with aPL-associated recurrent pregnancy loss and no thrombotic episodes. In two studies, aspirin associated with heparin, compared with aspirin alone, was beneficial in the prevention of fetal loss.[76,77] However, in a subsequent study, aspirin compared with placebo did not show any benefit.[78]

Subsets of patients received aspirin in the retrospective APAS studies reported in the previous section (see Table 13-3). In one study, aspirin was given to 23 patients for 37.8 years, including 10.3 patient-years of combined therapy with warfarin.

Of the 23 patients, 10 had 12 recurrences. Though the numbers are small, the events per year of follow-up were nonsignificantly higher in the aspirin-treated patients than in those receiving intermediate or high-intensity warfarin.[39] In another study, patients receiving low-dose aspirin (75 mg/day) had a lower rate of recurrence than untreated patients, but this effect was no longer statistically significant after adjustment for other risk factors for thrombosis.[34] Other authors found that when venous and arterial events were combined, patients taking aspirin alone appeared to have significantly fewer recurrences. However, they did not find any significant benefit of aspirin when analyzing arterial and venous events separately.[35]

Nevertheless, there is a rationale for the use of antiplatelet therapy in APAS. Although thrombocytopenia in this syndrome may be immune mediated,[79,80] it has been shown to respond to aspirin in some patients.[81] Thrombocytopenia has been ascribed in these cases to chronic consumption of platelets secondary to prolonged thrombotic activation. Aspirin may interfere with this phenomenon, thus ameliorating the thrombocytopenia. The use of anti-platelet drugs is therefore reasonable in the prevention of thrombosis in APAS.

Other antiplatelet agents or regimens shown to be beneficial in the prevention of atherosclerotic ischemic stroke, such as extended-release dipyridamole in association to aspirin,[82] clopidogrel,[83] or clopidogrel in association to aspirin,[84,85] have not been tested in APAS.

Antimalarial Drugs

Chloroquine and hydroxychloroquine are antimalarial drugs frequently used in the treatment of

Table 13-4. Hemorrhagic Complications in Retrospective Studies of Anticoagulation in APAS

Study	Patients (Total/Warfarin)	Bleeding Events	Rate per Patient-Year	Intensity
Khamashta et al.[34]	147/104	N = 29, 7 severe (2 peritoneal, 2 menorrhagia, 1 kidney, 1 subdural, 1 ovarian)	0.071 Severe: 0.017	INRs ≥ 3 in all cases
Krnic-Barrie et al.[35]	61/not stated	N = 4, 1 severe (death, intracerebral)	—	Prothrombin time ratio 2.3 in the severe case
Rosove and Brewer[39]	70/55	N = 5, 3 severe (2 subdural, 1 pulmonary)	0.031	INRs in the 3 severe cases: 26, unknown, 6.4

SLE and their beneficial effect has been documented.[86,87] Antimalarial drugs interrupt the generation and presentation of antigenic peptides by raising the pH within lysosomes, are platelet inhibitors, lower serum cholesterol and LDL lipoprotein levels, and may also decrease abnormal levels of cytokines.[88,89] In a recent experimental study, hydroxychloroquine was shown to reverse platelet activation induced by human IgG antiphospholipid antibodies.[90] Although they have not yet been tested in prospective studies, antimalarial drugs might therefore be useful in APAS patients with or without associated SLE.

Hydroxychloroquine has various side effects including gastrointestinal intolerance, pruritus, cutaneous eruptions, myopathy, and, especially, retinopathy. The incidence of retinopathy is low; it was seen once among 940 patients,[91] twice among 58 patients on long-term treatment (>6 years),[92] and in none of 82 patients treated for more than one year.[93] Retinal hyperpigmentation is typically present.[94] Retinal dysfunction may persist after discontinuation of the drug.[95] In pregnancy, the possible effect of hydroxychloroquine on the fetal eye has to be balanced against the risk of disease reactivation in case of discontinuation, which can also compromise pregnancy outcome. Data from Africa, where the drug is widely used, indicate that the drug is well tolerated during pregnancy.[96] Recent reports appear to confirm that it is safer to continue hydroxychloroquine during pregnancy rather than facing the risk of a flare-up of SLE.[97,98] It seems therefore reasonable to use antimalarial drugs as an adjunctive agent in APAS patients with recurrent thrombotic events who cannot undergo anticoagulation.

■ The Pros and Cons

This middle-aged woman with APAS has had an ischemic stroke, subsequently a pineal hemorrhage while taking warfarin, and then recurrent ischemic strokes, first while receiving aspirin, and later while receiving aspirin plus extended-release dipyridamole. No strokes have occurred since she was placed on hydroxychloroquine and aspirin.

The frequency of her thrombotic episodes has been variable. She suffered two ischemic strokes shortly after discontinuation of warfarin because of her pineal gland hemorrhage leading to acute obstructive hydrocephalus. This is in accordance with reported data showing that the rate of recurrence is highest during the first 6 months after the cessation of warfarin.[34]

Pineal gland hemorrhage is a rare complication of anticoagulation. It has been linked to underlying pineal cysts.[99,100] The nonenhanced T1-weighted MRI showed a hyperintense lesion in the pineal region extending to the upper aspect of the midbrain and obstructing the aqueduct, consistent with hemorrhage (see Figure 13-1). There was slight ring enhancement with contrast, and also some blood in the right posterior lateral ventricle (see Figures 13-2 and 13-3). The patient required a VP shunt because of hydrocephalus due to aqueductal obstruction (see Figure 13-4). The pineal region was not surgically explored, but no underlying pineal lesion was noted on a follow-up MRI (see Figure 13-5). We found no reports of her INR at the time of hemorrhage, which could have been beyond the therapeutic range.

The patient did not have a new stroke for 6 years while treated with the combination of aspirin and hydroxychloroquine. At present, the patient remains at high risk of recurrence of severely disabling or fatal ischemic stroke, with less risk of hemorrhage. Patients in whom anticoagulants are discontinued have a 50 percent probability of recurrent thromboembolism at 2 years and a 78 percent probability of recurrence at 8 years.[32]

Aspirin has so far not been shown to be clearly preventive in APAS.[34,35,39] In this patient, aspirin could perhaps be avoiding chronic consumption of platelets by her prothrombotic state, though she was not thrombocytopenic at the time aspirin was prescribed. Other antiplatelet agents or combinations in this syndrome have not been tested to date. There is therefore no evidence to consider them a valuable alternative to anticoagulation. Hydroxychloroquine has the added advantage of its immunomodulating effect[86–90] but, again, evidence of its clinical benefit in APAS is not available.

The patient could be followed by regular monitoring of platelet count and aPA, and perhaps be switched to anticoagulation in case of progressive thrombocytopenia or rising titers of aPA. But the relationship between platelet count, aPA titers, and clinical events is not clear, and there are reports of patients developing thrombotic episodes after becoming negative for antiphospholipid antibodies.[54]

Should the patient suffer a new ischemic stroke under her present medical treatment, she would probably have to be switched to warfarin under strict control of her INR. Warfarin should also be considered if she develops signs of thrombotic phenomena such as thrombocytopenia, venous thrombosis, or peripheral arterial events. So far, high-intensity long-term oral anticoagulation with warfarin has been shown to offer the best protection against recurrent thromboembolic events in APAS.[34,35,39] There would therefore be a rationale to reinitiate warfarin in this patient, at least at a low or standard-intensity (INR 2.0–3.0), in case of a recurrent thromboembolic event.

Another possibility is parenteral anticoagulation. Unfractionated heparin can cause thrombocytopenia.[56,57] Long-term unfractionated heparin treatment is not advisable because of the risk of heparin-induced osteoporosis[58–61] and aldosterone deficiency.[62–65] LMWH can be contemplated in case warfarin is considered too risky. In a prospective study LMWH was as beneficial as warfarin, although in 4 cases there were visual thrombotic events that remitted when patients were switched to warfarin, and relapsed when oral anticoagulation was again replaced by LMWH.[72] Nevertheless, the need for a long-term treatment in this case raises the concern about osteoporosis and other adverse effects that do occur also with LMWH. In addition, the fact that the patient should undergo daily subcutaneous injections must be taken into account.

Pregnancy would also increase the risk of thrombosis and add the risk of fetal loss. On the other hand, pregnancy facilitates a therapeutic decision on anticoagulation as it may be introduced on a fixed-term basis. As warfarin should be avoided because of its teratogenic risk, the best choice in this setting would be LMWH, which has been tested in pregnant women with APAS with good results.[72] Heparin is an alternative. It has been assessed alone and in combination with aspirin in antibody-positive pregnant women without thrombosis, with a high live-birth rate and good newborn outcome.[101,102]

Thrombolytic treatment with rt-PA within 3 hours of onset of ischemic stroke, if given intravenously in carefully selected patients, has been proven to reduce disability and improve clinical outcome at 3 months.[103,104] However, a prolonged clotting time (as observed in APAS), ongoing anticoagulation, or a history of intracranial hemorrhage are exclusion criteria for its use. Besides, intravenous rt-PA carries a 10-fold increase in risk of intracranial hemorrhage.[104] Although our patient was not anticoagulated at the time of admission, she did have the other contraindications for intravenous rt-PA administration.

■ The Main Points

- Antiphospholipid antibodies and APAS are strong risk factors for first and recurrent ischemic strokes.
- Antiphospholipid antibodies should be measured in all young patients with cryptogenic stroke under 45 years of age.
- Presence of antiphospholipid antibodies should be investigated in all women with a history of venous thrombosis and fetal loss.
- All isotypes of antiphospholipid antibodies should be tested, as well as their β_2 GPI binding dependency, when APAS is suspected.
- Evidence to date indicates that strictly controlled long-term high-intensity warfarin (INR ≥ 3) is the treatment of choice for APAS.
- Warfarin should be replaced by LMWH or unfractionated heparin during pregnancy.
- Though cerebral hemorrhage occurs more frequently with supratherapeutic anticoagulation, it may occasionally occur with therapeutic INR levels.
- Antiplatelet and antimalarial drugs can be used safely if anticoagulation is contraindicated, but there is no prospective evidence proving their clinical benefit.

■ References

1. Sokol DK, McIntyre JA, Short RA, Gutt J, Wagenknecht DR, Biller J, Garg B Henoch-Schönlein purpura and stroke: antiphosphatidylethanolamine antibody in CSF and serum. *Neurology* 2000; 55:1379–1381.

2. Wagenknecht DR, Sugi T, McIntyre JA. The evolution, evaluation and interpretation of antiphospholipid antibody assays. *Clin Immunol Newslett* 1995;15:28–38.

3. Kolominsky-Rabas PL, Weber M, Gefeller O, Neundoerfer B, Heuschmann PU. Epidemiology of ischemic stroke subtypes according to TOAST criteria: incidence, recurrence, and long-term survival in ischemic stroke subtypes: a population-based study. *Stroke* 2001; 32:2735–2740.

4. Hillen T, Coshall C, Tilling K, Rudd AG, McGovern R, Wolfe CD; South London Stroke Register. Cause of stroke recurrence is multifactorial: patterns, risk factors, and outcomes of stroke recurrence in the South London Stroke Register. *Stroke* 2003;34:1457–1463.

5. Petty GW, Brown RD Jr, Whisnant JP, Sicks JD, O'Fallon WM, Wiebers DO. Ischemic stroke subtypes: a population-based study of functional outcome, survival, and recurrence. *Stroke* 2000;31:1062–1068.

6. Angelini L, Ravelli A, Caporali R, Rumi V, Nardocci N, Martini A. High prevalence of antiphospholipid antibodies in children with idiopathic cerebral ischemia. *Pediatrics* 1994;94:500–503.

7. Baca V, Garcia-Ramirez R, Ramirez-Lacayo M, Marquez-Enriquez L, Martinez I, Lavalle C. Cerebral infarction and antiphospholipid syndrome in children. *J Rheumatol* 1996;23:1428–1431.

8. Campi A, Filippi M, Comi G, Scotti G. Recurrent acute transverse myelopathy associated with anticardiolipin antibodies. *AJNR Am J Neuroradiol* 1998;19:781–786.

9. Feldmann E, Levine SR. Cerebrovascular disease with antiphospholipid antibodies: immune mechanisms, significance, and therapeutic options. *Ann Neurol* 1995; 37(Suppl 1):S114–130.

10. Levine SR, Brey RL, Sawaya KL, Salowich-Palm L, Kokkinos J, Kostrzema Perry M, Havstad S, Carey J. Recurrent stroke and thrombo-occlusive events in the antiphospholipid syndrome. *Ann Neurol* 1995;38: 119–124.

11. Metz LM, Edworthy S, Mydlarski R, Fritzler MJ. The frequency of phospholipid antibodies in an unselected stroke population. *Can J Neurol Sci* 1998;25:64–92.

12. Provenzale JM, Barboriak DP, Allen NB, Ortel TL. Antiphospholipid antibodies: findings at arteriography. *AJNR Am J Neuroradiol* 1998;19:611–616.

13. Schoning M, Klein R, Krageloh-Mann I, Falck M, Bien S, Berg PA, Michaelis R. Antiphospholipid antibodies in cerebrovascular ischemia and stroke in childhood. *Neuropediatrics* 1994;25:8–14.

14. Takanashi J, Sugita K, Miyazato S, Sakao E, Miyamoto H, Niimi H. Antiphospholipid antibody syndrome in childhood strokes. *Ped Neurol* 1995;13: 323–326.

15. Tatlisumak T, Fisher M. Hematologic disorders associated with ischemic stroke. *J Neurol Sci* 1996;140: 1–116.

16. The Antiphospholipid Antibodies and Stroke Study Group (APASS). Anticardiolipin antibodies and the risk of recurrent thrombo-occlusive events and death. *Neurology* 1997;48:91–94.

17. Tietjen GE, Day M, Norris L, Aurora S, Halvorsen A, Schultz LR, Levine SR. Role of anticardiolipin antibodies in young persons with migraine and transient focal neurologic events: a prospective study. *Neurology* 1998;50:1433–1440.

18. Lie JT, Kobayashi S, Tokano Y, Hashimoto H. Systemic and cerebral vasculitis coexisting with disseminated coagulopathy in systemic lupus erythematosus associated with antiphospholipid syndrome. *J Rheumatol* 1995;22:2173–2176.

19. Martinez-Cordero E, Rivera Garcia BE, Aguilar Leon DE. Anticardiolipin antibodies in serum and cerebrospinal fluid from patients with systemic lupus erythematosus. *J Invest Allerg Clin Immunol* 1997;7: 596–601.

20. McCarty-Farid GA. Antiphospholipid antibodies in systemic lupus erythematosus. *Curr Opin Rheumatol* 1994;6:493–500.

21. Toubi E, Khamashta MA, Panarra A, Hughes GR. Association of antiphospholipid antibodies with central nervous system disease in systemic lupus erythematosus. *Am J Med* 1995;99:397–401.

22. Abuaf N, Laperche S, Rajoely B, Carsique R, Deschamps A, Rouquette AM, Barthet C, Khaled Z, Marbot C, Saab N, Rozen J, Girard PM, Rozenbaum W. Autoantibodies to phospholipids and to the coagulation proteins in AIDS. *Thromb Haemost* 1997;77: 856–861.

23. Dasgupta B, Almond MK, Tanqueray A. Polyarteritis nodosa and the antiphospholipid syndrome. *Br J Rheumatol* 1997;36:1210–1212.

24. Morelli S, Perrone C, Paroli M. Recurrent cerebral infarctions in polyarteritis nodosa with circulating antiphospholipid antibodies and mitral valve disease. *Lupus* 1998;7:51–52.

25. Zuckerman E, Toubi E, Shiran A, Sabo E, Shmuel Z, Golan TD, Abinader Yeshurun D. Anticardiolipin antibodies and acute myocardial infarction in non-systemic lupus erythmatosus patients: a controlled prospective study. *Am J Med* 1996;101:381–386.

26. Gatenby PA. Neurological and obstetric manifestations of the antiphospholipid syndrome. *Lupus* 1996;5: 170–172.

27. Cuadrado MJ, Hughes GRV. Antiphospholipid (Hughes) syndrome. *Rheum Dis Clin North Am* 2001;27;507–524.

28. Galli M, Confurius P, Massen C. Anticardiolipin antibodies directed not to cardiolipin but to a plasma protein cofactor. *Lancet* 1990;335:1544–1547.

29. Gonzales-Portillo F, McIntyre JA, Wagenknecht DR, Williams LS, Bruno A, Biller J. Spectrum of antiphospholipid antibodies (aPL) in patients with cerebrovascular disease. *J Stroke Cerebrovasc Dis* 2001;10: 222–226.

30. McNeil HP, Simpson RJ, Chesterman CN. Antiphospholipid antibodies are directed against a complex

antigen that includes a lipid-binding inhibitor of coagulation: β_2-glycoprotein I (apolipoprotein H). *Proc Natl Acad Sci USA* 1990;87:4120–4124.

31. Brey RL, Abbott RD, Curb JD, Sharp DS, Ross GW, Stallworth CL, Kittner SJ. β_2-Glycoprotein 1-dependent anticardiolipin antibodies and risk of ischemic stroke and myocardial infarction: the Honolulu heart program. *Stroke* 2001;32:1701–1706.

32. Derksen RH, de Groot PG, Kater L, Nieuwenhuis HK. Patients with antiphospholipid antibodies and venous thrombosis should receive long-term anticoagulant treatment. *Ann Rheum Dis* 1993;52:689–692.

33. Elezovic I, Miljic P, Antunovic P, Suvajdzic N, Sretenovic M, Colovic M. The management of antiphospholipid syndrome. *Vojnosanit Pregl* 1998;55(Suppl 2): 41–46.

34. Khamashta MA, Cuadrado MJ, Mujic F, Taub NA, Hunt BJ, Hughes GRV. The management of thrombosis in the antiphospholipid antibody syndrome. *N Engl J Med* 1995;332:993–997.

35. Krnic-Barrie S, O'Connor CR, Looney SW. A retrospective review of 61 patients with antiphospholipid syndrome: analysis of factors influencing recurrent thrombosis. *Arch Intern Med* 1997;157:2101–2108.

36. Petrovic R, Petrovic M, Novicic-Sasic D, Cirovic L, Damjanov N, Palic D. Anticardiolipin antibodies and clinical spectrum of antiphospholipid syndrome in patients with systemic lupus erythematosus. *Vojnosanit Pregl* 1998;55(Suppl 2):23–28.

37. Prandoni P, Simioni P, Girolami A. Antiphospholipid antibodies, recurrent thromboembolism, and intensity of warfarin anticoagulation. *Thromb Haemost* 1996; 75:859.

38. Rance A, Emmerich J, Fiessinger JN. Anticardiolipin antibodies and recurrent thromboembolism. *Thromb Haemost* 1997;77:221–222.

39. Rosove MH, Brewer PMC. Antiphospholipid thrombosis: clinical course after the first thrombotic event in 70 patients. *Ann Intern Med* 1992;117:303–308.

40. Ruiz-Irastorza G, Khamashta MA, Hunt BJ, Escudero A, Cuadrado MJ, Hughes GR. Bleeding and recurrent thrombosis in definite antiphospholipid syndrome: analysis of a series of 66 patients treated with oral anticoagulation to a target international normalized ratio of 3.5. *Arch Intern Med* 2002;162:1164–1169.

41. Schulman S, Svenungsson E, Granqvist S. Anticardiolipin antibodies predict early recurrence of thromboembolism and death among patients with venous thromboembolism following anticoagulant therapy. The Duration of Anticoagulation Study Group. *Am J Med* 1998;104:332–338.

42. Verro P, Levine SR, Tietjen GE. Cerebrovascular ischemic events with high positive anticardiolipin antibodies. *Stroke* 1998;29:2245–2253.

43. Zanon E, Prandoni P, Vianello F, Saggiorato G, Carraro G, Bagatella P, Girolami A. Anti-beta$_2$-glycoprotein I antibodies in patients with acute venous

thromboembolism: prevalence and association with recurrent thromboembolism. *Thromb Res* 1999;96: 269–274.

44. British Committee for Standards in Hematology. Guidelines on oral anticoagulation, third edition. *Br J Haematol* 1998;101:374–387.

45. Greaves M, Cohen H, Machin SJ, Mackie I. Guidelines on the investigation and management of the antiphospholipid syndrome. *Br J Haematol* 2000;109: 704–715.

46. Ginsberg JS, Wells PS, Brill-Edwards P, Donovan D, Moffatt K, Johnston M, Stevens P, Hirsh J. Antiphospholipid antibodies and venous thromboembolism. *Blood* 1995;86:3685–3691.

47. Ruiz-Irastorza G, Khamashta MA, Hughes GRV. Antiaggregant and anticoagulant therapy in systemic lupus erythematosus and Hughes' syndrome. *Lupus* 2001;10: 241–245.

48. Mohr JP, Thompson JL, Lazar RM, Levin B, Sacco RL, Furie KL, Kistler JP, Albers GW, Pettigrew LC, Adams HP Jr, Jackson CM, Pullicino P. A comparison of warfarin and aspirin for the prevention of recurrent ischemic stroke. *N Engl J Med* 2001;345:1444–1451.

49. Levine SR, Brey RL, Tilley BC, Thompson JLP, Sacco RL, Costigan TM, Rhine C, Murphy A, Levin B, Sciacca RR, Triplett DA, Mohr JP and the APASS investigators. Antiphospholipid Antibodies and Stroke Study (APASS). A collaborative study with WARSS. Abstract S38.001, AAN 54th Annual Meeting, Denver, April 2002.

50. Galli M, Barbui T. Antiprothrombin antibodies: detection and clinical significance in the antiphospholipid syndrome. *Blood* 1999;93:2149–2157.

51. Petri M. Management of thrombosis in antiphospholipid antibody syndrome. *Rheum Dis Clin North Am* 2001;27:633–642.

52. Schulman S, Rhedin AS, Lindmaker P, Carlsson A, Larfars G, Nicol P, Loogna E, Svensson E, Ljungberg B, Walter H. A comparison of six weeks with six months of oral anticoagulant therapy after a first episode of venous thromboembolism. Duration of Anticoagulation Trial Study Group. *N Engl J Med* 1995;332:1661–1665.

53. Piette JC, Wechsler B. Long term anticoagulant treatment in the antiphospholipid syndrome. *Ann Rheum Dis* 1994;53:355.

54. Derksen RHMW, de Groot PG, Kater L, Nieuwenhuis HK. Long term anticoagulant treatment in the antiphospholipid syndrome. *Ann Rheum Dis* 1994;53:355.

55. Khamashta MA. Management of thrombosis and pregnancy loss in the antiphopholipid syndrome. *Lupus* 1998;7(Suppl 2):S162–165.

56. Cancio LC, Cohen DJ. Heparin-induced thrombocytopenia and thrombosis. *J Am Coll Surg* 1998;186: 76–91.

57. Walenga JM, Bick RL. Heparin-induced thrombocytopenia, paradoxical thromboembolism, and other side

effects of heparin therapy. *Med Clin North Am* 1998; 82:635–658.

58. Bhandari M, Hirsh J, Weitz JI, Young E, Venner TJ, Shaughnessy SG. The effects of standard and low molecular weight heparin on bone nodule formation in vitro. *Thromb Haemost* 1998;80:413–417.

59. Lopez-Herce Cid JA, del Castillo Rueda A, Teigell Garcia L, Garrido Cantarero G, de Portugal Alvarez J. Osteoporosis in patients admitted to an internal medicine service of a university general hospital. *Ann Med Intern* 2001;18:121–123.

60. Schulman S, Hellgren-Wangdahl M. Pregnancy, heparin and osteoporosis. *Thromb Haemost* 2002;87:180–181.

61. Shaughnessy SG, Hirsh J, Bhandari M, Muir JM, Young E, Weitz JI. A histomorphometric evaluation of heparin-induced bone loss after discontinuation of heparin treatment in rats. *Blood* 1999;93:1231–1236.

62. Ford HC, Bailey RE. The effect of heparin on aldosterone secretion and metabolism in primary aldosteronism. *Steroids* 1966;7:30–40.

63. Kloppenborg PW, Casparie AF, Benraad TJ, Majoor CL. Inhibition of adrenal function in man by heparin or heparinoid Ro 1-8307. *Acta Med Scand* 1975;197:99–108.

64. Kutyrina IM, Nikishova TA, Tareyeva IE. Effects of heparin-induced aldosterone deficiency on renal function in patients with chronic glomerulonephritis. *Nephrol Dial Transplant* 1987;2:219–223.

65. Rospide C, Fustinoni O, Battilana N, Rodriguez Montero H. Findings on the antialdosteronic effect of heparin. *Prensa Med Argent* 1968;55:557–563.

66. Cailleux N, Moore N, Levesque H, Courtois H, Godin M. A low molecular weight heparin decreases plasma aldosterone in patients with primary hyperaldosteronism. *Eur J Clin Pharmacol* 1992;43:185–187.

67. Conn JW, Rovner DR, Cohen EL, Anderson JE Jr. Inhibition by heparinoid of aldosterone biosynthesis in man. *J Clin Endocrinol Metab* 1966;26:527–532.

68. Hunt BJ, Khamashta M, Lakasing L, Williams FM, Nelson-Piercy C, Bewley S, Hughes GR. Thromboprophylaxis in antiphospholipid syndrome pregnancies with previous cerebral arterial thrombotic events: is warfarin preferable? *Thromb Haemost* 1998;79:1060–1061.

69. Sanson BJ, Lensing AW, Prins MH, Ginsberg JS, Barkagan ZS, Lavenne-Pardonge E, Brenner B, Dulitzky M, Nielsen JD, Boda Z, Turi S, MacGillavry MR, Hamulyak K, Theunissen IM, Hunt BJ, Buller HR. Safety of low-molecular-weight heparin in pregnancy: a systematic review. *Thromb Haemost* 1999;81:668–672.

70. Nelson-Piercy C, Letsky E, de Swiet M. Low molecular weight heparin for obstetric thromboprophylaxis: experience of 69 pregnancies in 61 high risk women. *Am J Obstet Gynecol* 1997;176:1062–1068.

71. Shehata HA, Nelson-Piercy C, Khamashta MA. Management of pregnancy in antiphospholipid syndrome. *Rheum Dis Clin North Am* 2001;27:643–659.

72. Pauzner R, Dulitzki M, Langevitz P, Livnen A, Kenett R, Many A. Low molecular weight heparin and warfarin in the treatment of patients with antiphospholipid syndrome during pregnancy. *Thromb Haemost* 2001;86:1379–1384.

73. D'Angelo A, Valle PD, Crippa L. Monitoring therapy in patients with lupus anticoagulants. *Ann Intern Med* 1998;128:504.

74. Moll S, Ortel TL. Monitoring warfarin therapy in patients with lupus anticoagulants. *Ann Intern Med* 1997;127:177–185.

75. Lawrie AS, Purdy G, Mackie IJ. Monitoring of oral anticoagulant therapy in lupus anticoagulant positive patients with the antiphospholipid syndrome. *Br J Haematol* 1997;98:887–892.

76. Robert A, Le Querrec A, Delahousse B, Caron C, Houbouyan L, Boutière B, Horellou MH, Reber G, Sié P. Control of oral anticoagulation in patients with the antiphospholipid syndrome—influence of the lupus anticoagulant on International Normalized Ratio. Groupe "Méthodologie en Hémostase" du Groupe d'Etudes sur l'Hémostase et la Thrombose. *Thromb Haemost* 1998;80:99–103.

77. Castellino G, Cuadrado MJ, Godfrey T, Khamashta MA, Hughes GRV. Characteristics of patients with antiphospholipid syndrome with major bleeding after oral anticoagulant treatment. *Ann Rheum Dis* 2001;60:527–530.

78. Pattison NS, Chamley LW, Birdsall M, Zanderigo AM, Liddell HS, McDougall J. Does aspirin have a role in improving pregnancy outcome for women with the antiphospholipid syndrome? A randomized controlled trial. *Am J Obstet Gynecol* 2000;183:1008–1012.

79. Martinuzzo ME, Forastiero RR, Adamczuk Y, Pombo G, Carreras LO. Antiplatelet factor 4—heparin antibodies in patients with antiphospholipid antibodies. *Thromb Res* 1999;95:271–279.

80. Panzer S, Gschwandtner ME, Hutter D, Spitzauer S, Pabinger I. Specificities of platelet autoantiboies in patients with lupus anticoagulants in primary antiphospholipid syndrome. *Ann Hematol* 1997;74:239–242.

81. Alarcón-Segovia D, Sánchez-Guerrero J. Correction of thrombocytopenia with small dose aspirin in the primary antiphospholipid syndrome. *J Rheumatol* 1989;16:1359–1361.

82. Diener HC, Cunha L, Forbes C, Sivenius J, Smets P, Lowenthal A. European Stroke Prevention Study. 2. Dipyridamole and acetylsalicylic acid in the secondary prevention of stroke. *J Neurol Sci* 1996;143:1–13.

83. CAPRIE Steering Committee. A randomised, blinded, trial of clopidogrel versus aspirin in patients at risk of ischaemic events (CAPRIE). *Lancet* 1996;348:1329–1339.

84. Albers GW, Amarenco P. Combination therapy with clopidogrel and aspirin: can the CURE results be extrapolated to cerebrovascular patients? *Stroke* 2001;32:2948–2949.

85. Yusuf S, Zhao F, Mehta SR, Chrolavicius S, Tognoni G, Fox KK. Effects of clopidogrel in addition to aspirin in patients with acute coronary syndromes without ST-segment elevation. *N Engl J Med* 2001; 345:494–502.

86. Canadian Hydroxychloroquine Study Group. A randomized study of the effect of withdrawing hydroxychloroquine sulphate in systemic lupus erythematosus. *N Engl J Med* 1991;324:150–154.

87. Tsakonas E, Joseph L, Esdaile JM, Choquette D, Senecal JL, Cividino A, Danoff D, Osterland CK, Yeadon C, Smith CD. A long-term study of hydroxychloroquine withdrawal on exacerbations in systemic lupus erythematosus. The Canadian Hydroxychloroquine Study Group. *Lupus* 1998;7:80–85.

88. Fox RI, Kang HI. Mechanism of action of antimalarial drugs: inhibition of antigen processing and presentation. *Lupus* 1993;2(Suppl 1):S9–12.

89. Wallace DJ, Linker-Israeli M, Metzger AL, Stecher VJ. The relevance of antimalarial therapy with regard to thrombosis, hypercholesterolemia and cytokines in SLE. *Lupus* 1993;2(Suppl 1):S13–15.

90. Espinola RG, Pierangeli SS, Ghara AE, Harris EN. Hydroxychloroquine reverses platelet activation induced by human IgG antiphospholipid antibodies. *Thromb Haemost* 2002;87:518–522.

91. Avina-Zubieta JA, Galindo-Rodriguez G, Newman S, Suárez-Almazor ME, Russell AS. Long-term effectiveness of antimalarial drugs in rheumatic diseases. *Ann Rheum Dis* 1998;57:582–587.

92. Mavrikakis M, Papazoglou S, Sfikakis PP, Vaiopoulos G, Rougas K. Retinal toxicity in long term hydroxychloroquine treatment. *Ann Rheum Dis* 1996;55: 187–189.

93. Spalton DJ, Verdon Roe GM, Hughes GR. Hydroxychloroquine, dosage parameters and retinopathy. *Lupus* 1993;2:355–358.

94. Mazzuca SA, Yung R, Brandt KD, Yee RD, Katz BP. Current practices for monitoring ocular toxicity relayed to hydroxychloroquine therapy. *J Rheumatol* 1994;21: 59–63.

95. Weiner A, Sandberg MA, Gaudio AR, Kini MM, Berson EL. Hydroxychloroquine retinopathy. *Am J Ophthalmol* 1991;112:528–534.

96. Parke AL. Antimalarial drugs, systemic lupus erythematosus and pregnancy. *J Rheumatol* 1988;15: 607–610.

97. Parke A, West B. Hydroxychloroquine in pregnant patients with systemic lupus erythematosus. *J Rheumatol* 1996;23:1715–1718.

98. Parke AL, Rothfield NF. Antimalarial drugs in pregnancy—the North American experience. *Lupus* 1996; 5(Suppl 1):S67–69.

99. Apuzzo MLJ, Davey LM, Manuelidis EE. Pineal apoplexy associated with anticoagulant therapy. *J Neurosurg* 1976;45:223–226.

100. Erlich SS, Apuzzo MLJ. The pineal gland: anatomy, physiology, and clinical significance. *J Neurosurg* 1985;63:321–341.

101. Backos M, Rai R, Baxter N, Chilcott IT, Cohen H, Regan L. Pregnancy complications in women with recurrent miscarriage associated with antiphospholipid antibodies treated with low dose aspirin and heparin. *Br J Obstet Gynaecol* 1999;106:102–107.

102. Ruffatti A, Dalla Barba B, Del Ross T, Vettorato F, Rapizzi E, Tonello M, Suma V, Grella P, Gambari PF. Outcome of fifty-five newborns of antiphospholipid antibody-positive mothers treated with calcium heparin during pregnancy. *Clin Exp Rheumatol* 1998; 16:605–610.

103. Adams HP Jr, Adams RJ, Brott T, del Zoppo GJ, Furlan A, Goldstein LB, Grubb RL, Higashida R, Kidwell C, Kwiatkowski TG, Marler JR, Hademenos GJ. Stroke Council of the American Stroke Association: Guidelines for the early management of patients with ischemic stroke: a scientific statement from the Stroke Council of the American Stroke Association. *Stroke* 2003;34:1056–1083.

104. The National Institute of Neurological Disorders and Stroke rt-PA Stroke Study Group. Tissue plasminogen activator for acute ischemic stroke. *N Engl J Med* 1995;333:1581–1587.

Chapter 14

Intracranial Hemorrhage in Patients Using Warfarin

Eelco F. M. Wijdicks

A spontaneous or traumatic intracranial hemorrhage is one of the most serious complications associated with anticoagulation.[1] Comatose patients with an intracerebral hematoma and prior use of high-intensity anticoagulation (international ratio or INR >3), in particular, fair poorly, and this combination is typically fatal.[2] However, if the patient survives, resumption of anticoagulation with warfarin is at issue.[3–7] As frequently happens, in a certain number of patients the mere confrontation with a life-threatening hemorrhage results in a critical reconsideration of the true necessity of anticoagulation. This is supported by a recent study from Switzerland that suggested anticoagulation was not a straightforward indication in 38 percent of patients with intracranial hematoma.[8] Warfarin is often replaced with a combination of antiplatelet agents. Yet, in some patients, a prior history of recurrent arterial or venous occlusions or the presence of a mechanical heart valve would warrant resumption of warfarin without much debate. We estimate that major medical centers will be confronted approximately five times a year with these challenging cases.[7]

This chapter presents a clinical circumstance best summarized as a life-threatening complication of a required drug. But it counters the general clinical impression that a short interruption of anticoagulation is placing these patients at high risk.

■ The Patient

A 47-year-old attorney slips on the ice while intoxicated after a "spirited" dinner. He drives home, but a temporal headache appears, and the moment he parks his car in the garage he vomits. While undressing before going to bed, his wife notices a scalp hematoma and urges him to visit the emergency room. He has been on warfarin for an aortic St. Jude valve, and his INR values for some reason have been erratic. On arrival in the emergency room, he is slightly inebriated and jovial. Only a mild facial asymmetry is noted and a drift of the left arm. CT scan shows a large subdural hematoma with some mass effect and traumatic subarachnoid blood (Figure 14-1). INR is 4.2. About 30 minutes after arrival, when revisited to infuse plasma, he is much more drowsy. He opens his eyes only to pain and fends off pain stimuli accompanied by the use of a swear word. He receives fresh frozen plasma (3 units) and 2.5 mg vitamin K and undergoes craniotomy. Postoperatively, he recovers quickly. On the third postoperative day he develops atrial fibrillation for 4 hours, but it spontaneously reverts to sinus rhythm. The consulted cardiologist feels rapid anticoagulation is needed to prevent thrombosis of the prosthetic valve and to minimize systemic embolization. Two years prior, he needed an emergency embolectomy of a femoral artery embolus after anticoagulation was

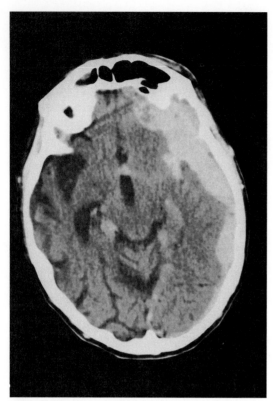

Figure 14-1. CT scan showing traumatic subdural hematoma and subarachnoid hemorrhage with some fluid-plasma levels typical of coagulopathy.

discontinued for one month as a result of a gastric hemorrhage.

■ The Problem

- How to reverse anticoagulation?
- What INR value is acceptable before evacuation of intracerebral or subdural hematoma?
- Who is at greatest risk of embolization after discontinuation of anticoagulation?
- When should one restart anticoagulation and with what agent?
- What are the long-term major risks of anticoagulation after a prior intracranial hemorrhage?

■ The Evidence

Anticoagulation of patients with nonneurological disorders (myocardial infarction, pulmonary embolus, peripheral vascular disease) is common and indications may be widening.[9] The use of warfarin is mandatory in patients with mechanical valves. Although debatable, the use of warfarin for severe occlusive nonsurgical cerebrovascular disease is prevalent, particularly with recurrent symptoms and "failed" antiplatelet trials. Indeed, anticoagulation of patients with prior noncardioembolic ischemic stroke may not be beneficial and may even be harmful, leading some experts to discourage its use.[10]

In order to appreciate the need for warfarin in patients with metallic heart valves—as in our patient example—it is useful to review some of the current knowledge on these devices. The beginning of heart valve replacement surgery marked a major feat in cardiac surgery by significantly improving functional class and cardiac physiology. Since then, several replacement valves have been manufactured using sophisticated mechanics (Figure 14-2). An alternative option is the use of cryopreserved bioprosthesis. This cryopreserved bioprosthesis (porcine or bovine pericardium) has advantages such as a much lower thrombogenicity. This allows for shorter anticoagulation targeting toward a lower INR goal and is possibly associated with less severe hemorrhages. However, due to structural deterioration, the durability of these valves is substantially less, making it a less attractive option for younger individuals. The decision by cardiovascular surgeons to use a particular type of heart valve is highly individualized, and surgical preference plays some role.

Outcome after prosthetic heart valve surgery has been good and results have been fairly consistent among published series and clinical trials. Mortality at 15 years, however, reaches 80 percent in those series biased toward older patients with significant comorbidity. Reoperation for valve structure deterioration is not common in mechanical valves, and this reduces mortality when compared with prosthetic metallic valves. Short-term outcome studies (<5 years) are unable to determine differences, and an advantage of one type of metallic heart valve over another is not apparent. However, comparison between observational surgical series is inherently flawed largely due to lack of reports of important baseline characteristics.[11,12] This makes it difficult to find discrepancies if they exist.

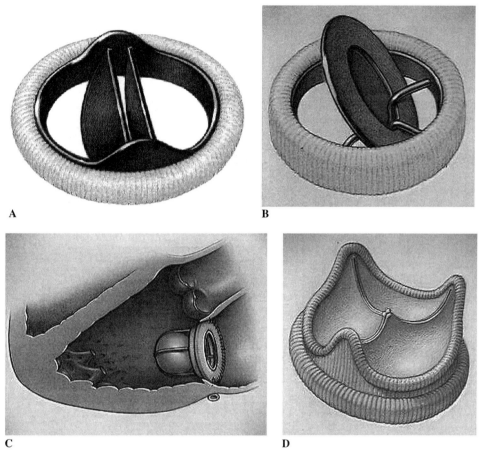

Figure 14-2. Metallic and prosthetic valves currently in use. (A) Bileaflet (two semicircular leaflets swinging apart with opening, e.g., St. Jude Medical). (B) Disk valve (e.g., design originally Björk, Shiley; now mostly manufactured by Hall Medtronic). (C) Ball valve (e.g., Starr Edwards). (D) Bioprosthetic valve (porcine).

Anticoagulation after valve replacement is generally regulated toward INR values of 3–4. Oral anticoagulation is dependent on the type and location of the valve and also the presence of atrial fibrillation. There is a common perception by experts seeing high volumes of patients that caged ball valves, a mitral position, and atrial fibrillation increase the embolic risk. Current standard recommendations (American College of Chest Physicians Consensus and British Society for Haematology) call for (1) INR range of 2–3 for bileaflet aortic valves (e.g., St. Jude medical) and no atrial fibrillation or abnormal ejection fraction on echocardiogram; (2) INR 2.5–3.5 for tilting disk and bileaflet valves in a mitral position and when a bileaflet valve is placed in the aorta position in a patient with coexisting atrial fibrillation; and (3) INR 2.5–3.5 for caged-ball valves. In patients with prior embolization, the INR values are targeted higher or combined with low-dose aspirin (80 mg).[13–15]

Clotting and Basic Pharmacology of Warfarin

Minimizing thromboembolism in patients with prosthetic valves using warfarin could be directed toward two targets. In patients with additional atrial fibrillation, intracardiac thrombi on the endocardium of the left atrium may form due to stasis or strands may appear on the artificial valve and bind platelet aggregates.[16] These thrombi may further mature into mixed platelet-fibrin-leucocyte particles catching plasma protein fragments, but they finally disintegrate, dislodge, and travel.

Warfarin is an antithrombotic agent closely linked to the so-called vitamin K cycle. The relationship between vitamin K and coagulation factors is complex but can be briefly summarized as follows. The important coagulation factors II, VII, IX, and X only become active after carboxylation of the glutamic acid residue incorporated in their chemical structure. This carboxylation requires vitamin KH_2, a reduced vitamin K form present in many food sources (particularly leafy vegetables). During the process of carboxylation, vitamin KH_2 oxidizes to vitamin KO which reduces to vitamin K_1, closing the vitamin K_1-vitamin KH_2-vitamin KO cycle. Warfarin predominantly blocks the formation of vitamin KH_2 and, hence, prevents activation of the above-mentioned clotting factors through this process of carboxylation. However, excess of vitamin K_1 intake (through dietary means or parenteral administration) can bypass this cycle through a pyridine nucleotide-dependent pathway which is not inhibited by warfarin.[17] Warfarin is rapidly absorbed through the gastrointestinal tract, has a high bioavailability and a half-life of 36–42 hours, and is bound to plasma albumin. Warfarin remains a complex drug to monitor, and its action is influenced by food high in vitamin K such as vegetables and lettuce more commonly consumed in the summer. Warfarin is also difficult to regulate when certain drugs are coadministered; most noticeable are aspirin, penicillins, oral contraceptives, and nonsteroidal anti-inflammatory drugs. Patients with prosthetic heart valves may also use "cardiac" drugs with established interactions (amiodarone, propranolol, propafenone). There is no inhibiting or potentiating effect of atenolol, felodipine, and metoprolol.

Age affects the pharmacokinetics of warfarin due to increased sensitivity, possibly a consequence of change in receptor affinity, and thus a lower daily dose of warfarin is needed. Consequently, elderly patients may possibly be at greater risk of bleeding with overdose. Liver disease additionally affects the synthesis of the four coagulant proteins inhibited by warfarin.

It is prudent to use fresh, frozen plasma or prothrombin concentrate and minimize the use of large doses of vitamin K (>5 mg). When using high doses of vitamin K, it may be difficult to rapidly attain a satisfactory INR in the weeks ahead due to warfarin resistance. Monitoring anticoagulation is

achieved using the prothrombin time. The prothrombin time (PT) is a reflection of reduction of factors II, VII, and X, with the most significant reduction in factor VII initially due to its short half-life. PT monitoring has been improved using a standard measure known as the International Normalized Ratio (INR).

Sudden discontinuation of warfarin in patients with intracranial hemorrhage may theoretically cause rebound hypercoagulability. Although there is no convincing clinical evidence of early embolization, laboratory studies have shown a factor VII rise favoring a procoagulant state.[18]

Diagnosis of Warfarin-Related Intracranial Hemorrhage

Treatment of patients with warfarin increases the risk for intracranial hematoma, and estimates based on patient populations studied in the 1980s and 1990s have suggested an 8–10-fold increase.[19] There are several predisposing factors. Established factors are prior INR with exponential increase with higher targets (Table 14-1), recent ischemic stroke with CT documentation of leukoaraiosis,[23] alcohol abuse, and liver disease. Traumatic brain injury (e.g., subdural hematoma) remains predominantly represented as a cause in published series.[8,24–26] The time exposed to warfarin may certainly be a factor, and some studies suggest the risk of intracranial hemorrhage is highest within the first 6 months[8] and even the first month.[27]

Most patients have a lobar hematoma, but in approximately one-third of patients the hematoma is localized in the basal ganglia while purely intraventricular hemorrhage occurs rarely (1 percent of patients).[23] Anticoagulated patients with intracranial hematomas are unstable neurologically. In the largest study to date, 47 percent of 106 initially surviving patients deteriorated clinically at a rate probably twice as high as in patients without anticoagulation.[28] Clinically, coma within hours of presentation is a poor prognosticating factor. Outcome is not only determined by size but also by ventricular extension, and horizontal shift of midline CT landmarks such as third ventricle, septum pellucidum, and pineal gland.[29] CT scan features of warfarin-related hemorrhage are blood sedimentation level (plasma–blood interface)[30,31]

Table 14-1. Relationship Between Anticoagulation Intensity and Bleeding in Patients with Prosthetic Heart Valves

Source	No. of Patients	Duration of Therapy	Target INR Range	Incidence of Bleeding (%)	P
Turpie et al. (1988)[20]	210	3 months	2.5–4.0 vs. 2.0–2.5	13.9 vs. 5.9	<0.002
Saour et al. (1990)[21]	247	3.5 years	7.4–10.8 vs. 1.9–3.6	42.4 vs. 21.3	<0.002
Altman et al. (1991)[22]*	99	11 months	3.0–4.5 vs. 2.0–2.9	24.0 vs. 6.0	<0.02

*Patients also given aspirin 300 mg daily, and dipyridamole 75 mg b.i.d.
Adapted and reprinted with permission from Hirsh J, Fuster V, Ansell J, Halperin JL. American Heart Association/American College of Cardiology Foundations guide to warfarin therapy. *Circulation* 2003;107:1692–1711.

and perhaps a proclivity to involve the vermis of the cerebellum.[27] Enlargement of its original size when the CT scan is repeated is common. This may occur despite normalization of the INR. Serial disruption of arterioles and venules surrounding an expanding pressured mass may lead to increasing volume. This mechanism would also better explain the early deterioration than other more protracted mechanisms involving inflammation or metalloprotease induction.

■ The Pros and Cons

Reversal of anticoagulation in a patient with intracerebral hematoma would seem obvious. However, the desired International Normalized Ratio (INR) level is unclear. Although not considered an alternative, there are no data to suggest that continuation of anticoagulation or correction to lower therapeutic INR would result in a worse outcome. There are no studies comparing levels of INR and growth of intracerebral hematoma over time. After the clot has reached to a certain size, further enlargement or rebleeding may not occur. There is some preliminary data to suggest enlargement of the hematoma completes within 12 hours.[32]

Reversal of the effects of warfarin can be achieved with fresh, frozen plasma and vitamin K. Traditionally, the INR should be below 1.5 when craniotomy is contemplated. In general, the vitamin K-dependent factors (II, VII, IX, and X) are usually at least 40 percent or higher when the INR is 1.4–1.5 or less. Based on the risk of bleeding for congenital isolated factor deficiency, most patients have normal or near-normal hemostasis when the factor level is 40 percent or higher.

By estimating plasma volume as $40\times$ body weight in mL (or using 15 mL/kg), in order to correct rapidly, full replacement of all coagulant factors would require 6–7 units of 200–250 mL of plasma.[33] The coagulation factor VII has a very short half-life (4–6 hours) but the half-lives of other procoagulant factors are longer (up to 2–4 days). Therefore, reversal of warfarin needs to be additionally managed with vitamin K (2.5 mg slow infusion IV). However, a recent review could not definitely establish the optimal dose and administration route of vitamin K in order to rapidly reverse warfarin.[34] Vitamin K alone adequately reverses oral anticoagulation but at a much slower pace (12–24 hours) and thus remains adequate in situations of elective surgery.

The volume load of fresh, frozen plasma is a serious concern in the elderly, and more recent studies have suggested using prothrombin complex concentrates containing all needed factors. Preliminary studies have demonstrated a more rapid increase in these procoagulant factors using prothrombin complex concentrate or very expensive factor VII concentrate.[35] Correction of INR can be achieved 3 times more quickly and within 15 minutes.[36] Although no large series of patients have been published, concentrates may be preferred in those unable to tolerate the volume load of plasma (e.g., patients with poor ventricular contractility) and in situations when INR is exceedingly high (>8).[37]

The decision to proceed with craniotomy is dependent on location, development of signs of brain herniation, and, to some extent, underlying comorbidity. When present in the cerebellum, evacuation of cerebellar hematoma is imperative when the clot is localized in the vermis and brainstem distortion or early hydrocephalus is present on admission CT. However, deterioration did not appear more common in previously anticoagulated patients with cerebellar hematomas.[38] Decisions on evacuation of intracranial hematomas are discussed in Chapter 16.

Another concern is the risk to the patient off anticoagulation (Table 14-2). The estimated aggregate value for annual probability of valvular thrombosis and embolization with a St. Jude valve and warfarin is quite low, respectively 0.001 and 0.01 percent.[43] Without anticoagulation, the risk of embolization increases almost fourfold[24] (risk of major stroke or death of 4 percent per year and risk of valve thrombosis of 1.8 percent per year). Embolization is also more common in patients with first-generation ball cage, tilting disk mitral prosthesis, double position prosthetic valves, atrial fibrillation, severe left ventricular dysfunction, prior embolic events, or another associated hypercoagulable state.[44]

The data on prevention of ischemic stroke in patients with atrial fibrillation using warfarin is robust. It has been eloquently summarized as follows: "Warfarin versus placebo translates into reducing the rate of thromboembolic event by 30 per 1000 person-years at the expense of 6 major hemorrhages per 1000 person-years."[45] This, however, only applies to patients older than 65 and with chronic or recurrent atrial fibrillation. Much less is known about the risk of discontinuation of warfarin in the setting of hemorrhage. In patients with prior stroke and atrial fibrillation, brief discontinuation of warfarin may be associated with a 3 percent risk of stroke recurrence.

The risk associated with short-term discontinuation in patients with atrial fibrillation alone seems quite low.[46,47] Blacker et al.[48] studied the risks of discontinuation for patients with atrial fibrillation and endoscopic procedures. The 30-day stroke risk in the total population undergoing endoscopy was low at 0.02 percent. A comparison with a population of 24,641 patients observed up to 36 days after general and vascular surgical procedures revealed a 0.08 percent risk of stroke.[47] In a subpopulation of patients with atrial fibrillation and adjusted anticoagulation, the observed risk of stroke was 1.06 percent. This is higher than that predicted by theoretical calculations[49] and substantially higher than the above-mentioned baseline risk.

In our patient example, restarting anticoagulation remains undisputed. Replacing it with antiplatelet agents could unnecessarily place our patient at risk. Wong et al. even calculated that changing to less effective antiplatelet agents could shorten life expectancy by 1.5 years.[43] One concern is the risk of rebleeding after resumption of warfarin. In addition, timing of resumption of warfarin may seem a major problem. Rebleeding after restarting heparin or warfarin is rarely seen, but the published experience is limited (see Table 14-2). We believe that aiming at a therapeutic INR 7–10 days after reversal of anticoagulation is a reasonable compromise while monitoring the size of hematoma or operation site with serial CT scanning. A recent advice of a waiting period of 4–6 weeks before restarting anticoagulation is unwarranted and not based on the data.[50]

Table 14-2. Studies on Intracerebral Hematoma and Prosthetic Valves

Author and Year	No. of Patients	Rebleeding*	Ischemic Stroke*	Restarting Anticoagulation (day)
Babikian et al. (1988)[39]	6	0	0	5–42 days (mean 19 days)
Butler and Tait (1998)[40]	13	1	3	Median 7 days
Wijdicks et al. (1998)[7]	26	0	0	Median 8 days
Bertram et al. (2000)[41]	15	3	3	60% within 7 days
Phan et al. (2000)[42]	52	0	1	Median 7 days

*Intrahospital event.

It may be prudent to serially image the valve in question with echocardiography, probably weekly. Most of the time, transthoracic echocardiogram can adequately image the prosthetic valve. When uncertainty persists, a transesophageal echocardiogram should be performed. Valve thrombosis usually is only detected on echocardiography and the appearance of strands can still be associated with a hemodynamic stable state. The emergence of spontaneous atrial contrast or strands should be considered an evolving thrombus. When valve thrombosis is diagnosed, thrombolysis is attempted first in most instances, but in this category of patients with an intracranial hematoma, replacement of the valve is needed if the mechanical function is compromised.

The starting day of warfarin can be arbitrarily set at day 5, aiming at a therapeutic INR between days 7 and 10 (Table 14-3). More aggressive resumption (within 3–7 days) should also be considered if only minor traumatic subarachnoid hemorrhage is present and follow-up CT has not documented later-appearing hemorrhagic contusions. Anticoagulation is gradually started using warfarin 5–10 mg orally. The use of low molecular weight heparins (LMWH) is ill advised. LMWH may seem comparable with unfractionated heparin[51] when used briefly. However, long-term use, as in pregnancy, has been unable to prevent valve thrombosis in up to 20 percent of cases.[52] Intravenous heparin is contraindicated when residual blood is seen on CT and should only be considered after

complete evacuation of an acute subdural hematoma in patients with perceived need for earlier anticoagulation or evidence of thrombus formation.

Long-term risk of recurrence after spontaneous intracranial hemorrhage without anticoagulation is low. In a study of 35 patients with median follow-up of 23.5 months, no recurrent hemorrhage was found.[53] The risk of recurrent hemorrhage in survivors from a cerebral hematoma after resumption of warfarin is not known, and data are obviously hard to obtain. In many patients, long-term outcome may not be available, or warfarin has been replaced by antiplatelet agents.

■ The Main Points

- Clinical deterioration in anticoagulated patients with intracranial hematoma occurs in at least half of the patients.
- Presentation with coma and CT evidence of tissue shift is a poor prognostic factor (see Chapter 16).
- Swift management in the neurological-neurosurgical intensive care unit is best characterized by aggressive reversal of anticoagulation with fresh frozen plasma, vitamin K, or use of prothrombin complex concentrate in patients with very high INR and poor cardiac function.
- Serial CT scan should be used to monitor expansion of hematoma. Craniotomy is only needed in clinically deteriorating patients.
- While the patient is recovering from the hemorrhage, echocardiogram should be performed weekly in an attempt to monitor the development of valve thrombus formation or valvular dysfunction.
- In most patients, aiming for a therapeutic INR 7 to 10 days after the hemorrhage conforms to a reasonable balance between the risk of new or worsening hemorrhage and the benefit of prevention of embolism.

Table 14-3. Useful Facts on Adjusting Warfarin

- Vitamin K_1 (>5 mg) may cause resistance to warfarin for one week.
- Vitamin K_1 could be administered in a slow intravenous infusion of 10 mg in patients with excessive INR (>20), but fresh, frozen plasma or prothrombin concentrate is also needed.
- Hepatic dysfunction potentiates response to warfarin (diminished available coagulation factors).
- Many drugs used in hospital inhibit clearance of warfarin.
- Heparin can be stopped when INR has been in therapeutic range for 2 days.

Reprinted with permission from Hirsh J, Fuster V, Ansell J, Halperin JL. American Heart Association/American College of Cardiology Foundations guide to warfarin therapy. *Circulation* 2003;107:1692–1711.[19]

■ References

1. Punthakee X, Doobay J, Anand SS. Oral-anticoagulant-related intracerebral hemorrhage. *Thromb Res* 2002; 108:31–36.
2. Nilsson OG, Lindgren A, Brandt L, Säveland H. Prediction of death in patients with primary intracerebral

hemorrhage: a prospective study of a defined population. *J Neurosurg* 2002;97:531–536.

3. Butler AC, Tait RC. Management of oral anticoagulant-induced intracranial haemorrhage. *Blood Rev* 1998; 12:35–44.

4. Gomez CR, Sandhu J, Mehta P. Resumption of anticoagulation during hypertensive cerebral hemorrhage with prosthetic heart valve. *Stroke* 1988;19:407.

5. Hacke W. The dilemma of reinstituting anticoagulation for patients with cardioembolic sources and intracranial hemorrhage: how wide is the strait between Skylla and Karybdis? *Arch Neurol* 2000;57:1682–1684.

6. Leker RR, Abramsky O. Early anticoagulation in patients with prosthetic heart valves and intracerebral hematoma. *Neurology* 1998;50:1489–1491.

7. Wijdicks EF, Schievink WI, Brown RD, Mullany CJ. The dilemma of discontinuation of anticoagulation therapy for patients with intracranial hemorrhage and mechanical heart valves. *Neurosurgery* 1998;42: 769–773.

8. Mattle H, Kohler S, Huber P, Rohner M, Steinsiepe KF. Anticoagulation-related intracranial extracerebral haemorrhage. *J Neurol Neurosurg Psychiatry* 1989; 52:829–837.

9. Ridker PM, Goldhaber SZ, Danielson E, Rosenberg Y, Eby CS, Deitch SR, Cushman M, Moll S, Kessler CM, Elliott CG, Paulson R, Wong T, Bauer KA, Schwartz BA, Miletich JP, Bounameaux H, Glynn RJ; PREVENT Investigators. Long-term, low-intensity warfarin therapy for the prevention of recurrent venous thromboembolism. *N Engl J Med* 2003;348:1425–1434.

10. Sandercock P, Mielke O, Liu M, Counsell C. Anticoagulants for preventing recurrence following presumed non-cardioembolic ischaemic stroke transient ischaemic attack. *Cochrane Database Syst Rev* 2003; (2):CD000248.

11. Byrne JG, Gudbjartsson T, Karavas AN, Mihaljevic T, Phillips BJ, Aranki SF, Rawn JD, Cohn LH. Biological vs. mechanical aortic root replacement. *Eur J Cardiothorac Surg* 2003;23:305–310.

12. Rahimtoola SH. Choice of prosthetic heart valve for adult patients. *J Am Coll Cardiol* 2003;41:893–904.

13. Ezekowitz MD. Anticoagulation management of valve replacement patients. *J Heart Valve Dis* 2002; 11(Suppl 1):S56–60.

14. Haemostasis and Thrombosis Task Force for the British Committee for Standards in Haemotology. Guidelines on oral anticoagulation, 3rd edition. *Br J Haematol* 1998;101:374–387.

15. Stein PD, Alpert JS, Bussey HI, Dalen JE, Turpie AGG. Antithrombotic therapy in patients with mechanical and biologic heart valves. *Chest* 2001;119: 220–227S.

16. Vongpatanasin W, Hillis LD, Lange RA. Prosthetic heart valves. *N Engl J Med* 1996;335:407–416.

17. Poller L, Hirsh J, eds. *Oral Anticoagulants*. London, Arnold; New York, Oxford University Press, 1996.

18. Schofield KP, Thomson JM, Poller L. Protein C response to induction and withdrawal of oral anticoagulant treatment. *Clin Lab Haematol* 1987;9: 255–262.

19. Hirsh J, Fuster V, Ansell J, Halperin JL. American Heart Association/American College of Cardiology Foundations guide to warfarin therapy. *Circulation* 2003;107:1692–1711.

20. Turpie AG, Gunstensen J, Hirsh J, Nelson H, Gent H. Randomised comparison of two intensities of oral anticoagulant therapy after tissue heart valve replacement. *Lancet* 1988;1:1242–1245.

21. Saour JN, Sieck JO, Mamo LA, Gallus AS. Trial of different intensities of anticoagulation in patients with prosthetic heart valves. *N Engl J Med* 1990;322: 428–432.

22. Altman R, Rouvier J, Gurfinkel E, D'Ortenicio O, Manzanel R, de La Fuente L, Favaloro RG. Comparison of two levels of anticoagulant therapy in patients with substitute heart valves. *J Thorac Cardiovasc Surg* 1991;101:427–431.

23. Franke CL, de Jonge J, van Swieten JC, Ope de Coul AA, van Gijn J. Intracerebral hematomas during anticoagulant treatment. *Stroke* 1990;21:726–730.

24. Cannegieter SC, Rosendaal FR, Briet E. Thromboembolic and bleeding complications in patients with mechanical heart valve prostheses. *Circulation* 1994;89:635–641.

25. Yasaka M, Minematsu K, Naritomi H, Sakata T, Yamaguchi T. Predisposing factors for enlargement of intracerebral hemorrhage in patients treated with warfarin. *Thromb Haemost* 2003;89:278–283.

26. Wintzen AR, de Jonge H, Loeliger EA, Bots GT. The risk of intracerebral hemorrhage during oral anticoagulant treatment. *Stroke* 1990;21:726–730.

27. Kase CS, Robinson RK, Stein RW, DeWitt LD, Hier DB, Harp DL, Williams JP, Caplan LR, Mohr JP. Anticoagulant related intracerebral hemorrhage. *Neurology* 1985;35:943–948.

28. Fujii Y, Takeuchi S, Sasaki O, Minakawa T, Tanaka R. Multivariate analysis of predictors of hematoma enlargement in spontaneous intracerebral hemorrhage. *Stroke* 1998;29:1160–1166.

29. Sjöblom L, Hardemark HG, Lindgren A, Norrving B, Fahlen M, Samuelsson M, Stigendal L, Stockelberg D, Taghavi A, Wallrup L, Wallvik J. Management and prognostic features of intracerebral hemorrhage during anticoagulant therapy: a Swedish multicenter study. *Stroke* 2001;32:2567–2574.

30. Ecker RD, Wijdicks EF. Footprints of coagulopathy. *J Neurol Neurosurg Psychiatry* 2002;73:534.

31. Ichikawa K, Yanagihara C. Sedimentation level in acute intracerebral hematoma in a patient receiving anticoagulation therapy: an autopsy study. *Neuroradiology* 1998;40:380–382.

32. Mayer SA. Ultra early hemostatic therapy for intracerebral hemorrhage. *Stroke* 2003;34:224–229.

33. Heit JA. Perioperative management of the chronically anticoagulated patient. *J Thromb Thrombolysis* 2001; 12:81–87.

34. Taylor CT, Chester EA, Byrd DC, Stephens MA. Vitamin K to reverse excessive anticoagulation: a review of the literature. *Pharmacotherapy* 1999;19: 1415–1425.

35. Yasaka M, Oomura M, Ikeno K, Naritomi H, Minematsu K. Effect of prothrombin complex concentrate on INR and blood coagulation system in emergency patients treated with warfarin overdose. *Ann Hematol* 2003;82:121–123.

36. Cartmill M, Dolan G, Byrne JL, Byrne PO. Prothrombin complex concentrate for oral anticoagulant reversal in neurosurgical emergencies. *Br J Neurosurg* 2000;14: 458–461.

37. Deveras RA, Kessler CM. Reversal of warfarin-induced excessive anticoagulation with recombinant human factor VIIa concentrate. *Ann Intern Med* 2002;137:884–888.

38. St Louis EK, Wijdicks EF, Li H. Predicting neurologic deterioration in patients with cerebellar hematomas. *Neurology* 1998;51:1364–1369.

39. Babikian VL, Kase CS, Pessin MS, Caplan LR, Gorelick PB. Resumption of anticoagulation after intracranial bleeding in patients with prosthetic heart valves. *Stroke* 1988;19:407–408.

40. Butler AC, Tait RC. Restarting anticoagulation in prosthetic heart valve patients after intracranial haemorrhage: a 2-year follow-up. *Br J Haematol* 1998;103: 1064–1066.

41. Bertram M, Bonsanto M, Hacke W, Schwab S. Managing the therapeutic dilemma: patients with spontaneous intracerebral hemorrhage and urgent need for anticoagulation. *J Neurol* 2000;247:209–214.

42. Phan TG, Koh M, Wijdicks EFM. Safety of discontinuation of anticoagulation in patients with intracranial hemorrhage at thromboembolic risk. *Arch Neurol* 2000;57:1710–1713.

43. Wong JB, Webb RK, Pauker SG. Double trouble: a patient with two prosthetic valves and two episodes of intracranial bleeding. *Med Decis Making* 1987;7:174–193.

44. Tiede DJ, Nishimura RA, Gastineau DA, Mullany CJ, Orszulak TA, Schaff HV. Modern management of prosthetic valve anticoagulation. *Mayo Clin Proc* 1998;73:665–680.

45. Diner BM. Anticoagulation or antiplatelet therapy for non-rheumatic atrial fibrillation and flutter. *Ann Emerg Med* 2003;41:141–143.

46. Carrel TP, Klingenmann W, Mohacsi PJ, Berdat P, Althaus U. Perioperative bleeding and thromboembolic risk during non-cardiac surgery in patients with mechanical prosthetic heart valves: an institutional review. *J Heart Valve Dis* 1999;8:392–398.

47. Parikh S, Cohen J. Perioperative stroke after general surgical procedures. *NY State J Med* 1993;93:162–165.

48. Blacker DJ, Wijdicks EFM, McClelland RL. Risk of stroke in anticoagulant patients with atrial fibrillation and endoscopic procedures. *Neurology* 2003;61:964–968.

49. Spandorfer J. The management of anticoagulation before and after procedures. *Med Clin North Am* 2001;85:1109–1116.

50. Crawley F, Bevan D, Wren D. Management of intracranial bleeding associated with anticoagulation: balancing the risk of further bleeding against thromboembolism from prosthetic heart valves. *J Neurol Neurosurg Psychiatry* 2000;69:396–398.

51. Montalescot G, Polle V, Collet JP, Leprince P, Bellanger A, Gandjbakhch I, Thomas D. Low molecular weight heparin after mechanical heart valve replacement. *Circulation* 2000;101:1083–1086.

52. Leyh RT, Fischer S, Ruhparwar A, Haverich A. Anticoagulant therapy in pregnant women with mechanical heart valves. *Arch Gynecol Obstet* 2003;268:1–4.

53. Vermeer SE, Algra A, Franke CL, Koudstaal PJ, Rinkel GJ. Long-term prognosis after recovery from primary intracerebral hemorrhage. *Neurology* 2002;59: 205–259.

Chapter 15
Spinal Epidural Metastases

David Schiff and Mark Shaffrey

Spinal epidural metastases (SEM) have the potential to occur with every systemic malignancy. The pathogenesis of at least 80 percent of cases begins with metastasis to the spinal canal, most commonly the vertebral body. Thus, it is not surprising that the most common tumors to metastasize to the spine are the most common causes of SEM. At autopsy, vertebral metastases have been described in 90 percent of patients with prostate cancer, 74 percent with breast cancer, 45 percent with lung cancer, 29 percent with lymphoma or renal cell carcinoma, and 25 percent with gastrointestinal cancers.[1] These figures parallel the frequency of these tumors producing SEM, with prostate cancer accounting for 24 percent, breast cancer 19 percent, and lung cancer 16 percent of SEM cases.[2] Perhaps 10 percent of SEM episodes are caused by the growth of paraspinal tumors through the neural foramen into the spinal canal. Patients with known paraspinal tumors, such as those with Pancoast tumors of the lung or lymphomas with retroperitoneal lymphadenopathy, are at greatest risk. The major concerns in management are discussed in this chapter.

■ The Patient

A 38-year-old woman with a family history of breast cancer was diagnosed with node-positive, estrogen and progesterone receptor-negative breast cancer 4 years earlier. She underwent lumpectomy, radiotherapy, and chemotherapy with cyclophosphamide, methotrexate, and fluorouracil. She now presents to her internist with progressive low back pain over 2 months that she attributed to lifting her 6-year-old child. The pain is localized to the lumbar region and initially responded well to anti-inflammatory drugs. She denies numbness, weakness, or urinary dysfunction.

■ The Problem

- Do cancer patients with back pain but no other neurological symptoms or signs require further workup?
- When a cancer patient has back pain and a corresponding bone metastasis on plain radiograph or radionuclide bone scan, what further radiological evaluation is necessary?
- Does the entire spine need to be imaged when cord compression is suspected, or is it adequate to image the symptomatic region?
- If this patient did not have a history of cancer, but had a destructive lesion seen on lumbar spine radiography, what would the next step be?
- If this patient has epidural metastasis, does she need corticosteroids? Should she undergo radiotherapy, chemotherapy, or surgery? Should asymptomatic epidural metastases be treated?
- If her epidural metastasis is treated, but recurs locally 2 years later, what treatment options are available?

■ The Evidence

The traditional teaching has been that compression of the spinal cord from SEM usually was anterior. This tenet was systematically examined in a recent MRI study that divided the circumference of the cord into four quadrants: anterior, posterior, and two lateral quadrants.[3] The authors studied 108 consecutive patients with SEM at 160 spinal levels. Remarkably, they found that isolated anterior compression with metastatic disease restricted to the vertebral body occurred in only 3 percent of episodes. Rather, coexisting structural involvement of both anterior and posterior spinal column was the rule, with bone involvement of both in 75 percent of cases and a soft tissue epidural component both anteriorly and posteriorly in 43 percent of cases. Circumferential soft tissue compression of the spinal cord occurred in 22 percent of cases. Nonetheless, vertebral body involvement was substantially more common than involvement of the posterior ring in SEM, suggesting that bony disease frequently progresses in an anterior to posterior direction. Hence, the presence of posterior vertebral involvement in spinal metastasis may predict impending SEM.

Which Patients with Isolated Back Pain Require Imaging?

Back pain is a common complaint in patients with cancer. The decision to perform radiological evaluation in patients with radiculopathy or myelopathy and back pain is relatively straightforward. A more difficult question is how to determine which cancer patients with isolated back pain require workup and when this workup should be performed. Determining that back pain is attributable to bone metastasis rather than a nonneoplastic cause may suffice to initiate palliative therapy such as radiotherapy without further workup. It has been common practice among oncologists to prescribe palliative fractionated radiotherapy to cancer patients with back pain once plain radiographs or radionuclide bone scan have demonstrated metastatic disease at a site corresponding to the pain. However, in some situations it may be important to know whether there actually is cord compression or isolated bone disease distinction.

This distinction requires the use of MR scanning or myelography which visualizes the spinal cord or thecal sac.

Several studies bear on the likelihood that a cancer patient with back pain but no evidence of radiculopathy or myelopathy has epidural tumor. Rodichok et al. prospectively studied 87 cancer patients with 93 episodes of back pain, some with radiculopathy or myelopathy, who were examined by a neurologist.[4] One subset of patients in this study had back pain and evidence of corresponding spinal metastasis on either radiographs or bone scan. All of these patients underwent myelography and 15/25 (60 percent) had epidural metastasis. Another subset of 17 patients had back pain but normal radiographs and bone scans. None of the patients in this group who underwent myelogram were found to have epidural disease. Thus, 25/42 (60 percent) of cancer patients with back pain but no radicular or myelopathic findings had abnormal radiography or bone scan, and at least 15/42 (36 percent) had epidural extension of metastasis. The same authors later published an expanded version of this series with similar findings.[5]

O'Rourke et al. prospectively studied 60 patients with cancer and a normal neurological examination but either back pain or a bone scan were positive for spinal metastases.[6] When plain radiographs were abnormal, patients always underwent myelogram. When plain radiographs were normal, results of spine CT were used to determine which patients required myelogram. Overall, 20/60 (33 percent) had epidural disease.

A study by Ruff and Lanska found markedly different results from these two studies.[7] The authors prospectively evaluated 97 male cancer patients with back pain. All patients were examined by a neurologist, all had plain films, and all but 2 underwent myelography. About 40 percent had myelopathy, 30 percent radiculopathy, and 30 percent isolated back pain. While half the patients in the radiculopathy group had SEM, no patient (0/29) with isolated back pain had epidural disease of any degree. The authors hypothesize that some of the difference might be related to differences in classification.

Results more consistent with Rodichok's and O'Rourke's studies were found in a retrospective study evaluating 41 cancer patients who had undergone plain x-rays, bone scan, and complete myelogram.[8] Thirty-three of 41 patients had pain without radiculopathy, myelopathy, or cauda equina syndrome on examination by a neurologist; the remaining 8 had radiculopathy. Twenty-eight patients had abnormal radiographs and 36 had abnormal bone scans. Epidural disease was detected on myelography at 86 percent of spinal levels in cases with abnormal radiographs and at 8 percent of spinal levels in cases with normal radiographs. Overall, 25/41 patients symptomatic with pain (with or without radiculopathy) had epidural disease on myelogram. Even if all 8 patients with radiculopathy had epidural disease, this means the incidence of epidural disease in patients with pain alone (without radiculopathy) was >50 percent. Admittedly, selection bias likely may have played a role in this population assessed with all three imaging modalities.

Kienstra et al. published another study providing sobering information to clinicians confident of accurately selecting cancer patients likely to have epidural disease.[9] They prospectively evaluated 170 patients with cancer and new back or radicular pain, excluding patients with known spinal metastases. All patients had standardized history and examination by a neurologist as well as whole spine radiography and MRI. Seventy-seven patients (45 percent) had normal neurological examination and 76 (44 percent) had evidence of radiculopathy. Overall, 80/170 (47 percent) had bony spinal metastases and 31/170 (18 percent) had SEM. Although their data do not reveal how many of the SEMs occurred in patients with radiculopathy versus isolated back pain, neither radicular pain nor radicular sensory loss was a statistically significant predictor of epidural disease. Since patients with known spinal metastases were excluded, it is not surprising that this figure is lower than in the studies by Portenoy, Rodichok, and O'Rourke. Importantly, no combination of historical features, findings on neurological examination, or radiograph results could discriminate patients with or without epidural metastases. The authors concluded that following neurological evaluation, spinal MRI was indicated in all patients while there was no role for plain radiographs.

In the most recent study relevant to this topic, Bayley et al. prospectively evaluated patients with prostate cancer, known vertebral metastases, no neurological symptoms, and normal neurological exam (generally not performed by a neurologist).[10] Sixty-eight patients were included, of whom 22 had back pain. All patients underwent spinal MR imaging. Sixty-five patients had vertebral metastasis on MRI. Twenty-two patients had clinically occult SEM on MRI, including 12 with subarachnoid space (SAS) compression without frank cord/cauda equina compression, and 10 had frank compression of spinal cord (SC) or cauda equina. Neither the presence of back pain nor the need for narcotic analgesics was predictive of occult SAS/SC compression; 9/22 (41 percent) with back pain had SAS/SC compression, as did 13/46 (28 percent) of those without back pain. Extent of disease (i.e., number of metastases) on bone scan and duration of continuous hormonal therapy were associated with increased risk of SAS/SC compression. The authors concluded that it is reasonable to consider all patients with extensive bone disease for MR scanning, especially those with more than 20 metastases on bone scan.

The bulk of evidence from these studies suggests that a substantial minority of cancer patients with isolated back pain, even without radiculopathy, will have epidural extension of tumor. The incidence is lower if patients with known spinal metastases are excluded and higher if restricted to patients with documented spinal metastases. In Portenoy et al.'s small study, no patient with isolated back pain and normal plain films and bone scan had epidural metastasis. However, this finding has not been confirmed, and in fact most cancer patients with back pain have spinal metastases. Moreover, although plain films without metastatic lesions decreased the risk of epidural disease in the study by Kienstra et al., plain spinal radiographs overall were not useful in identifying patients who could safely forgo MR scanning.

Are MRI or Myelography Necessary Before Radiation Therapy in Patients with Suspected Epidural Metastasis and Localizing Clinical or Radiological Signs?

As the above discussion suggests, this question might also be extended to include suspected spine metastasis without epidural extension, as these entities are not reliably distinguished clinically.

In their prospective evaluation of cancer patients with back pain, Rodichok et al. compared theoretical radiation ports based on plain radiographs to those constructed incorporating results of myelography.[5] In the case of myelography, ports extended two vertebral segments above and below the visualized epidural defect; ports based on plain radiographs included two segments above and below vertebrae in the symptomatic region that were radiographically abnormal. Of 78 patients with abnormal spine films and myelography, 15 had such diffuse vertebral disease that ports could not be constructed. Ports based on plain films would have adequately covered all symptomatic epidural disease seen on myelography in 50 of the remaining 63 patients (79 percent). Three of the 50 patients had second sites of asymptomatic epidural disease that would not have been covered with plain film-based ports. Thus, more than one-quarter of patients would have had potentially inadequate radiation ports if only plain radiographs had been utilized.

A retrospective study similarly compared ports based on clinical examination and radiographs with or without myelography in 24 patients with 29 episodes of neurological deficits from SEM related to solid tumor.[11] In 76 percent of episodes, radiographs revealed discrete bone lesions; 5 patients had diffuse bone disease and 2 had no bone lesions. The additional information provided by myelography altered radiation ports in 69 percent of episodes. Fifteen ports were increased and 2 decreased; myelography in one patient revealed disc herniation rather than SEM. In 2 patients, myelography revealed additional sites of SEM. The authors concluded that plain radiographs underestimated the extent of disease, and that myelography was essential for treatment planning.

Another study evaluated the contribution of spinal MR scanning to treatment planning.[12] One part of this retrospective study reviewed 100 patients with suspected metastatic spine disease (78 symptomatic and 22 asymptomatic with a positive bone scan). The authors found that 47 percent of patients had treatment changes based on MR scan results, most of which consisted of addition of or changes in radiation therapy. However, they did not specify how treatment would have been determined without the MR results, making it impossible to compare their study to the previous two. In the second part of this study, they prospectively studied 30 patients with cancer, suspected spinal metastatic disease, and symptoms of SEM. After patients underwent MRI, the ordering clinician completed a questionnaire addressing the utility of MRI. Medical records were then reviewed to determine whether MRI results altered therapy. In 12 of 30 cases (40 percent), MRI results altered therapy. While this study highlights the unquestionable utility of MRI, it does not prove that MRI is mandatory for treatment planning.

What Is the Optimal Form of Imaging?

The two definitive means of diagnosing SEM are MR scanning and myelography (often combined with CT scanning). Each images the thecal sac and can display indentations and encircling of the sac. MR imaging offers several potential advantages over myelography. It produces anatomically reliable images of the spinal cord and intramedullary pathology and is even more sensitive than radionuclide bone scans at identifying bony metastases.[13] Unlike myelography, it can image the entire thecal sac despite the presence of a complete subarachnoid block. Moreover, it spares the patient a lumbar puncture.

Myelography may be better tolerated by patients in considerable pain, since image quality in MR scanning is dependent on the ability to lie still. Myelography permits cerebrospinal fluid (CSF) analysis that, although not useful for the diagnosis of SEM, is the cornerstone of the diagnosis of leptomeningeal metastases. Postmyelogram CT scans at the level of thecal sac impingement provide additional anatomic information about the tumor and often demonstrate some rostral passage of contrast at the level of high-grade subarachnoid block not appreciated on the myelogram itself. Rarely, patients with complete subarachnoid block deteriorate neurologically when CSF pressure below the block has been reduced by the lumbar puncture. For this reason, it is frequently useful to have neurosurgical input when a myelogram is considered for suspected SEM. Other potential drawbacks of myelography in the cancer patient population include the small risks of cerebral herniation with brain metastasis and the risk of spinal subdural hematoma related to coagulopathy.

Several studies dating from the early years of spinal MR imaging compared MRI to CT myelogram for the diagnosis of SEM. The two technologies were roughly equivalent in sensitivity and specificity.[14–16] Given the convenience and widespread availability of MR imaging, it is doubtful that future comparative studies will be forthcoming. Nevertheless, there are occasional cases, particularly with laterally located lesions, in which CT myelogram demonstrates abnormalities not visualized on MR scanning. In addition, it is an alternative study in patients with mechanical valves, pacemakers, paramagnetic implants, and shrapnel.

How Much of the Spine Should be Imaged in Suspected SEM?

When the decision has been made to evaluate a patient for SEM with MRI, the question arises as to how much of the spine needs to be imaged. In the pre-MRI era, myelography typically delineated the entire thecal sac unless there was a complete subarachnoid block due to epidural tumor. In those cases, a second spinal puncture rostral to the block was generally performed with injection of radio-opaque dye to delineate the rostral extent of the block as well as any other lesions.

The ability of MRI to target specific spinal segments means that it is quite possible that the entire spine will not be imaged in a given patient. Careful MR scans of the cervical, thoracic, and lumbosacral spine may require 2 hours or more of machine time, a substantial burden in many facilities and to some patients. Although some institutions have protocols that include a sagittal screen of the entire spine before targeting the spinal segment of interest, such protocols are not universal and depend on clear communication between clinician, technologist, and radiologist.

One argument in favor of imaging the entire spine is that multiple SEMs are common. The incidence of multiple SEMs ranges from 22 to 44 percent of all patients with SEM in several large studies.[7,17–22] The incidence is higher in patients undergoing complete spinal imaging (32 percent) than in those having only a portion of their spine imaged (18 percent).[20] The only clinical or radiographic factor predicting the likelihood of detecting multiple SEMs was the presence of multiple vertebral metastases on plain radiographs or bone scan. All common tumor types were represented among patients with multiple SEMs, and the frequency of multiple SEMs did not differ significantly according to the primary tumor site. Rarely were multiple SEMs suspected clinically prior to myelography or MR scan. Asymptomatic "coincidental" SEM was rare in the cervical spine; failure to image the cervical spinal cord in patients with thoracic or lumbar SEM would have missed a second SEM in only 1 percent. However, failure to image either the thoracic or lumbosacral spine when epidural disease was found elsewhere was associated with a 21 percent chance of missing another epidural tumor deposit.

The second potentially compelling reason to image the spine beyond the suspected symptomatic site of SEM is the limitation of the history and examination in localizing the lesion. In one prospective study conducted in breast cancer patients with symptoms or signs of radiculopathy or myelopathy, neuro-oncologists correctly predicted the site of SEM within a margin of two vertebral bodies in only 58 (67 percent) of 87 SEMs.[23] Only half of the clinically mislocalized or unlocalized SEMs were asymptomatic. The mislocalized lesions could be grouped into four main categories: (1) patients with their anatomic lesion several levels rostral to their spinal sensory level (explainable on the basis of laminar organization of the sensory pathways);[24] (2) patients with signs of L3 radiculopathy with SEM at T8 or T10; (3) patients with findings of an L5 or S1 radiculopathy with a lesion at the conus; and (4) patients with an L4 or L5 SEM and psoas weakness suggesting more rostral pathology.[25]

The final issue influencing whether it is necessary to image the entire spine in cases of known or suspected SEM is the need to treat asymptomatic, incidentally detected SEMs. This topic is considered later.

What Is the Workup of Epidural Masses in Patients Not Known to Have Cancer?

Twenty percent of all cases of SEM arise in patients not previously recognized to have cancer. The majority of these patients do not have signs or symptoms suggesting systemic malignancy or the location of an underlying cancer. Typically, radiographs, CT, or MR scans demonstrate a destructive process suspicious for malignancy involving the vertebral column. Akin to the situation with suspected brain metastases of unknown primary, such patients often undergo extensive evaluation looking for the primary site of malignancy.

The causative tumors in SEM as the initial manifestation of malignancy differ substantially from the usual causes of SEM. Breast cancer is almost always detected before it produces SEM, and prostate cancer usually is as well. On the other hand, non-Hodgkin's lymphoma, multiple myeloma, and lung cancer commonly present with SEM.

A rational, cost-effective approach to diagnosing such patients depends on early radiologically guided needle biopsy of the epidural mass. Such biopsies are usually performed under CT or fluoroscopic guidance. Serious complications with percutaneous needle biopsies are rare but include pneumothorax with thoracic spine biopsy and damage to the great vessels with cervical spine biopsy. Consequently, CT is generally utilized for cervical and thoracic spine lesions, whereas fluoroscopy suffices for large lumbar lesions. Biopsies are diagnostic for malignancy in more than 90 percent of cases, and generally are conclusive at demonstrating the origin of hematological malignancies. When biopsy demonstrates carcinoma, immunostaining may suggest likely tissues of origin that can be pursued with further imaging studies like CT or endoscopy.[2]

The Value of Corticosteroids

The salutary effects of corticosteroids for epidural spinal cord compression were first reported anecdotally in 1968.[26] Rodent models of spinal cord compression confirmed the beneficial effects of dexamethasone improving and preserving neurological function.[27,28] As with brain metastases, although other corticosteroids also worked, dexamethasone was favored because of its low mineralocorticoid activity, long half-life, low cost, and long tradition. Based on extrapolation from an effective dose in rodent studies, studies from the Memorial Sloan-Kettering Cancer Center utilizing dexamethasone in conjunction with radiotherapy reported a favorable experience administering a 100 mg bolus of intravenous dexamethasone at diagnosis

followed by 24 mg every 6 hours.[29,30] If the patient was stable, dexamethasone was halved every 3 days. Given this institution's leading role in management of SEM, many clinicians adopted this dosing schedule.

What Is the Proper Dose of Corticosteroid?

One randomized controlled trial has confirmed the benefit of corticosteroids in SEM. Sorensen et al. randomized patients with solid tumors and myelographically confirmed SEM to radiation versus radiation plus high-dose dexamethasone. Pretreatment ambulatory status was a stratification factor, so the two groups were balanced on this important prognostic variable. A higher percentage of patients in the group receiving dexamethasone remained ambulatory both at the conclusion of radiotherapy and at 6 months.[31]

High-dose dexamethasone has significant side effects even when administered for 1 to 2 weeks. In Sorensen's trial, 11 percent of the patients in the dexamethasone group had serious steroid-related adverse events. Similarly, another report noted serious complications in 4 of 28 consecutive patients (14 percent) treated with this high-dose schedule.[32] After switching to a lower-dose regimen of 4 mg every 6 hours, equivalent therapeutic results were seen with no serious side effects in 38 consecutive patients.

Another study evaluated the effect of the initial dexamethasone bolus in SEM. This phase III trial randomized patients to a bolus of either 100 or 10 mg dexamethasone; all patients then received 4 mg every 6 hours in addition to standardized radiotherapy. There was no difference in neurological outcome or pain control between the two groups.[33]

Some patients have relative contraindications to corticosteroids, and the question arises whether it is ever reasonable to withhold corticosteroids in the management of SEM. Maranzano et al. studied 20 patients with either normal neurological exams or radiculopathy without significant weakness; none of the patients had massive spinal canal compromise. All received standard radiation without corticosteroids, and all improved or remained clinically stable throughout radiation. They concluded that in patients fulfilling these criteria, withholding of corticosteroids was justifiable.[34]

What Is the Preferred Radiation Dose and Schedule?

Since there have been no comparative studies of different dose-fractionation schemas for SEM, no optimal schedule has yet been identified.[35,36] The Radiation Therapy Oncology Group (RTOG) has compared different schedules for the palliation of symptomatic bone metastases. Initial analysis did not demonstrate any advantage to various schedules ranging from 300 cGy × 5 fractions to 400 cGy × 5 fractions to 500 cGy × 5 fractions to 300 cGy × 10 fractions to 270 cGy × 15 fractions.[36] Subsequent reanalysis using logistic regression suggested that increasing number of fractions led to improved pain control.[37] Nonetheless, single large fractions have been successfully used (particularly in England) to palliate pain from bony metastases and are convenient for patients. Single fractions have not been utilized for SEM.[38] One study evaluated a regimen of two fractions of 800 cGy given one week apart in 53 patients with SEM who had radioresistant tumors or a poor prognosis (e.g., poor performance status, paresis, paralysis), or a short life expectancy.[39] The outcome was similar to more standard courses, although more gastrointestinal side effects were observed with two large fractions. In another report, the two-fraction regimen was compared prospectively in patients with prostate cancer and SEM with a split course regimen of 1500 cGy in three fractions, 4 days of rest, and then 1500 cGy in five fractions.[40] The short course was used in 17 patients with a poor prognosis and the split course was used in 27 other patients. There were no differences in functional response or complications between the treatment regimens. Most commonly, radiation oncologists administer 2000 to 4000 cGy in 5 to 20 fractions, with 3000 cGy in 10 fractions being a particularly popular regimen.

How Quickly Should Treatment Be Started?

Numerous studies have shown that the single most important prognostic factor for neurological outcome following treatment for SEM is the level of neurological function when treatment is initiated.[29,41–47] Less important prognostic variables include the underlying radiosensitivity of the tumor,[42,48,49] the degree of spinal subarachnoid block[42,49] (less is better), and the rate at which motor deficits have developed (the slower the better).[50]

Analogous to the situation with traumatic spinal cord injury, in which glucocorticoids need to be initiated within 8 hours of injury to be beneficial,[51] neuro-oncologists have long suggested that treatment of SEM should begin as expeditiously as possible once the diagnosis has been made. A recently published study confirmed that recovery of ambulation depended on rapidity of treatment initiation. For the purposes of this study, initiation of treatment was defined as administration of the first dose of dexamethasone.[52] For patients who are nonambulatory at presentation, the initiation of treatment within 12 hours of loss of ambulation increased the likelihood of regaining ambulation with treatment by sevenfold compared with starting treatment more than 12 hours later.

What Is the Role of Surgery for SEM?

Surgical treatment of SEM may become necessary in patients with intractable pain, progression of neurological deficits, or spinal instability. The need for surgery in the first two instances, persistence of pain or neurological deficits, often reflects the failure of primary treatment modalities such as radiation therapy, corticosteroids, and bracing. Pain may persist due to disruption or compression of nerve roots, spinal cord, dura, periosteum, or the bony structures and articulations that provide spinal stability. Abrupt worsening of pain can be a sign of pathological fracture. Spinal instability may be present at the time of patient presentation due to advanced destruction of the vertebral column or present in a delayed fashion due to a combination of weakening bone from tumor involvement and the effects of radiation treatment, failure to halt the progression of radioresistant tumors (e.g., renal cell carcinoma), or tumor recurrence following initial treatment. Surgical management in all of these instances depends upon the anatomic level and location (anterior, posterior, or circumferential) of the lesion, the extent of bony involvement above and below the area of concern, and the prognosis of the patient.

Most of the early attempts at surgical treatment of SEM for patients with neurological deficits focused solely on posterior approaches via laminectomy. This approach represented a failure to recognize that generally there is substantial involvement of the vertebral body (with secondary extension into the epidural space) anterior to the spinal cord and that posterior spinal decompression could lead to further destabilization of the spine. A retrospective comparison of patients treated with laminectomy with or without radiation therapy versus radiotherapy alone did not demonstrate an advantage for this surgical approach.[53] Furthermore, a small randomized trial of laminectomy plus radiotherapy did not prove beneficial when compared with radiotherapy alone.[54]

Improvements in neuroimaging have lead to accurate assessments of the locations and extent of vertebral column and soft tissue involvement by SEM. The aforementioned "laminectomy" era depended largely upon spine x-rays or plain myelography for surgical planning. Now, MRI, CT, combined CT myelography, and nuclear medicine bone scans have allowed much more accurate anatomic assessment of spinal and systemic involvement of disease.

Anterior approaches to the cervical, thoracic (via thoracotomy), and lumbar spine (via retroperitoneal exposure) have been refined by spine surgeons to allow portals and, thereby, access to the entire vertebral body where compressive metastatic disease is most common. Surgical decompression of the pathological fracture of a vertebral body with extension of tumor and retropulsed bone fragments into the epidural spinal canal may now be achieved with vertebral corpectomy (vertebrectomy). This approach fulfills the basic principles of cancer surgery, often allowing extensive exposure for gross total removal of disease. Also, improvements in spinal instrumentation have permitted more aggressive tumor resection. Vertebrectomy is followed by arthrodesis (fusion) using autologous bone (e.g., iliac crest, fibula, rib, etc.), cadaveric bone, or synthetic cages packed with bone for strut grafting to help support axial load. Finally, internal fixation using instrumentation (usually titanium screws, plates, and rods) allows temporary stabilization while the bony fusion is maturing.

One of the tenets of successful fusion is that bone will only fuse to bone. Thus, it is of crucial importance that the adjacent vertebral bodies above and below the vertebrectomy are free of cancer. Solid bone fusion offers long-term stability, but radiotherapy must be delayed up to 6 weeks postoperatively so that the bone graft is not adversely affected by irradiation. Another alternative is the use of a quick-setting polymer, such as methylmethacrylate, for replacement of the vertebral body. Although this material is strong in resisting compressive forces and allows immediate radiotherapy, it is poor in resisting rotational and shearing forces that are common in the spine and therefore can lead to early failure of the construct. Thus, methylmethacrylate is only recommended in those circumstances in which surgical palliation is desirable and the life expectancy is short.

Although the vertebral body is most often affected by metastatic disease, involvement of the spinous processes and lamina with additional compression from a posterior direction are often underestimated.[55] A series of 100 patients with MRI evidence of spinal cord compression and known history of malignancy, reported coexisting anterior and posterior bony involvement in 75 percent of cases.[3] Circumferential soft tissue compression of the spinal cord occurred in 22 percent of cases. If tumor destruction involves both anterior and posterior elements (particularly the pedicles) of the vertebral column, a combination of anterior and posterior decompression and stabilization may be necessary.

Evidence suggests substantial benefit with aggressive surgical treatment of spinal metastases. One case series reported encouraging results for aggressive surgical treatment in 110 patients, 47 of whom had failed radiotherapy.[56] Prior to surgery, 48 patients were nonambulatory and 20 patients had severe paraparesis. Surgical treatment used anterior approach only in 30 percent, staged anterior and posterior resections in 48 percent, and an isolated posterior approach in 5 percent. Improvement was reported in 82 percent in terms of pain relief and ambulatory status. Median survival was 16 months, with 46 percent of patients alive at 2 years. These results are excellent despite frequent complications of wound breakdown, infection, stabilization failure, and hematomas. The substantial rate of complications is most likely related to the extensive nature of the surgery, the advanced age of the patient population, a high rate of prior treatment with steroids and radiation, poor nutritional status, and potential long periods of bed rest due to neurological deficits and surgical treatment.

Survival was not as prolonged in another report of 109 patients with thoracic spine metastases treated with surgical decompression and radiotherapy.[57] The median survival was 10 months. Patients who were ambulatory preoperatively survived longer than those who were nonambulatory or had sphincter incontinence. Survival was inversely correlated to the number of vertebral bodies involved with cancer. Survival was related to primary site of cancer. Patients with renal cell carcinoma survived the longest, followed by patients with breast, prostate, lung, and colon cancer, in descending order. A prospectively followed cohort of 139 patients with spinal epidural metastases confirmed the importance of functional status in predicting to survival.[52] Median length of survival was 104 weeks for ambulatory patients and 6 weeks for nonambulatory patients. Mean interval between loss of ambulation and death was approximately 4 weeks.

Examples of patients with SEM treated surgically are illustrated in Figures 15-1 to 15-3.

Should Asymptomatic Sites of SEM Be Irradiated?

Although most clinicians favor irradiating sites of epidural tumor even when asymptomatic, this issue remains unresolved. In the largest retrospective series, 108 of 337 patients with SEM had multiple epidural metastases.[20] In patients with multiple epidural deposits, an asymptomatic epidural deposit produced a higher degree of thecal sac compression than the symptomatic lesion in 11 percent, a similar degree in 28 percent, and a lesser degree in 62 percent of cases. The extent of thecal sac compression from the largest secondary epidural metastasis was 75–99 percent in 6 percent, 25–74 percent in 12 percent, 1–24 percent in 49 percent, and minimal in 32 percent. At least one asymptomatic epidural metastasis was included in radiation treatment ports in 93 percent of patients with multiple epidural metastases, suggesting that radiation oncologists generally believed it worthwhile to treat incidentally detected epidural metastases. Eleven patients developed recurrent epidural

metastasis in a previously irradiated port, while 30 patients developed a radiographically verified second episode of epidural metastasis in a previously unirradiated port. In 26/30 episodes, that side had been previously imaged and found to be free of epidural disease. The authors concluded that treatment of asymptomatic epidural metastases probably reduced subsequent episodes of spinal cord compression.

A smaller study found similar results, detecting 31 cases of multiple epidural metastases in 108 patients with spinal cord compression. All patients with multiple epidural metastases had all sites of disease irradiated. Two patients subsequently developed SEM at new, previously unirradiated sites, while one had local recurrence of SEM.[17] The authors favored treatment of symptomatic sites but proposed a phase III trial to address the issue more definitively.

Bayley et al. found that 9 of 22 patients with prostate cancer and epidural metastases had multiple epidural metastases at discontiguous cord levels.[10] They noted that some patients with subarachnoid space compression might not deteriorate if left untreated, particularly if they were hormone treatment-naïve or had limited life expectancy. However, all patients with frank cord compression and most with subarachnoid compression underwent radiotherapy. This decision was based on the high efficacy, low toxicity, and low cost of radiotherapy, compared to the high potential cost of a missed diagnosis.

One carefully conducted study yielded a different conclusion. Helweg-Larssen et al. followed 107 patients with myelographically confirmed epidural metastases.[19] Thirty-seven of the patients (35 percent) had multiple epidural metastases. Fourteen patients had all sites of epidural disease irradiated, while 23 patients had asymptomatic epidural metastases left untreated (the criteria for deciding which lesions would be treated were unspecified). Eight patients (7.5 percent) of the cohort developed a second occurrence of SEM, all at a new cord level. A second episode of SEM was found with the same frequency in patients with a single site of epidural disease and in those with multiple sites. The authors concluded that irradiation of asymptomatic epidural metastases was not indicated. However, they noted that 3 of 8 episodes of recurrent epidural metastasis in patients with multiple epidural metastases at

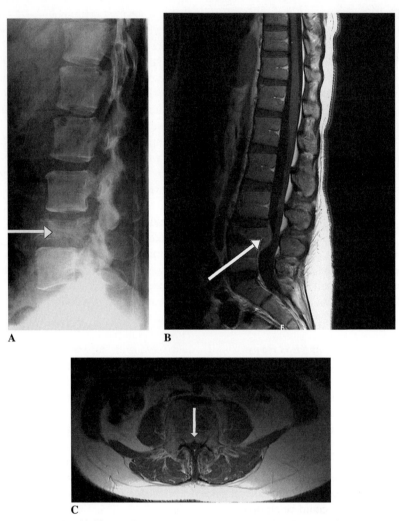

Figure 15-1. 38-year-old female with history of breast cancer. Due to extensive involvement of the L4 vertebral body and epidural space, anterior and posterior surgical approaches were necessary for decompression, instrumentation, and fusion. (A) A preoperative plain lumbar radiograph reveals an osteolytic pathological fracture of the L4 vertebral body (arrow). (B) Gadolinium-enhanced, sagittal, T1-weighted MR imaging demonstrates significant epidural disease and spinal canal compromise (arrow). (C) Gadolinium-enhanced, axial, T1-weighted MR imaging demonstrates diffuse vertebral body and pedicle involvement with spinal canal compromise.

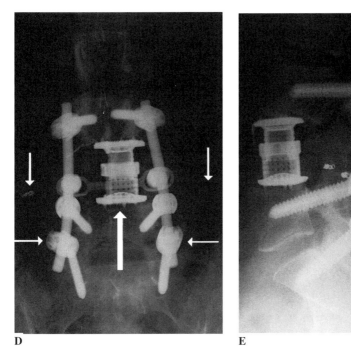

D   E

Figure 15-1.—*Cont'd*   (D) A postoperative AP lumbar radiograph reveals an expandable titanium cage placed following L4 vertebrectomy performed anteriorly (large block arrow) with titanium pedicle screw and rod instrumentation (horizontal line arrows) placed posteriorly. The tumor was very vascular on preoperative angiogram and preoperative coil embolization of bilateral feeding arteries was performed (vertical line arrows). (E) A postoperative lateral lumbar radiograph.

initial diagnosis occurred at sites with small epidural metastases on the original myelogram. Moreover, the median survival after diagnosis of SEM in this series was only 3.4 months, substantially lower than the 5–6 months more commonly reported. Since a sizable minority of the cases of recurrent SEM potentially could have been prevented by irradiating asymptomatic epidural metastases, and since more cases of recurrent SEM might have been seen if the population had lived longer, the conclusion of this study could be argued.

Is Chemotherapy Ever Useful in the Management of SEM?

Systemic chemotherapy reaches tumor in the epidural space unencumbered by the blood-spinal cord barrier, and thus may be an effective approach to treating SEM. Hormonal agents have been successfully employed against SEM from hormonally sensitive breast and prostate cancer. Small case series highlight the utility of chemotherapy in selected cases of

Hodgkin's disease, non-Hodgkin's lymphoma, germ cell tumors, and neuroblastoma producing SEM.[58] In general, chemotherapy is an attractive choice if the underlying tumor is likely to be extremely chemosensitive. Unfortunately, in most cases of SEM the responsible tumor is either not chemosensitive or has passed the stage of chemosensitivity. In such situations, radiation and surgery usually offer more hope of preserving neurological function.

Management of Recurrent Epidural Spinal Cord Compression

Epidural disease within a previously irradiated port arises in different settings. Sometimes the patient has not had previous bony metastasis, but the spinal cord was unavoidably included as part of the radiation field. In other situations, radiotherapy successfully treated vertebral metastasis months or years earlier, but the initially responsive tumor has now recurred. Finally, sometimes radiotherapy has been unsuccessfully utilized to treat a radioresistant bony

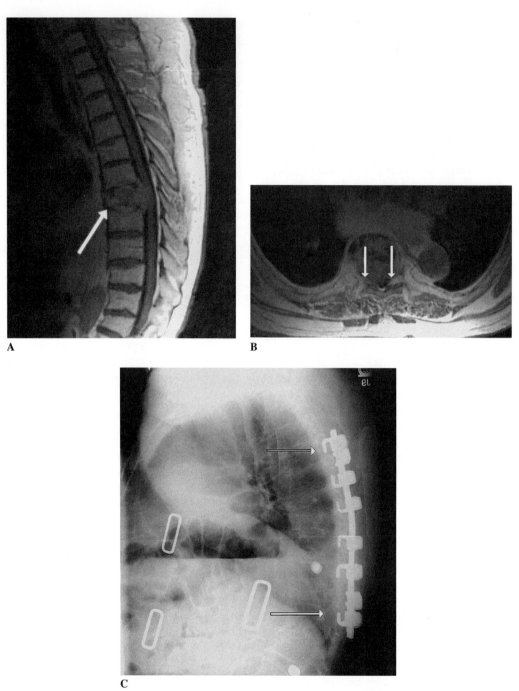

Figure 15-2. 77-year-old male with widely metastatic renal cell carcinoma presented with thoracic pain and progressive gait instability. (A) Preoperative, gadolinium-enhanced, sagittal, T1-weighted imaging reveals diffuse T8 vertebral body and epidural metastatic disease. (B) Preoperative, gadolinium-enhanced, axial, T1-weighted imaging demonstrates significant spinal canal compromise. (C) A postoperative, lateral thoracic radiograph reveals T5 to T11 posterior instrumentation and fusion (white arrows). A subtotal decompression of the T8 was performed only posteriorly due to the palliative nature of the procedure (to control pain and preserve ambulation) prior to completion of radiation treatments.

metastasis, and epidural metastasis is the inevitable consequence. Overall, incidence of local recurrence of spinal epidural metastasis has been estimated to occur in 0 percent[19,52] to 10 percent[21] of all patients with spinal epidural metastasis. It seems particularly common with breast cancer and particularly uncommon with lung cancer, perhaps reflecting the overall survival with each of these diseases.

Just as when epidural disease arises in a previously unirradiated region, all potential treatment options, including surgery, radiotherapy, and chemotherapy, must be considered. The criteria for surgery in this setting are similar to those described above, and surgery is particularly important to consider in patients who have failed radiotherapy for a radioresistant bony metastasis (e.g., from renal cell carcinoma). However, with certain tumors, including breast and prostate cancer and multiple myeloma, multiple spinal metastases are likely to be present. The presence of other involved regions of the spine diminishes the attractiveness of surgery both for technical reasons and because other levels may soon develop epidural metastases. Furthermore, by the time spinal metastases have recurred and progressed despite prior radiotherapy, visceral disease is frequently advanced, reducing life expectancy.

In this dire situation, it is worthwhile to consider the potential role of spinal reirradiation. The concern with reirradiating the spine is the risk of producing chronic progressive radiation myelopathy. Traditionally radiation oncologists have been willing to tolerate a 5 percent risk of radiation myelopathy at 5 years, which is thought to be associated with a dose of 4500–5000 cGy in 200 cGy fractions.[59] Nonetheless, radiation oncologists have sometimes been willing to reirradiate a spinal segment for epidural disease. A study of 54 such cases at the Mayo Clinic demonstrated that reirradiation resulted in preservation of ability to walk until death in 69 percent of patients, with only one patient developing possible radiation myelopathy.[60] In part, the rarity of radiation complications in this group may relate to the short expected survival following development of epidural metastasis; with a median survival of 5 months, patients may not have lived long enough to develop delayed radiation-induced myelopathy. The ability to repair sublethal radiation damage in the spinal cord may also be a factor; primate studies demonstrate that when animals are reirradiated 2 years after initial radiation, the dose required to produce radiation myelopathy suggests

that the effect of three-quarters of the previous radiation dose has been repaired over time.[61]

■ The Pros and Cons

In our patient, the possibility of SEM needs to be carefully considered even in the absence of clinical signs of radicular or spinal cord involvement. Vertebral metastases occur in up to three-quarters of patients with advanced breast cancer, and this cancer accounts for one-quarter of all cases of SEM. Humbling as it may be to neurologists, a normal neurological examination is all too compatible with spinal epidural metastasis. Therefore, MRI or myelogram should be used in this case to assess the extent of bony involvement and the integrity of the spinal cord and thecal sac. In our opinion, imaging of the spinal cord and epidural space to differentiate SEM from spinal metastasis restricted to bone should be performed prior to radiotherapy even in cases of back pain without other neurological symptoms or signs for optimal treatment planning.

Although myelography may be essential in certain clinical situations (e.g., patients with contraindications to have MRI, laterally located lesions that may escape detection by MRI), MRI has become the imaging modality of choice for patients with suspected SEM. It is widely available, safe (avoiding the risks of lumbar puncture), and it allows reliable visualization of the spinal cord, the spinal canal, and the bony elements. Since lesions are often multiple, imaging should include the thoracic and lumbosacral spine in every patient with a history of cancer presenting with low back pain.

Although no trial has been conducted to assess the relative efficacy of high- versus low-dose corticosteroids in patients with SEM, clinicians must balance concerns of steroid toxicity against the proven benefits of high doses for SEM. One arbitrary approach is to reserve high-dose dexamethasone (doses up to 100 mg bolus followed by 24 mg every 6 hours) for patients with weakness impairing ambulation. Patients with less severe compromise, such as our patient, may be treated with lower doses (e.g., 10 mg bolus and then 4 mg every 6 hours).

The ideal dose and schedule of radiation therapy will depend on the protocol used by the treating radiation oncologist. No ideal regimen can be identified by reviewing available evidence. The most

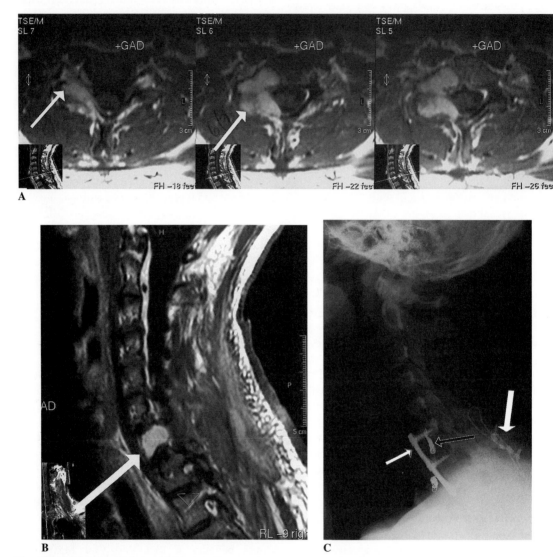

Figure 15-3. 58-year-old male with history of metastatic sarcoma. Extensive circumferential involvement of the C7 vertebral level required anterior and posterior decompression, instrumentation, and fusion. (A) Preoperative gadolinium-enhanced, axial, T1-weighted MR imaging demonstrates C7 level vertebral body, lateral mass, facet joint, lamina, and epidural space involvement with metastatic disease. There is significant compromise of the right C7 neural foramen which resulted in a clinical C7 radiculopathy (arrow). (B) Preoperative gadolinium-enhanced, sagittal, T1-weighted imaging reveals C7 vertebral body and epidural metastatic disease (arrow). (C) A postoperative lateral cervical radiograph demonstrating spinous process wiring with titanium cable (thick block arrow), titanium anterior cervical plating following vertebrectomy and autologous strut graft placement (thin block arrow), and coil embolization of the right vertebral artery to allow radical resection of the tumor (black line arrow).

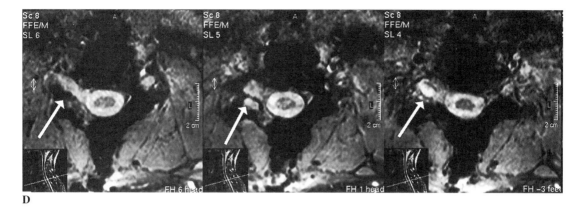

D

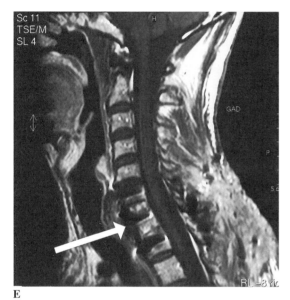

E

Figure 15-3.—*Cont'd*   (D) Postoperative axial, T2-weighted MR imaging demonstrating reopening of the neural foramen. (E) Postoperative gadolinium-enhanced, sagittal, T1-weighted imaging revealing replacement of the C7 vertebral body with an autologous iliac crest strut graft and titanium anterior cervical plate. Note the minimal amount of metallic artifact caused by the titanium instrumentation (arrow).

popular regimens administer 2000 to 4000 cGy in 5 to 20 fractions. The issue of how soon radiotherapy must be commenced (i.e., whether there is any harm in waiting until the following morning to initiate radiotherapy) remains undetermined. However, in the absence of data suggesting it is safe to defer radiotherapy even a few hours in patients who are rapidly deteriorating and are not surgical candidates, our policy has been to initiate radiation as rapidly as feasible.

Surgical treatment of spinal metastases may be indicated in patients with reasonable life expectancy and evidence of intractable pain, neurological deficits, or spinal instability. Although the surgery is rigorous and the chances of complications are high

due to trends toward advanced age, poor nutritional status, deconditioning from neurological deficits, and previous treatment with steroids and radiation, good results can be achieved with proper patient selection. Survival following surgery is best correlated with the preoperative ability to ambulate, maintenance of continence, and solitary spinal epidural deposits. The surgical plan depends on the extension of the disease and must be guided by the results of the imaging studies.

Chemotherapy has a very limited role in most cases of SEM. In patients with recurrence of SEM, spinal reirradiation seems to be both effective and safe, especially when treating tumors that have previously been radiosensitive.

■ The Main Points

- The absence of radiculopathy or myelopathy should not reassure the clinician that a patient with cancer and back pain does not have an epidural metastasis.
- When an epidural metastasis is suspected, the patient should have an MRI scan targeting the symptomatic region but also including at least sagittal images of the entire spinal column.
- In most cases, definitive treatment of epidural metastasis will include radiotherapy, surgery, or a combination of the two. Patients without advanced visceral metastases and a single epidural metastasis should be evaluated for possible resection.
- In patients with locally recurrent epidural disease who are not surgical candidates, a second course of spinal radiotherapy should be considered.

■ References

1. Abrams HL, Spiro R, Goldstein N. Metastases in carcinoma: analysis of 1000 autopsied cases. *Cancer* 1950;3:74–85.
2. Schiff D, O'Neill BP, Wang CH, O'Fallon JR. Neuroimaging and treatment implications of patients with multiple epidural spinal metastases. *Cancer* 1998;83:1593–1601.
3. Khaw FM, Worthy SA, Gibson MJ, Gholkar A. The appearance on MRI of vertebrae in acute compression of the spinal cord due to metastases. *J Bone Joint Surg—Br Vol* 1999;81:830–834.
4. Rodichok LD, Harper GR, Ruckdeschel JC, Price A, Roberson G, Barron KD, Horton J. Early diagnosis of spinal epidural metastases. *Am J Med* 1981;70: 1181–1188.
5. Rodichok LD, Ruckdeschel JC, Harper GR, Cooper G, Prevosti L, Fernando L, Baxter DH. Early detection and treatment of spinal epidural metastases: the role of myelography. *Ann Neurol* 1986;20:696–702.
6. O'Rourke T, George CB, Redmond J III, Davidson H, Cornett P, Fill WL, Spring DB, Sobel D, Dabe IB, Karl RD Jr. Spinal computed tomography and computed tomographic metrizamide myelography in the early diagnosis of metastatic disease. *J Clin Oncol* 1986;4:576–583.
7. Ruff RL, Lanska DJ. Epidural metastases in prospectively evaluated veterans with cancer and back pain. *Cancer* 1989;63:2234–2241. [Published erratum appears in *Cancer* 1990;66:935.]
8. Portenoy RK, Galer BS, Salamon O, Freilich M, Finkel JE, Milstein D, Thaler HT, Berger M, Lipton RB. Identification of epidural neoplasm: radiography and bone scintigraphy in the symptomatic and asymptomatic spine. *Cancer* 1989;64:2207–2213.
9. Kienstra GE, Terwee CB, Dekker FW, Canta LR, Borstlap AC, Tijssen CC, Bosch DA, Tijssen JG. Prediction of spinal epidural metastases. *Arch Neurol* 2000;57:690–695.
10. Bayley A, Milosevic M, Blend R, Logue J, Gospodarowicz M, Boxen I, Warde P, McLean M, Catton C, Catton P. A prospective study of factors predicting clinically occult spinal cord compression in patients with metastatic prostate carcinoma. *Cancer* 2001;92:303–310.
11. Calkins AR, Olson MA, Ellis JH. Impact of myelography on the radiotherapeutic management of malignant spinal cord compression. *Neurosurgery* 1986;19:614–616.
12. Colletti PM, Siegel HJ, Woo MY, Young HY, Terk MR. The impact on treatment planning of MRI of the spine in patients suspected of vertebral metastasis: an efficacy study. *Comput Med Imaging Graphics* 1996;20:159–162.
13. Ryan PJ, Fogelman I. The bone scan: where are we now? *Semin Nucl Med* 1995;25:76–91.
14. Godersky JC, Smoker WR, Knutzon R. Use of magnetic resonance imaging in the evaluation of metastatic spinal disease. *Neurosurgery* 1987;21:676–680.
15. Hagenau C, Grosh W, Currie M, Wiley RG. Comparison of spinal magnetic resonance imaging and myelography in cancer patients. *J Clin Oncol* 1987;5: 1663–1669.
16. Sarpel S, Sarpel G, Yu E, Hyder S, Kaufman B, Hindo W, Ezdinli E. Early diagnosis of spinal-epidural metastasis by magnetic resonance imaging. *Cancer* 1987;59:1112–1126.
17. Chamberlain MC, Kormanik PA. Epidural spinal cord compression: a single institution's retrospective experience *Neuro-Oncology* 1999;1:120–123.
18. Heldmann U, Myschetzky PS, Thomsen HS. Frequency of unexpected multifocal metastasis in patients with acute spinal cord compression: evaluation by low-field MR imaging in cancer patients. *Acta Radiol* 1997;38:372–375.
19. Helweg-Larsen S, Hansen SW, Sorensen PS. Second occurrence of symptomatic metastatic spinal cord compression and findings of multiple spinal epidural metastases. *Int J Radiat Oncol Biol Phys* 1995;33: 595–598.
20. Schiff D, Shaw EG, Cascino TL. Outcome after spinal reirradiation for malignant epidural spinal cord compression. *Ann Neurol* 1995;37:583–589.
21. van der Sande JJ, Boogerd W, Kroger R, Kappelle AC. Recurrent spinal epidural metastases: a prospective study with a complete follow up. *J Neurol Neurosurg Psychiatry* 1999;66:623–627.

22. van der Sande JJ, Kroger R, Boogerd W. Multiple spinal epidural metastases; an unexpectedly frequent finding. *J Neurol Neurosurg Psychiatry* 1990;53:1001–1003.

23. Boogerd W, van der Sande JJ, Kroger R. Early diagnosis and treatment of spinal epidural metastasis in breast cancer: a prospective study. *J Neurol Neurosurg Psychiatry* 1992;55:1188–1193.

24. Adams KK, Jackson CE, Rauch RA, Hart SF, Kleinguenther RS, Barohn RJ. Cervical myelopathy with false localizing sensory levels. *Arch Neurol* 1996;53:1155–1158.

25. Boogerd W, van der Sande JJ. Diagnosis and treatment of spinal cord compression in malignant disease. *Cancer Treat Rev* 1993;19:129–150.

26. Cantu RC. Corticosteroids for spinal metastases. *Lancet* 1968;2:912.

27. Delattre JY, Arbit E, Rosenblum MK, Thaler HT, Lau N, Galicich JH, Posner JB. High dose versus low dose dexamethasone in experimental epidural spinal cord compression. *Neurosurgery* 1988;22:1005–1007.

28. Ushio Y, Posner R, Posner JB, Shapiro WR. Experimental spinal cord compression by epidural neoplasm. *Neurology* 1977;27:422–429.

29. Greenberg HS, Kim JH, Posner JB. Epidural spinal cord compression from metastatic tumor: results with a new treatment protocol. *Ann Neurol* 1980;8:361–366.

30. Slatkin NE, Posner JB. Management of spinal epidural metastases. *Clin Neurosurg* 1983;30:698–716.

31. Sorensen PS, Helweg-Larsen S, Mouridsen H, Hansen HH. Effect of high-dose dexamethasone in carcinomatous metastatic spinal cord compression treated with radiotherapy: a randomised trial. *Eur J Cancer* 1994;30A:22–27.

32. Heimdal K, Hirschberg H, Slettebo H, Watne K, Nome O. High incidence of serious side effects of high-dose dexamethasone treatment in patients with epidural spinal cord compression. *J Neuro-Oncol* 1992;12:141–144.

33. Vecht CJ, Haaxma-Reiche H, van Putten WL, de Visser M, Vries EP, Twijnstra A. Initial bolus of conventional versus high-dose dexamethasone in metastatic spinal cord compression. *Neurology* 1989;39:1255–1257.

34. Maranzano E, Latini P, Beneventi S, Perruci E, Panizza BM, Aristei C, Lupattelli M, Tonato M. Radiotherapy without steroids in selected metastatic spinal cord compression patients: a phase II trial. *Am J Clin Oncol* 1996;19:179–183.

35 Bates T. A review of local radiotherapy in the treatment of bone metastases and cord compression [Review, 38 refs.]. *Int J Radiat Oncol Biol Phys* 1992;23:217–221.

36. Tong D, Gillick L, Hendrickson FR. The palliation of symptomatic osseous metastases: final results of the Study by the Radiation Therapy Oncology Group. *Cancer* 1982;50:893–899.

37. Blitzer PH. Reanalysis of the RTOG study of the palliation of symptomatic osseous metastasis. *Cancer* 1985;55:1468–1472.

38. Uppelschoten JM, Wanders SL, de Jong JM. Single-dose radiotherapy (6 Gy): palliation in painful bone metastases. *Radiother Oncol* 1995;36:198–202.

39. Maranzano E, Latini P, Perrucci E, Beneventi S, Lupattelli M, Corgna E. Short-course radiotherapy (8 Gy × 2) in metastatic spinal cord compression: an effective and feasible treatment. *Int J Radiat Oncol Biol Phys* 1997;38:1037–1044.

40. Maranzano E, Latini P, Beneventi S, Marafioti L, Piro F, Perrucci E, Lupattelli M. Comparison of two different radiotherapy schedules for spinal cord compression in prostate cancer. *Tumori* 1998;84:472–477.

41. Bach F, Larsen BH, Rohde K, Borgesen SE, Gjerris F, Boge-Rasmussen T, Agerlin N, Rasmusson B, Stjernholm P, Sorensen PS. Metastatic spinal cord compression: occurrence, symptoms, clinical presentations and prognosis in 398 patients with spinal cord compression. *Acta Neurochir* 1990;107:37–43.

42. Helweg-Larsen S, Johnsen A, Boesen J, Sorensen PS. Radiologic features compared to clinical findings in a prospective study of 153 patients with metastatic spinal cord compression treated by radiotherapy. *Acta Neurochir* 1997;139:105–111.

43. Kim RY, Spencer SA, Meredith RF, Weppelmann B, Lee JY, Smith JW, Salter MM. Extradural spinal cord compression: analysis of factors determining functional prognosis—prospective study. *Radiology* 1990;176:279–282.

44. Maranzano E, Latini P. Effectiveness of radiation therapy without surgery in metastatic spinal cord compression: final results from a prospective trial. *Int J Radiat Oncol Biol Phys* 1995;32:959–967 [see comments].

45. Maranzano E, Latini P, Checcaglini F, Perrucci E, Aristei C, Panizza BM, Ricci S. Radiation therapy of spinal cord compression caused by breast cancer: report of a prospective trial. *Int J Radiat Oncol Biol Phys* 1992;24:301–306.

46. Maranzano E, Latini P, Checcaglini F, Ricci S, Panizza BM, Aristei C, Perrucci E, Beneventi S, Corgna E, Tonato M. Radiation therapy in metastatic spinal cord compression: a prospective analysis of 105 consecutive patients. *Cancer* 1991;67:1311–1317.

47. Martenson JAJ, Evans RG, Lie MR, Ilstrup DM, Dinapoli RP, Ebersold MJ, Earle JD. Treatment outcome and complications in patients treated for malignant epidural spinal cord compression (SCC). *J Neuro-Oncol* 1985;3:77–84.

48. Helweg-Larsen S, Rasmusson B, Sorensen PS. Recovery of gait after radiotherapy in paralytic patients with metastatic epidural spinal cord compression. *Neurology* 1990;40:1234–1236.

49. Tomita T, Galicich JH, Sundaresan N. Radiation therapy for spinal epidural metastases with complete block. *Acta Radiol—Oncol* 1983;22:135–143.

50. Rades D, Karstens JH, Alberti W. Role of radiotherapy in the treatment of motor dysfunction due to metastatic

spinal cord compression: comparison of three different fractionation schedules. *Int J Radiat Oncol Biol Phys* 2002;54:1160–1164.

51. Bracken MB, Shepard MJ, Collins WF, Holford TR, Young W, Baskin DS, Eisenberg HM, Flamm E, Leo-Summers L, Maroon J. A randomized, controlled trial of methylprednisolone or naloxone in the treatment of acute spinal-cord injury: results of the Second National Acute Spinal Cord Injury Study. *N Engl J Med* 1990;322:1405–1411.

52. Zaidat OO, Ruff RL. Treatment of spinal epidural metastasis improves patient survival and functional state. *Neurology* 2002;58:1360–1366.

53. Findlay GF. Adverse effects of the management of malignant spinal cord compression. *J Neurol Neurosurg Psychiatry* 1984;47:761–768.

54. Young RF, Post EM, King GA. Treatment of spinal epidural metastases: randomized prospective comparison of laminectomy and radiotherapy. *J Neurosurg* 1980;53:741–748.

55. Healey JH, Brown HK. Complications of bone metastases. *Cancer* 2000;88:2940–2951.

56. Sundaresan N, Sachdev VP, Holland JF, Moore F, Sung M, Paciucci PA, Wu LT, Kelligher K, Hough L. Surgical treatment of spinal cord compression from epidural metastasis. *J Clin Oncol* 1995;13:2330–2335.

57. Sioutos PJ, Arbit E, Meshulam CF, Galicich JH. Spinal metastases from solid tumors: analysis of factors affecting survival. *Cancer* 1995;76:1453–1459.

58. Schiff D, O'Neill BP, Suman VJ. Spinal epidural metastasis as the initial manifestation of malignancy: clinical features and diagnostic approach. *Neurology* 1997;49:452–456.

59. Emami B, Lyman J, Brown A, Coia L, Goitein M, Munzenrider JE, Shank B, Solin LJ, Wesson M. Tolerance of normal tissue to therapeutic irradiation. *Int J Radiat Oncol Biol Phys* 1991;21:109–122.

60. Schiff D. Spinal metastases. In Schiff D, Wen PY, eds. *Cancer Neurology in Clinical Practice*. Totowa NJ, Humana Press, 2002:93–106.

61. Ang KK, Price RE, Stephens LC, Jiang GL, Feng Y, Schultheiss TE, Peters LJ. The tolerance of primate spinal cord to re-irradiation. *Int J Radiat Oncol Biol Phys* 1993;25:459–464.

Chapter 16
Surgery for Intracerebral Hematoma

Alejandro A. Rabinstein and Eelco F. M. Wijdicks

Rupture of an arterial branch inside the brain parenchyma may produce a sizable clot. It is unknown whether the formation and subsequent expansion of the hematoma results from blood dissecting tissue planes or simply from growing centrifugal pressure at its core. The observation that the hematoma usually tamponades against normal brain tissue within 6 to 8 hours is well established. Although at this stage homeostasis is maintained, cytotoxic products released from the clot may cause further damage to the surrounding brain.[1,2] The possibility of this additional injury has provided the strongest argument for early surgical evacuation of the hematoma. This approach is favored by quite a few neurosurgeons—predominantly in Asian countries—but its arbitrariness becomes evident when applied to patients who are barely symptomatic, are clinically stable, or seem to be actually improving from the initial deficits.

Recent studies have contributed to better define predictors of deterioration, and it may be argued that surgical intervention should be primarily restricted to those patients at high risk of clinical decline. The age of the patient, localization of the hematoma, and clinical course are important elements in decision-making. There is typically a reluctance to perform surgery in elderly patients and patients with a dominant-hemisphere hematoma. Meanwhile there is often a relatively low threshold to evacuate the clot when signs of cerebral herniation become evident. These and other physicians' biases have not been studied systematically but may explain the low recruitment rates to randomized trials.

The crucial question—when to operate in patients with intracerebral hematoma—has remained unanswered. This chapter will summarize and interpret the evidence available and point out the areas of persisting uncertainty.

■ The Patient

A 64-year-old man was found on the floor by his wife. He was unable to move his right limbs. On arrival at the emergency room, his blood pressure was 205/110 mmHg and he had a regular tachycardia. He was awake but confused and drifted off easily. He could name some simple objects but not others. During his naming attempts he showed some impersistence and verbal perseveration. He had left gaze preference and dense right hemiparesis with decreased muscle tone. Babinski sign was present on the right side. He was started on a nitroprusside drip to reduce his mean arterial pressure below 130 mmHg. A noncontrast CT scan of the brain obtained 5 to 6 hours after the onset of symptoms showed an extensive (50 cm³) left frontal intracerebral hemorrhage (ICH) with mild (<0.5 cm) midline shift (Figure 16-1).

The patient had no functional restrictions prior to this event. His medical background was remarkable for hypertension, diabetes mellitus type 2, hyperlipidemia, and smoking. His current medications were amlodipine, metformin, glyburide, and aspirin (81 mg/day).

The patient was admitted to the neurological intensive care unit for close monitoring. Over

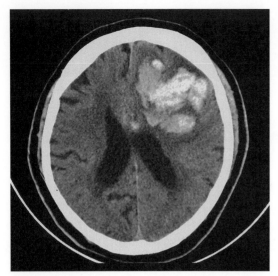

Figure 16-1. Presurgical noncontrast CT of the brain obtained 5 to 6 hours after the onset of symptoms. It shows an extensive left frontal intracerebral hemorrhage with mild (<0.5 cm) midline shift.

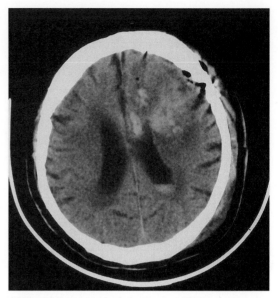

Figure 16-2. Postsurgical noncontrast CT of the brain showing nearly complete evacuation of the hematoma and resolution of the midline shift.

the course of the following 18 hours he became progressively more lethargic but remained able to open his eyes and follow simple commands to strong verbal call. A repeat CT scan of the brain showed minimal enlargement of the hematoma (60 cm³). During discussion of the treatment options with the patient's wife, she demanded that "everything possible should be done" to keep her husband alive. The patient was taken to the operating room and he underwent craniotomy for evacuation of the hematoma. The clot was evacuated almost entirely and intraoperative homeostasis could be achieved uneventfully.

After surgery, the patient remained stuporous and hemiplegic. Brain CT confirmed marked reduction in the volume of intracerebral blood with resolution of the midline shift (Figure 16-2). His postoperative course was complicated by ventilator-associated pneumonia that responded to antibiotic treatment. After 4 days, his level of alertness began to improve gradually. He was successfully extubated 8 days after the onset of symptoms and it became obvious that he had profound motor aphasia accompanied by milder comprehension deficits. On the ward, he received physical, occupational, and speech therapy, but his functional condition only improved minimally. He was transferred to a nursing home facility after 18 days of hospital stay.

Three months after the ictus, he remained fully dependent on basic activities of daily living.

■ The Problem

- Is surgical evacuation beneficial in patients with ICH?
- If so, when and for whom?
- Is surgery still of value once signs of brain herniation are present?
- Should we withhold surgery in patients with very poor prognosis?

■ The Evidence

The question of whether surgery is beneficial in patients with ICH defies straightforward answers. After many years of debate and despite several attempts at providing conclusive information through randomized trials, the uncertainty persists. The proportion of patients with ICH who are treated surgically remains substantial but the numbers vary greatly across different countries, centers, and even individual surgeons.[3] Yet more than 7000 patients with ICH per year are estimated to undergo hematoma evacuation in the United States, and surgery is even more frequently pursued in Germany and Japan.[4] These numbers are concerning for a treatment modality that is still awaiting scientific validation.

Surgical evacuation of a cerebral hematoma is intuitively justified, especially when signs of mass effect are present. The rationale for its indication is the prevention of complications caused by the blood clot, most notably mass effect and hydrocephalus. Mass effect can produce additional brain tissue damage directly by compressing surrounding structures and indirectly through the effects of raised intracranial pressure and herniation. Prevention of early hematoma enlargement was the driving hypothesis behind the proposition of ultra-early evacuation, but surgery within 4 hours of hematoma onset actually proved to be detrimental due to excessive postsurgical rebleeding.[5]

Randomized Trials

Seven randomized trials have compared surgical and conservative treatments for spontaneous ICH.[6–12] Unfortunately these trials have frequently mixed cases of ganglionic and lobar hemorrhage, two inherently different entities.

A landmark trial by McKissock et al.[6] was well designed but dates back to the pre-CT era. Therefore, despite the best efforts by the investigators, misdiagnosis at entry is likely to have occurred. Actually the authors recognized several misdiagnosed cases after randomization, reaching a known diagnostic error of 5 percent. The study randomized 180 patients to craniotomy for hematoma evacuation—as long as the hematoma could be localized and was accessible—or conservative management. The published data are insufficient to define how many patients randomized to surgery actually underwent craniotomy. Patients in the surgical group had a 28 percent increased mortality rate and an overall higher chance of death or dependency (odds ratio [OR] 2.0; 95 percent confidence intervals 1.04–3.86).

In the trial by Juvela et al., 52 patients were randomized to surgery or medical treatment within 48 hours of symptom onset.[8] Patients at entry were unconscious (but responsive to pain) or had severe hemiparesis or aphasia. Randomization was not

well balanced because patients allocated to surgical treatment had larger hematomas and significantly lower Glasgow coma scale (GCS) sum score at entry. Both mortality and functional dependence were slightly higher among surgically treated patients. The small number of patients precluded subgroup analysis. The authors concluded that spontaneous ICH should be treated conservatively.

Batjer et al. interrupted enrollment into their trial after only 21 patients had been randomized.[9] The therapeutic arms were best medical treatment (including routine use of steroids and mannitol), best medical treatment plus ventriculostomy for intracranial pressure monitoring, and surgical evacuation (with attempts to standardize the procedure using a predefined microsurgical technique). The reason for stopping the trial prematurely was the extremely poor outcome observed in each of the treatment groups. No differences among the groups were noted, but the very small number of patients studied impeded any meaningful comparison.

In the only randomized trial that solely used endoscopic aspiration for clot evacuation, Auer et al. reported favorable results with surgery. The investigators randomized 100 patients with symptomatic hematomas larger than $10\,cm^3$ within 48 hours of symptom onset[10] to partial endoscopic evacuation through a burr hole or medical treatment (including antifibrinolytic agents for 3 days). At 6 months, mortality was significantly lower and functional outcome was improved in the surgically treated patients. Subgroup analysis showed that the benefit afforded by surgery was restricted to patients younger than 60 years old who presented with lobar hematomas and were not stuporous at entry. The results of this trial have been questioned because outcome assessment was not blinded. However, this study remains the strongest evidence in favor of surgical treatment for spontaneous ICH.

The concept of early surgery has been tested in a few small, randomized studies. Zuccarello et al. randomized 20 patients (over a 2-year period) with ICH volume $>10\,cm^3$, focal neurological deficit, and GCS sum score >4 at the time of enrollment to either surgical evacuation (craniotomy or stereotactic aspiration as decided by the surgeon in each case) or medical treatment.[12] All patients were enrolled within 24 hours of symptom onset and operated within 3 hours of randomization. Median time from onset of symptoms to surgery was 8 hours and 35 minutes. Patients' neurological status at the time of randomization was better than that of patients enrolled into previous trials; median GCS sum score was 13 (range 11 to 14) in the surgical arm and 11 (range 6 to 13) in the medical arm ($p = 0.06$). At 3 months, there was a nonsignificant but well-defined trend toward better outcome in the surgically treated patients that was apparent on three different functional scales. Mortality was only minimally lower in the surgical group, but surgery afforded a significant reduction in residual neurological deficits assessed by the NIH stroke scale. The low recruitment rate in this study confirmed the difficulties faced by investigators dedicated to studying this matter.

A research group from the University of Texas has contributed to the field by completing two small but important studies focused on the value of early surgery for ICH. First, a single-center, pilot trial compared craniotomy within 12 hours of symptom onset versus best medical treatment.[11] Inclusion criteria required hematoma volume $\geq 10\,cm^3$ and presence of impairment of consciousness or severe hemiparesis. A total of 34 patients were randomized and at 6 months there was a trend toward lower mortality and better functional outcome in the surgical group. However, the authors do not mention any attempts to blind outcome assessment. The modest benefits observed with surgery in this pilot study understandably led the investigators to believe that shortening the time window to surgery could be more efficacious. Thus, a subsequent trial enrolled patients for craniotomy and clot evacuation within 4 hours of symptom onset to compare them with the patients randomized to the surgical and medical treatment arms within a 12-hour time window.[5] Median initial hematoma volume was $40\,cm^3$ (range 23 to $84\,cm^3$), and median GCS sum score was 12 (range 6 to 15). The trial had to be stopped prematurely after only 11 patients had been operated within 4 hours because of increased rate of rebleeding (40 percent compared with 12 percent among patients operated between 4 and 12 hours) and mortality (36 percent vs. 18 percent in patients operated between 4 and 12 hours, including 3 of 4 patients who rebled after ultra-early surgery). The investigators concluded that ultra-early craniotomy for hematoma evacuation cannot be recommended because it is complicated by rebleeding, most likely related to problems with homeostasis.

The results of a randomized, multicenter trial comparing stereotactic blood clot drainage after liquefaction with urokinase (instilled through a catheter into the hematoma every 6 hours for 2 days) with conservative treatment have just been released.[13] Seventy patients were enrolled within 72 hours of ICH onset. There were no differences in mortality and severe disability between the treatment groups. However, a significant ICH volume reduction was achieved by the neurosurgical intervention (10–20 percent, $P < 0.05$).

The salient features of the randomized trials on surgical versus medical treatment of ICH are summarized in Table 16-1.

Several meta-analyses have attempted to systematically review the data of these prospective randomized studies.[14-19] The results should be interpreted with caution because of the marked heterogeneity of the original trials, which have varied considerably in terms of diagnostic and inclusion criteria, surgical technique, outcome measures, and size of the population studied.

Older meta-analyses,[14-16] including the first four randomized trials,[6,8-10] concluded that craniotomy showed a tendency to be detrimental. Indeed, pooling the data from these trials ($n = 353$ patients), there is a nonsignificant increase in the odds of death and dependency at 6 months for patients treated surgically (OR 1.23; 95 percent CI 0.77–1.98). However, the positive results observed with endoscopic drainage in the study by Auer et al.[10] were highlighted as promising.

A subsequent meta-analysis[19] included the two more recent trials[11,12] as well as another previously overlooked Chinese study.[7] When all trials ($n = 533$ patients) were considered, there was still a trend toward greater chance of death and dependency among patients undergoing surgery (OR 1.20; 95 percent CI 0.83–1.74). However, the authors then decided to exclude the two trials with most notable methodological weaknesses. The trial by McKissock et al.[6] was excluded because of the high diagnostic error rate as a result of the unavailability of CT at the time the study was performed and the uncertainty about the number of patients allocated to surgery who actually underwent craniotomy. The study by Chen et al.[7] was removed from this restricted reanalysis due to concerns about markedly unbalanced randomization, inclusion of patients with cerebellar hematomas, and

Table 16-1. Summary of Published Randomized Trials Comparing Surgical and Medical Treatments for Patients with Intracerebral Hemorrhage (ICH)

Trial	Population	Surgical Technique	Results	OR (95% CI) of Death/Dependency
McKissock et al. (1961)[6]	n = 180 Clinical presentation/LP/angio consistent with ICH No defined time limit	Craniotomy	No significant difference Death S: 65% M: 51% Poor outcome S: 80% M: 66%	2.0 (1.0–3.9)
Juvela et al. (1989)[8]	n = 52 Unconscious or severe hemiparesis/dysphasia Ictus within 48 hr	Craniotomy	No significant difference Death S: 46% M: 38% Poor outcome S: 98% M: 66%	4.39 (0.8–23.6)
Auer et al. (1989)[10]	n = 100 ICH > 100 cm³, altered consciousness Ictus within 48 hr	Endoscopic aspiration	Significantly better Death S: 42% M: 70% Poor outcome S: 58% M: 74%	0.46 (0.2–1.0)
Batjer et al. (1990)[9]	n = 21 Putaminal ICH > 3 cm Altered consciousness or hemiparesis Ictus within 24 hr	Craniotomy	No significant difference Death S: 50% M: 85% Poor outcome S: 75% M: 85%	0.55 (0.1–4.9)

(Continued)

Table 16-1.—*Continued*

Trial	Population	Surgical Technique	Results	OR (95% CI) of Death/Dependency
Morgenstern et al. (1998)[11]	$n = 34$ ICH >9 cm^3, lobar or extending out of thalamus, GCS 5–15 Ictus within 12 hr	Craniotomy	No significant difference Death S: 24% M: 18% Poor outcome S: 69% M: 50%	0.46 (0.1–1.9)
Zuccarello et al. (1999)[12]	$n = 20$ ICH >10 cm^3, GCS >4, Ictus within 12 hr	Craniotomy/stereotactic aspiration	No significant difference Death S: 22% M: 27% Poor outcome S: 44% M: 64%	0.48 (0.1–2.7)
Teernstra et al. (2003)[13]	$n = 70$ ICH >10 cm^3, GEM 2–10 Ictus within 72 hr	Urokinase instillation and stereotactic drainage	No significant difference Death S: 56% M: 59% Poor outcome S: 75% M: 76%	0.52 (1.2–2.3)

LP, lumbar puncture; S, surgical; M, medical; GCS, Glasgow Coma Scale sum score; GEM, Glasgow Eye Motor Scale score. OR, odds ratio; CI, confidence interval.

possible incorporation into the surgical group of patients who only underwent ventricular drainage. This modified meta-analysis ($n = 227$) actually indicated a trend toward a reduction in the odds of death and dependency after surgery (OR 0.63; 95 percent CI 0.35–1.14).

The recruitment phase of the International Surgical Trial in Intracerebral Hemorrhage (ISTICH) has been completed.[11] This is a multi-center, randomized, controlled trial that randomized more than 1000 patients within 72 hours of hematoma onset to undergo immediate surgery versus medical treatment. The protocol indicated that there should be "clinical uncertainty" as to the need for surgical evacuation in the patients to be randomized. This has led some experts to express concerns about possible selection bias in patient enrollment.[1,20] Precise time limits for intervention were not defined in the protocol and a standardized surgical technique was not required. The results of this trial have been just reported in a platform presentation. Groups were well balanced with an overall median age of 62 years. Outcome assignment was based on a novel prognosis-based measure. There was no significant benefit from surgery in terms of neurological improvement or mortality. Subsequent subgroup analysis showed a trend towards a negative correlation between depth of hematoma location and benefit from surgery. These preliminary results seem unlikely to change current recommendations for treatment.

Nonrandomized Studies

Nonrandomized, controlled, retrospective studies comparing craniotomy versus medical treatment for ICH are difficult to group or juxtapose because they have assessed very different populations of patients. Nonetheless, their results generally indicate that medical treatment is superior to clot evacuation through craniotomy for patients with deep hematomas.[21,22] However, other authors contend that surgery may offer relatively good results for patients with putaminal hemorrhages, as long as surgery is performed promptly[23,24] and appropriate surgical candidates are carefully selected—basically excluding patients with coma, thalamic involvement, or mild symptoms and small hematoma size.[23–25]

Nonrandomized controlled series, case series, and abundant anecdotal experience consistently support the benefit of surgery (suboccipital craniotomy) for patients with cerebellar hemorrhage when the hematoma is large (>3 cm in horizontal diameter) or is causing brainstem compression or obstructive hydrocephalus.[26–29] However, one study found that neurosurgeons may be less enthusiastic about performing surgery in older patients (>70 years) with large cerebellar hematomas.[30] This bias could impact on outcome and complicate interpretation of retrospective studies.

Studies Testing Minimally Invasive Techniques

Various nonrandomized studies have also tested different methods to evacuate the hematoma through minimally invasive approaches. Since CT-guided stereotactic aspiration was first reported in 1978,[31] many innovative devices have been developed to facilitate endoscopic evacuation.[32–34] Ultrasound-guided evacuation has been pursued successfully in Japan,[35] and MRI-guided stereotactic drainage of ICH has also been recently introduced.[36] Instillation of thrombolytics into the hematoma has been used to facilitate subsequent drainage and aspiration of the clot.[13,37,38] This procedure seems to be particularly useful to remove intraparenchymal hematomas that are a few days old and large intraventricular clots.[39,40] Studies using aspiration after instillation of thrombolytics have reported similar rebleeding rates to studies using aspiration unaided by fibrinolytic agents.[41] As previously noted, a recently published randomized trial confirmed that stereotactic drainage after local treatment with urokinase can successfully reduce the size of the hematoma but failed to decrease the rate of death or severe disability.[13]

Current Management Guidelines

The current Guidelines for the Management of Spontaneous ICH approved by the American Heart Association state that "the decision about whether and when to operate remains controversial."[41] Nonetheless, based mostly on data from nonrandomized studies, surgery is cautiously recommended for young patients with large hematomas who are clinically deteriorating. The recommendation to evacuate cerebellar hematomas larger than 3 cm in patients with neurological worsening, obstructive hydrocephalus, or signs of brainstem compression is also largely empirical but widely accepted.

The recommendation not to pursue surgery in patients with hemorrhages <10 cm^3 or minimal neurological deficits is unquestionable. However, withholding surgery in deeply comatose (GCS sum score <5) patients with a cerebral hematoma is not beyond debate, as we shall discuss in our next section.

Emergency Craniotomy for Patients with Signs of Herniation

When patients with supratentorial hematomas show signs of clinical deterioration, evacuation of the hematoma is often pursued in daily practice. However, patients with clinical or radiological signs of herniation were typically excluded from randomized trials and most nonrandomized series. In fact, only one study has addressed the value of surgery in these most critical patients.[42] This retrospective study analyzed a population of 26 patients with evidence of brain tissue shift on their admission CT scan (>1 cm shift of the septum pellucidum) who underwent emergency craniotomy. Overall, the population studied was relatively young (median age 51 years; range 44–73 years) and most patients had right-sided lobar hematomas. Although mortality was high (54 percent), approximately a quarter of the patients regained functional independence after clot evacuation. Half of the survivors were severely disabled, but none remained in persistent vegetative state. Loss of upper brainstem reflexes was predictive of death or severe functional incapacity, but meaningful recovery was possible despite loss of pupillary reactivity. The presence of coma with loss of upper brainstem reflexes and extensor posturing invariably predicted death despite aggressive treatment. Therefore, this combination of clinical features indicating extensive pontomesencephalic destruction may define irreversibility. Radiological features failed to predict functional outcome. This suggests that decisions regarding emergency surgical evacuation should not be based solely upon CT

scan appearance, even if pronounced brain tissue shift is present.

Preconceived notions about futility of care could influence the decision to pursue surgery in some critical patients with ICH. This is apparent in the highly biased selection of surgical candidates that we observe in daily practice. However, it is unclear whether this selection is appropriately based on known prognostic factors or merely results from individual perceptions of most likely outcome.

Becker et al. designed a study aimed at determining how withdrawal of support and surgical intervention affect prognostic models for ICH in a single academic center.[43] In a population of 87 patients with ICH, the overall mortality was 34 percent and medical support was withdrawn in over three-quarters of patients who died. When withdrawal of support was included as a variable in the model predicting outcome, it negated the predictive value of all other variables. Withdrawal of support was uncommon among patients who had undergone surgery, and surgery was much less frequently performed in older patients and patients with left hemispheric hematomas. In addition, a survey of members of the Departments of Neurology and Neurosurgery at their institution revealed that the respondents tended to be overly pessimistic in prognosticating outcome. The investigators concluded that the level of medical support provided was the most important prognostic variable in determining outcome after ICH. According to the results of this study, withdrawal of support in patients deemed likely to have poor outcome could lead to self-fulfilling prophecies.

This provocative study has been the subject of much debate because of its potential implications. Limitations in outcome assessment and inability to retrospectively reconstruct the full set of factors that may have prompted withdrawal of support in each case (most notably the wishes of the patient and the family) may limit the validity of the results. However, the study clearly highlights the biases involved in the decision to operate on patients with ICH.

■ The Pros and Cons

In most cases, the decision about whether to evacuate a cerebral hematoma is complex. Many factors need to be weighed in the equation. In the absence of evidence from randomized trials proving its superiority over more conservative management, surgical treatment should be reserved for selected cases. How to appropriately select those cases remains problematic.

It is reasonable to consider surgery in patients with higher chances of deterioration and subsequent poor functional outcome if treated medically. Several prognostic factors have been validated by various studies. Low GCS sum score, older age, larger hematoma volume, deep hematoma location, intraventricular blood, shift of the septum pellucidum, effacement of contralateral ambient cistern, and contralateral hydrocephalus have been found to be predictive of worse outcome.[42,44–51] Therefore, the presence of these variables argues in favor of a more aggressive treatment plan. On the contrary, patients with none of these poor prognosticators may derive more harm than benefit from aggressive surgical intervention.

Treating more aggressively the sickest patients is intellectually and intuitively appealing, but the real conundrum is when to operate and how to identify those patients in whom any treatment will be futile. In young patients without major comorbidity and with good rehabilitation potential, we believe that surgery should be pursued as soon as clinical deterioration becomes evident and before herniation occurs. Ultra-early surgery to prevent hematoma enlargement should not be pursued because this practice has been shown to increase the risk of potentially fatal rebleeding.[5] Determining which patients have a hopeless functional prognosis is not simple. When reviewing the experience at our medical center, we found that even patients with advanced signs of radiological herniation who had already lost pupillary light reflex could regain functional independence after surgery.[42] Only comatose patients with loss of pontomesencephalic reflexes and extensor posturing invariably died.

Another thorny question is whether there is a role for surgery in the treatment of ganglionic hematomas and what should be the preferred surgical technique used for evacuation. Based on published and personal experience, we consider that in general ganglionic hemorrhages should not be evacuated through craniotomy. However, we recognize exceptions; it may be reasonable to operate on

a young and previously healthy patient with nondominant putaminal hemorrhage who presents with a good level of alertness and then deteriorates rapidly. Endoscopic aspiration may be an acceptable therapeutic option at centers with experience in the use of this technique. Stereotactic drainage aided by liquefaction of the hematoma through local instillation of a thrombolytic drug has been reported to be useful to treat large deep clots and extensive intraventricular hemorrhage, but experience with this method is limited outside of Japan. The value of external ventricular drainage in patients with ganglionic hematoma also remains unclear. Clotting inside the catheter is common (proving a rationale for the use of fibrinolytic agents) and intraventricular pressure is infrequently raised.[52] Ventriculostomy may only be beneficial in patients with thalamic or caudate hematomas who develop progressive hydrocephalus with clinical signs of deterioration. However, this clinical scenario is uncommon in clinical practice. Our proposed indications for surgical evacuation are summarized in Table 16-2.

In our patient, the decision to operate was questionable. The patient was not young, he had several comorbid conditions, and his hematoma involved eloquent regions of the dominant hemisphere. But he presented with progressive clinical deterioration and, despite the absence of hematoma enlargement or detectable changes in the degree of mass effect on CT scan, evacuation of the extensive clot could improve or at least stabilize his condition. The hematoma was surgically accessible and the patient had previously enjoyed a full level of function. And perhaps more importantly, the patient's wife adamantly demanded aggressive treatment. Even retrospectively, it is not easy to

Table 16-2. Proposed Indications for Surgery in Patients with ICH

- Cerebellar hematoma >3 cm with neurological deterioration, brainstem compression, or noncommunicating hydrocephalus.
- Young patient with signs of clinical deterioration secondary to moderate or large lobar hematoma in the nondominant hemisphere. In such cases, marked brain tissue shift on CT scan is not incompatible with meaningful functional recovery.
- Hematoma secondary to underlying structural lesion (tumor, vascular anomaly).

judge the appropriateness of the intervention. Although the functional outcome was unfavorable, surgery may have been this patient's only chance to regain meaningful function.

The outcome of patients with large ICH should not be assessed by survival only. Instead, it should be primarily focused on residual morbidity and functional recovery. A recent survey of British neurosurgeons showed that respondents had a wide range of opinions regarding what percentage reduction in poor outcome would justify surgery.[53] Nevertheless, we should all agree that a "lifesaving" craniotomy should not be performed if it will leave a patient with an apoplectic ICH in a destitute state.

■ The Main Points

- There is no established role for surgical evacuation in spontaneous ganglionic and lobar hematoma.
- Surgical evacuation of cerebellar hematoma is likely beneficial when clinical and radiological signs of mass effect are present.
- When suspecting an underlying lesion, surgical evacuation of the hematoma should be considered.
- Placement of ventriculostomy does not lead to improved outcome in patients with ganglionic hemorrhage.
- Clinical deterioration from a lobar hematoma is an indication for surgical evacuation in patients with good rehabilitation potential.
- The value of surgical evacuation on stable patients with lobar hematoma and mass effect remains unproven.
- Surgical evacuation in patients with expanding hematoma and loss of pontomesencephalic reflexes is likely futile.

■ References

1. Minematsu K. Evacuation of intracerebral hematoma is likely to be beneficial. *Stroke* 2003;34:1567–1568.
2. Felberg RA, Grotta JC, Shirzadi AL, Strong R, Narayana P, Hill-Felberg SJ, Aronowski J. Cell death in experimental intracerebral hemorrhage: the "black hole" model of hemorrhagic damage. *Ann Neurol* 2002;51:517–524.
3. Broderick J, Brott T, Tomsick T, Tew J, Duldner J, Huster G. Management of intracerebral hemorrhage in a large metropolitan population. *Neurosurgery* 1994;34:882–887.
4. Fayad PB, Awad IA. Surgery for intracerebral hemorrhage. *Neurology* 1998;51:S69–73.
5. Morgenstern LB, Demchuk AM, Kim DH, Frankowski RF, Grotta JC. Rebleeding leads to poor outcome in ultra-early craniotomy for intracerebral hemorrhage. *Neurology* 2001;56:1294–1299.
6. McKissock W, Richardson A, Taylor J. Primary intracerebral hemorrhage: a controlled trial of surgical and conservative treatment in 180 unselected cases. *Lancet* 1961;2:221–226.
7. Chen X, Yang H, Czherig Z. A prospective randomized trial of surgical and conservative treatment of hypertensive intracranial hemorrhage [in Chinese]. *Acta Acad Med Shanghai* 1992;19:237–240.
8. Juvela S, Heiskanen O, Poranen A, et al. The treatment of spontaneous intracerebral hemorrhage: a prospective randomized trial of surgical and conservative treatment. *J Neurosurg* 1989;70:755–758.
9. Batjer HH, Reisch JS, Allen BC, Plaizier LJ, Su CJ. Failure of surgery to improve outcome in hypertensive putaminal hemorrhage: a prospective randomized trial. *Arch Neurol* 1990;47:1103–1106.
10. Auer LM, Deinsberger W, Neiderkorn K, Gell G, Kleinert R, Schneider G, Holzer P, Bone G, Mokry M, Korner E, et al. Endoscopic surgery versus medical treatment for spontaneous intracerebral hematoma: a randomized study. *J Neurosurg* 1989;70:530–535.
11. Morgenstern LB, Frankowski RF, Shedden P, Pasteur W, Grotta JC. Surgical treatment for intracerebral hemorrhage (STICH): a single-center, randomized clinical trial. *Neurology* 1998;51:1359–1363.
12. Zuccarello M, Brott T, Derex L, Kothari R, Sauerbeck L, Tew J, Van Loveren H, Yeh HS, Tomsick T, Pancioli A, Khoury J, Broderick J. Early surgical treatment for supratentorial intracerebral hemorrhage: a randomized feasibility study. *Stroke* 1999;30:1833–1839.
13. Teernstra OP, Evers SM, Lodder J, Leffers P, Franke CL, Blaauw G. Stereotactic treatment of intracerebral hematoma by means of a plasminogen activator: a multicenter randomized controlled trial (SICHPA). *Stroke* 2003;34:968–974.
14. Hankey GJ, Hon C. Surgery for primary intracerebral hemorrhage: is it safe and effective? A systematic review of case series and randomized trials. *Stroke* 1997;28:2126–2132.
15. Prasad K, Shrivastava A. Surgery for primary supratentorial intracerebral hemorrhage [Cochrane review]. In *The Cochrane Library*, issue 4, 2000. Oxford, UK, Update Software.
16. Prasad K, Browman G, Srivastava A, Menon G. Surgery in primary supratentorial intracerebral hematoma: a meta-analysis of randomized trials. *Acta Neurol Scand* 1997;95:103–110.

17. Saver J. Surgical therapy. In Feldmann E, ed. *Intracerebral Hemorrhage.* Armonk, NY, Futura Publishing Co., 1994:303–332.

18. Saver JL, Hankey G, Hon C. Surgery for primary intracerebral hemorrhage: meta-analysis of CT-era studies. *Stroke* 1998;29:1477–1478 [letter and response].

19. Fernandes HM, Gregson B, Siddique S, Mendelow AD. Surgery in intracerebral hemorrhage: the uncertainty continues. *Stroke* 2000;31:2511–2516.

20. Donnan GA, Davis SM. Surgery for intracerebral hemorrhage: an evidence-poor zone. *Stroke* 2003; 34:1569–1570.

21. Brambilla GL, Rodriguez y Baena R, Sangiovanni G, Rainoldi F, Locatelli D. Spontaneous intracerebral hemorrhage: medical or surgical treatment. *J Neurosurg Sci* 1983;27:95–101.

22. Waga S, Yamamoto Y. Hypertensive putaminal hemorrhage: treatment and results. Is surgical treatment superior to conservative one? *Stroke* 1983;14:480–485.

23. Kaneko M, Koba T, Yokoyama T. Early surgical treatment for hypertensive intracerebral hemorrhage. *J Neurosurg* 1977;46:579–583.

24. Kaneko M, Tanaka K, Shimada T, Sato K, Uemura K. Long-term evaluation of ultra-early operation for hypertensive intracerebral hemorrhage in 100 cases. *J Neurosurg* 1983;58:838–842.

25. Bolander HG, Kourtopoulos H, Liliequist B, Wittboldt S. Treatment of spontaneous intracerebral haemorrhage: a retrospective analysis of 74 consecutive cases with special reference to computertomographic data. *Acta Neurochir (Wien)* 1983;67:19–28.

26. van Loon J, Van Calenbergh F, Goffin J, Plets C. Controversies in the management of spontaneous cerebellar haemorrhage: a consecutive series of 49 cases and review of the literature. *Acta Neurochir (Wien)* 1993;122:187–193.

27. Firsching R, Huber M, Frowein RA. Cerebellar haemorrhage: management and prognosis. *Neurosurg Rev* 1991;14:191–194.

28. Da Pian R, Bazzan A, Pasqualin A. Surgical versus medical treatment of spontaneous posterior fossa haematomas: a cooperative study on 205 cases. *Neurol Res* 1984;6:145–151.

29. Kase C. Cerebellar hemorrhage. In Kase C, Caplan L, eds. *Intracerebral Hemorrhage.* Boston, Butterworth-Heinemann, 1994:425–443.

30. Wijdicks EF, St Louis EK, Atkinson JD, Li H. Clinician's biases toward surgery in cerebellar hematomas: an analysis of decision-making in 94 patients. *Cerebrovasc Dis* 2000;10:93–96.

31. Backlund EO, von Holst H. Controlled subtotal evacuation of intracerebral haematomas by stereotactic technique. *Surg Neurol* 1978;9:99–101.

32. Nguyen JP, Decq P, Brugieres P, Yepes C, Melon E, Gaston A, Keravel Y. A technique for stereotactic aspiration of deep intracerebral hematomas under computed tomographic control using a new device. *Neurosurgery* 1992;31:330–334.

33. Iseki H, Amano K, Kawamura H, Tanikawa T, Kawabatake H, Notani M, Shiwaku T, Iwata Y, Taira T, Nagao H, et al. A new apparatus for CT-guided stereotactic surgery. *Appl Neurophysiol* 1985;48:50–60.

34. Niizuma H, Suzuki J. Stereotactic aspiration of putaminal hemorrhage using a double track aspiration technique. *Neurosurgery* 1988;22:432–436.

35. Kanaya H, Kuroda K. Development in neurosurgical approaches to hypertensive intracerebral hemorrhage. In Kauffman H, ed. *Intracerebral Hematomas.* New York, Raven Press, 1992:197–210.

36. Tyler D, Mandybur G. Interventional MRI-guided stereotactic aspiration of acute/subacute intracerebral hematomas. *Stereotact Funct Neurosurg* 1999;72: 129–135.

37. Schaller C, Rohde V, Meyer B, Hassler W. Stereotactic puncture and lysis of spontaneous intracerebral hemorrhage using recombinant tissue-plasminogen activator. *Neurosurgery* 1995;36:328–333.

38. Montes JM, Wong JH, Fayad PB, Awad IA. Stereotactic computed tomographic-guided aspiration and thrombolysis of intracerebral hematoma: protocol and preliminary experience. *Stroke* 2000;31:834–840.

39. Findlay JM, Grace MG, Weir BK. Treatment of intraventricular hemorrhage with tissue plasminogen activator. *Neurosurgery* 1993;32:941–947.

40. Naff NJ, Carhuapoma JR, Williams MA, Bhardwaj A, Ulatowski JA, Bederson J, Bullock R, Schmutzhard E, Pfausler B, Keyl PM, Tuhrim S, Hanley DF. Treatment of intraventricular hemorrhage with urokinase: effects on 30-day survival. *Stroke* 2000;31:841–847.

41. Broderick JP, Adams HP Jr, Barsan W, Feinberg W, Feldmann E, Grotta J, Kase C, Krieger D, Mayberg M, Tilley B, Zabramski JM, Zuccarello M. Guidelines for the management of spontaneous intracerebral hemorrhage: a statement for healthcare professionals from a special writing group of the Stroke Council, American Heart Association. *Stroke* 1999;30:905–915.

42. Rabinstein AA, Atkinson JL, Wijdicks EF. Emergency craniotomy in patients worsening due to expanded cerebral hematoma: to what purpose? *Neurology* 2002;58:1367–1372.

43. Becker KJ, Baxter AB, Cohen WA, Bybee HM, Tirschwell DL, Newell DW, Winn HR, Longstreth WT Jr. Withdrawal of support in intracerebral hemorrhage may lead to self-fulfilling prophecies. *Neurology* 2001;56:766–772.

44. Juvela S. Risk factors for impaired outcome after spontaneous intracerebral hemorrhage. *Arch Neurol* 1995;52:1193–1200.

45. Schwarz S, Jauss M, Krieger D, Dorfler A, Albert F, Hacke W. Haematoma evacuation does not improve outcome in spontaneous supratentorial intracerebral hemorrhage: a case-control study. *Acta Neurochir (Wien)* 1997;139:897–904.

46. Lampl Y, Gilad R, Eshel Y, Sarova-Pinhas I. Neurological and functional outcome in patients with supratentorial hemorrhages: a prospective study. *Stroke* 1995;26:2249–2253.

47. Hardemark HG, Wesslen N, Persson L. Influence of clinical factors, CT findings and early management on outcome in supratentorial intracerebral hemorrhage. *Cerebrovasc Dis* 1999;9:10–21.

48. Flemming KD, Wijdicks EFM, St Louis EK, Li H. Predicting deterioration in patients with lobar hemorrhages. *J Neurol Neurosurg Psychiatry* 1999;66:600–605.

49. Flemming KD, Wijdicks EFM, Li H. Can we predict poor outcome at presentation in patients with lobar hemorrhage? *Cerebrovasc Dis* 2001;11:183–189.

50. Broderick JP, Brott TG, Duldner JE, Tomsick T, Huster G. Volume of intracerebral hemorrhage: a powerful and easy-to-use predictor of 30-day mortality. *Stroke* 1993;24:987–993.

51. Diringer MN, Edwards DF, Zarzulia AR. Hydrocephalus: a previously unrecognized predictor of poor outcome from supratentorial intracerebral hemorrhage. *Stroke* 1998;29:1352–1357.

52. Adams RE, Diringer MN. Response to external ventricular drainage in spontaneous intracerebral hemorrhage with hydrocephalus. *Neurology* 1998;50:519–523.

53. Fernandes HM, Mendelow AD. Spontaneous intracerebral hemorrhage: a surgical dilemma. *Br J Neurosurg* 1999;13:389–394.

Chapter 17
Chemotherapy for Brain Tumors

Warren P. Mason

Primary brain tumors likely originate from glial cells or their precursors. Most primary brain tumors are of astrocytic or oligodendroglial origin, and range from low-grade neoplasms such as the astrocytoma, to extremely high-grade, the most common of which is the glioblastoma multiforme. High-grade tumors such as the glioblastoma multiforme can arise from successive de-differentiation of a low-grade neoplasm, or develop de novo.[1]

The current management of high-grade glial neoplasms consists of surgery followed by focal radiotherapy, and chemotherapy. Despite aggressive treatment, these tumors are incurable. The most common primary brain tumor, the glioblastoma, has a dismal prognosis for survival of approximately one year, with only 15–20 percent of patients surviving more than 2 years.[2] For this reason, the search for effective medical therapies including chemotherapeutic drugs has been a focus of neuro-oncology for several decades. The administration of chemotherapy for patients with brain tumors has been fraught with many challenges, including the absence of truly effective drugs despite preclinical evidence of activity. Many reasons exist for the limited efficacy of chemotherapy for most brain tumors, including the presence of a blood-brain barrier that restricts drug entry into the central nervous system. Furthermore, drug resistance may develop, in part due to the genetic heterogeneity and instability of these neoplasms.[3]

Chemotherapy for primary high-grade brain tumors can be administered immediately after radiotherapy (adjuvant chemotherapy), or at the time of recurrence. The timing of chemotherapy is a major controversy in neuro-oncology, and the value of adjuvant chemotherapy for high-grade neoplasms is unproved despite decades of clinical trials where adjuvant chemotherapy did not alter outcome for the majority of patients who received it. Nonetheless, patients with high-grade glial neoplasms continue to receive adjuvant chemotherapy because there appears to be a small but consistent fraction of patients, perhaps 10–15 percent, who do benefit from adjuvant chemotherapy in terms of delayed time to progression and survival. In fact, most long-term survivors of glioblastoma multiforme have received adjuvant chemotherapy.[2] Thus it would appear that there is a minority of patients with glioblastoma multiforme who have chemosensitive tumors and who benefit from receiving chemotherapy sooner rather than later. These tumors likely have unique genetic derangements that make them susceptible to the effects of cytotoxic drugs. A major challenge in neuro-oncology is to understand the nature of this chemosensitivity, and discover ways to identify these patients so that chemotherapy can be incorporated early into the management of their diseases.

The current most commonly used drugs used to treat high-grade glial tumors consist of intravenous carmustine (BCNU); the combination chemotherapy regimen consisting of procarbazine, lomustine (CCNU), and vincristine (PCV regimen); and recently the oral drug temozolomide. These agents all have good central nervous system penetration and modest efficacy against gliomas. Monotherapy appears to be as effective as and generally less toxic than combination chemotherapy regimens for high-grade gliomas,[4] except for anaplastic oligodendroglial tumors, where PCV chemotherapy has been a standard treatment.[5] Temozolomide is very well tolerated and is becoming the most used agent for primary brain tumors, although data regarding its use in the adjuvant setting are not available.[6,7]

■ **The Patient**

A 52-year-old man was brought to the emergency room after a colleague found him unresponsive in his office. When examined in the emergency department, he was alert and oriented but looked tired. He did not have any traumatic bruises or cuts, and had not been incontinent of urine or stool. His neurological examination was completely normal without any evidence of focal neurological deficits or papilledema. He had experienced three similar episodes of unexplained loss of consciousness in the past 10 months but had been otherwise well. An MR scan of his brain was performed that day disclosing a heterogeneously enhancing mass in the anterior right temporal lobe suggestive of a high-grade glial neoplasm (Figure 17-1). He was placed on phenytoin and dexamethasone.

A craniotomy with gross total excision of the brain tumor was performed (Figure 17-2). The patient recovered uneventfully after surgery. Pathological review of his tumor disclosed a glioblastoma multiforme with areas of prominent oligodendroglial differentiation (Figure 17-3). Molecular genetic studies were performed on the tumor specimen, and loss of heterozygosity of chromosomes 1p was detected.

Following surgery, conventional radiotherapy using the parallel pair method was administered to a dose of 5000 cGy in 25 fractions. The patient tolerated radiotherapy well and was able to taper and discontinue dexamethasone. The patient returned to work and continued taking phenytoin without further episodes of loss of consciousness. Following completion of radiotherapy, the patient started adjuvant chemotherapy with lomustine at a dosage of 130 mg/m^2 every 6 weeks. It followed a discussion with his oncologist about the value of initiating chemotherapy for glioblastoma at this stage in his illness when there was no evidence of tumor progression. He was also interested in novel anticancer therapies and with the agreement of his treating physician commenced thalidomide and sulindac based on preliminary evidence of their potential

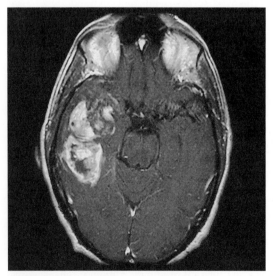

Figure 17-1. T1-weighted MR scan of the brain following gadolinium-DTPA administration discloses a large complex enhancing mass with areas of necrosis suggesting a high-grade primary brain tumor.

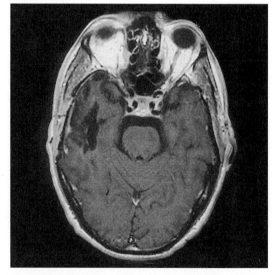

Figure 17-2. T1-weighted MR scan of the brain following gadolinium-DTPA administration after complete resection of a glioblastoma multiforme. There is no residual enhancement at the resection site, suggesting a gross total excision of the tumor.

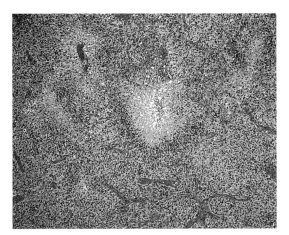

Figure 17-3. Photomicrograph of a section of tissue stained with hematoxylin and eosin disclosing a glioblastoma multiforme with areas of necrosis, high cellularity, pseudopallisading, and neovascularization (magnification × 400). There are areas where cells and nuclei are rounded, suggesting a degree of oligodendroglial differentiation.

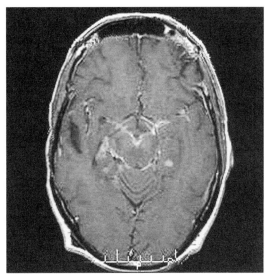

Figure 17-4. T1-weighted MRI of the brain following gadolinium-DTPA administration revealing abnormal nodular enhancement in the mesial temporal lobes, and overlying membranes of the brainstem and basal cisterns. These findings are consistent with a diagnosis of leptomeningeal gliomatosis. Note the absence of enhancement at the site of tumor resection where disease is controlled.

antiangiogenic activity. After completing five cycles of chemotherapy without evidence of clinical or radiographic progression, the patient decided to stop chemotherapy because of persistent fatigue. Chemotherapy was otherwise well tolerated without significant myelosuppression or pulmonary toxicity.

Three months after stopping chemotherapy, the patient's family noticed gradually increasing confusion, diminished memory, and disorientation. He had episodes of urinary incontinence. When examined, he had an impaired mental status and was ataxic. An MRI of his brain revealed communicating hydrocephalus with new enhancement of the leptomeninges of the basal cisterns. The appearance of the surgical cavity and overlying membranes was stable without evidence of local recurrence (Figure 17-4). A lumbar puncture showed an opening pressure of 28 cm H_2O and elevated CSF protein (4 g/dL) but no cytological evidence of malignancy.

With the presumptive diagnosis of leptomeningeal gliomatosis, the patient had a ventriculoperitoneal shunt inserted. His symptoms improved dramatically, and he was able to return to work. Systemic temozolomide chemotherapy at a dosage of 200 mg/m^2/day for 5 days every 28 days was started for leptomeningeal dissemination of his glioblastoma.

He was stable clinically and radiographically for 4 months on temozolomide therapy until he began to experience increasing somnolence, confusion, and disorientation. Temozolomide chemotherapy was stopped because of clinical progression, and the patient received one cycle of irinotecan at a dosage of 150 mg/m^2/day for 3 days. He continued to deteriorate and died of progressive leptomeningeal disease while receiving palliative whole-brain radiotherapy. Necropsy was not performed.

■ The Problem

- Chemotherapy has a limited and palliative role in the management of glioblastoma and other glial neoplasms. When should this man have received chemotherapy?
- He received three different chemotherapeutic agents in addition to other unconventional agents of questionable activity. Which agents should have been used to treat his disease?

■ The Evidence

Approximately 17,000 Americans are diagnosed annually with primary brain tumors, and half of these are classified as high-grade cancers such as glioblastoma multiforme and anaplastic astrocytoma.[8] Although rare, primary brain tumors represent a challenge to the clinician because of their associated morbidity and mortality, and the limited therapeutic options available for their management. The prognosis for patients with newly diagnosed glioblastoma is grim, with median survival in the range of 9 to 12 months, and a survival rate of approximately 10 percent at 2 years.[9] Cytoreductive surgery followed by postoperative radiotherapy is the cornerstone of management, with chemotherapy having a limited and controversial role.[10]

Adjuvant Chemotherapy for High-Grade Astrocytomas

Malignant gliomas recur locally and rarely metastasize. Gliomas are infiltrative diseases, and total surgical resection is impossible.[11] For these reasons, postoperative therapies such as cranial irradiation and chemotherapy are administered in an attempt to delay tumor progression. Chemotherapy that is administered postoperatively without clinical or radiographic evidence of tumor progression is called adjuvant chemotherapy. Historically, the nitrosoureas have been the most effective agents against malignant glioma, and these agents have been studied extensively as adjuvant treatment for these cancers.[9,10] In 1978, the results of a clinical trial conducted under the auspices of the Brain Tumor Study Group where patients with newly diagnosed high-grade glial neoplasms were randomized to receive best conventional supportive care or treatment with radiotherapy and BCNU chemotherapy alone or in combination were reported.[12] In this trial, patients receiving only supportive care survived a median of 14 weeks, with patients receiving BCNU alone surviving 18 weeks, radiotherapy alone 36 weeks, and radiotherapy plus BCNU 35 weeks. Although the survival curve for patients treated with radiotherapy alone was virtually identical to that for patients receiving both radiotherapy and chemotherapy, the latter group did have a statistically significant

survival advantage at 18 months, at which time 10 percent in the combined modality arm were alive compared with only 4 percent in the arm that received only radiotherapy. A similar phase III study reported by the Brain Tumor Study Group in 1980 confirmed these results, including a statistically significant survival advantage at 18 months or longer for patients who received both chemotherapy and radiotherapy.[13] This "tail on the curve," that is, the patients who had improved survival on adjuvant chemotherapy, which has been a consistent feature of many phase III studies, was interpreted to mean that some patients benefit from adjuvant chemotherapy but most do not. This has formed the basis for the recommendation of adjuvant chemotherapy.[14,15]

Since these initial studies, numerous investigators have explored the role of adjuvant chemotherapy with often conflicting results (Table 17-1). In 1990, the Northern California Oncology Group reported the results of a phase III trial comparing BCNU with the drug combination of procarbazine, lomustine, and vincristine (PCV) for patients with newly diagnosed glioblastoma multiforme and anaplastic glioma.[19] Patients in both histological groups receiving the PCV combination therapy survived longer than those randomized to monotherapy with BCNU, but the difference was statistically significant only for patients who had anaplastic glioma. For patients with this favorable histology, median survival in the PCV arm was 157.1 weeks compared with 82.1 weeks in the BCNU arm. The study is the basis for the recommendation to use adjuvant chemotherapy for patients with anaplastic astrocytomas. Moreover, this and other trials have demonstrated no advantage of multi-agent chemotherapy over single-agent chemotherapy with nitrosourea for glioblastoma multiforme.[10,17,18,20] However, this conclusion is limited by the inclusion of patients with tumors that had oligodendroglial features in addition to patients with pure anaplastic astrocytomas.[21] A recent phase III study conducted by the Medical Research Council randomizing patients 70 years of age or younger to adjuvant radiation therapy versus radiation therapy plus PCV chemotherapy has demonstrated no difference in median survival between both treatment arms for both glioblastoma multiforme and anaplastic astrocytoma histologies.[18] Furthermore, the results of this study reinforced the belief that radiotherapy alone

Table 17-1. Selected Phase III Trials Evaluating Adjuvant Chemotherapy for Malignant Glioma

Reference	Treatment	Total No. of Patients	% GBM	Results
Walker et al.[12]	Surgery alone RT BCNU + RT BCNU	222	n.a.	BCNU increased survival from 4% to 18% at 18 months
Walker et al.[13]	MeCCNU alone RT alone RT + BCNU RT + MeCCNU	358	84	BCNU increased survival at 18 months
Chang et al.[14]	RT alone RT + boost RT + BCNU RT + MeCCNU + DTIC	535	83	BCNU improved survival to 43 weeks in patients aged 40 to 60
Green et al.[15]	RT + mPred RT + BCNU RT + PCB RT + BCNU + mPred	527	87	BCNU improved survival from 40 to 50 weeks
Levin et al.[16]	RT + HU + BCNU RT + HU +PCV	148	50	PCV significantly improves survival for patients with AA
Shapiro et al.[17]	RT + BCNU RT + BCNU + PCB RT + BCNU + HU + PCB + VM-26	510	80	No difference
Medical Research Council[18]	RT alone RT + PCV	674	67	No difference

AA, anaplastic astrocytoma; GBM, glioblastoma multiforme; RT, radiotherapy; BCNU, carmustine; MeCCNU, methylCCNU; mPred, methylprednisolone; HU, hydroxyurea; PCB, procarbazine; PCV, procarbazine, lomustine, vincristine.

remains a standard and appropriate first-line therapy for high-grade astrocytic neoplasms.

The route of chemotherapy administration was evaluated in a study comparing intra-venous BCNU with intra-arterial BCNU with or without intravenous 5-fluorouracil for patients with high-grade gliomas following radiotherapy in a randomized phase II study reported in 1992.[22] In this trial, intravenous BCNU was superior to intra-arterial BCNU largely because the latter arm suffered serious and disproportionate toxicity in the form of irreversible encephalopathy and visual loss ipsilateral to the infused carotid artery. For this reason, patients with anaplastic astrocytoma randomized to receive intra-arterial chemotherapy had a reduced survival when compared to the arm receiving intravenous chemotherapy. The addition of 5-fluorouracil had no impact on survival.

Although the alkylating agent temozolomide is increasingly becoming the favored chemotherapeutic agent for malignant gliomas, no agents have been

shown superior to nitrosoureas as adjuvant treatment for glioblastoma multiforme.[7,23] A recent phase II study using the alkylating agent temozolomide as radiosensitizer (a drug that enhances the effect of radiotherapy) and adjuvant chemotherapy for patients with newly diagnosed glioblastoma multiforme has produced impressive preliminary data with median survival of 16 months and 1- and 2-year survival rates of 58 and 31 percent, respectively.[24] A recently completed phase III study conducted by the European Organization for the Research and Treatment of Cancer and the National Cancer Institute of Canada randomizing patients with newly diagnosed glioblastoma multiforme to radiotherapy alone versus radiotherapy with this temozolomide regimen has completed accrual, with preliminary results expected in approximately 2 years.

The value of chemotherapy administered following surgery but before radiotherapy (neoadjuvant chemotherapy) has not been extensively studied.[20,25]

There are obstacles to conducting such studies, largely because radiotherapy alters the radiographic appearance of gliomas, and consequently makes evaluation of response difficult. However, a number of ongoing phase III studies are addressing this issue, and results are anticipated in the near future.

A meta-analysis of 16 studies published between 1975 and 1989 has concluded that adjuvant chemotherapy does provide a survival advantage for a minority of patients with high-grade gliomas.[26] Nonetheless, the role of adjuvant chemotherapy for high-grade gliomas remains controversial and continues to be limited because the majority of patients who receive such treatment experience no benefit in terms of survival.[3] However, perhaps more importantly, these studies have identified a number of prognostic variables associated with favorable outcome including histology, younger age, minimal residual disease following surgical resection, and good performance status.[11,27–30] Histology is perhaps the most important variable, with glioblastoma multiforme patients surviving approximately half as long as those with anaplastic astrocytoma.[19]

Chemotherapy for Recurrent High-Grade Astrocytomas

Patients with recurrent high-grade astrocytomas have limited therapeutic options, and chemotherapy is often administered at this point, usually with disappointing results. A number of agents have been tested in phase II studies, where responses are uncommon and often of short duration (Table 17-2). As with most phase III studies in glioma, most phase II studies have indiscriminately enrolled patients with glioblastoma and anaplastic astrocytoma, and have used variable response criteria, making interpretation of results and comparisons between studies difficult.[10,20] Nitrosoureas have been the most commonly prescribed agents for recurrent glioblastoma multiforme and anaplastic astrocytoma, with response rates varying from 21 to 31 percent.[31,32] However, nitrosoureas are frequently not administered at recurrence because many patients have had prior exposure to these agents in the adjuvant setting. As a consequence, a number of chemotherapeutic agents have been tested in patients with recurrent astrocytic tumors, with procarbazine, platinum analogs, irinotecan, and most recently temozolomide being the agents most commonly used.[23,33–43]

Procarbazine has often been employed for high-grade astrocytoma and glioblastoma multiforme at recurrence. A phase II study published by Rodriguez et al. reported a response rate of 28 percent to single-agent procarbazine in a series of 99 patients with recurrent high-grade gliomas.[41] Although platinum analogs continue to be used alone or in combination with other chemotherapies in the setting of recurrence, activity is minimal with reported objective responses in the range of 11 to 21 percent. The topoisomerase I inhibitor irinotecan has been tested in patients with recurrent disease with some evidence of activity. A study involving 60 patients with recurrent

Table 17-2. Selected Phase II Trials for Progressive Malignant Glioma

Reference	Treatment	Tumor Histology	% Response + Stable Disease	Median Time to Progression (weeks)
Rosenblum et al.[31]	CCNU	GBM + AA	42	23
Wilson et al.[32]	BCNU	GBM	29	22
Newton et al.[33]	Procarbazine	GBM	31	40
Gutin et al.[34]	PCV	GBM	45	15
Friedman et al.[35]	Irinotecan	GBM/AA	43/70	18/12
Yung et al.[36]	Carboplatin	GBM/AA	40/57	61
Jeremic et al.[67]	Carboplatin + Vp-16	GBM/AA	21/32	42.5
Yung et al.[6]	Temozolomide	GBM/AA	40/66	11/22

AA, anaplastic astrocytoma; GBM, glioblastoma multiforme; BCNU, carmustine; CCNU, lomustine; PCV, procarbazine, lomustine, vincristine; Vp-16, etoposide.

high-grade gliomas reported a partial response rate of 15 percent.[35] However, because the use of concurrent anticonvulsants enhances the metabolism of irinotecan, the activity of this agent may have been diminished because many patients were treated at subtherapeutic doses.

Most recently, temozolomide has emerged as the most promising agent for the management of recurrent anaplastic astrocytoma and glioblastoma multiforme. This oral alkylating agent is particularly interesting because it depletes methylguanine methyltransferase, the enzyme responsible for the development of resistance to alkylating agents, and because it can be administered for prolonged duration without significant or cumulative myelosuppression.[44] Preliminary studies using temozolomide in phase II studies for recurrent glioma after radiotherapy reported a radiographic response rate of 25 percent.[45] Moreover, temozolomide has been evaluated separately for recurrent glioblastoma multiforme and anaplastic astrocytoma at recurrence with favorable results.[38,43] A phase III study randomized patients with recurrent glioblastoma multiforme following nitrosourea failure to receive either procarbazine or temozolomide. Patients receiving temozolomide had a partial response rate of 4.7 percent at 85 days, and patients receiving procarbazine had a 3 percent response rate at 99 days. There was no difference in median and overall survival between the arms, but patients receiving temozolomide had a statistically significant improvement in progression-free survival and quality of life while on therapy. A phase II study evaluating temozolomide in 162 patients with recurrent anaplastic astrocytoma or oligoastrocytoma at first relapse reported a progression-free survival of 46 percent at 6 months, and an overall survival of 75 percent and 56 percent at 6 months and one year, respectively. The overall response rate was 35 percent, with 8 percent having a complete radiographic response and 27 percent having a partial response. Based on these data, temozolomide has been approved in the United States for treating recurrent anaplastic astrocytoma and in Europe and Canada for the treatment of recurrent anaplastic astrocytoma and glioblastoma multiforme. Ongoing studies are exploring the role of this agent over a prolonged duration or intensified dose, or in combination with other chemotherapeutic agents or novel therapies.[7]

In addition to conventional approaches to the delivery of chemotherapeutic agents, there has been growing interest in interstitial chemotherapy using controlled release of biodegradable polymers impregnated with nitrosoureas. A recently reported placebo-controlled study randomized patients with recurrent glioblastoma to receive BCNU wafers inserted at the time of surgery for re-resection of tumor.[46] Patients receiving BCNU wafers had a 64 percent 6-month survival compared with 44 percent in the placebo-treated arm, but there was no statistically significant difference in median and overall survival. Nonetheless, a multiple regression analysis model demonstrated a beneficial effect of the BCNU wafer in recurrent glioblastoma. Further studies are evaluating this novel delivery system in newly diagnosed disease, and trials incorporating agents other than BCNU are in progress.

While chemotherapy continues to have a role in the management of recurrent anaplastic astrocytoma and glioblastoma, responses are brief and treatment remains palliative. The majority of patients with recurrent disease receive little or no benefit from available chemotherapies, and new drugs need to be developed if there is to be any meaningful change in the prognosis of these diseases.

Chemotherapy for Anaplastic Oligodendroglioma and Oligoastrocytoma

Malignant tumors of oligodendroglial lineage have been shown recently to be highly chemosensitive tumors. In 1988, a series of 8 patients with recurrent anaplastic oligodendrogliomas that responded to chemotherapy, namely the PCV regimen (procarbazine, lomustine, and vincristine), was reported.[47] Subsequently, these same investigators demonstrated that newly diagnosed aggressive oligodendrogliomas are also highly chemosensitive neoplasms, and can respond with objective reduction in tumor bulk to nitrosourea-based chemotherapy regimens prior to treatment with radiotherapy.[48] These preliminary studies formed the basis for a subsequent phase II study evaluating the role of PCV chemotherapy for newly diagnosed or recurrent anaplastic oligodendroglioma.[5] Of 24 eligible patients, 18 responded (including 9 who had complete radiographic responses), 4 had stable disease, and 2 had early progression on therapy. Median time to progression was related to the extent of the response and was at least 25 months for complete responders.

Anaplastic oligodendrogliomas have been shown subsequently to be responsive to a variety of chemotherapeutic agents, including vincristine and cisplatin, melphalan, thiotepa, paclitaxel, and temozolomide.[49–53] Moreover, anaplastic tumors of mixed histology, having both oligodendroglial and astrocytic features, have also been shown to respond to chemotherapy, usually in a less dramatic and durable way.[54,55] Furthermore, less malignant oligodendrogliomas, including aggressive (enhancing, expanding, and symptomatic oligodendrogliomas that are not histologically anaplastic) and low-grade oligodendrogliomas, can also respond to chemotherapy, particularly the PCV regimen.[56,57] Chemotherapy for low-grade oligodendroglial tumors is currently under exploration as a means of delaying or avoiding cranial irradiation and its delayed toxicities. Although no pathological or clinical features have been demonstrated to be predictive of a response to chemotherapy, recent reports indicate that allelic loss of heterozygosity of chromosomes 1p and 19q is predictive of radiographic response and improved prognosis for patients with anaplastic oligodendrogliomas. Thus, molecular diagnostic techniques may be used to identify a subset of patients with oligodendroglial neoplasms who might benefit from earlier chemotherapy.[58,59]

Despite the impressive and predictable responses of oligodendroglial tumors to a variety of chemotherapeutic agents, the role and timing of chemotherapy for these tumors remains under investigation. A large intergroup study randomizing patients with pure and mixed anaplastic oligodendrogliomas to receive radiotherapy alone or in combination with four cycles of an intensive PCV regimen has recently completed accrual; once available, the results of this study may provide important information to resolve this question.

■ The Pros and Cons

Patients with high-grade brain tumors present difficult challenges to the clinician because these cancers are aggressive, and treatment options are few. The standard treatments of surgery and radiotherapy control these diseases for durations seldom longer than one year, and for this reason, additional treatments that might delay progression and prolong survival are desperately sought. Available chemotherapeutic agents have very limited efficacy, and studies to date have not provided clear guidelines about which agents should be administered and when. The trials that have recommended adjuvant chemotherapy were conducted in an era when accurate radiographic evaluation was not available, and included patients with a variety of histologies. Moreover, radiographic response criteria, which remain a subject of controversy today, were not standardized at the time these studies were conducted, and for this reason they are probably not reliable.[60]

Given these constraints, it is difficult to recommend adjuvant chemotherapy to most patients with glioblastoma multiforme and anaplastic astrocytoma because the studies that support adjuvant chemotherapy are flawed methodologically and have shown little, if any, benefit of early treatment. Nevertheless, most large studies exploring the role of adjuvant chemotherapy for high-grade glial neoplasms have consistently demonstrated that a minority of patients, possibly as many as 15 percent, benefit from adjuvant chemotherapy in terms of extended long-term survival.[13,15] It was this observation that accounted for early enthusiasm for adjuvant chemotherapy for these diseases. Clinicians were prepared to treat many for the benefit of a few. However, more recently, enthusiasm for adjuvant chemotherapy has waned in the neuro-oncological community. Today, clinicians may be more inclined to withhold adjuvant chemotherapy, thereby preventing the majority from experiencing the unpleasant and potentially harmful toxicities of a treatment without benefit, while denying a minority a treatment that would be beneficial.[61]

A challenge facing neuro-oncologists today is how to identify patients who would respond to adjuvant chemotherapy. There is no dispute that gliomas can respond, sometimes impressively and for prolonged durations, to chemotherapy, but responses cannot be predicted reliably. From innumerable phase II and III studies, prognostic factors have been identified that help the clinician to select patients who may respond to aggressive strategies that include early chemotherapy. These factors include histology, younger age, history of a low-grade glioma, maximal surgical resection with minimal residual disease, and good performance status.[11,27–30] Selecting only patients with favorable prognostic factors may be a facile way to increase the likelihood of response to adjuvant chemotherapy, but this strategy would exclude others who do not fit these profiles but might also benefit from such treatment. For instance, DeAngelis et al. have shown that enhanced 18-month survival in the original Brain Tumor Study Group trials was not attributable to contamination of these studies by patients with chemosensitive oligodendrogliomas, thus excluding this explanation for "the tail on the survival curve."[21] While clinicians can continue to rely on prognostic factors to help guide treatment recommendations, the real challenge is how to select chemosensitive gliomas for treatment with chemotherapy, and to understand why this subset of tumors is responding.

There has been some progress in understanding the determinants of chemoresponsiveness in glial tumors, and much of this work has derived from careful study of the most chemosensitive of all glial tumors, the anaplastic oligodendroglioma. Tumors of oligodendroglial lineage respond to a variety of chemotherapeutic agents that exert their toxic effects by a variety of mechanisms. Moreover, responses are observed in low-grade, mixed, and anaplastic tumors containing oligodendroglial elements, although the responses are variable and influenced by the clinical, radiographic, and pathological characteristics of the neoplasm.[62] Molecular genetic analysis of glial tumors has identified a variety of alterations unique to tumors of oligodendroglial lineage, including abnormalities of chromosomes 1p and 19q and intact p53 genes.[58,63] Specifically, recent work by Cairncross et al. has shown that loss of heterozygosity of chromosome 1p in anaplastic oligodendroglioma predicts response to chemotherapy and improves overall survival.[5] The reason underlying this association remains elusive, and is the focus of ongoing intensive research.[64] Nonetheless, this discovery represents a first step in understanding the molecular genetic determinants of chemosensitivity, and serves as a model for future endeavors. While approximately 80 percent of all anaplastic oligodendrogliomas harbor this unique genetic signature, a small minority of other glial neoplasms,

including mixed glioma, anaplastic astrocytoma, and glioblastoma, have this genetic alteration and do respond to chemotherapy.[65–67] Whether these tumors that do not appear histologically oligodendroglial are in fact oligodendrogliomas is not clear at this point. Moreover, whether glioblastomas with 1p loss of heterozygosity are as chemosensitive as anaplastic oligodendrogliomas with the same alteration is not known. Importantly, there are other subsets of chemosensitive astrocytomas that do not have oligodendroglioma-like genetic alterations, and identifying these tumors and understanding why they too are chemosensitive is critical.

We do not know why most astrocytic tumors are resistant to chemotherapy while a few respond. The answer may relate to intrinsic drug resistance or limited central nervous system penetration of most agents. However, the answer is probably to be found at the molecular level. Indeed, at the molecular level, not all glioblastomas and astrocytomas are the same.[1,68] For example, inactivation of the p53 gene and epidermal growth factor receptor (EGFR) amplification are mutually exclusive genetic alterations.[69] Approximately one-third of glioblastomas harbor p53 mutations and another third have EGFR amplification.[1,70,71] Generally, glioblastomas with p53 mutations occur in younger patients and evolve from low-grade astrocytomas, so-called secondary glioblastomas, whereas those with EGFR amplification occur in older patients and typically arise de novo.[72] We know that younger patients who have glioblastomas that have evolved from a low-grade neoplasm are more likely to respond to chemotherapy than an older individual with a rapid presentation of a glioblastoma, and likely genetic alterations, possibly related to p53, play a crucial role here. Recently, the Children's Cancer Group has reported an inverse association between survival and overexpression of p53 in children with a variety of primary brain tumors, suggesting that this gene plays a critical role in pediatric brain tumors as well.[73]

In addition to these genetic alterations, nearly all glioblastomas suffer inactivation of the cell-cycle control pathway that includes p16, cyclin-dependent kinase 4 (cdk4), and the retinoblastoma protein (pRb).[74,75] Tumors with deletion of the p16 gene have proliferative indices that are twice those of other glioblastomas.[76] Perhaps proliferation rates influence the response of gliomas to cytotoxic drugs and may influence why some gliomas are more sensitive to chemotherapy than others. The response of gliomas to chemotherapy is likely a predictable phenomenon governed by specific molecular alterations. Understanding these alterations is an urgent issue in neuro-oncology because it will help the clinician provide appropriate therapy to patients with gliomas. Patients with chemosensitive gliomas should receive chemotherapy, as they will likely respond and derive survival benefit from the treatment. It is in this subset of patients that questions surrounding the optimal timing of chemotherapy, doses, schedules, and methods of delivery should be tested. Patients who have tumors that are predictably resistant to available chemotherapies should be spared the toxicity of these drugs. These patients should receive novel therapies such as antiangiogenic agents and signal transduction inhibitors early on. Clearly, a detailed understanding of the molecular genetic alterations that define subsets of gliomas has the potential to tailor therapy in a way that maximizes benefit, and this goal should become a primary focus in neuro-oncology.

■ The Main Points

- The role of chemotherapy in the management of high-grade astrocytic neoplasms, including glioblastoma multiforme, remains poorly defined. Clearly, current chemotherapeutic agents have very limited activity against these tumors.
- There is a subset of patients with gliomas responsive to chemotherapy that significantly benefits from the treatment. Responsive tumors are often oligodendroglial in lineage, but other subsets of glial tumors, including some cases classified histologically as anaplastic astrocytoma and glioblastoma multiforme, may also respond to chemotherapy.
- The challenge is identifying these chemosensitive astrocytic tumors. Molecular genetics is likely to play a prominent role in this effort.
- At present, because the benefit of adjuvant chemotherapy for patients with high-grade astrocytic tumors is so small, it cannot be recommended as part of standard initial therapy for all patients. Patients who may benefit from adjuvant or early chemotherapy include those who conserve a high level of function and harbor tumors with the following characteristics: previously low-grade, oligodendroglial features, favorable genetics such as 1p and 19q loss of heterozygosity, and minimal postoperative residual disease.

- For most patients with high-grade astrocytic neoplasms, delaying chemotherapy until there is evidence of disease progression remains a reasonable strategy. Current therapies for most high-grade gliomas remain inadequate, and novel and more effective treatments are required to achieve meaningful improvement in patient survival.

■ References

1. Louis DN, Gusella JF. A tiger behind many doors: multiple genetic pathways to malignant glioma. *Trends Genet* 1995;11:412–415.
2. Scott J, Rewcastle N, Brasher P, et al. Which glioblastoma multiforme patient will become a long-term survivor? A population-based study. *Ann Neurol* 1999;46:183–188.
3. Mason W, Lewis DN, Cairncross JG. Chemosensitive gliomas in adults? Which ones and why? *J Clin Oncol* 1997;15:3423–3426.
4. Prados M, Scott C, Curran WJ, et al. Procarbazine, lomustine, and vincristine (PCV) chemotherapy for anaplastic astrocytoma: a retrospective review of Radiation Therapy Oncology Group protocols comparing survival with carmustine or PCV adjuvant chemotherapy. *J Clin Oncol* 1999;17:3389–3395.
5. Cairncross G, Macdonald D, Ludwin S, Lee D, Cascino T, Buckner J, Fulton D, Dropcho E, Stewart D, Schold C Jr, et al. Chemotherapy for anaplastic oligodendroglioma. *J Clin Oncol* 1994;12:2013–2021.
6. Yung A, et al. Randomized trial of temodal (TEM) vs procarbazine (PCB) in glioblastoma multiforme (GBM) at first relapse. *Proc Am Soc Clin Oncol* 1999;18:139A.
7. Yung W. Temozolomide in malignant glioma. *Semin Oncol* 2000;27:27–34.
8. Greenlee R, Murray T, Bolden S, et al. Cancer statistics, 2000. *CA Cancer J Clin* 2000;50:7–33.
9. Lesser GJ, Grossman S. The chemotherapy of high-grade astrocytomas. *Semin Oncol* 1994;21:220–235.
10. Fine H. The basis for current recommendations for malignant gliomas. *J Neurooncol* 1994;20:111–120.

11. Devaux BC, O'Fallon JR, Kelly P. Resection, biopsy, and survival in malignant glial neoplasms: a retrospective study of clinical parameters, therapy, and outcome. *J Neurosurg* 1993;78:267–275.

12. Walker M, Alexander E, Hunt W, et al. Evaluation of BCNU and/or radiotherapy in the treatment of anaplastic gliomas. *J Neurosurg* 1978;49:333–343.

13. Walker M, Green S, Byar D, et al. Randomized comparison of radiotherapy and nitrosoureas for the treatment of malignant glioma after surgery. *N Engl J Med* 1980;303:1323–1329.

14. Chang C, Horton J, Schoenfeld D, et al. Comparison of postoperative radiotherapy and combined postoperative radiotherapy and chemotherapy in the multidisciplinary management of malignant gliomas. *Cancer* 1983;52:997–1007.

15. Green SB, Byar DP, Walker MD, et al. Comparisons of carmustine, procarbazine, and high-dose methylprednisolone as additions to surgery and radiotherapy for the treatment of malignant glioma after surgery. *Cancer Treat Rep* 1983;67:121–132.

16. Levin VA, Wara WM, Davis RL, Vestnys P, Resser KJ, Yatsko K, Nutik S, Gutin PH, Wilson CB. Phase III comparison of BCNU and the combination of procarbazine, CCNU, and vincristine administered after radiotherapy with hydroxyurea for malignant gliomas. *J Neurosurg* 1985;63:218–223.

17. Shapiro W, Green S, Burger P, et al. Randomized trial of three chemotherapy regimens and two radiotherapy regimens in postoperative treatment of malignant glioma. *J Neurosurg* 1989;71:1–9.

18. Medical Research Council Brain Tumour Working Party. Randomized trial of procarbazine, lomustine, and vincristine in the adjuvant treatment of high-grade astrocytoma: a Medical Research Council trial. *J Clin Oncol* 2001;19:509–518.

19. Levin VA, Silver P, Hannigan J, et al. Superiority of post-radiotherapy adjuvant chemotherapy with CCNU, procarbazine, and vincristine (PCV) over BCNU for anaplastic gliomas: NCOG 6G61 final report. *Int J Radiat Oncol Biol Phys* 1990;18:321–324.

20. Galanis E, Buckner J. Chemotherapy for high-grade gliomas. *Br J Cancer* 2000;82:1371–1380.

21. DeAngelis L, Burger P, Green S, et al. Adjuvant chemotherapy for malignant glioma: who benefits? *Ann Neurol* 1996;40:491–492.

22. Shapiro WR, Green SB, Burger PC, et al. A randomized comparison of intraarterial versus intravenous BCNU, with or without intravenous 5-fluorouracil, for newly diagnosed patients with malignant gliomas. *J Neurosurg* 1992;76:772.

23. Macdonald DR. Temozolomide for recurrent high-grade glioma. *Semin Oncol* 2001;28:3–12.

24. Stupp R, Dietrich P-Y, Kralijevic SO, et al. Promising survival for patients with newly diagnosed glioblastoma multiforme treated with concomitant radiation plus temozolomide followed by adjuvant temozolomide. *J Clin Oncol* 2002;20:1375–1382.

25. Grossman SA, Wharam M, Sheidler V, et al. Phase II study of continuous infusion carmustine and cisplatin followed by cranial irradiation in adults with newly diagnosed high-grade astrocytoma. *J Clin Oncol* 1997;15:2596–2603.

26. Fine HA, Dear KBJ, Loeffler JS, et al. Meta-analysis of radiation therapy with and without adjuvant chemotherapy for malignant gliomas in adults. *Cancer* 1993;71:2585–2597.

27. Chandler KL, Prados MD, Malec M, Wilson CB. Long-term survival in patients with glioblastoma multiforme. *Neurosurgery* 1993;32:716–720.

28. Grant R, Liang B, Page M, et al. Age influences chemotherapy response in astrocytomas. *Neurology* 1995;45:929–933.

29. Winger M, Macdonald D, Cairncross J. Supratentorial anaplastic gliomas in adults: the prognostic importance of extent of resection and prior low-grade glioma. *J Neurosurg* 1989;71:487–493.

30. Wong E, Hess K, Gleason M, et al. Outcomes and prognostic factors in recurrent glioma patients enrolled onto phase II clinical trials. *J Clin Oncol* 1999;17:2572–2578.

31. Rosenblum ML, Reynolds JAF, Smith KA, et al. Chloroethyl-cyclohexyl-nitrosourea (CCNU) in the treatment of malignant brain tumors. *J Neurosurg* 1973;39:306–314.

32. Wilson CB, Gutin PH, Boldrey EB, et al. Single-agent chemotherapy of brain tumors: a 5-year review. *Arch Neurol* 1976;33:739–744.

33. Newton HB, Junck L, Bromberg J, Page MA, Greenberg HS. Procarbazine chemotherapy in the treatment of recurrent malignant astrocytomas after radiation and nitrosourea failure. *Neurology* 1990;40:1743–1746.

34. Gutin P, Wilson C, Kumar A. Phase II study of procarbazine, CCNU and vincristine combination chemotherapy in the treatment of malignant brain tumors. *Cancer* 1975;32:1398–1404.

35. Friedman H, Petros W, Friedman A, et al. Irinotecan therapy in adults with recurrent or progressive malignant glioma. *J Clin Oncol* 1999;17:1516–1525.

36. Yung WK, Mechtler L, Gleason MJ. Intravenous carboplatin for recurrent malignant glioma: a phase II study. *J Clin Oncol* 1991;9:860–864.

37. Smith JS, Perry A, Borell TJ, Lee HK, et al. Alterations of chromosome arms 1p and 19q as predictors of survival in oligodendrogliomas, astrocytomas, and mixed oligoastrocytomas. *J Clin Oncol* 2000;18: 636–645.

38. Yung WKA, Albright RE, Olson J, et al. A phase II study of temozolomide versus procarbazine in patients with glioblastoma multiforme at first relapse. *Br J Cancer* 2000;85:588–593.

39. Brandes AA, Ermani M, Pasetto L, Amista P, et al. Temozolomide in high grade gliomas at second relapse: a phase II study (Abstract 646). *Proc Am Soc Clin Oncol* 2000.

40. Buckner JC, Brown L, Cascino T. Phase II evaluation of infusional etoposide and cisplatin in patients with recurrent astrocytoma. *J Neurooncol* 1990;9:349–354.

41. Rodriguez LA, Prados M, Silver P. Reevaluation of procarbazine for the treatment of recurrent malignant central nervous system tumors. *Cancer* 1989;64: 2420–2423.

42. Warnick RE, Prados MD, Mack EE, et al. A phase II study of intravenous carboplatin for the treatment of recurrent gliomas. *J Neurooncol* 1994;19:69–74.

43. Yung WKA, Prados MD, Yaya-Tur P, Rosenfeld SS, Brada M, Friedman HS, et al. Multicenter phase II trial of temozolomide in patients with anaplastic astrocytoma or anaplastic oligoastrocytoma at first relapse. *J Clin Oncol* 1999;17:2762–2771.

44. Newlands ES, Stevens MFG, Wedge S, et al. Temozolomide: a review of its discovery, chemical properties, preclinical development and clinical trials. *Cancer Treat* 1997;23:35–61.

45. Newlands ES, Blackledge GRP, Slack JA, et al. The Charing Cross Hospital experience with temozolomide in patients with gliomas. *Eur J Cancer* 1996;32A: 2236–2241.

46. Brem H, Piantadosi S, Burger P, Walker M, Selker R, Vick NA, Black K, Sisti M, Brem S, Mohr G, et al. Placebo-controlled trial of safety and efficacy of intraoperative controlled delivery by biodegradable polymers of chemotherapy for recurrent gliomas. *Lancet* 1995;345:1008–1012.

47. Cairncross JG, Macdonald DR. Successful chemotherapy for recurrent malignant oligodendroglioma. *Ann Neurol* 1988;23:360–364.

48. Macdonald DR, Gaspar L, Cairncross J. Successful chemotherapy for newly diagnosed aggressive oligodendroglioma. *Ann Neurol* 1990;27:573–574.

49. Brown M, Cairncross J, Vick N, et al. Differential response of recurrent oligodendrogliomas versus astrocytomas to intravenous melphalan. *Neurosurgery* 1990;40:397–398.

50. Cairncross G, Swinnen L, Stiff P, Rosenfeld S, Vaughan W, Paleologos N, et al. High-dose thiotepa with hematopoietic reconstitution (deferring radiation) for newly diagnosed aggressive oligodendroglioma (Abstract 1386). *Proc Am Soc Clin Oncol* 1997;16:388a.

51. Chamberlain M, Kormanik P. Salvage chemotherapy with paclitaxel for recurrent oligodendrogliomas. *J Clin Oncol* 1997;15:3427–3432.

52. Chinot O-L, Honore S, Dufour H, et al. Safety and efficacy of temozolomide in patients with recurrent anaplastic oligodendroglioma after standard radiotherapy and chemotherapy. *J Clin Oncol* 2001;19: 2449–2455.

53. Peterson K, Paleologos N, Forsyth P, et al. Salvage chemotherapy for oligodendroglioma. *J Neurosurg* 1996;85:597–601.

54. Glass J, Hochberg FH, Gruber ML, et al. The treatment of oligodendrogliomas and mixed oligodendroglioma-astrocytomas with PCV chemotherapy. *J Neurosurg* 1992;76:741–745.

55. Kyritsis A, Yung W, Bruner J, Gleason M, Levin V. The treatment of anaplastic oligodendrogliomas and mixed gliomas. *Neurosurgery* 1993;32:365–371.

56. Mason WP, Krol GS, DeAngelis LM. Low-grade oligodendroglioma responds to chemotherapy. *Neurology* 1996;46:203–207.

57. Paleologos N, Macdonald D, Vick N, Cairncross J. Neoadjuvant procarbazine, CCNU, and vincristine for anaplastic and aggressive oligodendroglioma. *Neurology* 1999;53:1141–1143.

58. Cairncross JG, Ueki K, Zlatescu MC, Lisle DK, Finkelstein DM, Hammond RR, Silver JS, Stark PC. Specific genetic predictors of chemotherapeutic response and survival in patients with anaplastic oligodendrogliomas. *J Natl Cancer Inst* 1998;90: 1473–1479.

59. Ino Y, Betensky R, Zlatescu M, et al. Molecular subtypes of anaplastic oligodendroglioma: implications for patient management at diagnosis. *Clin Cancer Res* 2001;7:839–845.

60. Grant R, Liang BC, Slattery J, et al. Chemotherapy response criteria in malignant glioma. *Neurology* 1997;48:1336–1340.

61. Postma T, van Groeningen C, Witjes R, et al. Neurotoxicity of combination chemotherapy with procarbazine, CCNU and vincristine (PCV) for recurrent glioma. *J Neurooncol* 1998;38:69–75.

62. Fortin D, Cairncross GJ, Hammond RR. Oligodendroglioma: an appraisal of recent data pertaining to diagnosis and treatment. *Neurosurgery* 1999;45:1279–1291.

63. Reifenberger J, Reifenberger G, Liu L, et al. Molecular genetic analysis of oligodendroglial tumors shows preferential allelic deletions on 19q and 1p. *Am J Pathol* 1994;145:1175–1190.

64. von Deimling A, Louis D, von Ammon K, et al. Evidence for a tumor suppressor gene on chromosome 19q with human astrocytomas, oligodendrogliomas and mixed gliomas. *Cancer Res* 1992;52:4277–4279.

65. Kraus J, Koopmann J, Kaskel P, et al. Shared allelic losses on chromosomes 1p and 19q suggest a common origin of oligodendroglioma and oligoastrocytoma. *J Neuropathol Exp Neurol* 1995;54:91–95.

66. Maintz D, Feidler K, Koopman J, et al. Molecular genetic evidence for subsets of oligoastrocytomas. *J Neuropathol Exp Neurol* 1997;56:1098–1104.

67. Jeremic B, Grujicic D, Jevremovic S, et al. Carboplatin and etoposide chemotherapy regimen for recurrent malignant glioma: a phase II study. *J Clin Oncol* 1992;10:1074–1077.

68. Louis D. A molecular genetic model of astrocytoma histopathology. *Brain Pathol* 1997;7:755–764.

69. Watanabe K, Tachibana O, Sato K, et al. Overexpression of the EGF receptor and p53 mutations are mutually exclusive in the evolution of primary and secondary glioblastomas. *Brain Pathol* 1996;6:217–223.

70. Louis D, von Deimling A, Chung R, et al. Comparative study of p53 gene and protein alterations in human astrocytomas. *J Neuropathol Exp Neurol* 1993;52:31–38.

71. Louis DN. The p53 gene and protein in human brain tumors. *J Neuropathol Exp Neurol* 1994;53:11–21.

72. Reifenberger J, Ring C, Gies U, et al. Analysis of p53 mutation and epidermal growth factor receptor amplification in recurrent gliomas with malignant progression. *J Neuropathol Exp Neurol* 1996;55:822–831.

73. Pollack IF, Finkelstein SD, Woods J, et al. Expression of p53 and prognosis in children with malignant gliomas. *N Engl J Med* 2002;346:420–427.

74. He J, Olson JJ, James CD. Lack of p16^{INK4} or retinoblastoma protein (pRb), or amplification-associated overexpression of cdk4 is observed in distinct subsets of malignant glial tumors and cell lines. *Cancer Res* 1995;55:4833–4838.

75. Ueki K, Ono Y, Henson J, et al. CDKN2/p16 or RB alterations occur in the majority of glioblastomas and are inversely correlated. *Cancer Res* 1996;56:150–153.

76. Ono Y, Tamiya T, Ichikawa T, et al. Malignant astrocytomas with homozygous CDKN2/p16 gene deletions have higher Ki-67 proliferation indices. *J Neuropathol Exp Neurol* 1996;55:1026–1031.

Chapter 18
Acute Poisoning from Tropical Fish

Carmen D. Cirstea, Robert G. Feldman*, and Daniel S. Sax

Humans may eat infected fish at the end of the food chain cascade, which begins with smaller fish that contain the toxin of the dinoflagellate *Gambierdiscus toxicus*. Consuming large predatory fish from tropical reef ecosystems might be not only a delightful gastronomic experience but sometimes also a hazardous one. Among these prized gourmet species are mackerel, barracuda, red snapper, coral trout, grouper, amberjack and moray eels[1] (Figure 18-1). Consumption of any of the 400 species of tropical reef fish has been implicated in causing ciguatera poisoning.[2] Among these species, Barracuda is one of the most ciguatoxic fish, causing it to be banned from sale in Puerto Rico.[2] Rare cases have been reported after the ingestion of temperate fish, including farm-raised salmon, which presumably acquired the toxin from eating contaminated food.[3] However, in general, ciguatera toxic illness from nontropical fish is extremely rare. Ciguatera poisoning has almost never been associated with cold-water fish.[3,4]

Ciguatera intoxication is not an infectious disease and there is no specific therapy. Ciguatoxins are among the most potent biological toxins known. This dramatic intoxication may be encountered in nontropical countries around the world given the extensive international commerce in exotic frozen fish, which is making it a global health problem and a real challenge for the clinician.[1] The incidence of ciguatera toxin illness is also expected to increase in association with global

warming and widespread bleaching and death of coral.[4] Increased awareness of marine biotoxins and their peculiar neurotropic effects is needed in arriving at an early diagnosis. This in turn will ensure an earlier treatment and a shorter convalescence. Consequently the early identification of this intoxication in sentinel cases has the potential to reduce the number of subsequent cases in cluster outbreaks.[1]

Maintaining a high degree of suspicion about the role of environmental and often occupational neurotoxins in certain neurological illnesses is very important. For this reason, this fascinating and mysterious subject is included in this monograph.

■ The Patient

A 79-year-old man was seen in the emergency room at Boston Medical Center 2 weeks after vacationing in St. Martin, West Indies. He complained of nausea, vomiting, diarrhea, myalgias, fever, chills, generalized weakness, and prominent sensory disturbances. Distressing limb paresthesias, sensation of hot/cold reversal, perioral numbness, and unpleasant taste to all foods were additionally mentioned.

The history revealed that the patient initially developed these symptoms while in St. Martin 3 days after having eaten red snapper fish at a local restaurant. The patient's complaints caused a local physician to diagnose dengue fever. Quinine was

---

*Deceased.

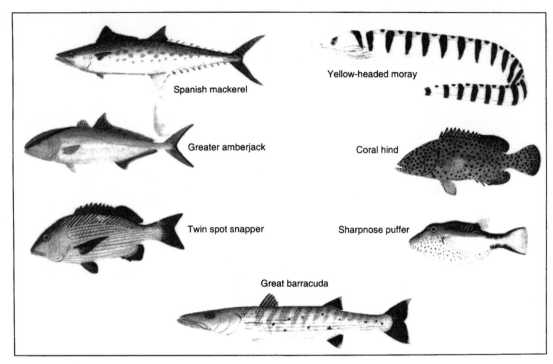

Figure 18-1. Examples of neurotoxic tropical fish. (From Lieske E, Myers R, *Coral Reef Fishes from the Caribbean, Indian Ocean and Pacific Ocean Including the Red Sea.* Princeton, NJ, Princeton University Press, 1996. Reprinted with permission of Princeton University Press.)

prescribed. After increasing the dose of quinine, the patient developed severe nausea, tinnitus, decreased hearing, dizziness, and confusion.

He was admitted to the medical intensive care unit with a diagnosis of probable quinine toxicity. On general medical examination he was an elderly, tired-looking man in mild respiratory distress. His temperature was 99.4°F, blood pressure 133/75 mmHg, pulse 120/minute, and respiratory rate 18/minute. Examination of the cardiovascular and respiratory systems showed jugular venous distension, diffuse, coarse rales bilaterally, and irregularly irregular rhythm with a 1/6 holosystolic murmur.

Neurological examination revealed bilateral facial palsy with decreased eye blink frequency and flattened facial expression. The gag reflex was decreased. Over the entire body, including the face, cutaneous sensation of light touch was intact, but pinprick was reduced inconsistently with unpleasant sensations consistent with hyperpathia. Sensory testing showed impaired vibration and joint position sense in both legs. Tendon reflexes were symmetric

and brisk. Mild end point tremor was noted on finger-to-nose to finger testing. The patient was able to take a few steps with slightly broad base, but he could not be tested further because of the sensation of imminent fecal release he experienced when standing.

Laboratory investigations yielded an increased quinine level of 10.6 μmol/L. Normal tests included complete blood count, BUN and creatinine, ANA screen, plasma zinc level, haptoglobin, transferrin, TSH, B_{12}, folate, CK, and RPR. Stool studies were negative for ova and parasites, leukocytes, *Salmonella, Shigella, Campylobacter jejuni*, and *Yersinia*. Serum antibody titers were negative for *Mycoplasma, Legionella*, and influenza A and B.

Lumbar puncture was performed and the CSF analysis was normal including protein, glucose, and IgG index. Oligoclonal bands and myelin basic protein were absent; routine microbiology, VDRL, and RPR were negative. MRI of the brain, and cervical, thoracic, and lumbar spine was normal. SPECT scan of the head was negative. EEG was normal.

However, somatosensory evoked potentials of the median nerves and the posterior tibial nerves were abnormal bilaterally. Nerve conduction studies revealed reduced right sural sensory potential amplitude and slowed nerve conduction velocity. Right peroneal distal motor latency was prolonged (7.1 msec). Motor conduction in the right leg was slowed. The evoked amplitude was markedly reduced at all levels and the F-wave response was prolonged. An absent right posterior tibial H-reflex latency was found. The F-wave response was prolonged. The left ulnar nerve distal motor latency was 3.1 msec. Electromyography showed acute partial denervation in the right distal lower extremity muscles. The electrophysiological studies of the peripheral nerves were interpreted as showing evidence of a mixed sensory-motor predominantly demyelinating peripheral neuropathy affecting the lower limb more than the upper limb. These neurophysiological findings, persistence of sensory symptoms, and the history of a red snapper fish meal suggested a marine neurotoxin-induced disorder. The features in this case indicated ciguatera fish poisoning (Table 18-1).

The hospitalization course was complicated by pulmonary edema and aspiration pneumonia requiring intubation. The patient improved slowly with aggressive physical therapy and eventually was able to ambulate with a walker.

On outpatient follow-up examination several weeks after discharge, the patient had persistent burning and itching sensation in his feet, and numbness and tingling in his hands, associated with mild tremulousness and weakness. Also he complained of perineal numbness and impotence. He noticed that at times he felt warm and then cold. The facial diplegia gradually improved. The patient had bothersome urinary retention requiring straight catheterization for 2 months but resolving eventually.

One year later the patient developed cardiac failure after a laparoscopic cholecystectomy. At that time he again noticed that food tasted bad to him and he experienced the same symptoms of unpleasant dysesthesias and sensation of hot/cold reversal that he had experienced when he returned from St. Martin. Approximately 3 years later he had a second electrophysiological study done which continued to show evidence of chronic sensorimotor neuropathy of axonal type.

■ The Problem

- How is a diagnosis of a marine neurotoxin-induced illness made, given the fact that many of the symptoms are similar to other neurological conditions?
- Are there therapies that reduce severity or duration of symptoms?
- What is the long-term outcome?

■ The Evidence

The Diagnostic Challenge and Mimicking Illnesses

A diagnosis of ciguatera toxin illness was made in our patient based on the history of tropical fish intake in an endemic area in conjunction with characteristic clinical manifestations. The temporal progression of symptoms was that of an acute process. Exposure to the toxin was temporally related to the onset of the clinical symptoms. The patient experienced initially gastrointestinal symptoms (nausea, vomiting, diarrhea) soon after a tropical fish meal, then generalized weakness and bothersome paresthesias in the feet and perioral numbness followed by painful and burning sensations triggered by cold stimuli. The decreased muscle tone and hypoactive reflexes suggested neuromuscular disease. A mixed sensorimotor neuropathy was noted on electrophysiological studies.

The differential diagnostic considerations in a case such as ours with acute onset of neuropathy include Guillain-Barré syndrome, metallic toxic neuropathies (e.g., arsenic, lead, thallium), Lyme disease, botulism, transverse myelitis, and other poisonings by marine biotoxins (e.g., puffer fish, shellfish, and other dinoflagellate organisms).

Many features of the Guillain-Barré syndrome were present in our patient. The antecedent event could have been the gastrointestinal illness, which was followed by progressive weakness in both legs and arms over days to weeks, cranial nerve involvement with facial palsy, and autonomic dysfunction. The deep tendon reflexes, which were initially brisk, became hypoactive over days. What was unusual was that the sensory symptoms and signs

Table 18-1. Characteristic Features of Neurotoxins Present in Fish

Neurotoxin	Clinical Findings	Mechanism of Action	Clinical Management	Prognosis
Tetrodotoxin Found in puffer fish, porcupine fish, sunfish, japanese ivory shell, trumpet shell	Gastroenteritis, paresthesias, ataxia, muscle weakness, sweating, hypersalivation, cardiac arrhythmias, hypotension, occurring within 30 min to 1 hour after exposure, followed by persistent sensory and motor neuropathy	Reversible disruption of neurotransmission by blocking voltage-gated sodium channels in myelinated and unmyelinated peripheral nerves	Supportive measures, syrup of ipecac or endoscopic removal of contaminated fish; mechanical ventilation with respiratory failure IV edrophonium or IM neostigmine	Patients who survive acute illness usually recover within 4 to 7 days; no persistent clinical manifestations have been reported
Saxitoxin/Brevetoxin (Paralytic shellfish poisoning) Found in bivalve shellfish, muscles, clams, scallops	Nausea, vomiting, abdominal cramping, headache, dizziness, dysarthria, ataxia, muscle weakness, respiratory paralysis	Blockage of voltage-gated sodium channels by binding to sodium channel receptors	Supportive measures; syrup of ipecac, fluids, electrolytes	Recovery is typically complete, with no long-term sequelae
Ciguatoxin Found in large, bottom-dwelling reef fish, such as barracuda, sturgeon, grouper, sea bass, red snapper	Muscle cramps, pain, weakness, ataxia, tremor, hypotension, bradycardia, paresthesias, dysesthesias, respiratory distress seizures	Abnormal prolongation of sodium channels, with increase in membrane excitability	Syrup of ipecac, endoscopic removal of fish, IV mannitol, mechanical ventilation with respiratory failure	Neuropathy recovers within months Symptoms may recur during periods of acute stress, months to years after exposure
Stonustoxin Found in stonefish from South Pacific	Pain, erythema, swelling around the site of spine stab; hypotension is prominent; cardiac arrhythmias, paresthesias, muscle weakness, paralysis, neuropathy, seizures, respiratory failure	Interference with nitric oxide pathway; increases release of acetylcholine; impairs cholinergic transmission	IM antivenom; adrenaline for hypersensitive reactions to antivenom	Neurological symptoms may persist for several weeks but typically resolve spontaneously within several days after cessation of exposure

Modified from Feldman RG. Biological toxins and the nervous system. In Johnson RT, Griffin JW, McArthur JC, eds. *Current Therapy in Neurologic Disease*. Philadelphia, Mosby, 2002: 343–353.[5]

were prominent in the clinical picture, whereas in the typical GBS these are mild and transient and there is often no fever by the time neurological symptoms appear. Also, loss of reflexes from one day to the next is almost diagnostic of Guillain-Barré syndrome, and this was not seen in our case.

The evolution of neurological signs over a period of hours to days after a gastrointestinal illness is also suggestive of botulism. Botulism develops after consumption of contaminated food, with gastrointestinal symptoms, mainly constipation, and with prominent ophthalmoparesis and bulbar weakness. The absence of prominent dryness of mouth and throat and constipation, which are typical of the early stage of botulism, and the presence of fever, argue clinically against the diagnosis. Nerve conduction studies reveal in these cases low-amplitude compound muscle potentials. High-frequency repetitive nerve stimulation or maximal voluntary contraction leads to an incremental response that is typical for presynaptic neuromuscular transmission defect, and is quite different from the results found in our patient.

There were other considerations. Spinal cord compression or postinfectious transverse myelitis may present a diagnostic challenge before upper motor neuron signs develop and before electrodiagnostic and CSF studies are available. The early urinary and sensory abnormalities in our patient called for an MRI of the spine, even though there was no sharply demarcated sensory level on examination. Sensorimotor neuropathies with axonal and demyelinating features may also be paraneoplastic neuropathies, which often precede the diagnosis of tumor by years and are immunologically mediated. This diagnosis is made when none of the following etiologies are found: metabolic or nutritional deficits, infiltration of nerves or spinal roots by the tumor, or a side effect of chemotherapy. In our patient, the lack of weight loss and other signs of malignancy argued against this diagnosis.

Any acute cranial nerve deficit and perioral numbness demands a consideration of diseases in the brainstem, especially infarction from occlusion of the basilar artery in an elderly patient. This alternative was excluded by MRI of the brain in our patient.

Other neuropathic causes of rapidly progressive generalized weakness, such as hypophosphatemic neuropathy, severe renal failure, Lyme disease, and diphtheria, were incompatible with the history and clinical features of this case.

Demographics of Ciguatera Fish Poisoning

Ciguatera fish intoxication is the most common tropical fish food poisoning. About 25,000 cases are reported annually worldwide, with the highest rates occurring in endemic tropical and subtropical areas between 35°N latitude and 35°S latitude, including the Caribbean Sea and the South Pacific Ocean[6,7] where the incidence may approach 10 percent of the population annually.[1] Cases of ciguatera toxicity are found in temperate regions because of the increasing number of tourists. Fish exportation from these areas may bring contaminated fish to unlikely locales. Isolated outbreaks have also been reported in temperate countries (e.g., the United States, Canada, Europe). Most cases in the United States occur in Hawaii and in southeastern Florida, with occasional cases reported from Texas, California, and the inland states.[8] Clinical observations on ciguatera toxin illness between 1964 and 1977 on 3009 patients from South Pacific islands revealed a variation in symptoms according to the locale.[9] Neurological symptoms predominate in the Pacific Ocean, while in the Caribbean Sea gastrointestinal symptoms dominate the clinical picture, suggesting that different ciguatoxins may be present in Pacific and Caribbean waters.[10] Also, repeated poisonings with this toxin appeared to result in a clinically more severe illness compared with the symptoms expressed upon a single or initial encounter.[9]

Many ciguatera toxin cases are not reported and increased awareness of this disease is needed. It is estimated that 50 million people from developed nations travel to tropical countries each year, and more than 50 percent of individuals will have health problems as the result of travel.[11] Consequently, primary care providers and neurologists practicing in developed countries diagnose and treat patients with tropical diseases as a result of travel and returning tourists. For us, it should always be kept in mind that the travel history is a key element in every patient who is evaluated for seemingly common and otherwise unexplained neurological symptoms.[11]

The Marine Toxin

The name ciguatera comes from an eighteenth-century Portuguese biologist's description of symptoms following ingestion of *cigua* (the Spanish name for turban fish).[6] The ingested fish is not poisonous unless it is infected by dinoflagellates (*Gambierdiscus toxicus*). Other dinoflagellates are known to produce neurotoxic effects. Among them, *Pfiesteria* is a newly described marine toxin under intense current scientific scrutiny.[12] A number of toxins are produced by these dinoflagellates, which are unicellular algae-like organisms growing on and around coral reefs.[6] They had been isolated previously in the Gambier Islands in French Polynesia from toxic biodetritus covering dead corals.[13] The direct and reproducible relationship between the number of *G. toxicus* cells and the toxin concentration in the biodetritus, and the capacity of the *G. toxicus* cultured cells to produce ciguatera toxin complex, confirmed the dinoflagellate as the responsible agent.[13]

"Ciguatoxin" is a complex of at least three chemically distinct toxins: ciguatoxin, maitotoxin, and scaritoxin.[14] An interesting fact is that uninfected fish from one part of an island can be harmless while fish from the other side of a coral reef can be deadly. Only certain genetic strains of *G. toxicus* are toxic.[4] The presence of algae blooms and consequently of the toxic fish in subtropical and tropical waters is sporadic, patchy, and unpredictable. The environmental triggers for blooms of *G. toxicus* are uncertain.[10] This makes it impossible to determine whether a fish, caught from a specific area at a specific time, may be safe to eat or not without the use of scientific testing.[8]

These potent ciguateric neurotoxins are heat-stable, lipid-soluble polyethers that accumulate through the food chain, as mentioned earlier. Herbivorous fish eat *G. toxicus,* a marine dinoflagellate living in association with microalgae on the dead coral or in the biodetritus on the sea floor, and the toxin concentrates in viscera and flesh. Larger carnivorous fish consume the herbivorous fish and further concentrate the toxins, which appear to be harmless to the fish themselves.[4,15] There are more than 20 precursor gambiertoxins and ciguatoxins identified in *G. toxicus* and in herbivorous and carnivorous fish.[4]

The toxins become more polar as they undergo oxidative metabolism and pass up the food chain (Figure 18-2). The more oxidized forms are up to 10-fold more toxic than the ciguatoxins produced by *G. toxicus.*[10] The ciguatoxin P-CTX-1 found in carnivorous fish in the Pacific Ocean causes ciguatera toxicity at levels of 0.1 µg/kg in the flesh of fish.[10] The main Caribbean ciguatoxin C-CTX-1 is less polar and 10-fold less toxic than P-CTX-1.[10]

Structural elucidation of the toxin requires first its isolation, which has proven extremely difficult because of its high potency (LD_{50}, 0.45 µg/kg),[14] low concentration in toxic fish, and toxin instability during purification.[16]

Clinical Manifestations

Ciguatera fish poisoning is suspected in patients who present with an acute characteristic combination of gastrointestinal, cardiovascular, and neurological symptoms occurring after ingestion of

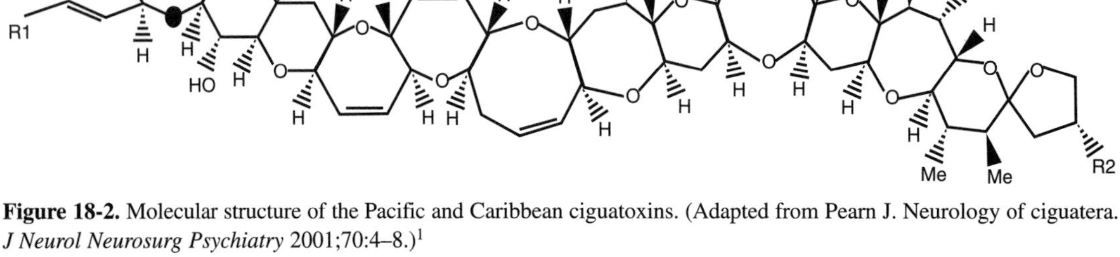

Figure 18-2. Molecular structure of the Pacific and Caribbean ciguatoxins. (Adapted from Pearn J. Neurology of ciguatera. *J Neurol Neurosurg Psychiatry* 2001;70:4–8.)[1]

Table 18-2. Symptoms of Acute Ciguatera Intoxication

Gastrointestinal symptoms
  Nausea, vomiting, diarrhea, abdominal pain
Cardiovascular symptoms
  Bradycardia
  Hypotension
Neurological symptoms
  Paresthesias of extremities and circumoral
  Dysesthesias
  Hot/cold temperature sensation reversal
  Weakness
  Cerebellar signs, tremor
Other constitutional symptoms
  Arthralgias, myalgias
  Dental pain, sensation of loose teeth
  Blurred vision, headache
  Chills, diaphoresis

---

tropical fish (Table 18-2). Gastrointestinal symptoms are often the first to appear, usually within the first 12 hours after eating contaminated fish.[17] Vomiting and diarrhea may be severe enough to cause serious dehydration, though gastrointestinal symptoms usually last only 1 or 2 days.[17] Fever is present only rarely.[18] Cardiovascular symptoms include bradycardia, cardiac arrhythmias, hypotension, and abnormalities of T wave on the electrocardiogram. Blood pressure may fall significantly even to shock levels[17] and later may change to tachycardia and hypertension.[18] Cardiovascular symptoms may persist for several weeks, but usually resolve in 48 hours.[18] Neurological effects may appear up to 3 days after ingestion of contaminated fish and comprise a bizarre constellation of symptoms including perception of perioral numbness and tingling sensation, painful or loose teeth, itching which might increase with exposure to cold, paresthesias,[6] hyperesthesia, cranial nerve palsies, metallic taste, ataxia, vertigo, tremors, muscle weakness, arthralgia, and myalgia.[18] A common complaint is extreme muscle weakness.[18] Reversal of the perception of sensation of hot and cold temperatures is often encountered.[18] This peculiar feature of "cold reversal," which means that cold stimuli are being felt as painful and hot, is considered almost pathognomonic for ciguatera intoxication.[19] The basis of this interesting paradoxical reversal of temperature perception commonly described in ciguatera poisoning was linked to an exaggerated and intense nerve depolarization occurring in peripheral small A-delta myelinated and, in particular, C-polymodal nociceptive fibers.[20]

Both peripheral and central nervous systems are affected. Autonomic dysfunction leads to orthostatic hypotension, bradycardia, hypersalivation, laryngeal spasm, mydriasis, or miosis.[1] We presume that in our patient urinary and fecal abnormalities were autonomic manifestations of his neuropathy. Fatalities related to ciguatera toxin illness may be due to cardiovascular collapse or respiratory failure.[18] The fatality rate is low possibly because fish rarely accumulate levels of ciguatoxin sufficient to be lethal for humans at a single meal.[10] The neurological symptoms typically persist for a few days to a few weeks and in 20 percent of cases for months, with fewer than 2 percent persisting for years.[21] Our case illustrates the persistence of neurological symptoms that occurs in some patients, with exacerbations usually triggered by a later intercurrent illness. Victims of ciguatera intoxication may experience sensitization with recurrence of the typical symptoms even years after the first attack, usually following the ingestion of canned fish, meat, chicken, eggs, alcohol, and especially nontoxic reef fish.[17]

The long-term consequences of ciguatera toxin illness have been recognized. More than half of the patients intoxicated with Caribbean ciguatoxins had chronic dysesthesias with a median duration exceeding 2 weeks after initial poisoning in studies carried out in the U.S. Virgin Islands.[1] Fatigue, myalgias, and sleep and mood disturbances are part of the syndrome. Its similarities with the poorly defined chronic fatigue syndrome are notable.

It was demonstrated by pharmacological analysis that the ciguatoxin acts in part by neuromuscular junction blockage, probably presynaptically since muscle contractions after direct muscle stimulation remain unaffected. Demyelination in peripheral nerves and the central nervous system has also been reported in ciguatera poisoning.[22] Our case is interesting from this point of view because the initial presentation was with electrophysiological evidence of demyelination, which evolved in time to the axonal type of neuropathy.

Ciguatoxin increases mainly the voltage-dependent sodium channel permeability in excitable membranes, acting at receptor site 5 of the sodium channel and causing membrane depolarization.[14,16]

Evidence suggests that the neurotoxin binds to the sodium channel receptor sites of somatic and autonomic nerves, causing voltage-gated opening of sodium channels in cell membranes, thus producing cell membrane excitability and instability, and consequently triggering membrane depolarization.[1] Maitotoxin, another ciguatera-associated toxin, increases calcium ion influx through excitable membranes and causes release of norepinephrine.[14] Scaritoxin increases the permeability of sodium channels and causes norepinephrine and acetylcholine release.[14] Tetrodotoxin blocks ciguatoxin-induced depolarization.[16] The changes in membrane excitability triggered by depolarization are antagonized by increased extracellular Ca ion concentration.[16]

Electrophysiological studies done in the acute stage show significant slowing of conduction velocity and prolongation of the absolute refractory, relative refractory, and supernormal periods. These electrophysiological findings indirectly suggest that ciguatoxin causes an abnormally prolonged sodium channel opening in nerve membranes, in contrast with other fish toxins.[23]

The pathophysiological mechanism of neuropathy associated with ciguatera toxin is described as an "axonal channelopathy." Abnormalities of peripheral nerve sodium and potassium channels result in clinical and electrophysiological manifestations unrelated to axonal degeneration or demyelinization. Prolonged sodium channel activation results in repetitive firing.[11,24] By this action, intracellular water and sodium influx could increase and induce neuronal edema.[25] Ciguatoxin provokes in vitro nodal swelling and a large increase in internodal length and volume, which are possibly linked to changes in membrane sodium current.[25] Slowing of nerve conduction could be explained by both nodal swelling and prolonged activation. In ciguatera toxicity, edema of the Schwann cell cytoplasm compresses the axon in vivo.[15] Increased endoneurial fluid pressure induced by edema might reduce nerve blood flow, and either direct compressive effects or endoneurial fluid pressure could induce nerve blood supply deficiency. Edema may also lead to further axonal ischemic disturbances. Neuronal edema may need to be managed as a neurological emergency[26] and the administration of mannitol is effective in the treatment of this edematous response.[27] The recurrence of ciguatera symptoms may be explained by at least two mechanisms: ciguatoxin binding to voltage-dependent sodium channels in the cell membranes of excitable tissues such as nerves and muscles, leading to physical damage to the cells, or an autoimmune mechanism.[21] Lipid storage and slow release of toxin has been also proposed as the cause for the persistence and recurrence of the symptoms. Relapse of symptoms may be triggered not only by alcohol but also by ingestion of chicken or pig meat from animals fed with fishmeal. Such commercial meat stocks contain ciguatoxins in otherwise subclinical concentrations.[1]

Diagnostic Tests

Simple inspection, taste, and smell cannot detect ciguatoxin-infected fish, which look, taste, and smell normal.[4] Currently, there is no practical laboratory test with sufficient sensitivity and specificity to detect ciguatoxin in human blood or urine, whereas various types of assays have been developed to detect ciguatoxin in contaminated fish.[21] A variety of assay techniques can test fish for ciguatoxin—in vivo bioassays in animals such as mouse, cat, and mongoose and in vitro assays such as immunoglobulin immunoassays—but these tests have limited clinical benefit as most institutions do not have the ability to perform either; also none of these tests has the sensitivity and specificity necessary for routine testing in the laboratory.[14,28]

The most widely used detection method of ciguatoxin in fish is the mouse bioassay, which requires purification of fish extracts before injection in mouse.[4] All bioassay methods are subjective, cumbersome, time-consuming, and expensive.[18]

A radioimmunoassay (RIA) was the first successful detection method of ciguatoxin directly from contaminated fish tissue, using a sheep antibody prepared with purified moray eel ciguatoxin conjugated to human serum albumin as carrier.[29] RIA was effective and has been utilized to distinguish the toxic fishes in human ciguatera poisoning outbreaks from the nontoxic fishes, but its complexity and the use of expensive isotope-counting instruments made the search for a simpler alternative necessary.[28,29]

The next refined method, easier to run and used extensively in surveys for endemic areas of ciguatera poisoning, was the stick-enzyme immunoassay

(S-EIA) using sheep anti-ciguatoxin and Mab-ciguatoxin coupled to horseradish peroxidase.[29] An improved technique used colored polystyrene particles coated with Mab-CTX as markers for direct detection of ciguatoxin and was called solid-phase immunobead assay (SPIA).[29] Another upgraded technique, the membrane immunobead assay (MIA), used for detecting ciguatoxin (CTX) and related polyethers directly from fish tissue, is based on the same immunological principles used to develop SPIA.[29] Monoclonal antibody to CTX antigen attaches to colored immunobeads (colored latex particles) on the membrane portion of the membrane stick. A visible color change will announce a positive sample whereas negative samples will not change color; the intensity of color is proportional to the concentration of ciguatoxin attached to the membrane.[29] The claimed specificity of the MIA is 85.7 percent and the sensitivity is 92.3 percent; the suboptimal specificity is the result of closely related low-potency toxins that cross-react with monoclonal antibodies to CTX.[4]

A recently developed neuroblastoma cell bioassay that detects seafood toxins active at the sodium voltage-gated channel, which measures the toxin plasma concentrations expressed in brevetoxin-1 equivalents, has emerged as a potential diagnostic tool for acute ciguatera intoxication.[2] Brevetoxins cause the paralytic shellfish poisoning associated with red tides and apparently are not causative of ciguatera intoxication.[2] Brevetoxins share structural similarities with ciguatoxins, are also produced by dinoflagellates, and selectively target a common binding site at the voltage-gated sodium channel.[2] Brevetoxins have the advantage of being commercially available in pure form; therefore, given the similarities with ciguatoxin, they can be used as a substitute for ciguatoxin in ciguatera diagnostic techniques.[2] Such a plasma assay capable of detecting toxins would be useful in confirming the diagnosis of marine toxin intoxication.[2]

■ The Pros and Cons

The Illness

It is pertinent to ask ourselves what would we have done differently if we had been the first ones to evaluate a particular case and whether we would have done better in managing a certain case. Obviously it is easier to discuss decisions in retrospect when things look different, crooked lines look straight, and unusual and bizarre symptoms start to make sense. Initial presentation with fever in the patient described in this chapter pointed toward an infectious illness, leading the doctor in the Caribbean to treat the patient with quinine for dengue fever, which is a mosquito-borne disease and one of the tropical viral hemorrhagic fevers. The clinical presentation is dominated in this infectious disease by headache, sore throat, myalgias, ecchymoses, and gingival or gastrointestinal bleeding,[11] which is quite different from the presentation that our patient had. Perhaps our patient's symptoms could have been attributed to another foodborne illness, such as botulism, which is potentially curable if treated early enough. A knowledgeable practitioner would argue correctly that the absence of prominent dryness of mouth and throat and constipation, which are typical of early stage of botulism, and the presence of fever, were clinical arguments against this diagnosis, although atypical presentations are often reported.

To Treat or Not to Treat

The only undoubtedly effective treatment for ciguatera poisoning is to avoid eating reef fish, particularly the viscera (i.e., liver, gonads, intestines).[6,18] The indigenous populations in the Western Pacific use traditional remedies for treating ciguatera toxin illness. Scientific foundations for their use have not been established.[30] Ethnocentric methods in the various locales where marine toxins are found are used to detect a potentially contaminated fish. The fish is laid down on the sand to see if ants are attracted to it. If the ants are attracted, the fish is safe to eat; if they stay away, it is assumed there is a possible fish toxin present.[31] Fishermen in tropical areas also use another simple test to determine whether a fish is safe to eat: if their gums tingle after rubbing fish organs on them, then the fish is not fit for consumption.[6,17] Cooking, boiling, steaming, baking, smoking, salting, pickling, frying, drying, or freezing do not destroy the ciguatoxin.[6,8,18] It is therefore wise to follow local advice when eating fish from tropical waters. Teaching patients to reduce or eliminate from the diet alcohol, nuts, fish, shellfish, and nut oils minimizes recurrent episodes in those persons previously intoxicated.[8]

Simple treatments like mannitol or gabapentin have been reported to reduce the severity and duration of acute symptoms. Mannitol given intravenously at a dose of 10 mL/kg of a 20 percent solution infused slowly over 30–45 minutes, within the first 48 hours, reduces neurological symptoms.[1] Most case series reports showed that more than 60 percent of victims have symptoms reversed by mannitol infusion when this treatment is given early after onset of symptoms; this benefit has been ascribed to beneficial effects on axonal edema.[1] A report that supports this treatment involves a Queensland family of four (including a pregnant woman) with severe ciguatera intoxication, confirmed by bioassay of the fish. All four recovered after treatment with intravenous mannitol. At birth, the infant appeared to be symptom-free.[32] However, a double-blind randomized trial of mannitol therapy concluded that mannitol was not superior to normal saline in relieving symptoms and signs of ciguatera intoxication at 24 hours and had more side effects such as discomfort along the vein used for infusion.[19] Two cases of ciguatera poisoning treated with gabapentin responded to this drug. The patients had rapid amelioration of symptoms with recurrence after stopping the drug.[33] Atropine has been effective in treating symptomatic bradycardia and gastrointestinal symptoms related to excess cholinergic stimulation in the early stages of the poisoning.[14,17] Activated charcoal, which may bind the toxin in the gastrointestinal tract, was found to be rarely useful given the delay in onset of symptoms.[14] In the acute phase of intoxication, intravenous rehydration with crystalloid and electrolyte replacement is necessary because of the dehydration; antiemetics such as droperidol, prochlorperazine, and metoclopramide proved to be beneficial too.[14]

Other drugs have been used to ameliorate chronic symptoms of depression, insomnia, and chronic fatigue in ciguatera fish poisoning. Amitriptyline has been most extensively used; its mechanism of action is thought to be related to sodium channel modulation as well as anticholinergic activity.[17,34] Tocainide, mexiletine, phenytoin, and carbamazepine were tried because of their pharmacological effects on sodium channels.[34] Lidocaine given intravenously may also have a local

anesthetic therapeutic effect by selectively blocking those sodium channels, which have been chronically altered by ciguatoxin.[35] Finally, nifedipine, a calcium channel antagonist, has been used because of its ability to counteract the cellular uptake of calcium.[14]

EDTA (calcium disodium edetate) was administered within 24 hours of the poisoning with inconclusive results, and corticosteroids were ineffective in ameliorating symptoms.[36] The combination of intravenous electrolytes, calcium gluconate, and vitamin B complex, in addition to a high-protein diet and supplemental vitamin C, provided satisfactory results following the acute period and seemed to lessen the duration of the illness.[36]

■ The Main Points

- Ciguatera intoxication is not an infectious disease, and there is no specific therapy.
- Currently, there is no standardized and definitive treatment approach in ciguatera intoxication, therapy being primarily symptomatic and supportive.
- Mannitol and gabapentin have been used, but their value is uncertain.
- Ciguatera toxin illness is usually self-limiting. Supportive measures are successful in relieving acute symptoms and avoiding complications. A small percentage of patients die as a result of shock or respiratory failure.

■ References

1. Pearn J. Neurology of ciguatera. *J Neurol Neurosurg Psychiatry* 2001;70:4–8.
2. Matta J, Navas J, Milad M, Manger R, Hupka A, Frazer T. A pilot study for the detection of acute ciguatera intoxication in human blood. *J Toxicol Clin Toxicol* 2002;40:49–57.
3. DiNubile MJ, Hokama Y. The ciguatera poisoning syndrome from farm-raised salmon. *Ann Intern Med* 1995;122:113–114.
4. Lehane L. Ciguatera update. *Med J Aust* 2000;172:176–179.
5. Feldman, RG. Biological toxins and the nervous system. In Johnson RT, Griffin JW, McArthur JC, eds. *Current Therapy in Neurologic Disease*. Philadelphia, Mosby, 2002:343–353.

6. Caplan CE. Ciguatera fish poisoning. *Can Med Assoc J* 1998;159:1394.

7. Goodman A, Williams TN, Maitland K. Ciguatera poisoning in Vanuatu. *Am J Trop Med Hyg* 2003; 68:263–266.

8. Gollop JH, Pon EW. Ciguatera: a review. *Hawaii Med J* 1992;51:91–99.

9. Bagnis R, Kuberski T, Laugier S. Clinical observations of 3009 cases of ciguatera in the South Pacific. *Am J Trop Med Hyg* 1979;28:1067–1073.

10. Lewis JR. The changing face of ciguatera. *Toxicon* 2001;39:97–106.

11. Del Brutto OH, Carod Artal FJ, Roman GC, Senanayake N. Tropical neurology. *Continuum* 2002; 8:7–10.

12. Samet J, Bignami GS, Feldman RG, Hawkins W, Neff J, Smayda T. *Pfiesteria*: review of the science and identification of research gaps. Report for the National Center for Environmental Health, Centers for Disease Control and Prevention. *Environ Health Perspect* 2001;109 (Suppl 5):639–659.

13. Bagnis R, Chanteau S, Chungue E, Hurtel JM, Yasumoto T, Inoue A. Origins of ciguatera fish poisoning: a new dinoflagellate, *Gambierdiscus toxicus* Adachi and Fukuyo, definitively involved as a causal agent. *Toxicon* 1980;18:199–208.

14. Clark RF, Williams SR, Nordt SP, Manoguerra AS. A review of selected seafood poisonings. *Undersea Hyperbar Med* 1999;26:175–185.

15. Allsop JL, Martini L, Lebris H, Pollard J, Walsh J, Hodgkinson S. Les manifestations neurologiques de la ciguatera. trois cas avec étude neurophysiologique et examen d'une biopsie nerveuse. *Rev Neurol (Paris)* 1986;142:590–597.

16. Kaplan GJ. Ciguatoxin. *Clin Toxicol* 2002;40: 386–390.

17. Swift AE, Swift TR. Ciguatera. *J Toxicol Clin Toxicol* 1993; 31:1–29.

18. Hui YH, Gorham JR, Murrell KD, Cliver O. Fish toxins. In Hui YH, ed. *Foodborne Disease Handbook*, vol 3. New York, Marcel Dekker, 1994:473–496.

19. Schnorf H, Taurarii M, Cundy T. Ciguatera fish poisoning: a double-blind randomized trial of mannitol therapy. *Neurology* 2002;58:873–880.

20. Cameron J, Capra MF. The basis of the paradoxical disturbance of temperature perception in ciguatera poisoning. *J Toxicol Clin Toxicol* 1993;31:571–579.

21. Pearn JH. Chronic fatigue syndrome: chronic ciguatera poisoning as a differential diagnosis. *Med J Aust* 1997;166:309–310.

22. Goetz CG. Animal poisons and venoms. In Goetz CG, *Neurotoxins in Clinical Practice.* New York, Spectrum Publications, 1985:148–159.

23. Cameron J, Flowers AE, Capra MF. Electrophysiological studies on ciguatera poisoning in man. Part II. *J Neurol Sci* 1991;101:93–97.

24. Derouiche F, Cohen E, Rodier G, Boulay C, Courtois S. Ciguatera et neuropathie périphérique: un cas. *Rev Neurol (Paris)* 2000;156:514–516.

25. Benoit E, Juzans P, Legrand AM, Molgo J. Nodal swelling produced by ciguatoxin-induced selective activation of sodium channels in myelinated nerve fibers. *Neuroscience* 1996;71:1121–1131.

26. Gilles A, Sabine R. Serious neurological manifestations of ciguatera: is the delay unusually long? *J Neurol Neurosurg Psychiatry* 1998;64:688–694.

27. Pearn JH, Lewis JR, Ruff T, Tait M, Quinn J, Murtha W, King G, Mallet A, Gillespie CN. Ciguatera and mannitol: experience with a new treatment regimen. *Med J Aust* 1989;151:77–80.

28. Hokama Y, Banner AH, Boylan DB. A radioimmunoassay for the detection of ciguatoxin. *Toxicon* 1977;15:317–325.

29. Hokama Y, Takenaka WE, Nishimura KL, Ebesu SM, Bourke R, Sullivan PK. A simple membrane immunobead assay for detecting ciguatoxin and related polyethers from human ciguatera intoxication and natural reef fishes. *J AOAC Int* 1998;81: 727–735.

30. Bourdy G, Cabalion P, Amade P, Laurent D. Traditional remedies used in the Western Pacific for the treatment of ciguatera poisoning. *J Ethnopharmacol* 1992;36:163–174.

31. Irving AM. Ciguatera fish poisoning. *Can Med Assoc J* 1999;160:1127.

32. Fenner JP, Richard JL, Williamson AJ, Michael LW. A Queensland family with ciguatera after eating coral trout. *Med J Aust* 1997;166:473–475.

33. Perez CM, Vasquez PA, Perret CF. Treatment of ciguatera poisoning with gabapentin. *N Engl J Med* 2001;344:692–693.

34. Lange WR, Snyder FR, Fudala PJ. Travel and ciguatera fish poisoning. *Arch Intern Med* 1992;152: 2049–2053.

35. Cameron J, Flowers EA, Capra FM. Modification of the peripheral nerve disturbance in ciguatera poisoning in rats with lidocaine. *Musc Nerv* 1993;16: 782–786.

36. Findlay ER. Ciguatera poisoning: a report of 35 cases. *Toxicon* 1975;13:383–385.

Chapter 19
Crises in Myasthenia Gravis

Ji Chong and Stephan A. Mayer

There has been good progress over the last decades in the management of a patient with myasthenic crisis. Intensive care management with positive pressure ventilation and aggressive pulmonary care has played a large role, but other more specific treatments have had an effect.[1]

Most conspicuously, mortality from myasthenia gravis has decreased. In a study of hospitalized patients with myasthenia gravis followed over a 45-year period, mortality was examined in different time periods when different interventions were available.[2] The authors looked at the periods 1940 to 1957, 1958 to 1965, and 1966 to 1985. During the first period, patients were being treated with anticholinesterase medications, negative pressure ventilation, and antibiotics. In the middle period, positive pressure and volume-controlled ventilation were available. In the last period, corticosteroids were routinely used. Mortality in patients who reached their worst disease severity during the first time period was 31 percent, in the second 14 percent, and in the third, 7 percent.

Cohen and Younger also studied mortality retrospectively but in a large number of patients (period between 1960 and 1980). Positive pressure ventilators and intensive care units were available after 1962 at Presbyterian Hospital. In a total of 447 patients, mortality from crisis decreased from 42 percent at the beginning of this period to 6 percent at the end.[3] Thomas et al. conducted a follow-up study at the same institution from 1985 to 1994 and found no further reduction in mortality. These reviews suggest that primary goals of care could be minimizing the duration of crisis and optimizing functional outcome at discharge (Figure 19-1).[4]

Crises in myasthenia gravis (although not precisely defined) introduce several treatment dilemmas and uncertainties. Current practices may differ and several institutions have adopted protocols for management when these patients present in the ICU. In this chapter we present our management protocol and experience.

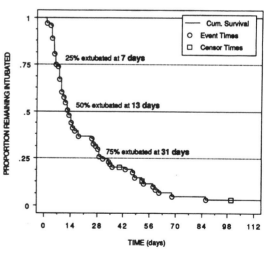

Figure 19-1. Survival curve depicting duration of mechanical ventilation in 73 patients with myasthenic crisis. (Reprinted with permission from Thomas CE, Mayer SA, Gungor Y, Swarup R, Webster EA, Chang I, Brannagan TH, Fink ME, Rowland LP. Myasthenic crisis: clinical features, mortality, complications, and risk factors for prolonged intubation. *Neurology* 1997;48:1253–1260.)[4]

■ The Patient

A 42-year-old Jehovah's Witness with a history of myasthenia gravis presented to the emergency room with progressive weakness and shortness of breath.

She was diagnosed with generalized myasthenia gravis at the age of 18. She had a transcervical thymectomy at the age of 32. She continued to require pyridostigmine and prednisone after the thymectomy, and on a computerized tomography (CT) scan of the chest a year after the thymectomy, was found to have residual thymus. The patient, being a Jehovah's Witness, refused a transsternal thymectomy because she was anemic and did not want blood transfusions. She had also refused non-corticosteroid immunosuppressive agents.

Despite being on a suboptimal medical regimen, she had not required intubation and mechanical ventilation since her thymectomy. Exacerbations had been treated with increased prednisone doses. She was being maintained on pyridostigmine 120 mg every 3 hours and prednisone 40 mg/day.

She was at her baseline, performing all activities of daily living, fully ambulatory, but primarily housebound due to fear of fatiguing while out of the house, until one week prior to presentation. She had noted progressive dysphagia, diplopia, and generalized weakness. Although she had refused blood products in the past, she agreed to an outpatient trial of intravenous gamma-globulins (IVIG) for this exacerbation. She received one dose on the day prior to presentation. That day, she developed severe diffuse headache and neck pain. She had no fevers or cough but had profuse diarrhea. She developed worsening dysphagia and nasal regurgitation of liquids. She also became progressively short of breath, leading to her presentation to the emergency room.

In the emergency room she was afebrile, tachycardic, and had a normal blood pressure. She was drowsy but oriented when fully aroused. She had bilateral lateral rectus and right superior rectus weakness as well as bilateral ptosis. Pupillary light reactivity was normal. She had bifacial weakness and muscle strength in the limbs was MRC 4/5+ throughout. Her bedside vital capacity was 1000 mL. Her initial room air arterial gas was pH 7.38, P_{CO_2} 47, P_{O_2} 97, HCO_3 28. She became more lethargic in the emergency room and, after a brief trial of BiPAP, was intubated due to evolving hypercarbia.

In the neurological intensive care unit (NICU), she was evaluated for an infectious source of her exacerbation. A lumbar puncture revealed evidence of aseptic meningitis. After cultures remained sterile, this was attributed to her IVIG. She was treated with plasmapheresis and experienced a rapid recovery of strength. She was extubated within a week and the remainder of her hospital course was uncomplicated.

■ The Problem

- When is there a need for mechanical ventilation and what is the potential for BiPAP?
- What type of mechanical ventilation is needed and for how long? What is the best weaning method? When is it optimal to proceed with a tracheostomy?
- Which immunomodulatory therapy should be used? Are corticosteroids indicated?

■ The Evidence

Myasthenia gravis is an autoimmune disorder caused by antibodies to the acetylcholine receptor at the neuromuscular junction. It causes weakness that may involve only the extraocular muscles, but commonly is generalized. When weakness involves respiratory muscles and mechanical ventilation is necessary, the patient is considered "in crisis."[5] Fifteen to 20 percent of patients with generalized myasthenia gravis develop crisis.[6] One-third of patients who survive an initial crisis will experience a second one.[4]

Although there are no large, prospective, randomized trials to evaluate the efficacy of the many different types of interventions used to treat myasthenic crisis, there have obviously been improvements in management. However, because of limited data, many controversies still exist.

Respiratory Support

Frequent bedside monitoring of vital capacity may be helpful in deciding when to intubate. Normal vital capacity is 65 mL/kg. Reduction to 30 mL/kg is associated with a poor cough, and patients with vital capacity below 15 mL/kg usually

Table 19-1. Criteria for Intubation

Vital capacity less than 15 mL/kg
Po_2 less than 70 mmHg on room air
Pco_2 greater than 50 mmHg associated with acidosis
   (pH less than 7.35)
Severe oropharyngeal paresis with inability to protect
   the airway

Table 19-2. Criteria for Initiating Spontaneous Breathing Trials

Vital capacity greater than 15 mL/kg
Peak inspiratory pressure greater than 25 cm H_2O
PEEP = 5 cm H_2O
Po_2 greater than 80 mmHg on 40 percent oxygen
No adverse medical conditions: infection, fever,
   hypotension, anemia, gastric distention, volume
   overload, or cardiac arrhythmias

requires intubation.[6] However, pulmonary function tests in myasthenia gravis typically fluctuate, as do the patient's subjective feeling of dyspnea and level of distress. Although the predominant view is that intubation should be performed before significant blood gas abnormalities occur (Table 19-1), in practice this seems to be surprisingly difficult to accomplish.

The route of intubation is arbitrary (see Chapter 7). Nasotracheal intubation is preferred by some over oral endotracheal intubation because it may be more comfortable and less likely to be displaced;[6] the main disadvantage of this approach is an increased risk of sinusitis. Once intubated, ventilation is usually initiated with a volume-cycled ventilator with 100 percent inspired O_2, and the FiO_2 is then gradually reduced to ensure a PaO_2 of 80 to 100 mmHg. Typically, positive end expiratory pressure (PEEP) of 3 to 5 cm H_2O is given, with a tidal volume of 8–12 mL/kg and a respiratory rate of 12. Based on the observation that atelectasis occurs frequently after intubation and is associated with prolonged crisis, some have advocated a "high pressure, high volume" ventilator strategy, employing generous levels of PEEP (5–15 cm H_2O) and larger tidal volumes (12–15 mL/kg) with lower respiratory rates.[7] Others have described a respiratory management protocol for myasthenic crisis which focuses on the use of ventilator sighs (150 percent of the baseline tidal volume) every 15–30 minutes, airway suctioning every 1–4 hours, chest physiotherapy (percussion or vibration with postural drainage) every 4–6 hours, the liberal application of PEEP (5–10 cm H_2O), and turning in bed every 2 hours.[8] Whether these or other respiratory care interventions can reduce the duration of crisis or frequency of complications remains to be determined.

The patient can start to be weaned off the ventilator when he or she is medically and hemodynamically stable, oxygenating well, and showing signs of improved respiratory muscle strength (Table 19-2). The process of weaning involves initiating a spontaneous breathing trial with little or no respiratory assistance. If the patient is intubated, continuous positive airway pressure (CPAP) with a pressure support level of 5 cm H_2O is a standard starting point (Table 19-3). The level of pressure support should be adjusted at the start of the trial to maintain the respiratory rate <30 and the tidal volume (TV) >300 mL.

Table 19-3. Columbia Spontaneous Breathing Trial Protocol

Begin the weaning trial by switching the ventilator mode
   from SIMV to CPAP with PS of 5 cm H_2O.
At the start of the trial, adjust the level of PS to maintain
   RR <30 and TV >0.3 L.
Record the RR/TV ratio (rapid shallow breathing index,
   RSBI) hourly on a flow sheet.
If the level of pressure support is >5 cm H_2O, every
   2–4 hours it may be decreased by 1–2 cm H_2O if the
   patient remains comfortable and the RSBI is <100.
The weaning trial should be stopped if the following occur:

- RSBI >100
- Oxygen saturation <94 percent
- Heart rate >120
- Signs of respiratory distress

An arterial blood gas at this time may be helpful.
When the weaning trial is over, return to SIMV mode
   overnight. Adjust the rate to maintain minute ventilation
   between 6–10 L/min.
Repeat daily with the goal of matching or increasing the
   duration of the trial from the day before, and reducing
   the level of pressure support.
The ability to remain overnight on CPAP with a PS of
   5 cm H_2O indicates a high likelihood of successful
   extubation.

CPAP, continuous positive airway pressure; SIMV, synchronized
   intermittent mandatory ventilation; PS, pressure support;
   RR, respiratory rate.

The endpoint of the trial is the duration of spontaneous breathing until the patient tires, which is usually reflected by a rapid shallow breathing index (rate divided by TV in liters) of greater than 100.[9] Tracheostomy is usually performed if intubation is expected for more than 2 weeks. BiPAP can be used to complete weaning.[10]

A retrospective review of patient charts identified certain predictors of prolonged intubation.[4] In this study, the median duration of crisis was 13 days and the median ICU stay was 14 days. 25 percent of patients were extubated at 7 days, 50 percent at 13 days, and 75 percent at 31 days (see Figure 19-1). Baseline risk factors for prolonged intubation were: age greater than 50, best vital capacity less than 25 mL/kg within 6 days of intubation, and a preintubation serum bicarbonate level greater than 30 mg/dL. The risk of experiencing a crisis longer than 2 weeks in duration was approximately 10 percent with none of the risk factors, 25 percent with one, 50 percent with two, and 90 percent with all three.

Endotracheal intubation is the standard of care in myasthenic crisis, but noninvasive ventilatory support is an option that needs further study. A review of the literature examining noninvasive positive pressure ventilation (NPPV) in acute respiratory failure found favorable effects on survival, need for intubation, and length of hospital stay for some conditions.[11] Use of noninvasive negative pressure cuirass ventilation has been reported in a child with myasthenic crisis.[12] Cuirass ventilation may help patients with myasthenia gravis by increasing tonic activity of the diaphragm and intercostal muscles.[13] A recent preliminary study in 9 patients in myasthenic crises found a trial of BiPAP worthwhile to prevent intubation. BiPAP was not successful in patients with hypercarbia ($PaCO_2$ >50 mmHg). Its use for several hours—while monitoring the patient's respiratory frequency, blood gases, and comfort level—should be considered. It may bridge the time to improvement from IVIG or plasma exchange.[14]

There are also different options for tracheostomy. Nomori and Ishihara used a minitracheostomy tube (MTT) for patients with Duchenne muscular dystrophy and myasthenia gravis.[15] MTT does not allow volume-controlled ventilation because of its small size, but pressure-controlled ventilation may be used. The small size of the tube theoretically allows speaking and eating. They tested this device in 5 patients with MG after a mean of 8 days with a conventional endotracheal tube. All patients could speak with the MTT, but none could eat secondary to poor bulbar function. Blood gases were similar to those obtained with conventional tubes. Its use is not established in myasthenia gravis, and experts have expressed concerns because of blocking of the airway and sudden death.[16-18]

Acetylcholinesterase Inhibitors

There are some data that acetylcholinesterase inhibitors may help in myasthenic crisis but more compelling arguments against their routine use. One report has described a 10-year-old boy who had been on oral pyridostigmine and prednisolone.[19] He was admitted with an acute exacerbation that did not respond to IVIG and increased corticosteroids. He continued to require ventilatory support and increasing doses of pyridostigmine. He was eventually placed on continuous intravenous neostigmine up to 0.012 mg/kg/hr after which he improved. The infusion was continued for 9 days and then changed to an oral regimen. The authors found this regimen to be safe and without cholinergic side effects.

Another report describes 2 patients who were treated with continuous pyridostigmine.[20] One patient did not respond to increased steroids and plasmapheresis. He improved on continuous pyridostigmine 4 mg/hr, along with continued corticosteroids and plasmapheresis. A second patient developed pulmonary edema during plasmapheresis. He was intubated and placed on pyridostigmine 3 mg/hr with prompt response and extubation. The authors concluded that the short half-life of intravenous pyridostigmine makes a drip easier to titrate and administer. They suggested that continuous pyridostigmine may help patients who have an established response to the oral drug.

In addition to these case reports, a large population-based retrospective study lends some support to the use of continuous anticholinesterase drugs. This study compared continuous pyridostigmine, pyridostigmine plus prednisolone, and plasmapheresis in myasthenic crisis.[21] Of 63 crises, 24 were treated with pyridostigmine 1–2 mg/hr; 18 with pyridostigmine 1–2 mg/hr with prednisolone

100 mg over 5 days; and 21 with plasmapheresis for 1–5 exchanges (7 of these patients also received prednisolone, azathioprine, or IVIG). They found the outcome to be the same in all three groups. The average duration of mechanical ventilation was 9 days (median 5, range 2–51). The 3-month outcome in terms of the degree of severity of myasthenic symptoms was also the same. The rate of asystolic arrest was surprisingly high in this series, which may have been related to excessive cholinergic effects at the sinoatrial node.[22]

For years, justification for stopping anticholinesterase medications has been based on the concept that these medications can exacerbate myasthenic weakness. Ferguson et al. reported an influential retrospective study of precipitating factors of ventilatory failure in 31 patients with myasthenia gravis.[23] They defined four categories of crisis. "Myasthenic" crisis occurred in the setting of generalized weakness. In the 12 patients in this category, 6 had respiratory infections. "Cholinergic" crisis developed in patients whose weakness corresponded with an increase in anticholinesterase intake. Eight patients were placed in this category, and they had side effects of colic, diarrhea, and increased secretions, but only one had miosis and bradycardia. "Steroid-induced" crisis was defined as developing respiratory difficulty after receiving steroids. The average time to crisis was 5.8 days after starting steroids. "Brittle" crisis was alternating myasthenic and cholinergic crisis, and these were often compounded by chest infection.

The whole concept of cholinergic crisis is questionable. It is thought that increased acetylcholinesterase inhibition causes worsening neuromuscular blockade and may precipitate respiratory muscle failure. Acetylcholinesterase inhibitors may produce increased bronchial secretions as well as bronchospasm, which may cause problems in patients with myasthenia, but "cholinergic crisis" is a different pathological process. Cholinergic crisis is the direct effect of acetylcholinesterase inhibitors causing weakness. In cholinergic crisis, there should theoretically be immediate improvement once the medication has been stopped. However, Rowland reports never having seen any patient improve immediately after stopping medications.[1]

The effects of large amounts of neostigmine on patients with myasthenia has been studied[24] by examining strength in 4 patients with myasthenia gravis while being given continuous intravenous infusions of neostigmine. Significant weakness was produced. But the doses were at levels unlikely to be given by mouth. The doses of neostigmine were equivalent to 960 to 2400 mg pyridostigmine. Cholinergic crisis can potentially occur, but only at very high doses that are not typically given to patients.

Cholinergic medications administered during a crisis can cause problems with ventilation and cholinergic effects on bronchial smooth muscle may aggravate crisis.[25] This concern was supported after examining lung function in patients on pyridostigmine.[26] There was significant increase in airway resistance in 8 of 21 patients, and this resistance was reversible with ipratropium bromide. The patients who had high airway resistance on anticholinesterase drugs were more likely to have a history of smoking, atopy, or a family history of respiratory problems.

Standard practice at our center is to stop cholinergic medication when a myasthenic patient is on a ventilator, for the simple reason that they can drastically increase the production of tracheobronchial secretions. Left unchecked, mucous plugging can lead to increased work of breathing, atelectasis, and even segmental and lobar collapse. In our view, cholinergic medications should be used to improve a quality of life in stable myasthenic patients. The disease itself should be adequately under control to permit breathing without mechanical ventilation before cholinergic agents are restarted following a crisis.

Corticosteroids

Corticosteroids are useful for attaining long-term immunosuppression, controlling the overall severity of myasthenia, and preventing crisis. For several reasons, however, it is unlikely that their routine use can shorten the duration of crisis. First, their immunosuppressive properties can take weeks to take effect. Second, they can actually increase myasthenic weakness in the short term. Third, they can increase the frequency of infection, promote hyperglycemia, impair wound healing, and cause acute confusional state and a host of other longterm problems. For these reasons, some experts suggest to reserve corticosteroids (1 mg/kg of prednisone) for patients in crisis when they have been on the ventilator for 2 weeks despite plasma exchange, and it is clear that aggressive disease control is necessary.[6]

One study provided further insights. It reported 9 patients with a total of 42 courses of methylprednisolone (60 mg IM for 10 days)[27] while anticholinesterase drugs were continued. A decrease in strength was seen in 30 of the 42 courses of treatment (70 percent). This decrease was seen on the 1st to 6th day (mean 1.8 days) of steroid treatment and was maximal at the 3rd to 10th days (mean 4.1 days). Progressive improvement was seen in 90 percent. Maximal strength was recorded between day 1 and 13 after stopping corticosteroids.

These results were confirmed by a nonblinded, uncontrolled study in which 15 patients were given high-dose IV methylprednisolone.[28] Although this was not a study of the use of corticosteroids in crisis, 13 had severe generalized myasthenia, and 8 required mechanical ventilation. Patients were given a single 2 g dose of methylprednisolone. If no improvement was seen in 5 days, a second dose was given, and 5 days later a third dose if needed. The degree of weakness, functional status, and vital capacities were reported. Improvement began at a mean of 3 days after the first infusion. Improvement occurred in 12 of the 15 patients. Three patients had transient decrease in strength at day 1, which lasted 3 days, and peak improvement occurred at 14 days. Side effects included gastrointestinal bleeding, herpes zoster, infection and psychosis.

Immunomodulatory Treatment of Myasthenic Crisis

There is only one prospective randomized trial evaluating the efficacy of plasmapheresis versus IVIG in myasthenic crisis.[29] There are no large prospective trials to assess other types of treatment and the retrospective studies and case series have provided conflicting results. Furthermore, some question whether immune treatment has any effect on the length of crisis. For example, a retrospective chart review of 35 patients with crisis[30] found that plasmapheresis used in 24 episodes resulted in a median time on mechanical ventilation of 20 days. In the other 11 patients, no plasmapheresis was performed because of early spontaneous improvement.

Median time on the ventilator in these patients was 5 days. This finding points to the difficulty of analyzing retrospective data to evaluate these treatments.

On the other hand, there are many reports of the beneficial effects of plasmapheresis. One study of 16 patients with refractory generalized myasthenia, randomized patients into control and plasmapheresis groups.[31] These patients had not responded to anticholinesterase drugs, steroids, and IVIG treatment. Plasmapheresis was performed every other day until a total volume of 12,000 mL was exchanged. All 9 patients in the treatment group improved versus none in the control group. Four control patients required plasmapheresis early, and the other 3 had plasmapheresis after the preset 40 days. Age, sex, severity of disease, and antibody titer did not predict response. Eventually 75 percent of all the patients improved.

A retrospective chart review of 32 patients treated for crisis with plasmapheresis showed significant improvement in all cases. The authors defined crisis as bulbar or respiratory weakness requiring assistance with feeding and clearing of secretions; only 13 of these patients were intubated. All patients were successfully extubated and all returned to precrisis status after treatment with plasmapheresis.[32]

Another study evaluated 32 patients with onset of myasthenia after age 50.[33] The mean duration of crisis in these older patients was 33 days. Crisis was shortest (18 days) in patients treated with plasma exchange and prednisone.

Gajdos et al. conducted a prospective, randomized, nonblinded study to assess efficacy of IVIG versus plasmapheresis in acute myasthenic exacerbation.[29] They compared plasmapheresis (3 exchanges) with two different IVIG regimens (400 mg/kg/day for 3 or 5 days). These were patients with exacerbations defined as difficulty in swallowing, acute respiratory failure, or major functional disability. Therefore, this was not strictly a study of patients in myasthenic crisis. The outcome measures were muscle strength scores. Follow-up, however, was only for 15 days. Both groups had similar degrees of disease severity, presence of antibodies, treatment with steroids, and number requiring mechanical ventilation. A sample size of 86 was used to detect a 50 percent difference in mean strength score between day 0 and day 15. In this study, plasmapheresis and IVIG in either dose were equally efficacious. However, more adverse events occurred with plasmapheresis (14 events versus 1 in IVIG). Improvement rates were 66 percent with plasmapheresis, 61 percent with IVIG for 3 days, and 39 percent with IVIG for 5 days (not statistically significant).

A retrospective chart review compared IVIG and plasmapheresis in patients with myasthenia gravis and respiratory decompensation.[34] Fifty-four patients with a vital capacity <1000 mL, maximal inspiratory force <−20 cm H_2O, or intubation were given either IVIG or plasmapheresis. Plasmapheresis was performed for 5–6 exchanges and IVIG was given at 400 mg/kg/day for 5 days. Twenty-six episodes were treated with IVIG and 28 with plasmapheresis. The investigators found that plasmapheresis improved ventilatory status at 2 weeks and functional outcome in 1 month. But there were higher rates of cardiovascular and infectious complications with plasmapheresis. They concluded that IVIG may be a good alternative in patients at risk of hemodynamic complications or who do not respond to plasmapheresis.

In summary, it seems that plasmapheresis and IVIG probably offer similar benefits and that the selection of one over another should be based primarily on consideration of their side effects. Further evidence-based analysis is available in the Cochrane Library.[35,36]

Supportive Medical Care

Medical complications are the most common cause of morbidity and mortality in patients with myasthenic crisis and its treatment may be the best means of improving outcome. The most common medical complications during myasthenic crisis are fever (69 percent), pneumonia (51 percent), and atelectasis (40 percent).[4] Complications that significantly increased the duration of myasthenic crisis were atelectasis, anemia requiring transfusion, *C. difficile* colitis, and congestive heart failure. Generous application of PEEP, aggressive blood transfusion, and avoidance of unnecessary antibiotics have been proposed as possible ways to minimize these complications.[4]

Mortality from myasthenic crisis also primarily results from medical complications. A chart review

of 447 patients with myasthenia gravis at Presbyterian Hospital between 1960 and 1980 showed the two major causes of death during crisis were primary cardiac events in 33 percent and pneumonia in 25 percent.[3] A population-based study in Denmark focused on mortality in myasthenia during the period from 1975 to 1989 also found that the most common cause of death was cardiovascular disease (31 percent).[37]

Because neuromuscular disease and prolonged intubation are risk factors for nosocomial infection, a randomized, double-blind, placebo-controlled trial was performed to determine if selective decontamination of the digestive tract reduces morbidity and mortality in neurological patients on long-term ventilation.[38] Forty patients received intravenous cefotaxime for 72 hours. One group then received placebo, and the other received an oral gel containing amphotericin B, polymyxin E, and tobramycin. Antibiotics were continued until 48 hours after extubation. Surveillance cultures of oropharynx, trachea, stomach, stool, and urine were followed. Effective decontamination was documented, but there was no decrease in infections, ICU stay, or hospital stay.

Many drugs have been implicated in worsening myasthenic symptoms.[39,40] Drugs with neuromuscular blocking effects should be avoided (Table 19-4).

Table 19-4. Drugs That Can Exacerbate Weakness in Myasthenia Gravis

Antibiotics
Aminoglycosides (gentamycin, streptomycin, others)
Peptide antibiotics (polymyxin B, colistin)
Tetracyclines (tetracycline, doxycycline, others)
Erythromycin
Clindamycin
Ciprofloxacin
Ampicillin
Antiarrhythmics
Quinidine
Procainamide
Lidocaine
Neuromuscular junction blockers
Vecuronium
Pancuronium
Quinine
Corticosteroids
Thyroid hormones
Beta blockers
Phenytoin

■ The Pros and Cons

Although there are few or no randomized controlled trials to support the different aspects of management for a patient with myasthenic crisis, after weighing the available evidence, we have designed a standardized treatment protocol in our institution.

A patient who appears to be approaching respiratory failure should be monitored closely in an intensive care unit. Frequent bedside vital capacity measurements should be performed, and in general, a patient should be intubated and mechanically ventilated according to the criteria displayed in Table 19-1. BiPAP should be considered in appropriate patients (i.e., patients without excessive secretions and no hypercarbia). Concurrently, one must search for a precipitant of myasthenic crisis, particularly infection.

When a patient is intubated, we stop all anticholinesterase medications to prevent the problems of increased secretions and secondary mucous plugging. Aggressive chest physical therapy and suctioning is performed every 1–4 hours while the patient is on positive pressure ventilation to maximize lung ventilation. Fiber-optic bronchoscopy is used to further improve pulmonary toilet when evidence of air space loss is found on chest radiography. We use antibiotics with caution. One must avoid antibiotics and other medications that may worsen neuromuscular transmission and restrict antimicrobial use to limit the risk of causing *C. difficile* colitis.

We treat patients with either plasmapheresis or IVIG depending on other comorbid conditions. For instance, patients with renal insufficiency, leukopenia, polycythemia, or cardiomyopathy may not be good candidates for IVIG. IVIG may also cause aseptic meningitis and serum sickness. Plasmapheresis, on the other hand, may be difficult to administer safely in patients with poor vascular access, coagulopathy, or those who cannot tolerate pronounced fluid shifts.

We carefully monitor the patient for other medical problems, especially since cardiac complications are the most frequent cause of death during myasthenic crisis. Metabolic abnormalities are aggressively corrected, particularly deficiencies of potassium and phosphate, which can exacerbate muscle weakness. Nutrition, fever, metabolic derangements, and fluid overload must be addressed before weaning is attempted.

If the patient's respiratory status improves and there are no complications of fever or pulmonary infection, we wean mechanical ventilation using the protocol outlined in Table 19-3. We advocate early tracheostomy if intubation time is expected to exceed 14 days. This prevents the development of laryngomalacia and allows for easier tracheal care.

We generally reserve corticosteroid therapy only for patients who have severe disease refractory to plasmapheresis or IVIG, and who have been intubated for at least 10 days with no immediate prospects for recovery.

■ The Main Points

- Intubate sooner rather than later, and use a "high-pressure, high-volume" ventilator strategy.
- Consider BiPAP in patients with marginally decreased mechanical pulmonary function but no hypercarbia.
- Use aggressive pulmonary toilet, including bronchoscopy when needed.
- Stop anticholinesterase inhibitors while the patient is mechanically ventilated.
- Treat with plasmapheresis or IVIG depending on comorbid conditions.
- Limit antibiotics to those patients with demonstrated infection.
- Avoid drugs that may worsen neuromuscular weakness.
- Perform early tracheostomy if the anticipated duration of mechanical ventilation exceeds 2 weeks.
- Reserve corticosteroids for patients who remain intubated after 10–14 days.
- Interrupt sedation daily and move aggressively to spontaneous breathing trials.

■ References

1. Rowland LP. Controversies about the treatment of myasthenia gravis. *J Neurol Neurosurg Psychiatry* 1980;43:644–659.
2. Grob D, Arsura EL, Brunner NG, Namba T. The course of myasthenia gravis and therapies affecting outcome. *Ann NY Acad Sci* 1987;505:472–499.

3. Cohen MS, Younger D. Aspects of the natural history of myasthenia gravis: crisis and death. *Ann NY Acad Sci* 1981;377:670–677.

4. Thomas CE, Mayer SA, Gungor Y, Swarup R, Webster EA, Chang I, Brannagan TH, Fink ME, Rowland LP. Myasthenic crisis: clinical features, mortality, complications, and risk factors for prolonged intubation. *Neurology* 1997;48:1253–1260.

5. Drachman DB. Myasthenia gravis. *N Engl J Med* 1994;330:1797–1810.

6. Fink ME. Treatment of the critically ill patient with myasthenia gravis. In Ropper AH, ed. *Neurological and Neurosurgical Intensive Care*, 3rd ed. New York, Raven Press, 1993:351–362.

7. Mayer SA. Intensive care of the myasthenic patient. *Neurology* 1997;48(Suppl 5):S70-75.

8. Varelas PN, Chua HC, Natterman J, Barmadia L, Zimmerman P, Yahia A, Ulatowski J, Bhardwaj A, Williams MA, Hanley DF. Ventilatory care in myasthenia gravis crisis: assessing the baseline adverse event rate. *Crit Care Med* 2002;30:2663–2668.

9. Yavagal DL, Mayer SA. Respiratory complications of rapidly progressive neuromuscular syndromes: Guillain-Barré syndrome and myasthenia gravis. In Hill, NS, ed. *Pulmonary Complications of Neuromuscular Diseases. Sem Resp Crit Care Med* 2002;23:221–229.

10. Rabinstein AA, Wijdicks EF. Weaning from the ventilator using BiPAP in myasthenia gravis. *Muscle Nerve* 2003;27:252–253.

11. Keenan SP, Brake D. An evidence-based approach to noninvasive ventilation in acute respiratory failure. *Crit Care Clin* 1998;14:359–372.

12. Chisakuta A, Tasker RC. Respiratory failure in myasthenia gravis and negative pressure support. *Pediatr Neurol* 1998;19:225–226.

13. Meessen NE, van der Grinten PM, Luijendijk SC, Folgering HT. Continuous negative airway pressure increases tonic activity in diaphragm and intercostal muscles in humans. *J Appl Physiol* 1994;77:1256–1262.

14. Rabinstein AA, Wijdicks EF. BiPAP in acute respiratory failure due to myasthenic crisis may prevent intubation. *Neurology* 2002;59:1647–1649.

15. Nomori H, Ishihara T. Pressure-controlled ventilation via a mini-tracheostomy tube for patients with neuromuscular disease. *Neurology* 2000;55:698–702.

16. Ryan EW. Minitracheostomy: a new, simple technique for treating patients with retention of sputum. *Br Med J* 1990;300:958–959.

17. Reynolds JE, Mendell JR. Another approach to ventilatory failure in neuromuscular disease. *Neurology* 2000;55:611–612.

18. Bach JR. Intubation and tracheostomy paradigm paralysis. *Neurology* 2000;55:613–614.

19. Briassoulis G, Hatzis T, Liakopoulou T, Youroukos S. Continuous neostigmine infusion in post-thymectomy juvenile myasthenic crisis. *J Child Neurol* 2000;15:747–749.

20. Saltis LM, Martin BR, Traeger SM, Bonfiglio MF. Continuous infusion of pyridostigmine in the management of myasthenic crisis. *Crit Care Med* 1993;21:938–940.

21. Berrouschot J, Baumann I, Kalischewski P, Sterker M, Schneider D. Therapy of myasthenic crisis. *Crit Care Med* 1997;25:1228–1235.

22. Mayer SA, Thomas CE. Therapy of myasthenic crisis. *Crit Care Med* 1998;26:1136–1137.

23. Ferguson IT, Murphy RP, Lascelles RG. Ventilatory failure in myasthenia gravis. *J Neurol Neurosurg Psychiatry* 1982;45:217–222.

24. Rowland LP, Korengold MC, Jaffe IA, Berg L, Shy GM. Prostigmine-induced muscle weakness in myasthenia gravis patients. *Neurology* 1955;5:89–99.

25. Ringqvist I, Ringqvist T. Changes in respiratory mechanics in myasthenia gravis with therapy. *Acta Med Scand* 1971;190:509–518.

26. Shale DJ, Lane DJ, Davis CJ. Air-flow limitation in myasthenia gravis: the effect of acetylcholinesterase inhibitor therapy on air-flow limitation. *Am Rev Respir Dis* 1983;128:618–621.

27. Brunner NG, Namba T, Grob D. Corticosteroids in management of severe, generalized myasthenia gravis. *Neurology* 1972;22:603–610.

28. Arsura E, Brunner NG, Namba T, Grob D. High-dose intravenous methylprednisolone in myasthenia gravis. *Arch Neurol* 1985;42:1149–1153.

29. Gajdos P, Chevret S, Clair B, Tranchant C, Chastang C. Clinical trial of plasma exchange and high-dose intravenous immunoglobulin in myasthenia gravis. *Ann Neurol* 1997;41:789–796.

30. Chang I, Fink ME. Plasmapheresis in the treatment of myasthenic crisis. *Neurology* 1992;42(Suppl 3):242.

31. Kornfeld P, Ambinder EP, Mittag T, Bender AN, Papatestas AE, Goldberg J, Genkins G. Plasmapheresis in refractory generalized myasthenia gravis. *Arch Neurol* 1981;38:478–481.

32. Mahalati K, Dawson RB, Collins JO, Mayer RF. Predictable recovery from myasthenia gravis crisis with plasma exchange: thirty-six cases and review of current management. *J Clin Apheresis* 1999;14:1–8.

33. Sellman MS, Mayer RF. Treatment of myasthenic crisis in late life. *South Med J* 1985;78:1208–1210.

34. Quereshi AI, Choudhry MA, Akbar MS, Mohammad Y, Chua HC, Yahia AM, Ulatowski JA, Krendel DA, Leshner RT. Plasma exchange versus intravenous immunoglobulin treatment in myasthenic crisis. *Neurology* 1999;52:629.

35. Gajdos P, Chevret S, Toyka K. Plasma exchange for myasthenia gravis. *Cochrane Database Syst Rev* 2002;(4):CD002275.

36. Gajdos P, Chevret S, Toyka K. Intravenous immunoglobulin for myasthenia gravis. *Cochrane Database Syst Rev* 2003;(2):CD002277.

37. Christensen PB, Jensen TS, Tsiropoulos I, Sorensen T, Kjaer M, Hojer-Pederson E, Rasmussen MJ, Lehfeldt E. Mortality and survival in myasthenia gravis: a Danish population based study. *J Neurol Neurosurg Psychiatry* 1998;64:78–83.

38. Hammond JM, Potgieter PD. Neurologic disease requiring long-term ventilation: the role of selective decontamination of the digestive tract in preventing nosocomial infection. *Chest* 1993;104: 547–551.

39. Bedlack RS, Sanders DB. How to handle myasthenic crisis: essential steps in patient care. *Postgrad Med* 2000;107:211–222.

40. Jenkins RB, Witorsch P, Smyth NP. Aspects of treatment of crisis in myasthenia gravis. *South Med J* 1970;63:1127–1130.

Chapter 20
Fulminant White Matter Disease

Brian G. Weinshenker and Claudia F. Lucchinetti

Rapidly progressive white matter disease may present with symptoms and signs consistent with long tract involvement (hemiplegia, hemisensory impairments), or with other typical symptoms of white matter disease, such as optic neuritis and internuclear ophthalmoplegia. However, less specific symptoms such as encephalopathy or coma may dominate the clinical picture, and long tract signs may be mild or nonexistent. Patients may present with focal "cortical" findings, such as aphasia, apraxia, and cortical blindness. Patients may even present with spells of neurological dysfunction due to ephaptic transmission of ectopically generated activity in demyelinated tracts (e.g., paroxysmal tonic spasms, paroxysmal ataxia, and dysarthria). Often, involvement of white matter primarily is first suggested by radiological findings, especially by magnetic resonance imaging (MRI). However, not every acute "white matter" selective disease represents inflammatory demyelinating disease of the central nervous system. Radiological findings are generally nonspecific with regard to etiology. Neoplasms and vascular and inflammatory diseases can all result in rapidly progressive white matter disease. Occasionally, gray matter cerebral neurodegenerative disorders may be accompanied by substantial evidence for "secondary" white matter involvement. The management of these patients is difficult. The first and most important challenge is to achieve an accurate diagnosis. This is the main focus of this chapter.

■ The Patient

A 39-year-old woman presents to the emergency room with a rapidly developing quadriparesis. She had been in good health aside from an episode of right optic neuritis, which occurred 3 years prior to her current presentation. At that time, she developed severe visual loss in the right eye associated with pain with eye movement over 2 days. She was investigated with an MRI scan of the head, which was normal aside from gadolinium enhancement and increased T2 signal over the length of the right optic nerve. She was treated with intravenous methylprednisolone and recovered substantially, but was left with a residual central scotoma and a visual acuity of 20/100 in that eye.

Her current problem began 3 days prior to admission, at which time she developed burning pain and numbness over the left side of the neck and the left shoulder. Subsequently, she developed urine retention, which was rapidly followed by weakness of both legs and subsequently of both arms, worse on the right. Neurological examination revealed a severe flaccid quadriparesis; strength was Medical Research Council 1–2/5 range in most muscle groups of the right limbs and 3–4/5 in muscle groups of the left limbs. There were bilateral Babinski signs. There was a sensory level to pinprick at T1. The patient was unable to sit or stand independently.

MRI scan of the spine revealed a gadolinium-enhancing lesion extending from the lower medulla to C3 (Figure 20-1). MRI scan of the head was otherwise normal.

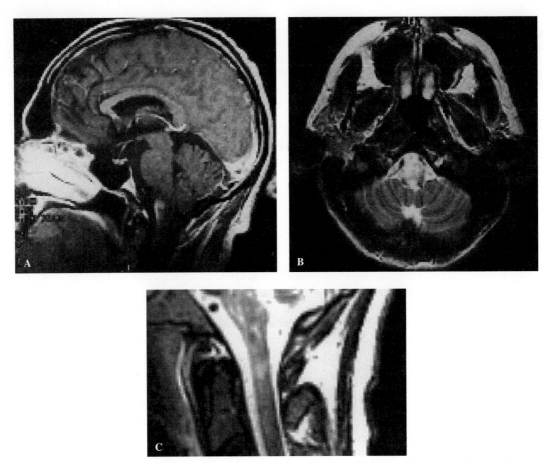

Figure 20-1. Sagittal midline (A) and axial T1 (B) post gadolinium infusion MRI images showing an enhancing lesion in the medulla that is contiguous with a cord lesion that extends through much of the cervical cord (C) in a patient with respiratory failure resulting from neuromyelitis optica.

The patient was treated with intravenous methylprednisolone 1 g/day for 7 days, but in spite of treatment, the patient did not improve, and in fact her respiratory function deteriorated. Chest x-ray revealed bilateral elevation of the diaphragms, and intubation was required because of respiratory failure due to hypoventilation.

After failing intravenous methylprednisolone therapy, the patient was treated with 7 treatments of plasma exchange, 1.0–1.5 plasma volumes per exchange replacing with 5 percent albumin in saline, every other day for 2 weeks. Within 24 hours of the first treatment, obvious improvement was evident in strength and after the third course of plasma exchange, respiratory function improved to the extent that she could be extubated. By the end

of the seventh course of plasma exchange she was able to bear weight, and within one month of concluding plasma exchange she could walk 50 feet without walking aids.

■ The Problem

- There are atypical features for multiple sclerosis (the longitudinally extensive lesion, the lack of other lesions on MRI scan of the head and respiratory failure). Is there an alternative diagnosis?
- Does it matter in terms of acute therapy whether a diagnosis of multiple sclerosis or other inflammatory demyelinating disease

is made? Does it matter in terms of long-term therapy, assuming that the patient survives?

- What are the therapeutic options for inflammatory demyelinating disease in a patient who has failed treatment with high-dose corticosteroids?
- What is the prognosis? Do the prognosis and optimal treatment vary depending on the specific type of demyelinating disease?

■ The Evidence

This case was chosen because it has features that would be atypical for multiple sclerosis (MS), including respiratory failure from an acute attack. However, the relapsing-remitting nature of the illness, and some of the symptoms, such as optic neuritis, clearly suggest that the patient has a demyelinating disease. She has failed standard therapy for an acute attack, and until recently there was no established therapeutic alternative to manage her underlying illness aside from symptomatic therapy. Her case indicates the heterogeneity of fulminant white matter disease, and the final diagnosis is one that likely mandates therapy that differs from that which would be suggested to prevent future attacks of MS.

The most precise diagnosis for this patient is neuromyelitis optica (NMO—probably synonymous with Devic's disease; opticospinal variant of MS; Asian-type MS). While historically diagnosed in the setting of bilateral optic neuritis and myelitis occurring either simultaneously or within a short interval of one another, the diagnostic criteria have recently been expanded to recognize that most patients have a relapsing rather than a monophasic course of disease.[1] Typically, the myelitis of NMO is severe, and is associated with a longitudinally extensive lesion on MRI of the cord affecting the central portion of the cord. Respiratory failure occurs in approximately one-third of patients with relapsing illness and a lesser percentage of patients with monophasic illness. Unlike MS, there are usually no parenchymal lesions on the initial MRI of the brain, no elevation of IgG index or oligoclonal bands in the cerebrospinal fluid. However, there is extensive deposition of immunoglobulin associated with complement activation in the brain.[2]

The differential diagnosis is very broad, and in many instances, noninvasive tests do not provide a definitive diagnosis. Biopsy is a recent approach to the diagnosis in cases where the radiology and other noninvasive investigations do not yield a confident diagnosis. There are a broad variety of inflammatory demyelinating disease types, but for almost all, the therapeutic approaches to arrest the acute disease process are the same at the present time. However, some inflammatory diseases (e.g., vasculitis and sarcoidosis) may require different approaches, and neoplastic and vascular disorders often require very different therapies. For acute management, it is more important to precisely classify the right category of disease process (e.g., inflammatory demyelinating disease) than to define the specific syndrome (e.g. MS, Marburg's variant of MS, neuromyelitis optica), the specific categorization of which may become evident only with follow-up.

The spectrum of presentations of white matter disease is broad. The commonest presentations may be classified as follows: multifocal cerebral and/or long tract involvement; coma or encephalopathy (confusion); focal cerebral disorder, with or without signs of raised intracranial pressure; brainstem disorder, with involvement of long tracts or consciousness, without or with cranial nerve involvement; optic neuritis; and rapidly progressing myelopathy affecting long tracts.

The differential diagnosis of acute white matter disease depends in part on the presenting syndrome. The differential diagnosis is different for cerebral versus spinal cord versus combined disorders. The differential diagnosis of cerebral disorders is given in Table 20-1. Idiopathic inflammatory demyelinating disease (IIDD) will be considered in the following section. The most common diagnoses aside from IIDDs are neoplasms (lymphoma, including intravascular lymphoma; gliomatosis cerebri), sarcoidosis, vasculitis, and vasculopathies. The differential diagnosis of rapidly progressive myelopathy is given in Table 20-2. IIDD, specifically acute transverse myelitis, acute partial myelitis, and recurrent myelitis (as occurs in the setting of neuromyelitis optica), is also an important cause of rapidly worsening myelopathy. However, other causes, including vascular causes (venous hypertension often secondary to an underlying dural arteriovenous fistula, embolic disease, dissection),

Table 20-1. Differential Diagnosis of Acute Leukoencephalopathy

Inflammatory
  Idiopathic inflammatory demyelinating disease
    Fulminant multiple sclerosis, including
      Marburg's variant of MS
    Tumefactive cerebral demyelinating lesions,
      including Balo's concentric sclerosis
  Drug-induced inflammatory demyelinating
    disease (5FU/levamisole;* TNF-alpha
    scavengers)
  Behçet's syndrome
  Hashimoto's (autoimmune) encephalopathy*
  Other (e.g., SLE, Sjögren's syndrome)
  Neurosarcoidosis
Ischemic/Vascular
  Thromboembolic (cardiac, arterial, paradoxical)
  Vasculopathy
    Moya Moya
    Retinocochlear vasculopathy of Susac*
    CADASIL
  Vasculitis
    Systemic
    Primary CNS
    Drug-induced
    Infection-associated
  Venous infarction due to venous sinus
    thrombosis
  Other
    Degos disease*
Metabolic/Nutritional
  Mitochondrial encephalomyelopathy
  Vitamin B_{12} deficiency
  Central pontine myelinolysis
  Methylene tetrahydrofolate deficiency*
  Ketotic hyperglycinemia*
Infectious
  Cerebritis/abscess
  Viral encephalitis
  Lyme disease
  Tuberculosis
  Progressive multifocal leukoencephalopathy
  Whipple's disease*
  HIV
    Primary infection
    Opportunistic infection
  Cysticercosis
  SSPE and other slow viral illnesses*
  Neurosyphilis
Postinfectious
Radiation-induced
Toxic
  Chemotherapy
    Methotrexate
    Nitrous oxide (produces acute B_{12} deficiency)

  Solvents
  Carbon monoxide
  Clioquinol*
  Lead
Genetic
  Mitochondrial encephalopathy
  CADASIL*
Oncological
  Neoplastic
    Gliomatosis cerebri
    Primary CNS lymphoma
    Intravascular lymphoma (neoplastic
      angioendotheliomatosis)
  Paraneoplastic
    Limbic encephalitis
    Progressive spasticity and dementia associated
      with anti-amphiphysin antibodies*
    Brainstem encephalitis
Miscellaneous
  Reversible posterior leukoencephalopathy
    (associated with hypertensive encephalopathy
    or immunosuppressive drugs such as tacrolimus or
    cyclosporine)

SLE, systemic lupus erythematosus; CADASIL, cerebral autosomal dominant arteriopathy with subcortical ischemic
  leukoencephalopathy; CNS, central nervous system;
  HIV, human immunodeficiency virus; SSPE, subacute
  sclerosising panencephalitis; 5FU, 5-fluorouracil.
*Entities currently felt to be very rare, though many are
  recently recognized and accurate estimates of their occurrence are unavailable.

infectious myelitis (typically viral), and structural/compressive etiologies are also common.

The key to the correct diagnosis is to consider the following five items:

1. The setting in which the disease occurs—patients with idiopathic IIDDs typically are previously healthy, or have had prior attacks suggestive of demyelinating disease; in the setting of patients with immunosuppression, consider opportunistic infection or lymphoma; in the setting of patients with cerebrovascular disease risk factors, consider stroke; in hypercoagulable states, consider embolism or venous thrombosis.

2. The specific clinical findings—certain clinical features may suggest certain disorders, such as cortical blindness and reversible posterior leukoencephalopathy that may be associated with hypertension or cyclosporine treatment;

Table 20-2. Differential Diagnosis of Rapidly Progressive Myelopathy

Compression
   Tumor
      Extradural or intradural
      Intraparenchymal
   Abcess
      Bone—with or without fracture/instability
        of the spine
      Epidural lipomatosis
Idiopathic transverse myelitis
Neuromyelitis optica
Multiple sclerosis
Viral myelitis
Postviral or associated with acute disseminated
   encephalomyelitis*
Radiation-induced
Vascular—especially dural arteriovenous fistula
   with venous hypertension
Associated with connective tissue disease—i.e.,
   lupus, anticardiolipin antibodies
Vasculitis
Paraneoplastic myelopathy

*Difficult to distinguish from idiopathic transverse myelitis.

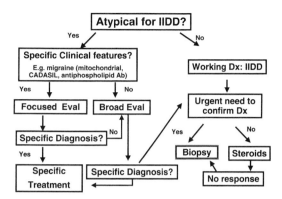

Figure 20-2. Algorithm outlining approach to a patient with a suspected idiopathic inflammatory disease of the central nervous system. IIDD, idiopathic inflammatory demyelinating disease.

a complete transverse myelitis completely sparing the dorsal columns suggests a vascular lesion.

3. The presence of associated systemic disease—generally patients with IIDDs do not have other systemic symptoms; livedo reticularis should suggest antiphospholipid antibody syndrome and pleuritis should suggest an underlying systemic inflammatory disease such as lupus.

4. Radiological findings—IIDDs typically have enhancing lesions with relatively little mass effect, and may show an "open ring" enhancement pattern, wherein the border of the lesion abutting the deep white matter enhances, but not the margin abutting against the cortex. Toxic and metabolic white matter disease and certain infections, such as progressive multifocal leukoencephalopathy, do not enhance with gadolinium.

5. Response to empirical treatment, typically with corticosteroids—while a favorable response may occur in patients with diverse inflammatory and some noninflammatory diseases, notably lymphoma, persistent resolution of gadolinium-enhancing lesions following corticosteroid

treatment generally suggests an inflammatory disorder.

The way in which these considerations can be integrated into the clinical evaluation of the patient is illustrated in Figure 20-2.

The Spectrum of Idiopathic Inflammatory Demyelinating Disorders

Multiple sclerosis (MS) was first pathologically described over 160 years ago; however, the classic clinicopathological pattern of chronic MS represents only one member of a family of closely related idiopathic inflammatory demyelinating diseases (IIDDs) that include acute MS (Marburg variant), Balo's concentric sclerosis, acute disseminated encephalomyelitis (ADEM), and neuromyelitis optica (Devic's disease). Although the clinical and pathological characteristics of these diseases are diverse, the presence of transitional forms suggests a spectrum of inflammatory diseases that may share a pathogenic relationship and may therefore respond to similar treatment strategies.[3]

Marburg Variant of MS

Acute MS was recognized as a subtype of the disease by Otto Marburg in 1906.[4] This entity is clinically characterized by rapid progression and an exceptionally severe course, which typically leads to death within one year from presentation. The course is generally monophasic and relentlessly progressive, with death usually secondary to brainstem involvement or cerebral herniation. There are no MRI series that illustrate the radiographic spectrum of this variant, likely due to its rarity. Cerebrospinal fluid (CSF) results are variable, and often oligoclonal bands are absent, possibly due to the fulminant and relatively short course of the illness. Although the extent of necrosis, axonal injury, and demyelination distinguishes the Marburg variant of MS from ADEM, it is often difficult to distinguish between these entities on clinical grounds, especially in cases with disease duration of several weeks. The fulminant nature of these lesions makes them very difficult to treat, and patients are typically managed with supportive care, occasionally requiring measures to reduce raised intracranial pressure. Although high doses of intravenous steroids are considered the first line of therapy, they are often of limited benefit. Several reports suggest a role for plasma exchange in those patients who do not respond to a course of corticosteroids (see next section). This supports recent neuropathological observations suggesting a potential role for demyelinating antibodies in disease pathogenesis.[5,6]

Balo's Concentric Sclerosis

Balo's concentric sclerosis is another acute variant of MS that is distinguished by its unique concentric pathology characterized by alternating rims of myelin preservation and loss giving the lesions the macro- and microscopic structure of onion bulbs.[7] Similar to the Marburg variant, the clinical course is typically fulminant, with an acute monophasic progressive course over weeks to months that often ends in death within one year, usually due to cerebral herniation or pneumonia. Occasionally the course may be subacute and there are rare reports of long-term survival. Patients often present with predominantly cerebral symptoms including headache, disturbances in consciousness, aphasia, cognitive decline, psychiatric symptoms, seizures, and signs of raised intracranial pressure. Most cases of Balo's concentric sclerosis are diagnosed postmortem; however, recent MRI reports demonstrating characteristic concentric rings of demyelination have suggested

the potential for antemortem diagnosis.[8-10] The CSF resembles that of other MS patients and patients often have oligoclonal bands with evidence of increased IgG production. There are reports of therapeutic responsiveness to glucocorticoids, immunosuppressives, and plasma exchange.[11] Several investigators argue that Balo's concentric sclerosis is a rare variant of MS, since transitional forms have been observed where the presence of both concentric lesions and MS plaques are found within the same patient, underscoring the difficulty in classification of the IIDDs.

Perivenous Encephalomyelitis

Several syndromes can be grouped under the term perivenous encephalomyelitis. These include acute disseminated encephalomyelitis (ADEM), postinfectious encephalomyelitis, postvaccinial encephalomyelitis, and the more severe hyperacute syndrome, acute hemorrhagic leukoencephalomyelitis (AHLE).[12,13]

ADEM is generally a monophasic disorder that begins within 6 days to 6 weeks following an antigenic challenge. At least 70 percent of patients report a precipitating event (infection or vaccine) during the prior few weeks. However, the only epidemiologically and pathologically proven association is with the rabies vaccination.[14] ADEM can occur at any age but is more common in childhood. The clinical course is rapidly progressive leading to focal or multifocal neurological deficits. A prodrome of headache, low-grade fever, myalgias, and malaise often precedes the onset of ADEM by a few days. Headache, fever, seizures, myelopathy, optic neuritis, and brainstem or cerebellar disturbances are common. Drowsiness and lethargy are frequent and may progress to coma. The overall mortality in ADEM is 10–25 percent. Although ADEM is considered a monophasic disorder, there are rare cases of this disorder relapsing up to 18 months following an infection. The limited extent and perivenular pathological pattern of demyelination help distinguish ADEM from MS lesions. However, as in the other IIDDs, there are also transitional cases with histological features of both ADEM and MS, suggesting that these conditions may represent a continuous spectrum of inflammatory demyelinating disease.

Neuromyelitis Optica (Devic's Disease)

The most recent retrospective review defined NMO as a monophasic or relapsing disorder characterized by severe transverse myelitis associated with either unilateral or bilateral optic neuritis.[1] Approximately 35 percent of NMO patients have a monophasic illness, and 55 percent develop relapses restricted to the optic nerves and spinal cord. Rarely patients may have a relentlessly progressive course to death. The monophasic course is more common in younger patients with no sex predilection, whereas the relapsing form is more common in women. Patients with relapsing NMO typically have a very aggressive disease with frequent and severe exacerbations, and a poor prognosis.

MRI of the brain may demonstrate optic nerve or chiasm enlargement, T2 signal change, and enhancement. Increased T2 signal in the medulla is not uncommon and usually is continuous with a high cervical cord lesion. Cerebral white matter lesions on brain MRI develop in about 25 percent of cases on follow-up. Spine MRI usually shows cord swelling, signal changes, and enhancement over the length of three or more contiguous vertebral segments. This appearance may resemble a spinal cord tumor and lead to consideration of biopsy. A minority of patients with NMO have normocellular CSF during the acute phase. A marked pleocytosis is often present, sometimes exceeding 100 cells/μL. Moreover, neutrophils are commonly seen in the CSF and may even predominate. The protein concentration is often very high and in nearly half of patients exceeds 100 mg/dL. Despite the intense inflammatory response, oligoclonal bands are often absent. Relapsing NMO is often associated with autoimmune disorders. These patients frequently have an elevated ESR and nonspecific elevation of autoantibodies including ANA, anti-extractable nuclear antigens (such as SS-A and SS-B), and antiphospholipid antibodies.

Anecdotal reports indicate that glucocorticoids, azathioprine, IVIG, and plasma exchange have been associated with a beneficial response.[15] Supportive care is the mainstay of therapy. Mechanical ventilation is occasionally necessary to treat respiratory failure, which carries a very poor prognosis.[1]

The pathogenesis of NMO is not well understood. It is still a matter of debate whether NMO represents a variant of MS. However, based upon the generally restricted topography of the lesions, atypical CSF findings, MRI abnormalities, associated autoantibodies, clinical course, prognosis, and pathology, most argue that NMO (Devic's disease) is a distinct nosological entity. Recent immunohistochemical studies suggest that NMO has a humoral and complement-mediated basis targeting CNS perivascular regions.[2]

Acute Treatment

Treatment depends on the etiology. It is beyond the scope of this chapter to consider therapy for each of the entities that may mimic inflammatory demyelinating disease presented in Table 20-1. Supportive therapy (protection of airway and ventilation, management of agitation and confusion, prevention of aspiration, decubitus ulcers, and deep venous thrombosis, and bladder and bowel management) is the same for rapidly progressive white matter disease as for other acute neurological disorders and will not be considered in detail.

There are two aspects to the management of these disorders. The first is salvage from the acute disability and restoration of function. That is the immediate problem that faced the clinicians caring for the patient described. The second aspect is maintenance therapy, if necessary, to prevent continuing or recurrent inflammatory demyelinating disease activity.

Corticosteroids are universally regarded as the treatment of choice.[16] Surprisingly few data are available that document the effectiveness of this treatment for acute catastrophic attacks of demyelinating disease and the proportion of patients who are unresponsive to treatment in this setting. While widely accepted as treatment of choice for virtually all acute attacks of IIDD, there are no controlled trials of corticosteroids in neuromyelitis optica for acute treatment. Virtually all controlled data emerge from the study of corticosteroids in attacks of MS, the prototypic inflammatory demyelinating disease of the central nervous system.

Kurtzke et al. studied the outcome of MS in 527 U.S. World War II veterans hospitalized during the war.[17] Eighteen of 527 (3.4 percent) had attacks sufficiently severe to render them nonambulatory (EDSS 7–9), one measure of an attack of catastrophic proportion. As military recruits, it would be expected that most had little if any disability before enrollment in the military service. Eight of the 18 patients (44 percent) improved by greater than 1 EDSS point at discharge (mean interval of 105 days following admission); therefore, 10 of 18 (56 percent) had severe residual neurological deficits. Most reported cases with the Marburg variant of MS have been fatal,[18,19] likely reflecting a very poor outcome, even if this dismal prognosis reflects some degree of reporting bias. Survivors, however, may subsequently follow a course typical of relapsing-remitting MS. The prognosis for recovery from acute transverse myelitis was poor in 16/31 cases in one series,[20] and these results seem to be representative of other reports in the literature. Similarly, a high proportion of patients with neuromyelitis optica who typically develop longitudinally extensive myelitis have a poor outcome from either their initial or subsequent attacks.[1]

Plasma exchange has been assessed as a treatment for patients with MS since 1980 in a series of uncontrolled reports including both cases with acute attacks and patients with progressive MS with variable degrees of benefit. The most promising results were reported in the small number of patients with acute, catastrophic attacks.[21] A controlled clinical trial reported in 1989 failed to convincingly show benefit when plasma exchange was studied as an adjunct to adrenocorticotropic hormone (ACTH) and cyclophosphamide for acute attacks of MS.[22] However, this study included patients with attacks of variable degrees of severity and included patients with both relapsing-remitting and progressive forms of MS. A modest short-term benefit was reported for patients who had relapsing-remitting MS only.

Shortly thereafter, Rodriguez et al. reported their uncontrolled results in 6 patients with acute severe attacks of multiple sclerosis that suggested a high response rate with rapid and dramatic recovery.[23] All patients in this case series were quadriplegic, hemiplegic, or paraplegic. Additionally, 2 patients were aphasic and 2 required artificial ventilation. In these corticosteroid-refractory patients, plasma exchange was administered as a monotherapy. All patients in this series responded to treatment and 5 had experienced excellent results. Improvement began within days of initiation of treatment. The therapeutic benefit was sustained on follow-up.

The previous controlled trial failed to adequately address the uncontrolled observations by Rodriguez et al. and other groups. Accordingly, between 1995 and 1998, we conducted a randomized clinical trial of plasma exchange in the setting of acute, severe attacks of MS or other idiopathic inflammatory demyelinating diseases.[24] Enrolled patients had failed to respond to corticosteroid therapy. We enrolled 22 patients over 4 years. The trial was designed to give 80 percent power to detect a significant difference in the proportion of patients experiencing functionally important recovery, assuming a success rate of 20 percent in the sham-treated group and 70 percent in the active-treated group. While the sample size was relatively small, it was expected to be sufficient to detect such a major difference in the frequency of functionally important improvement between sham therapy and active therapy.

Patients included in the trial had either clinically definite MS ($n = 12$) or other inflammatory demyelinating diseases ($n = 10$), most commonly acute transverse myelitis. Two patients were enrolled with a diagnosis of neuromyelitis optica. All patients had acute attacks of major proportion of at least 3 weeks duration and failed to improve a minimum of 2 weeks after having received methylprednisolone therapy at a minimum dose of 500 mg/day. We did not intend to investigate plasma exchange as an alternative treatment, but rather as a rescue treatment for patients who failed treatment with corticosteroids. We recognized that corticosteroid therapy was safe, effective, and widely accepted. All patients enrolled had quadriplegia, paraplegia, or hemiplegia as a "targeted neurological deficit." In addition, one patient with a clinical diagnosis of acute disseminated encephalomyelitis was comatose, and 2 patients who had cerebral hemisphere lesions were aphasic. The spectrum of neurological deficits of patients enrolled in this controlled trial was typical of those of the patients previously reported in the series of Rodriguez et al.

The study was conducted using a crossover design. However, only patients who failed to improve in the first treatment period crossed over. This approach was feasible because the improvement in responders was evident very early in the course of treatment and was unlikely to occur subsequent to crossover related to the first course of treatment. This approach guaranteed access to the active treatment to all patients who had not improved, which was the only ethical and feasible way that a sham-controlled trial could be conducted in this setting. Furthermore, we suspected that this approach might enhance the power of the study, as patients who failed sham treatment and subsequently were responders to active treatment would be particularly informative.

The treatment administered was standard plasma exchange by continuous-flow centrifugation. On average, 1.1 plasma volumes (54 mL/kg) were exchanged every other day for 7 treatments and replaced with a mixture of 5 percent albumin and saline. In the sham-treated patients, blood was separated in an identical fashion into the cell and plasma fractions but then recombined and returned to the patient unchanged. The endpoint was moderate-to-marked (functionally important) improvement in the targeted neurological deficit without any worsening in any other existing deficit and without any newly developing neurological deficit. This endpoint allowed the decision about success to be individualized to the patient's specific attack-related neurological deficit.

Five of the 11 patients undergoing active plasma exchange in the first treatment period improved versus 1 out of 11 who received sham therapy. None of the 6 treatment failures in the active treatment first group improved after crossover. However, 3 out of 8 surviving treatment failures in the sham treatment first group improved to a moderate-to-marked degree after crossover. There were 2 patients who died in the study, both of whom received only sham exchange. One died of progressive increased intracranial pressure and herniation. The clinical diagnosis for that patient was acute disseminated encephalomyelitis, which was confirmed at autopsy. The second patient died of a presumed pulmonary embolus in the setting of heparin-associated thrombocytopenia syndrome.

Overall, 8 of 19 individuals (42.1 percent) receiving active treatment were treatment successes versus 1 of 17 (5.9 percent) who received sham treatment. A novel, but simple, statistical approach applicable to a crossover study in which only treatment failures cross over was developed for this trial. The differences between active and sham treatment were significant ($p = 0.01$). Blinding was entirely satisfactory both for physicians and patients, as anticipated considering that specific clinical adverse effects or laboratory abnormalities were not expected based on whether active or sham treatment was administered.

Adverse effects related to treatment were very few, the most common being significant anemia, which developed in most patients and in 4 of 22 patients was severe (hemoglobin <8.0). The anemia was invariably asymptomatic and corrected within one month. Central intravenous catheters were necessary in 13 of 22 patients, but insertion was accomplished without sequelae. There were no other common serious adverse effects. A number of incidental side effects unrelated to the specific treatment also occurred.

A long-term benefit from the treatment was not anticipated, and was not the primary endpoint of the study. In fact, 4 of 8 patients who received active treatment and were treatment successes had recurrent attacks during the 6-month follow-up period. However, the remaining 4 patients have been free of subsequent relapses with follow-up as long as 4 years, presumably reflecting the natural course of their illness. They would have been unable to live independently had their apparently fixed neurological deficit at the time of enrollment persisted.

The mechanism of action was unclear from this study. However, the success of plasma exchange as a monotherapy could suggest that a humoral factor is responsible for sustaining disability in at least 40 percent of patients with acute catastrophic attacks. Considerable evidence has recently emerged that suggests a role for humoral autoimmunity in MS[5,25] and more recently in NMO.[2] The nature of the humoral factor or factors remains elusive. Plasma exchange is selective in that it targets only humoral factors but nonselective in that it removes all components of plasma. Further studies to identify clinical and serological factors that might predict treatment success are underway. However, some patients may have not responded either because they did not have the specific humoral components or perhaps because they sustained such severe axonal injury that they were unable to benefit from treatment, which may complicate subsequent analysis of serum components for association with clinical benefit.

Ten of 12 patients who were treatment failures failed to recover over 6 months of follow-up, though 2 out of 12 did meet the criteria for moderate improvement at 6 months. These data suggest but do not prove that the patients who were selected for this clinical trial were unlikely to experience spontaneous improvement in the absence of treatment.

Based on these results, plasma exchange should be used in the following circumstances:

1. For severe attacks of idiopathic inflammatory demyelinating disease.
2. After exclusion of other disorders that might mimic such inflammatory demyelinating diseases.
3. In patients who fail to achieve significant improvement after high-dose intravenous methylprednisolone.

The American Society for Apheresis has recognized the results of this study and has recently upgraded the indication of plasma exchange for acute demyelinating diseases unresponsive to corticosteroids as a category II indication (generally accepted in a supportive role).[26]

Rensel et al. have also reported good results with the use of plasma exchange in treating acute attacks of neuromyelitis optica.[27] Keegan et al. have recently reviewed their complete experience at the Mayo Clinic with the use of plasma exchange for acute attacks of demyelinating disease. They have confirmed that the response rate in their uncontrolled experience, using a similar definition of success as was used in the randomized trial described above, was virtually identical at approximately 44 percent. Included in that series were 10 patients with acute attacks of neuromyelitis optica, and the success rate was 60 percent in that subgroup, which was somewhat (though not significantly) better than that seen in other IIDDs, perhaps in part due to the important role of humoral factors in this disorder.[28]

Long-Term Management

Acute IIDDs may be monophasic, and perhaps this is more often the case with fulminant presentations, such as acute disseminated encephalomyelitis, Marburg's variant of MS, and acute tumefactive demyelinating lesions. However, any or all of these conditions may be the harbinger of a recurrent IIDD that may lead to stepwise accumulation of disability. Often, as is the case in patients with MS, the accumulation of axonal injury may be subclinical until a threshold of neurological injury is reached, beyond which progressive axonal loss, even without continuing evidence of active inflammation, may occur. However, for many individuals with MS or other IIDDs, many if not most attacks of MS may lead to cumulative symptoms and signs, which over months to years may lead to major impairment and disability. The full spectrum of long-term management of MS is beyond the scope of this review, and we shall concentrate here on the management of relatively rapid, stepwise deteriorating MS and other IIDDs.

There have been no controlled clinical trials strictly targeting patients with fulminant, rapidly worsening MS. Lublin and Reingold have classified MS according to the temporal course,[29] as suggested by McAlpine et al.[30] Within this classification, Lublin and Reingold included a second tier of classification based on outcome: benign MS and malignant MS. The latter was defined as "a disease with a rapid progressive course leading to significant disability in multiple neurological systems or death in a relatively short time after disease onset." This definition was left, perhaps deliberately, qualitative. The authors did not clarify whether the result could occur as a result of a single acute severe attack. Furthermore, the authors did not indicate whether failure of standard therapy was necessary to meet this definition. Weinstock-Guttman et al. added certain qualifiers to operationalize this definition for the purposes of a prospective study. They defined fulminant MS as "rapid, continuous neurological decline to a level of severe neurological disability manifested by at least a 1.5 worsening on the EDSS during 3–6 months of observation with no response to corticosteroid therapy."[31] However, undoubtedly, such patients have participated in other trials of secondary-progressive MS, the category that applies to the majority of these patients. Furthermore, a placebo-treated control group would likely be unacceptable both for patients and Institutional Review Boards, and consequently a placebo-controlled trial is unlikely to occur in this circumstance.

In smaller, uncontrolled studies, it has been difficult to identify the number of patients who might satisfy the criteria for fulminant MS or to know what their specific outcome might have been in the absence of treatment. However, one study reported experience in 17 patients ascertained over 27 months at the Cleveland Clinic, a practice that saw 800 new and 8000 follow-up patients per year over that interval.[31] Even if we were to assume that there was no selection bias in their practice and that all of the cases came from within the newly evaluated patients, the frequency of fulminant MS would be approximately 1 percent over 27 months if all eligible cases were enrolled. Given the assumptions, this is likely an overestimate of the frequency. Of the 17 enrolled patients, 8 were men and 9 were women with mean disease duration of 9 ± 7.4 years (range 1–25 years). Ten of 17 patients had EDSS scores ≥8.0, and all had scores of ≥6.0. All but one patient had secondary-progressive MS; the other patient had primary-progressive MS. The occurrence of some patients with fulminant inflammatory disease who have a primary-progressive course illustrates the limitation of the current classification of this subgroup. Typically, patients with primary-progressive MS have insidiously progressive myelopathies with relatively few brain MRI lesions.[32] However, occasional patients with fulminant cerebral and cord involvement but without clinical relapses and remissions may also satisfy the current criteria for primary-progressive MS.

Weinstock-Guttman et al. treated patients with intravenous cyclophosphamide ($500\,mg/m^2$) and intravenous methylprednisolone (1 g) daily for 5 days with appropriate hydration and treatment of nausea with metoclopramide.[31] This was followed by a tapering dose of oral steroids for 5 days. Adverse effects were as expected: nausea, leukopenia, and alopecia. One patient developed fever that was associated with a urinary tract infection and recovered. Patients were followed for 24 months. At 12 months, 4 of 17 (23.5 percent) were stable and 9 of 17 (53 percent) had improved by ≥1.0 EDSS point. At 24 months, 4 of 13 (31 percent) were stable and 5 of 13 (38 percent) were improved. Of 10 patients with EDSS ≥8.0 (nonambulatory), 5 (50 percent) became ambulatory (EDSS ≤6.5). The highest proportion in the "improved" category was observed at 3 months. One patient improved by 3.5 EDSS points (6.5 to 3.0), but others improved by at most 1.5 EDSS points. Similar favorable results in patients

with MS who are resistant to other first-line immunomodulatory agents such as interferon beta and glatiramer acetate have been reported by others[33] and these results have been supported by rapid reduction in contrast-enhancing lesion frequency and T2 lesion load on MRI.[34]

Other induction strategies that have been proposed, although not specifically studied in this setting, include treatment with other immunosuppressive drugs such as cladribine[35] and mitoxantrone.[36,37] The FDA has recently approved mitoxantrone for this indication. The adverse effects include nausea, myelosuppression, alopecia, menstrual dysfunction, amenorrhea, and cardiotoxicity. The usual dose suggested is $12\,mg/m^2$ and the drug is given typically every 3 months. The maximum cumulative dose recommended is $140\,mg/m^2$. Careful attention must be paid to avoid cumulative cardiotoxicity by baseline assessment and ongoing monitoring of cardiac function. Patients should have a cardiac reassessment including a measure of ejection fraction when a cumulative dose of $100\,mg/m^2$ is reached, and a significant reduction in ejection fraction or an ejection fraction of <50 percent should preclude further treatments. Preexisting cardiac disease, prior mediastinal radiotherapy, and other strong risk factors for cardiac disease are contraindications. Therefore, this drug seems to be an appropriate alternative to consider given its new official status in the United States.

More aggressive strategies have been attempted to achieve longer-term success in suppressing inflammatory disease activity. Stem cell transplantation has also been recently used in this setting and guidelines for its study have been published. The rationale is essentially the same as for cyclophosphamide, which has previously been advocated for patients with chronic progressive multiple sclerosis, namely to achieve rapid global immunosuppression.[38,39] Stem cell transplantation, particularly with T-cell depletion of the graft, may produce more profound and long-lasting immunosuppression, but the strategy is essentially similar to the strategy underlying other chemotherapeutic agents. There have been a limited number of publications on the results of this treatment, and all suffer from relatively short follow-up. However, pilot uncontrolled studies from both Greece ($n=23$),[40] the United States ($n=9$)[41] and Spain ($n=14$)[42]

suggest that patients with aggressive, rapidly worsening primary- or secondary-progressive MS can stabilize (and occasionally improve slightly) over follow-up periods of less than 2 years. The Greek results suggest a 78 percent response rate overall, but a low rate of response in primary-progressive MS. The 3-year progression-free survival is 92 percent for secondary-progressive MS and 39 percent for primary-progressive MS in the Greek study. The most optimistic findings from the American and Spanish studies are that follow-up MRI studies during followup of several years have not revealed new lesions, suggesting near-total suppression of the disease. It is not yet clear whether differences in patient selection and follow-up or methodology for ablation of the immune system and depletion of the graft explain the differences between these two series.

Controlled clinical trials have not been performed specifically targeting other demyelinating diseases such as neuromyelitis optica. However, there is a general impression that interferon beta, which is the standard drug utilized for prophylaxis of attacks of MS, is not very effective in the prophylaxis of attacks of neuromyelitis optica. For this condition, generalized immunosuppression has been suggested, largely on the basis of anecdotal clinical experience, to be the most effective agent; specifically, azathioprine combined with corticosteroids is considered the first drug of choice to suppress the disease when it is clear that continuing attacks are likely.[43]

■ The Pros and Cons

Is it important to achieve a definite diagnosis before initiating therapy, to the extent of proceeding to brain biopsy, or is empirical therapy reasonable?

Pros. In general, the more precise the diagnosis, the more clearly a prognosis can be given and the more appropriately can treatment be prescribed. An extreme example is the differentiation of glioma from tumefactive demyelination. The clinical principles discussed above (setting, symptoms, radiology, etc.) can be useful. Generally, IIDDs occur in healthy, young persons. Radiologically, demyelinating lesions are associated with relatively little mass effect; specific findings such as the open ring sign may be very helpful at suggesting

a demyelinating lesion. Nonetheless, unequivocal clinical differentiation between these diagnoses is often very difficult in the absence of biopsy evidence. Inappropriate treatment with radiotherapy may prove catastrophic in patients with demyelinating disease.[44]

Cons. The principal arguments against the use of brain or cord biopsy are the following: (1) significant morbidity resulting from the biopsy; (2) biopsy results, while perhaps increasing the precision of the diagnosis, often do not alter management; (3) brain biopsy samples may be misinterpreted and lead to inappropriate treatment.

In terms of the risk of biopsy, the morbidity from brain biopsy is low, typically in the range of 1 percent.[45] Patients for whom such biopsies are being considered have substantial neurological impairment, and one could reasonably argue that the small risk of biopsy is minuscule compared to the risk of missing adequate treatment. The major risk is cerebral hemorrhage, particularly with stereotactic biopsies. In the absence of coagulopathy, the risk is minimal, although one should carefully consider whether amyloid angiopathy is a plausible explanation for the clinical syndrome and whether it is suggested by the MRI scan (multiple foci of hemosiderin suggesting prior subclinical brain hemorrhage). Cord biopsy is considerably more difficult to accomplish without morbidity, as is brainstem biopsy, and greater discretion should be applied about the need for biopsies when the relevant lesions to be biopsied are intramedullary.

Neurologists discussing biopsy with a neurosurgeon are often rightfully asked to justify how biopsy might alter treatment. Whether the cause of an acute leukoencephalopathy is demyelinating, vasculitis, or sarcoidosis, corticosteroids are standard therapy. Regardless of the specific subtype of demyelinating disease, corticosteroids remain the primary first therapy. In fact, for patients failing corticosteroid therapy who have demyelinating disease, we recommend plasma exchange regardless of the specific subtype of demyelinating disease. Favorable responses seem to occur in patients with a variety of acute demyelinating diseases, though larger experience using plasma exchange for the spectrum of these acute diseases is necessary before one might reasonably conclude that there are no important differences in response between subtypes.

An empirical course of corticosteroid treatment can be justified for most patients even when the diagnosis is uncertain. While a favorable response clinically and radiologically is nonspecific and may occur even in the setting of glioma and lymphoma, the long-term course will usually answer the question. Empirical treatment with steroids is an appropriate approach unless the patient is rapidly deteriorating, has life-threatening complications (e.g., impending cerebral herniation), or deteriorates in the face of corticosteroid treatment or after stopping corticosteroid treatment. In those situations, biopsy for definitive diagnosis is most appropriate. For acute demyelinating diseases, a brief course of corticosteroids may induce a sustained remission, whereas for infiltrative corticosteroid-responsive conditions, such as sarcoidosis, or for vasculitis, prolonged corticosteroid therapy over months to years is typically necessary. In these conditions, there typically will be either no or a short-lived response to a brief course of high-dose corticosteroids.

Brain biopsy interpretation is difficult, particularly on limited samples. For some diseases, such as vasculitis, sampling bias may preclude a definitive diagnosis. However, even when a specific diagnosis is not possible, it is generally possible to exclude many diagnoses (e.g., neoplasia, granulomatous diseases, or infarction) and to suggest a certain category of diagnoses. For example, cerebral infarcts are occasionally detected when demyelinating disease is clinically suspected. When infarcts are detected on biopsy, the diagnostic approach often changes toward tests to rule out vasculopathies or vasculitis. Brain biopsies from patients with demyelinating disease are occasionally misinterpreted as showing glioma. However, in reviewing such cases, the diagnosis could have been appropriately made on the original specimen when reviewed by an experienced neuropathologist. The key findings on biopsy that indicate inflammatory demyelinating disease are the presence of histiocytes, characteristically absent in tumors, intimately admixed with reactive astrocytes. Certain findings in reactive astrocytes (e.g., clumped chromatin in "Creutzfeldt cells," which may be interpreted as mitotic figures) may lead to misdiagnosis as glioma.

In patients who fail corticosteroid therapy with acute severe demyelinating syndromes, what is the optimal therapy—plasma exchange or immunosuppression?

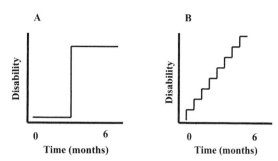

Figure 20-3. Classification of time course of fulminant demyelinating disease. (A) Acute severe attack, for which corticosteroids, if necessary, followed by plasma exchange, is the suggested treatment. (B) Stepwise progressive deterioration, for which immunosuppression is the preferred treatment approach.

Plasma Exchange. Plasma exchange is the only treatment that has been studied in a controlled phase II study specifically for this purpose. Plasma exchange has also independently been reported as effective in multiple anecdotal reports both preceding and following the controlled trial. It tends to work rapidly, and if benefit is going to occur, substantial improvement is usually evident within 3–5 treatments.

Immunosuppression. Many investigators feel that immunosuppression is an appropriate treatment for acute severe attacks based on anecdotal experience, though few reports exist that document acute improvement in this setting. Largely, the favorable experience with immunosuppression has occurred in patients with stepwise, relatively rapidly worsening multiple sclerosis. Figure 20-3 illustrates the two scenarios of rapidly worsening demyelinating disease. Plasma exchange is advised for the scenario in Figure 20-3A, and immunosuppression for the scenario in Figure 20-3B.

■ The Main Points

- Based on clinical features, the demographic characteristics, and the radiological findings, a reasonable hypothesis can be reached about the diagnosis of a patient with acute leukoencephalopathy or myelopathy.
- When it is unlikely that a patient has an inflammatory demyelinating disease, a thorough

evaluation for other etiologies is appropriate. If a specific clinical feature makes a specific diagnosis very likely, a more focused evaluation is possible and preferable.

- Consider an empirical trial of corticosteroids when inflammatory disorders are suspected. Rapidly achieved, sustained resolution of a lesion makes glioma quite unlikely and may avert the need for biopsy.
- When a patient is in dire condition, continues to deteriorate, or when steroid therapy fails, seriously consider biopsy of the brain. Reconsider if the only lesion is in the brainstem or the spinal cord.
- Do not expect definitive results from each biopsy. Biopsy may direct further investigations, i.e., pathology suggestive of infarct rather than demyelination may prompt further investigation for an underlying vasculopathy or vasculitis.
- Be aware of the pitfalls of incorrect diagnosis based on the biopsy.
- Consider plasma exchange for patients with severe deficits due to acute demyelinating disease who fail to respond to corticosteroids.
- Consider aggressive immunosuppression for patients with rapid stepwise worsening of an idiopathic inflammatory demyelinating disease.

■ References

1. Wingerchuk DM, Hogancamp WF, O'Brien PC, Weinshenker BG. The clinical course of neuromyelitis optica (Devic's syndrome). *Neurology* 1999;53: 1107–1114.
2. Lucchinetti CF, Mandler RN, McGavern D, et al. A role for humoral mechanisms in the pathogenesis of Devic's neuromyelitis optica. *Brain* 2002;125:1450–1461.
3. Krucke W. On the histopathology of acute hemorrhagic leukoencephalitis, acute disseminated encephalitis, and concentric sclerosis. *International Symposium on Aetiology and Pathogenesis of the Demyelinating Diseases*. 1973:11–27.
4. Marburg O. Die sogenannte "akute Multiple Sklerose." *J Psychiatric Neurol* 1906;27:211–312.
5. Storch MK, Piddlesden S, Haltia M, Livanainen M, Morgan P, Lassmann H. Multiple sclerosis: in situ evidence for antibody- and complement-mediated demyelination. *Ann Neurol* 1998;43:465–471.
6. Lucchinetti CF, Bruck W, Parisi J, Scheithauer B, Rodriguez M, Lassmann H. Heterogeneity of multiple sclerosis lesions: implications for the pathogenesis of demyelination. *Ann Neurol* 2000;47:707–717.
7. Balo J. Encephalitis periaxalis concentrica. *Arch Neurol* 1928;19:242–263.
8. Kastrup O, Stude P, Limmroth V. Balo's concentric sclerosis: evolution of active demyelination demonstrated by serial contrast-enhanced MRI. *J Neurol* 2002;249:811–814.
9. Kastrup O, Stude P, Limmroth V. Balo's concentric sclerosis demonstrated by contrast MRI. *Neurology* 2001;57:1610.
10. Karaarslan E, Altintas A, Senol U, et al. Balo's concentric sclerosis: clinical and radiologic features of five cases. *AJNR Am J Neuroradial* 2001;22: 1362–1367.
11. Louboutin J, Elie B. Treatment of Balo's concentric sclerosis with immunosuppressant drugs followed by multimodality evoked potentials and MRI. *Muscle Nerve* 1995;18:1478–1480.
12. Kesselring J, Miller DH, Robb SA, et al. Acute disseminated encephalomyelitis: MRI findings and the distinction from multiple sclerosis. *Brain* 1990; 113:291–302.
13. Hart M, Earle K. Haemorrhagic and perivenous encephalitis: a clinical-pathological review of 38 cases. *J Neurol Neurosurg Psychiatry* 1975;38:585–591.
14. Chau NV, Hien TT, Sellar R, Kneen R, Farrar JJ. "Can't you use another vaccine?" Postrabies vaccination encephalitis. *J Neurol Neurosurg Psychiatry* 1999;67:555–556.
15. Mandler RN, Davis LE, Jeffery DR, Kornfeld M. Devic's neuromyelitis optica: a clinicopathological study of 8 patients. *Ann Neurol* 1993;34:162–168.
16. Kinkel R. Methylprednisolone. In Rudick R, Goodkin D, eds. *Multiple Sclerosis Therapeutics*. London, Martin Dunitz, 1999:349–370.
17. Kurtzke JF, Beebe GW, Nagler B, Auth TL, Kurland LT, Nefzger MD. Studies on the natural history of multiple sclerosis. 7. Correlates of clinical change in an early bout. *Acta Neurol Scand* 1973;49:379–395.
18. Mendez MF, Pogacar S. Malignant monophasic multiple sclerosis or "Marburg's disease." *Neurology* 1988;38:1153–1155.
19. Johnson MD, Lavin P, Whetsell WO Jr. Fulminant monophasic multiple sclerosis, Marburg's type. *J Neurol Neurosurg Psychiatry* 1990;53:918–921.
20. Kalita J, Misra U, Mandal S. Prognostic indicators of acute transverse myelitis. *Acta Neurol Scand* 1998;98:60–63.
21. Weinshenker BG. Therapeutic plasma exchange for multiple sclerosis. In Rudick RA, Goodkin DE, eds. *Multiple Sclerosis Therapeutics*. London, Martin Dunitz, 1999:323–333.
22. Weiner HL, Dau PC, Khatri BO, et al. Double-blind study of true vs. sham plasma exchange in patients treated with immunosuppression for acute attacks of multiple sclerosis. *Neurology* 1989;39:1143–1149.

23. Rodriguez M, Karnes WE, Bartleson JD, Pineda AA. Plasmapheresis in acute episodes of fulminant CNS inflammatory demyelination. *Neurology* 1993;43: 1100–1104.

24. Weinshenker BG, O'Brien PC, Petterson TM, et al. A randomized trial of plasma exchange in acute central nervous system inflammatory demyelinating disease. *Ann Neurol* 1999;46:878–886.

25. Genain CP, Cannella B, Hauser SL, Raine CS. Identification of autoantibodies associated with myelin damage in multiple sclerosis. *Nature Med* 1999;5: 170–175.

26. Weinstein R. Therapeutic apheresis in neurological diseases. *J Clin Apheresis* 2000;15:74–128.

27. Rensel MR, Weinstock-Guttman B, Kinkel R, Rudick R, Jacobs L. Clinical experience with plasma exchange for severe relapse in patients with Devic's disease. *Neurology* 2000;54(Suppl 3):A23 (abstract).

28. Keegan M, Pineda AA, McClelland RL, Darby CH, Rodriguez M, Weinshenker BG. Plasma exchange for severe attacks of CNS demyelination: predictors of response. *Neurology* 2002;58:143–146.

29. Lublin FD, Reingold SC. Defining the clinical course of multiple sclerosis: results of an international survey. *Neurology* 1996;46:907–911.

30. McAlpine D, Compston N, Lumsden C. *Multiple Sclerosis*. Edinburgh, Livingstone, 1955.

31. Weinstock-Guttman B, Kinkel R, Cohen J, et al. Treatment of fulminant multiple sclerosis with intravenous cyclophosphamide. *Neurologist* 1997;3: 178–185.

32. Thompson AJ, Polman CH, Miller DH, et al. Primary progressive multiple sclerosis. *Brain* 1997;120: 1085–1096.

33. Khan OA, Zvartau-Hind M, Coan C, et al. Effect of monthly intravenous cyclophosphamide in rapidly deteriorating multiple sclerosis patients resistant to conventional therapy. *Multiple Sclerosis* 2001;7: 185–188.

34. Gobbini MI, Smith ME, Richert ND, Frank JA, McFarland HF. Effect of open label pulse cyclophosphamide therapy on MRI measures of disease activity in five patients with refractory relapsing-remitting multiple sclerosis. *J Neuroimmunol* 1999; 99:142–149.

35. Rice GPA, for the Cladribine Clinical Study Group, Filippi M, Comi G, for the Cladribine MRI Study Group. Cladribine and progressive MS: clinical and MRI outcomes of a multicenter controlled trial. *Neurology* 2000;54:1145–1155.

36. Edan G, Miller D, Clanet M, et al. Therapeutic effect of mitoxantrone combined with methylprednisolone in multiple sclerosis: a randomized multicenter study of active disease using MRI and clinical criteria. *J Neurol* 1997;62:112–118.

37. Hartung HP, Gonsette R, Konig N, et al. Mitoxantrone in progressive multiple sclerosis: a placebo-controlled, double-blind, randomised, multicentre trial. *Lancet* 2002;360:2018–2025.

38. Hauser SL, Dawson DM, Lehrich JR, et al. Intensive immunosuppression in progressive multiple sclerosis: a randomized, three-arm study of high-dose intravenous cyclophosphamide, plasma exchange, and ACTH. *N Engl J Med* 1983;308:173–180.

39. Carter JL, Hafler DA, Dawson DM, Orav J, Weiner HL. Immunosuppression with high-dose i.v. cyclophosphamide and ACTH in progressive multiple sclerosis: cumulative 6-year experience in 164 patients. *Neurology* 1988;38:9–14.

40. Fassas A, Anagnostopoulos A, Kazis A, et al. Autologous stem cell transplantation in progressive multiple sclerosis—an interim analysis of efficacy. *J Clin Immunol* 2000;20:24–30.

41. Burns W, Burt R. Hematopoietic stem cell transplantation. In Rudick R, Goodkin D, eds. *Multiple Sclerosis Therapeutics*. London, Martin Dunitz, 1999: 371–378.

42. Saiz A, Blanco Y, Carreras E, et al. Clinical and MRI outcome after autologous hematopoietic stem cell transplantation in MS. *Neurology* 2004;62:282–284.

43. Mandler RN, Ahmed W, Dencoff JE. Devic's neuromyelitis optica: a prospective study of seven patients treated with prednisone and azathioprine. *Neurology* 1998;51:1219–1220.

44. Peterson K, Rosenblum M, Powers J, Alvord E, Walker R, Posner J. Effect of brain irradiation on demyelinating lesions. *Neurology* 1993;43:2105–2112.

45. Davis DH, Kelly PJ, Marsh WR, Kall BA, Goerss SJ. Computer-assisted stereotactic biopsy of intracranial lesions. *Appl Neurophysiol* 1987;50:172–177.

Chapter 21

The Unstable Spine after Trauma

Aaron A. Cohen-Gadol, Cormac O. Maher,
and William E. Krauss

There are more than one million acute injuries to the spine each year in the United States with approximately 50,000 of these resulting in fractures to the bony spinal column.[1] In decreasing order, many injuries occur due to motor vehicle accidents, falls or diving, violence, and sport-related activities.[2] Under these circumstances, when patients are approached by bystanders or emergency medical services, the suspicion of spine injury should be very high. At the scene of accident, immobilization of the spine immediately has one of the highest priorities. Use of rigid backboards, cervical collars, and sandbags will immobilize the spine during transport. The improvements in spinal stabilization have possibly reduced the progression of incomplete spinal cord injuries to complete injury. Faster transport using helicopters has allowed a more timely management in the appropriate centers. This has decreased the percentage of patients with complete spinal cord injury (SCI) presenting to tertiary care facilities from 65 percent in the late 1960s to about 40 percent in the late 1990s. However, 10–25 percent of patients may still undergo additional damage from inadequate early immobilization.[3]

There is often a significant uncertainty about the definition of an "unstable spine." Lack of consensus has frequently complicated the discussion of whether or not a fracture needs further intervention. Generally, clinical spinal stability has been defined as "the ability of the spine under physiologic loads to maintain relationship between vertebrae, so that there is neither initial nor subsequent neurologic deficit, no major deformity, and no severe pain."[4]

Instability may not be evident from initial studies and a high index of suspicion is required, which is often based on recognition of certain fracture patterns.

This is a considerable unease with physicians—including trauma surgeons and neurologists—when a spine injury is suspected. This is a simple result of the complexity of radiological evaluation (so-called "clearing of the spine") and an instinctive distrust in any initial preliminary assessment. Certain viewing protocols are more reliable than random assessment of the radiological studies.[5] This chapter provides some of the essentials in spine evaluation after considerable trauma. It provides an update of current consensus among experts in this field.

■ The Patient

A 56-year-old male was brought to the emergency room department (ED) after a motor vehicle accident. He was an unrestrained driver who fell asleep while driving, steered off the road, and rolled over into a ditch. He did not remember the details of the accident. At the time of the ED admission, he was complaining of bilateral arm weakness and neck pain. Neurological examination was remarkable for bilateral arm weakness (left > right and proximal > distal). His sensory exam revealed decreased sensation in C5–T1 dermatome to pinprick. Reflexes in these distributions were slightly increased. The remaining neurological examination was unremarkable.

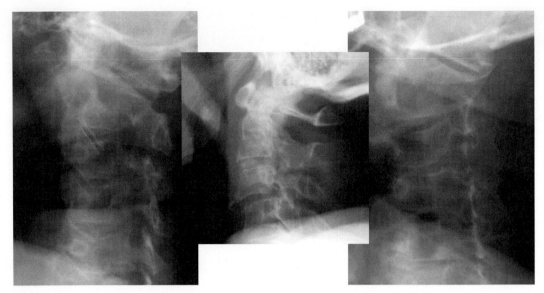

Figure 21-1. Cervical spine x-ray series (odontoid, lateral, and oblique views) demonstrated anterolisthesis (anterior dislocation) of C3 on C4 and unilateral (left) C3 on C4 locked facet.

Thorough evaluation by the trauma service did not demonstrate other injuries. A four-view (odontoid, lateral, and two oblique views) cervical spine x-ray series demonstrated anterolisthesis (anterior dislocation) of C3 on C4 and unilateral (left) C3 on C4 locked facet (Figure 21-1). There were also small, displaced fractures at the anterior superior corner of C4 and inferior corner of C4 vertebral bodies. A CT scan of the cervical spine with sagittal and coronal reconstructions additionally disclosed a unilateral locked left facet at C3 on C4 and left pedicle fractures at these levels. There was anterior vertebral body dislocation of C3 on C4 associated with 40 percent narrowing of the spinal canal (Figure 21-2).

The presence of the above neurological deficits and complex fractures prompted an MRI of the cervical spine to assess the degree of cord compression (suspected) due to disk fragments in the canal and to help estimate the extent of the posteriorligamentous injury. MRI revealed an extruded disk fragment causing moderate compression of the spinal cord. Increased T2-signal spinal cord changes were noted consistent with cord contusion (Figure 21-3).

After intravenous infusion of methylprednisolone, the patient was taken to the operating room emergently for removal of the anterior compressing disk fragment. Closed reduction of the locked facet was deferred since this maneuver may cause further spinal cord compression by "dragging" the extruded disk fragment posteriorly into the spinal canal, causing more neuronal injury. Following an anterior neck approach and disk removal, an instrumented fusion of the C3–4 levels was performed (Figures 21-4 and 21-5). Muscle strength improved postoperatively.

■ The Problem

- What x-ray views of the spine are adequate and when is further imaging (CT or MRI) indicated?
- What are surgical options for major types of bone and ligamentous injury?
- How can we additionally protect the spinal cord?

■ The Evidence

This case illustrates some of the important details in the management of cervical spine trauma associated with spinal cord injury. Closed reduction has to be considered with caution; and if neurological

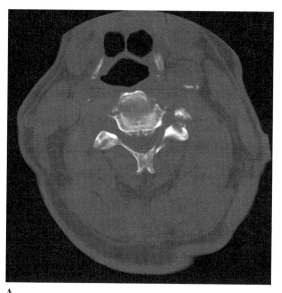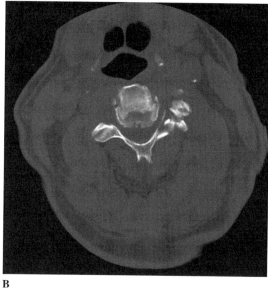

A   B

Figure 21-2. An axial CT scan of the cervical spine disclosed a unilateral locked left facet at C3 on C4 and left pedicle fractures at these levels. There was anterior vertebral body dislocation of C3 on C4 associated with 40 percent narrowing of the spinal canal.

deterioration is noted during or immediately after closed reduction, emergent MRI is necessary to exclude spinal cord compression. If such compression is discovered, decompressive surgery is urgently indicated. The choice of anterior, posterior, or circumferential stabilization procedure is often a matter of debate. If significant anterior and posterior spinal column disruption (bony or ligamentous) is present, circumferential stabilization procedures may be necessary. In selected cases, one may proceed with only an anterior or posterior fusion.

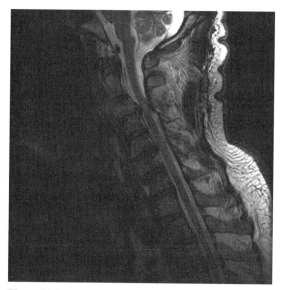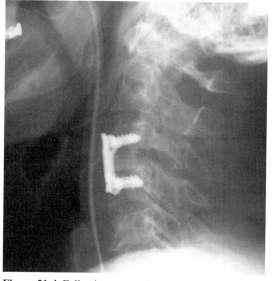

Figure 21-3. MRI verified an extruded disk fragment causing moderate compression of the spinal cord. Increased T2-signal spinal cord changes were noted consistent with cord contusion.

Figure 21-4. Following an anterior neck approach and disk removal, an instrumental fusion of the C3–4 levels was performed.

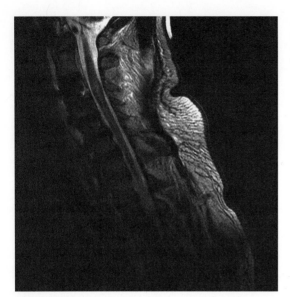

Figure 21-5. A postoperative MRI reveals adequate decompression.

In this case, the presence of the posterior arch (lamina and facet) fractures is another evidence for posterior ligamentous injury. However, since an anterior stabilization procedure was accomplished, he did not undergo a posterior fusion. The patient was regularly followed for early evidence of deformity by serial imaging.

Initial Evaluation in Emergency Department

Patients who are suspected to have a traumatic spine injury should be evaluated through a thorough neurological exam with special attention to posterior spine tenderness or stepoff. However, altered level of consciousness due to concurrent severe head injury or drug intoxication may limit the exam. Full spine precautions should be maintained. The patient may be turned using the log-roll technique. A thorough review of the mechanism of injury and symptoms noted at the time of injury is required. It is important to review interval changes in symptoms. These include the changes in neck or arm pain, motor, sensory, and bowel or bladder function since the trauma.

One should assume that early treatment of hypotension (systolic blood pressure less than 90 mmHg) could prevent secondary ischemic injury to the already compromised spinal cord. Trauma patients may be hypotensive due to dehydration or injury to other organs. Severe cord injury can decrease the sympathetic outflow from the CNS with peripheral vasodilatation or bradycardia further worsening this hypotensive state. This secondary insult to the injured cord due to hypoperfusion will affect spinal cord recovery. Therefore, a normotensive state must be maintained with an expeditious use of volume expanders or vasopressors. A vigilant search for the possible source of bleeding (mostly abdomen) should be undertaken.

Patients with a high cervical spinal cord injury, or severe head or chest trauma, may not ventilate adequately. Similarly, one should assume that severe hypoxia can exacerbate the spinal cord injury cascade and adversely affect the outcome, and early intubation may be necessary. The use of sedative drugs to control agitation in the acute period may cause hypotension or respiratory depression and therefore should be kept to a minimum.

Radiographic Evaluation

In cases of major trauma, a three-view cervical spine x-ray series (anteroposterior, lateral, and odontoid views) should be reviewed prior to obtaining axial imaging, obliques, or flexion/extension films. Lateral cervical spine x-ray must adequately evaluate the cervicothoracic junction. Oblique radiographs may add to the specificity of diagnosis. Inspection of the x-ray cervical films for rotational malalignment, offsets in the anterior body, dorsal body, or spinal laminar line are all critical (see Figure 21-4). Facet injuries can elude the inexperienced reviewer on the survey lateral cervical spine x-rays. Their recognition has been enhanced by the advent of computerized tomography (CT) using reconstruction views. Radiographic imaging, however, needs to be combined with clinical evaluation of the patient. Specifically, the posterior column needs to be assessed to avoid missed injuries. Facet injuries include a wide spectrum of ligamentous or osseous findings.

Widening of the spinous processes may be evident in unilateral and bilateral cervical facet injuries. The "bow-tie" sign seen in the lateral film is caused by visualization of both subluxed facets at the level of the injury.[6] Anterior subluxation of 3–5 mm (about 25 percent of vertebral body width) on lateral imaging is generally associated with unilateral facet dislocation. A displacement greater than 5–7 mm (about 50 percent) suggests bilateral facet dislocation. Facet fractures can be mobile and may reduce spontaneously in the supine position. Attention to the significant degree of soft tissue injury associated with these radiographic findings is critical.

Routine evaluation of the thoracolumbar spine is controversial. However, any localized tenderness or stepoff warrants imaging. Up to 5–30 percent of spine fractures are multiple and detection of one fracture requires radiographic evaluation of the entire spine. CT may be used to further investigate a suspicious finding or fracture pattern observed on plain x-rays. With its axial and three-dimensional capability to elucidate osseous anatomy, CT provides valuable data regarding treatment options. It also provides important information regarding operative decompression and selection of the appropriate instrumentation hardware for fracture fixation.

Magnetic resonance imaging (MRI) adds a superior visualization of the neural elements, disks, and ligaments in multiple planes.[7] It is typically conducted in a subacute setting to discern the cause of a neurological deficit, to detect a disc herniation, or to evaluate the integrity of posterior ligaments. Obviously, it is not a part of the routine emergency room evaluation, but it can provide information about timing and planning of surgical intervention. MRI may identify previously unrecognized unstable ligamentous injury and herniated disks that require emergency decompression.

The major vectors of force responsible for spine column injury are flexion, axial compression, extension, rotation, shear, distraction, or their combinations.[8] The history and complete imaging will help elucidate the true measure of the impact and the main vectors of force causing injury (Table 21-1). This will allow selection of proper interventions directed specifically at the disrupted elements.

Cervical Spine Injuries

Direct trauma, acceleration, or deceleration moments may briefly displace the cervical spine outside its normal range. Neurological injury may occur

Table 21-1. Trauma scenario suspicious for C-Spine Injury

Fall from ≥1 meter/5 stairs
Axial load to head (e.g., diving)
Motor vehicle high speed rollover, ejection
Motorized recreational vehicles
Bicycle collision
Hit by bus or truck
Hit by high-speed vehicle

Adapted from The Canadian C-spine rule for radiography in alert and stable trauma patients. *JAMA* 2001;286: 1841–1848.[9]

from the initial cord deformation or later instability. The initial force to the spine and resulting translation of bony elements into the canal and neural foramen may determine the neurological features. Trauma can also result in ligamentous disruption and instability, leading to progressive deformity. The premorbid dimensions of the spinal canal play an important role in the degree of neural injury after trauma. Patients with congenital narrow canals are at a greater risk of developing radiculopathy, myelopathy, or combinations even if the trauma was relatively trivial. Unilateral facet injuries may be difficult to recognize because they may present only as persistent neck pain without any obvious radiographic findings. Actually, delayed diagnosis of an asymptomatic unilateral cervical facet subluxation has occurred in up to 40 percent of patients.[10]

Trauma victims with cervical spine injuries should be managed with immobilization and closed reduction to attain anatomical alignment. Treatment will depend on the degree of neurological deficit and severity of the deformity. For example, closed reduction of dislocated facets provides the most expedient means to restore canal diameter and reverse ongoing cord compression. In a patient who has a complete or incomplete spinal cord injury, this should be done most expeditiously in the emergency room with the use of a halo or Gardner-Wells tongs. Initial manual in-line traction supplemented by weights starting at 5 to 10 lb is performed to provide axial traction in slight flexion without any attempt at rotation.

Weights are added incrementally with periodic reexamination of the patient clinically as well as radiographically. Reduction may require up to 10 lb per segment cephalad to the injury. For example, in a C5–6 bilateral facet dislocation, less than 50 lb of weight is often required. If at any time during closed reduction neurological deterioration occurs, emergent imaging is obtained. Closed reduction is indicated in an awake and alert patient whose neurological status is carefully monitored. Successful closed reduction may be followed with elective operative stabilization. Rizzolo et al. reported 40 percent and 80 percent rates of disc injury in unilateral and bilateral facet dislocations, respectively.[11] This high rate of disc injury becomes an important factor in the closed reduction of these injuries. The displaced disc may cause further narrowing of the canal during reduction under anesthesia. If closed reduction is considered in a patient with unreliable neurological examination, prereduction MRI may detect the presence of a displaced disc.

If closed reduction cannot be attained safely, open reduction with anterior diskectomy and fusion or posterior facetectomy and fusion may be considered. In this case, a preoperative MRI can exclude the presence of a ruptured disc. This prevents the above-mentioned neurological complication during intraoperative reduction of the anesthestized patient. An anterior decompressive procedure is considered if a ruptured disc is found on imaging.

Ligamentous Injuries

The principal ligaments injured in cervical trauma are interspinous or supraspinous ligaments, facet capsules, and occasionally the ligamentum flavum. These injuries are especially common in distractive flexion mechanisms of trauma. Posterior spine pain or tenderness is suggestive of this ligamentous disruption. Flexion x-rays may show evidence of spinous process divergence or vertebral body malalignment. These injuries tend to reduce spontaneously in extension.

A partial ligamentous disruption may be present when there is widening of the spinous processes on flexion/extension views and limited vertebral body translation of less than 3–5 mm. In these cases a course of nonoperative immobilization with a hard

collar may be initially attempted. The patient should be later reevaluated with flexion/extension films after a minimum of 8–12 weeks. If further instability or malalignment is noted, posterior fusion to reestablish the posterior tension band is warranted.

More severe ligamentous disruptions may result in unilateral or bilateral subluxed ("perched") facets. In the more common mechanism of distractive flexion, up to two-thirds of patients will present with neurologic deficits.[6] Detailed baseline neurological evaluation is followed by infusion of the methylprednisolone protocol in the setting of cord injury. Expeditious use of Gardner-Wells tongs for early closed reduction is also warranted.

When compared to bilateral facet dislocations, unilateral dislocations are less likely successfully treated with closed reduction. The rate of complete reduction in unilateral injuries has been as low as 25 percent.[10] On the other hand, bilateral facet injuries have been successfully reduced in up to 50–75 percent of cases.[12] This difference may be explained by several factors. Unilateral facet injuries tend to be diagnosed in a more delayed fashion than their bilateral counterparts, making closed reduction more problematic. Bilateral facet subluxations are associated with greater ligamentous disruptions, decreasing the resistance against which traction works to cause reduction.

Unilateral and bilateral facet subluxations are primarily ligamentous injuries. The inter/supraspinous ligaments and facet capsules are markedly disrupted in these cases. Attempts to maintain reduction in a halo have not been associated with an adequate success rate. Operative stabilization after closed reduction is strongly recommended.

Thoracic and Lumbar Fractures

Approximately 15,000 major thoracolumbar injuries occur annually in the United States, and 15–20 percent of these have neurological deficits, most commonly at T12–L1.[13,14] The Denis three-column model has been commonly used for the evaluation of instability in thoracolumbar fractures. In this model the columns are defined as *anterior*, composed of anterior longitudinal ligament, anterior

Table 21-2. Column Failure in Four Common Types of Major Thoracolumbar Fractures[13]

Fracture Type	Anterior Column	Middle Column	Posterior Column
Compression	Compression	Intact	Intact, or distraction if severe
Burst	Compression	Compression	Intact
Seat belt (Chance fracture)	Intact or mild compression	Distraction	Distraction
Fracture dislocation	Compression, rotation, shear	Distraction, rotation, shear	Distraction, rotation, shear

half of the disc, and vertebral body; *middle*, includes posterior longitudinal ligament, posterior half of vertebral body, and disc; and *posterior*, consisting of facets, posterior bony arch, and posterior ligaments (Table 21-2).

Injuries to the posterior column alone may not cause instability. However, significant injury to two or more columns is associated with instability. This instability may cause further neurological deficits or progressive deformity and warrants thorough evaluation by a spine surgeon for stabilization. Surgical indications for treatment of thoracic and lumbar fractures are controversial since few prospective studies of different modalities have been performed. The goals of surgery are to provide a functional alignment of the spine, to maximize neurological recovery, and to allow early patient mobility. Nonsurgical treatment is indicated for many of the compression fractures, burst fractures with no change in neurologic findings and some cases of Chance (seat belt) fractures.[15]

Compression fractures of the upper lumbar spine typically occur in elderly patients with profound osteoporosis, or may be the first presenting symptom of a metastatic disease. Anterior compression fractures are caused by axial loading in flexion. If the anterior loss of vertebral body is less than 50 percent and there is no significant deformity (<11° angulation at the injury site), these fractures are generally treated in a thoracolumbosacral orthosis. This is a single-column injury, and patients are typically neurologically intact. However, if the anterior height loss is more than 50 percent, the likelihood of concurrent posterior column injury is significant.[16] Surgical treatment may be considered if kyphosis at the fracture level is more than 40°, multiple contiguous compression fractures are evident and overall kyphosis of more than 60°, or if deformity is progressive.

Axial loading with or without flexion or extension components may cause anterior and middle column injuries; this is commonly referred to as a burst fracture. The retropulsed fractures may enter the canal producing variable degrees of neurological findings. Up to half of these patients present with significant neurological deficits. These injuries may require operative fixation. The rib cage provides additional elements of stability for thoracic spine fractures, and the Denis three-column model utilized for lumbar fractures may not adequately explain instability in these cases.

A lap belt may act as a fulcrum during high-speed automobile deceleration accidents, causing hyperflexion injury and tension failure of the upper lumbar spine.[17] This is known as a Chance fracture.[18] The fracture proceeds from the anterior to posterior direction, involving all three columns. This mechanism of trauma with its variable disruption of osseous and ligamentous structures can cause vertebral body translation, resulting in a very unstable fracture.[19] Concurrent intra-abdominal injuries must be ruled out. As a guideline, purely osseous injuries may heal in a brace; however, ligamentous injuries do not and require operative intervention.

Failure of all three columns as a result of compression, tension, rotation, or shear forces can cause the most unstable injury pattern, a fracture dislocation. This fracture pattern is frequently accompanied by significant neurological findings and operative stabilization is indicated.

In some poorly classified fractures it remains uncertain if they are stable or unstable; in such cases, the treatment plan is arbitrary and the problems of prolonged recumbency and hospitalization costs must be weighed against the risks associated with major spine surgery.

The surgical approach in thoracolumbar and other spinal fractures is controversial and is affected by factors such as mechanism of injury, fracture pattern, extent of bony and ligamentous injury, level of injury, presence of neurological deficits, other associated injuries, surgical approach, and perhaps also surgeon's experience, and type of instrumentation. Application of posterior instrumentation often "reverses" the mechanism of injury. Utilization of pedicle screws, a hook-rod, or a hybrid of these will cause distraction and allow immobilization of the affected segments to facilitate bony fusion. Any instrumentation will fail with time if solid fusion does not form. Vertebrectomy and diskectomy will allow anterior decompression of the spinal cord. Strut grafting with placement of an anterior plate in these cases will restore the alignment of the spine, especially in the case of burst fractures. Some of the more unstable injuries (three-column) may require a combined anterior and posterior approach for adequate stabilization.

Gunshot Wounds to the Spine

Upon admission, patients with gunshot wound to their spine should receive broad-spectrum antibiotics and tetanus prophylaxis. In cases with cord symptoms, methylprednisolone is considered. Coexisting abdominal injuries take precedence. Patients with SCI may not complain of their intra-abdominal injuries and a high index of suspicion is required.

Gunshot wounds to the spine by civilian handguns create a direct injury from the bullet. On the other hand, military weapons in addition create extensive injury by shock waves and cavitation. For this reason, civilian injuries often do not cause instability requiring stabilization procedures.[20] Decompression and removal of the bullet from the spinal canal is controversial. Available studies have shown contradictory results regarding surgical treatment of these cases.[21-24] Evidence of a persistent CSF leak and deteriorating neurological exam are indications for surgical exploration.

■ The Pros and Cons

Important quandaries are how and when to protect or decompress the spinal cord. The pharmacological treatment options for acute spinal cord injury have been tested and include two corticosteroids (methylprednisolone and trilizad mesylate), naloxone, and GM1 ganglioside. These drugs may have the potential to maintain integrity of the blood-spinal cord barrier, therefore reducing vasogenic edema, increasing blood flow, and most importantly decreasing inflammatory response to injury.[25] However, the precise mechanisms of action of these agents remain incompletely elucidated.

In the acute setting, evidence of spinal cord trauma may merit the use of methylprednisolone. As recommended after the results of the third National Acute Spinal Cord Injury Study (NASCIS III) became available, methylprednisolone is given as a bolus of 30 mg/kg body weight over 15 minutes followed by a drip at 5.4 mg/kg/hr for the subsequent 23 hours for patients who receive methylprednisolone bolus within 3 hours of injury. When the protocol is initiated 3 to 8 hours after injury, infusion should continue for 48 hours.[26]

However, the first National Acute Spinal Cord Injury Study (NASCIS I)[27] reported no difference in motor or sensory outcome between the two groups treated with low but different doses of methylprednisolone at one-year follow-up.[28] A multicenter NASCIS II trial compared a much higher dose of methylprednisolone (30 mg/kg as a bolus and then 5.4 mg/kg/hr infusion for 23 hours) with naloxone or placebo. This study demonstrated significant improvement in the motor function at 6-month follow-up associated with the administration of methylprednisolone within 8 hours of injury.[29] The one-year follow-up of the patients in this report also revealed improvement in motor scores.[30] However, the one-year follow-up results of the NASCIS III trial demonstrated no significant difference in functional outcome in any treatment group.[26] Thus, significant clinical benefit from the administration of methylprednisolone after acute spinal cord injury has not been conclusively demonstrated despite its widespread use. In fact, a recent appraisal of the members of the committee of the Canadian Spine Society and Canadian Neurological Society clearly expressed the view that the use of methylprednisolone after acute spinal cord injury was not the standard of care.[31] In addition, risk of sepsis, pneumonia and hyperglycemia was cited.[31] Whether methylprednisolone should be used to treat acute SCI, remains unresolved and debatable.

Another controversial issue surrounds relief of spinal cord compression. Improvement of long-term neurological and functional outcome has been claimed. The most appropriate timing of decompressive surgery is not known and is influenced by the neurological status of the patient and severity of the associated injuries.

Timely spinal cord decompression in animal models has enhanced the potential for neurological recovery.[32,33] Obviously, such models may not reproduce the same conditions that occur in human spinal trauma. However, there is evidence for neurological recovery among patients with neurological deficits who underwent early decompressive surgery.[34,35] But there are other conflicting studies, and randomized, controlled human trials have not been performed. Some authors have demonstrated a higher rate of delayed neurological deterioration among patients with acute spinal cord injury who underwent surgery early and therefore recommended delayed surgery.[36] Others have recommended surgery as soon as possible (within 1–3 days post-injury) with the understanding that there is no evidence to support any of these approaches.

Generally, other life-threatening injuries are managed first and urgent spine surgery is considered when the patient is deemed stable for a long procedure. Urgent spine surgery is usually performed within 48 hours of injury. There is no proven evidence that early surgery alters the neurological deficit of a patient with complete cord injury.[37] We feel that the only accepted indication for emergent decompressive surgery is progressive neurological deterioration, which may occur in about 1–2 percent of patients with thoracolumbar fractures.[38,39]

■ The Main Points

- The role of steroids in the treatment of acute spinal cord injury remains unsettled and significant functional recovery has not been consistently documented.
- Early relief of cord compression is controversial, and the best timing of decompressive surgery is not well established.
- For cervical fractures, closed reduction has to be considered with caution. If neurological deterioration is noted during or immediately after closed reduction, emergent MRI is necessary to document spinal cord compression. Emergent decompressive surgery is then indicated.
- The choice of anterior, posterior, or circumferential stabilization procedure is often based on the surgeon's preference. If significant anterior and posterior spinal column disruption (bony or ligamentous) is present, circumferential stabilization procedures may be necessary.
- Isolated osseous fractures may heal well with adequate immobilization, but ligamentous injuries typically require open surgery.
- Unilateral and bilateral facet subluxations are primarily ligamentous injuries, and in those cases inter/supraspinous ligaments and facet capsules are markedly disrupted. Attempts to maintain reduction with a halo are inefficient, and operative stabilization after closed reduction is needed.
- For lumbar fractures, injuries to posterior elements alone may not cause instability. More significant injury may be associated with instability and subsequent deformity.

■ References

1. Connelly P, Abitol J, Martin R. *Spine Trauma*. Rosemont, IL, American Academy of Orthopedic Surgeons, 1997.
2. Henson S. *Spinal Trauma*. American Association of Neurological Surgeons, 1998.
3. Amar P, Levy M. Contemporary management of spinal cord injury. *Contemp Neurosurg* 23, 2001.
4. White A, Panjabi M. *Clinical Biomechanics of the Spine*, 2nd ed. Philadelphia, JB Lippincott, 1990.
5. Bandiera G, Stiell IG, Wells GA, Clement C, De Maio V, Vandemhenn KL, Greenberg GH, Lesiuk H, Brison R, Cass D, Dreyer J, Eisenhauer MA, Macphail I, McKnight RD, Morrison L, Reardon M, Schull M, Worthington J; Canadian C-Spine and CT Head Study Group. The Canadian C-spine rule performs better than unstructured physician judgment. *Ann Emerg Med* 2003;42:395–402.
6. Andreshak J, Dekutoski M. Management of unilateral facet dislocations: a review of the literature. *Orthopedics* 1997;20:917–926.
7. Haba H, Taneichi H, Kotani Y, Terae S, Abe S, Yoshikawa H, Abumi K, Minami A, Kaneda K. Diagnostic accuracy of magnetic resonance imaging for detecting posterior ligamentous complex injury associated with thoracic and lumbar fractures. *J Neurosurg* 2003;99(1 Suppl):20–26.

8. Eismont F, Garfin S, Abitol J. *Thoracic and Lumbar Spine Injuries*. Philadelphia, WB Saunders, 1987.

9. The Canadian C-spine rule for radiography in alert and stable trauma patients. *JAMA* 2001;286:1841–1848.

10. Rorabeck C, Rock M, Hawkins R. Unilateral facet dislocation of the cervical spine: an analysis of the results of treatment in 26 patients. *Spine* 1987;12:23–27.

11. Rizzolo SJ, Piazza MR, Cotler JM, Balderston RA, Schaefer D, Flanders A. Intervertebral disc injury complicating cervical spine trauma. *Spine* 1991;16 (6 Suppl):S187–189.

12. Sonntag V. Management of bilateral locked facets of the cervical spine. *Neurosurgery* 1981;8:150–152.

13. Denis F. The three column spine and its significance in the classification of acute thoracolumbar spine injuries. *Spine* 1983;8:817–831.

14. Riggins R, Kraus J. The risk of neurological damage with fractures of the vertebrae. *J Trauma* 1977;17:126.

15. Anderson P. Nonsurgical treatment of patients with thoracolumbar fractures. *Instr Course Lect* 1995; 44:57.

16. Maiman D, Pintar F. Anatomy and clinical biomechanics of the thoracic spine. *Clin Neurosurg* 1992; 38:296–324.

17. Anderson P, Henley M, Rivara F, Maier RV. Flexion-distraction and Chance injuries to the lumbosacral spine. *J Orthop Trauma* 1991;5:153–160.

18. Chance C. Note on a type of flexion fracture of the spine. *Br J Radiol* 1948;21:452–453.

19. Triantafyllou S, Bertzbein S. Flexion distraction injuries of the thoracolumbar spine: a review. *Orthopedics* 1992;15:357–363.

20. Meyer P, Apple O, Bahlman, HH. Symposium: Management of fractures of thoracolumbar spine. *Contemp Orthop* 1989;16:57–86.

21. Benzel E, Hadden T, Coleman J. Civilian gunshot wounds to the spinal cord and cauda equina. *Neurosurgery* 1987;20:181–185.

22. Heiden J, Weiss M, Rosenberg A. Penetrating gunshot wounds of the cervical spine in civilians: a review of 38 cases. *J Neurosurg* 1975;42:575–579.

23. Stauffer E, Wood R, Kelly E. Gunshot wounds of the spine: the effects of laminectomy. *J Bone Joint Surg Am* 1982;61:1244–1245.

24. Venger B, Simpson R, Narayan R. Neurosurgical intervention in penetrating spinal trauma with associated visceral injury. *J Neurosurg* 1989;70:514–518.

25. Amar P, Levy M. Pathogenesis and pharmacological strategies for mitigating secondary damage in acute spinal cord injury. *Neurosurgery* 1999; 44:1027–1040.

26. Bracken M, Shepard M, Holford T, Leo-Summers L, Aldrich EF, Fazl M, Fehlings MG, Herr DL, Hitchon PW, Marshall LF, Nockels RP, Pascale V, Perot PL Jr, Piepmeier J, Sonntag VK, Wagner F, Wilberger JE, Winn HR, Young W. Methylprednisolone or tirilazad mesylate administration after acute spinal cord injury: 1-year follow-up. Results of the Third National Acute Spinal Cord Injury Randomized Controlled Trial. *J Neurosurg* 1998;89:699–706.

27. Bracken M, Collins W, Freeman D, Shepard MJ, Wagner FW, Silten RM, Hellenbrand KG, Ransohoff J, Hunt WE, Perot PL Jr, et al. Efficacy of methylprednisolone in acute spinal cord injury. *JAMA* 1984; 251:45–52.

28. Bracken M, Shepard M, Hellenbrand K, Collins WF, Leo LS, Freeman DF, Wagner FC, Flamm ES, Eisenberg HM, Goodman JH, et al. Methylprednisolone and neurological function 1 year after spinal cord injury. Results of the National Acute Spinal Cord Injury Study. *J Neurosurg* 1985;63:704–713.

29. Bracken M, Shepard M, Collins W, Holford TR, Young W, Baskin DS, Eisenberg HM, Flamm, E. Leo-Summers L, Maroon J, et al. A randomized-controlled trial of methylprednisolone or naloxone in the treatment of acute spinal cord injury. Results of the Second National Acute Spinal Cord Injury Study (NASCIS-2). *N Engl J Med* 1990;322:1405–1411.

30. Bracken M, Shepard M, Collins W Jr, Holford TR, Baskin DS, Eisenberg HM, Flamm E, Leo-Summers L, Maroon JC, Marshall LF, et al. Methylprednisolone or naloxone treatment after acute spinal cord injury: 1-year follow-up data. Results of the Second National Acute Spinal Cord Injury Study. *J Neurosurg* 1992;76:23–31.

31. Hugenholtz H, Cass DE, Dvorak MF, Fewer DH, Fox RJ, Izukawa DM, Lexchin J, Tuli S, Bharatwal N, Short C. High-dose methylprednisolone for acute closed spinal cord injury—only a treatment option. *Can J Neurol Sci* 2002;29:227–235.

32. Bohlmann H, Bahniuk E, Raskulinecz G. Mechanical factors affecting recovery from incomplete cervical cord injury: a preliminary report. *Johns Hopkins Med J* 1979;145:115.

33. Delamarter R, Bohlmann H, Dodge L. Experimental lumar spinal stenosis: analysis of cortical evoked potentials, microvasculature, and histopathology. *J Bone Joint Surg Am* 1990;72:110.

34. Clohisy Y, Behooz A, Bucholz R. Neurologic recovery associated with anterior decompression of spine fractures at the thoracolumbar junction (T12–L1). *Spine* 1992;17(Suppl):S325.

35. Krengel W, Anderson P, Henley M. Early stabilization and decompression for incomplete paraplegia due to a thoracic-level spinal cord injury. *Spine* 1993;18:2080.

36. Marshall L, Knowlton S, Garfin S. Deterioration after spinal cord injury: a multicenter study. *J Neurosurg* 1987;66:400.

37. Bohlmann H, Freehafer A, Dejak J. The results of treatment of acute injuries of the upper thoracic spine with paralysis. *J Bone Joint Surg Am* 1985;6:360.

38. Chapman J, Anderson P. Thoracolumbar spine fractures with neurological deficit. *Orthop Clin North Am* 1994;25:595–612.

39. Spivak J, Vaccaro A, Colter J. Thoracolumbar spine trauma. II. Principles of management. *J Am Acad Orthop Surg* 1995;3:353.

Chapter 22

The Clinical Diversity of Traumatic Head Injury

Lawrence F. Marshall and Henry E. Aryan

The advances in neurotraumatology brought about by the ability to image the brain, monitor its function, and respond to increased intracranial pressure have altered the management of patients with traumatic head injury. But as a result of these opportunities, a whole host of potentially new quandaries have been introduced into specific aspects of the management of these patients. However, traumatic brain injury represents a spectrum of disease with widely varying outcomes. Primarily, comatose patients after traumatic brain injury are likely to suffer persistent functional deficits. But for many others less affected by the initial impact to the brain, the predominant sequelae pertain to the problematic and ambiguous domain of cognitive and behavioral disorders. The decision-making with regard to early intervention for cortical contusions and intracerebral hemorrhages is also very complex and often open to question.

In comatose patients with devastatingly severe brain injuries, the role of early decompressive surgery, hyperventilation, and cerebral perfusion pressure-directed therapy are controversial and represent vigorously debated areas despite the appearance of an emerging consensus from a number of expert groups. The answers to these many questions can only come from further well-orchestrated, comparative clinical trials in large numbers of more or less homogeneous groups of patients. None of these are available or even remotely planned at present.

Patients with head injury are routinely classified with regard to severity using the Glasgow Coma Scale (GCS) (see Chapter 1) as mild, minor, moderate, and severe. It is appropriate to examine these categories first. Also, it is important to emphasize that the most challenging problem is a patient who appears not to be severely injured initially, but in whom additional information (e.g., neuroimaging) suggests grave risk of worsening and additional morbidity. (This was succinctly noted by Klauber and associates 15 years ago.[1]) These cases present a major management dilemma due to the often unclear balance between the benefit from surgical intervention to prevent neurological deterioration and the risk of further brain damage that may be caused by the surgery itself. In this chapter, we shall illustrate these dilemmas and present some of the major controversies. The use of hyperventilation, osmotic diuretics, and corticosteroids has been discussed in Chapter 8.

■ The Patient

Case 1. A child was brought to the emergency department by his parents after falling from a skateboard. He presented with a GCS score of 13. CT scan initially showed a small extradural hematoma (Figure 22-1A). Routine laboratory studies were ordered, including coagulation studies. Based on the CT scan results, the neurosurgeon

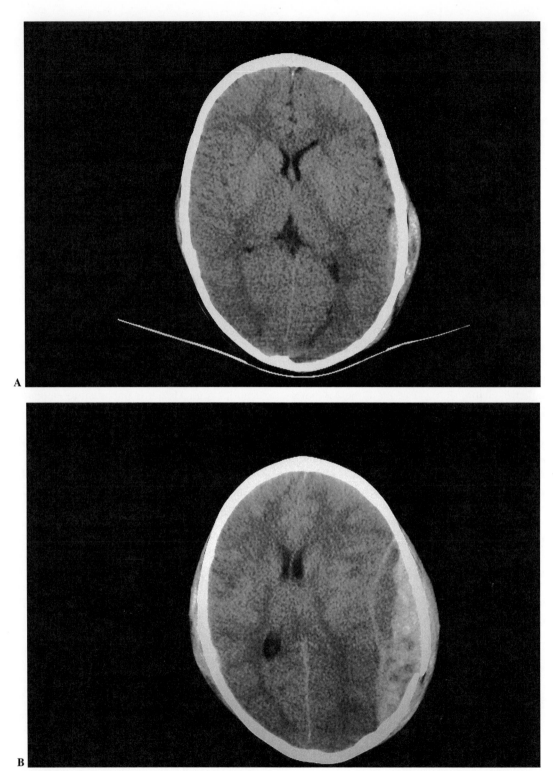

Figure 22-1. (A) CT scan of the head showing epidural hematoma in a child. (B) Repeat CT scan of the head showing substantial increase in the size of the epidural hematoma. (Note hyperlucent areas indicating ongoing bleeding)

decided to admit and observe the child. Several hours later, however, the child deteriorated clinically and underwent an emergent second CT scan. This study demonstrated a much larger extradural hematoma (Figure 22-1B). Surprisingly, the INR was greater than 3 but for some reason it was reported late to the clinicians caring for the child. By the time the abnormality was recognized and treatment initiated, the clot had expanded leading to catastrophic and long-term brain damage.

Case 2. A 29-year-old man traveling at a speed of approximately 40 miles/hour was involved in a motorcycle crash. He was not wearing a helmet at the time of the accident. The patient was evacuated by helicopter to the emergency room at a regional level I trauma center. On admission he was withdrawing to pain, without eye opening or moaning. Both pupils were 4 mm and reactive to light. He was intubated for airway protection. He had a mild left-sided hemiparesis but was difficult to assess because he was sedated and paralyzed at the time of intubation prior to the arrival of the neurosurgeon. An emergency CT scan of the head demonstrated a right frontotemporal contusion with horizontal shift (Figure 22-2A). The neurosurgeon requested to hyperventilate the patient to drive the $PaCO_2$ down to a level of 30–34 mmHg, but the emergency room physician, having read recent guidelines indicating that "hyperventilation is harmful to patients with severe brain injury," refused.[2,3] The flabbergasted neurosurgeon immediately transferred the patient to the neurosurgical intensive care unit (ICU) where he initiated hyperventilation. An intracranial pressure (ICP) monitor was placed and the initial ICP ranged between 15 and 20 mmHg. The neurosurgical resident suggested surgical evacuation because "this pressure was too high for a patient with a temporal lobe lesion."[4] The attending neurosurgeon countered that, because they had managed to control the ICP below 20 mmHg with hyperventilation and mannitol, operation would be necessary only if the pupils changed. The attending neurosurgeon also indicated that he wanted the mean arterial blood pressure to be greater than 90 mmHg and that the patient should be "cooled as per the recommendation of Clifton's group."[5]

Using albumin and substantial quantities of saline along with a vasopressor, the intravascular volume was expanded and temperature was reduced to 34°C. Twelve hours after admission the ICP was fluctuating between 20 and 25 mmHg, and a repeat CT scan was obtained. The intracranial hematoma had doubled in size, with a midline shift of 6 mm (Figure 22-2B). The neurosurgical attending was called but again instructed the resident to hold off surgical intervention until changes in the pupil size and light response became apparent. In addition, he recommended that the mean arterial pressure be raised further with the use of pressors aiming at a mean arterial pressure of at least 100–110 mmHg. The resident, while unhappy with the decision, reluctantly followed the attending's instructions. Two hours later the patient developed acute uncal herniation signs (see Chapter 1). The patient was rushed to the operating room for evacuation of his hematoma, resulting in a postoperative reduction of ICP. However, the patient exhibited postoperative extensor posturing and 3 months post injury remains in a minimally conscious state.

■ The Problem

- What are the major differences of opinion with regard to comprehensive management of severe head injury?
- What are the criteria for surgical intervention and which patients need a high level of surveillance?
- What are the main causes of deterioration in patients with initially normal consciousness?

■ The Evidence

Patients with head injury can be arbitrarily separated into four categories: mild for those with an admission GCS score of 15, minor for those with an admission GCS score of 13–14, moderate with an admission GCS of 9–12, and severe for patients with a GCS score from 8 to 3. This is a workable classification given that the frequency of deterioration and long-term sequelae is much lower in patients who are awake and have a GCS score of 15.

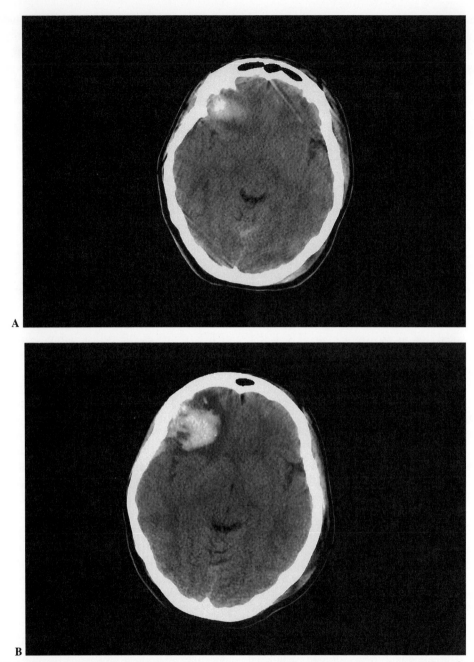

Figure 22-2. (A) CT scan of the head showing right frontotemporal contusion measuring approximately 12 cm^3 with a right to left shift of approximately 3–4 mm. (B) Repeat CT scan of head showing intracranial hematoma now larger, with midline shift of 6 mm and clot now measuring approximately 25 cm^3.

The population of patients with a minor head injury and a GCS score of 13–14 is of particular concern because CT abnormalities are not that uncommon, and approximately 10 percent of these patients will deteriorate.[6] However, given the initial clinical absence of significant structural brain damage, a neurosurgeon would understandably prefer to intervene before these patients deteriorate and thus suffer irreversible damage from an expanding hematoma. In case 1 a significant coagulation abnormality was not recognized. More stringent surveillance and the administration of fresh frozen plasma might have led to earlier intervention and a better long-term outcome.

The risk of sequelae for patients with moderately severe brain injury, defined as admission GCS score of 9–12, has been grossly underestimated. The need for very close observation and, often, surgical intervention in such patients has been generally unrecognized. The biphasic clinical course of initial improvement followed by deterioration (even resulting in brain death as an all too common occurrence) is well appreciated by experienced neurosurgeons. These patients obviously have severe injuries, and many of them have been categorized separately and are now best known as the "talk and deteriorate" category.[7] In these patients with moderately severe injury, deterioration is usually secondary to expansion of a cortical contusion or intraparenchymal hemorrhage. There is much to be said for the argument that a high level of surveillance combined with established criteria for surgical intervention may make it possible to operate on many of these patients before further irreversible brain damage develops.

Some of these concerns have been recognized, and the Brain Trauma Foundation[2,3] and the European Brain Injury Consortium[8] have specifically developed standardized protocols for the care of these patients.

Neurocognitive and behavioral sequelae can occur in the absence of loss of consciousness and are age-related.[9] Persistent neurocognitive sequelae are exceedingly rare in teenagers with head injury and no loss of consciousness; but in elderly patients, these symptoms are not infrequently (5–10 percent) elicited by history and confirmed by neurocognitive testing one year or more following their injury.[10] It is therefore important for the clinician to appreciate that the patient's age and not only the presence or absence of loss of consciousness or the length of post-traumatic amnesia are important predictive factors of cognitive sequelae. Depression clearly affects cognitive function and, while in this population it is unlikely that the depression is secondary to direct tissue injury, it nevertheless can complicate assessment. In some patients with persistent neurobehavioral symptoms, not only the circumstances of the accident must be well understood but also a history of prior symptoms of depression should be investigated. The term "postconcussive syndrome" has been used for these symptoms, but there are major uncertainties surrounding this designation, and it is shrouded by compensation claims with unclear evidence of its relevance. Some studies have noted development of brain atrophy.[11] A comprehensive discussion is outside the scope of this monograph of acute neurology, but excellent reviews on this topic can be found in the literature.[12,13]

Mild Head Injury

If one separates alert patients with a GCS of 15 from those with GCS scores of 13–14, one has identified a patient group in which there is the least likelihood of acute deterioration (best estimates being less than 1/1000). The signs and symptoms in these patients are primarily due to the primary brain injury.

Even in this group of patients, it is a challenge to distinguish patients who truly have sequelae from their brain injury weeks or months after the injury from those who malinger or have symptom exaggeration. Headache is not infrequent in the first few months but is much less common (<5 percent) at one year. Persistent headache should suggest the possibility of a preexisting condition, such as migraine, or that the complaint has no clear structural basis.

Minor Head Injury

It has been argued that classifying patients with a GCS scale score of 13–14 separately from those patients with a GCS of 15 is reasonable because they have a much greater likelihood of having suffered parenchymal damage and of developing long-term sequelae. This separation somewhat serves to illustrate the spectrum of traumatic brain injury. There are dramatic differences in outcome between these patients and those who have a GCS score of less than 8. Nonetheless, one must anticipate the overlapping nature of clinical outcomes in patients with similar but not identical GCS scores.

In patients with minor head injury, post-traumatic symptoms include difficulties with recent memory and concentration, and these deficits are more frequent and persistent than in patients with mild head injury. In a landmark study of patients with minor traumatic brain injury with no evidence of structural brain damage and hospitalized for a minimum of 24 hours, Levin and colleagues[14] described sequelae over the first several months. Over 50 percent of the patients had evidence of residual dysfunction in one or more cognitive domains. A small group, which Levin et al.[14] termed the "miserable minority," had cognitive sequelae for years. Such symptomatology is not limited to the domains of recent memory, attention, and concentration. Patients may also have behavioral sequelae that interfere with married life, interactions with children, and particularly stress in the workplace.

Profound behavioral problems, particularly impatience and intemperate outbursts, are also more common than in patients with mild injury. Depression is not at all uncommon and in patients with minor head injury it may in part reflect structural tissue injury, with microscopic brain damage to regions involved in mood control. Overall recovery takes longer when compared with mild head injury. The likelihood of long-term sequelae is not insubstantial, although the great majority eventually recover to their premorbid state. Despite these facts, the currently used classification in the literature of mild and minor head injury is often problematic and perhaps misleading. For most clinicians, it may be impossible to strictly define clear boundaries between these two categories.

Moderate and Severe Head Injury

Moderate head injury occurs in approximately 10 percent of all patients suffering head injury and affects disproportionately the older members of society.[15] It has been demonstrated that 40 percent of patients with moderate head injury over 60 years of age were in nursing care facilities 3 months or more after their injuries, indicating the substantial disability caused by these injuries in the elderly population.[15] Some of these patients will require surgical intervention for intracranial hematomas. Patients with coagulation disturbances are particularly at risk, although this can also be a consequence of injury itself because brain tissue is rich in thromboplastin, resulting in a cascade which ultimately produces disseminated intravascular coagulopathy. An aggressive search for clotting abnormalities must be carried out and when such abnormalities are present, they must be immediately corrected.[16]

The presence of an intracranial hematoma on the initial CT scan is an important predictor of clinical deterioration. If a sizable clot is in the epidural space or in the brain parenchyma, there is a 1 in 10 chance that these lesions will expand. However, small acute subdural hematomas rarely expand and usually disappear on follow-up scanning.[16]

Patients with intracerebral hemorrhages in the dominant hemisphere are perhaps the most challenging as a group. Neurosurgeons are reluctant to operate on patients with posterior frontal and temporal lobe hematomas who, despite a considerable risk of herniation, may develop additional surgical damage to language centers. In these cases, the neurosurgeon is often tempted to operate if there is mass effect, but frequently delays surgery for fear of producing more brain damage. Obviously, the problem with delaying surgery in such patients is that once brainstem compression has occurred, it always results in major sequelae.

It is our contention and that of Becker et al.[17] that such patients are at much greater risk of death or serious morbidity from herniation and brainstem compression than from meticulous evacuation of the clot. We feel that surgery should be carried out expeditiously in patients with temporal lobe lesions of $15\,cm^3$ or greater or with lesions in the posterior frontal region greater than $25\,cm^3$. There is evidence indicating that such hematomas will expand by approximately 40–50 percent in the first 24 hours.[18] In addition, we demonstrated that compression of the third nerve is relatively uncommon in high parietal and occipital lesions at ICPs below 30–35 mmHg.[4] Lesions adjacent to the brainstem may result in third nerve compression and transtentorial herniation at pressures well under 20 mmHg. Thus, delaying operative evacuation in patients with posterior frontal and temporal lesions is unwise. Our indications for surgical intervention are shown in Table 22-1.

The likelihood of neurobehavioral sequelae in this population is quite high and the family should be advised that patients with these injuries rarely recover completely to normal. However, their deficits can often be coped with through judicious planning and counseling. It is critically important to explain to the families what problems the

Table 22-1. Indications for Surgical Intervention in Acute Head Injury

Skull Fracture	Epidural Hematoma (EDH)	Subdural Hematoma (SDH)	Intracerebral Hematoma (ICH)	Cerebral Edema
Depressed open skull fracture	Any size symptomatic EDH and certainly those larger than 25 cm^3	Symptomatic SDH larger than 25 cm^3 with >1 cm thickness (5 mm in children)	Focal contusion with clot measuring >25 cm^3 except in the temporal lobe where lesions >15 cm^3 should be evacuated	Decompressive craniectomy; no clear benefit has been reported in an adequately designed prospective multicenter trial
Depressed fracture >1 cm with dural laceration	Asymptomatic EDH with >1 cm thickness (5 mm in children)			

patients are likely to encounter and to emphasize that slowing of intellectual processing and intemperate and inappropriate emotional behavior are actually more common and problematic than hemiparesis. Neurosurgeons and rehabilitation physicians need to counsel patients that they may have substantial difficulties in returning to the workplace and provide support in finding alternatives. Vocational rehabilitation may be helpful in some cases. Patients need to be encouraged to maintain as many of their previous activities as possible and not to become reclusive despite easy fatigability during the first months following injury. Patients with moderate brain injury who have often been hospitalized for significant periods of time should begin a program of regular exercise as early as possible. For the elderly, involvement in physical activity at a senior center or in more traditional physical therapy and rehabilitation environments should be a high priority. Family members, particularly grandchildren for seniors, and spouses and children should be encouraged to interact positively with the individual and instructed on the best way to provide support to the patient.

■ **The Pros and Cons**

In the first patient, insufficient attention was paid to initial abnormalities in clotting studies. While it is true that many patients with acute head injury have such abnormalities, and that they may be self-limited, clotting abnormalities are obviously concerning if the patient has an identified intracranial hemorrhage. In such cases, we seriously consider the administration of fresh frozen plasma to correct prolonged coagulation times or platelet infusion if the patient has thrombocytopenia. This decision will depend on the size of the initial hemorrhage on CT scan, and the severity of the coagulation abnormalities.

Case 2 illustrates many of the current dilemmas and some of the misunderstandings faced by the neurotraumatologist. A number of concerns can be raised about the care in the second case. This includes the choice of hyperventilation; the reluctance of the attending neurosurgeon to evacuate the right frontotemporal hematoma; the use of "cerebral perfusion pressure (CPP)-guided therapy"[9,19] in a patient who already had an intracranial hematoma; and finally, the use of hypothermia in light of a recent national study that failed to demonstrate efficacy and was even associated in some of the participating institutions with a substantially higher mortality in the treated group. The recommendation that hyperventilation should be avoided is based on one randomized controlled study of a relatively small number of patients[20] that has been challenged.[21] There is evidence that hyperventilation may interfere with brain perfusion and oxygenation,[22,23] but this evidence is so far limited and studies have produced conflicting results. Studies using PET scanning failed to demonstrate that hyperventilation results in brain ischemia, suggesting that the dangers of hyperventilation may have been exaggerated.[24]

Brain metabolism is coupled to blood flow, so when flow is reduced by hyperventilation, metabolism slows. Moreover, in patients with defective autoregulation, which is very common in this population, hyperventilation may have a positive effect by reducing intracranial volume with little or no effect on perfusion in damaged areas. Oertel and colleagues have also demonstrated that hyperventilation is effective in the treatment of intracranial hypertension. In their study comparing hyperventilation, elevation of the cerebral perfusion pressure, and metabolic suppression using propofol infusion, they found that hyperventilation was the most consistently effective therapy for the control of intracranial hypertension.[25] Thus, hyperventilation is effective in reducing elevated intracranial pressure in patients with head injury,[26,27] and the evidence claiming adverse consequences of hyperventilation in this population is not totally compelling. A definitive conclusion with regard to the risk and benefit of judicious hyperventilation is not available, but it would be incorrect to totally dismiss this measure. Brief moderate hyperventilation may be particularly useful as a "bridge" to decompressive surgery in patients with acute intracranial hypertension from a post-traumatic mass lesion. (See also Chapter 8 for further insights.)

Of particular interest in this case of severe head injury was the utilization of "CPP therapy," as has been advocated by Rosner.[9,19,28] A contrasting approach has been that of Nordström, also known as the "Lund concept" of post-traumatic brain edema therapy.[29] Here, the CPP is strictly controlled and the emphasis is on the treatment of edema and reduction of cerebral blood volume rather than on raising the CPP. A detailed analysis in a large number of patients entered into a multicenter international trial for the treatment of head injury found no positive effect of CPPs above 60 mmHg. This study indicated that treatment protocols for the management of severe head injury should rather emphasize the reduction of ICP to less than 20 mmHg and not control of the CPP.[30]

Further evidence arguing against "CPP therapy" comes from a study by Robertson et al., who demonstrated an increased frequency of adult respiratory distress syndrome (ARDS) in patients who were volume expanded as a result of "CPP-guided therapy."[31]

The choice to target ICP rather than CPP is based on the observations from our own unit as well as others.[30,31] In Juul's study, no benefit of a CPP of greater than 60 mmHg could be demonstrated, suggesting that it is illogical to push the blood pressure to extreme limits to increase CPP to 80–90 mmHg. In a number of patients in San Diego, delayed brain swelling was observed, beginning on the fourth to sixth day in patients in whom CPP-guided therapy had been utilized. This suggests that blood-brain barrier breakdown, which begins to occur on the third to fourth days, may make patients vulnerable to substantial elevations of the systolic blood pressure. Thus, based on our own observations and those of the Lund group, we believe that the primary target of therapy for severe brain injury, where continuous monitoring of the ICP is employed, should be the ICP. This does not mean that the blood pressure should be ignored. Rather, one should accept as a basic principle of treatment that the blood pressure will be adequately maintained with volume and with vasopressors if necessary. However, the CPP in some ways is an arbitrary calculation because the brain is perfused in systole. Thus, in patients with a wide pulse pressure, the mean arterial pressure, which is utilized in the calculation of CPP, really inadequately reflects brain perfusion. Although there have been advocates for using the systolic blood pressure to calculate CPP, this has not been the methodology utilized to date. Thus, a threshold level of 60 mmHg for the CPP when one uses the mean arterial pressure for its calculation builds in a satisfactory margin of safety.

Also, the adverse consequences of vasopressors have been underestimated. We have had a number of patients, during the time when CPP therapy was "en vogue," who developed significant ischemia of the peripheral vasculature. In one instance, a hand had to be amputated and in a number of other patients renal failure developed.

The final issue raised in the case of this severely injured patient was the use of hypothermia. In a recently completed multicenter trial, no overall benefit of hypothermia was demonstrated and, in some centers, there was an increased risk of mortality and morbidity.[5] A subgroup of patients who were younger and had hyperthermia prior to admission showed some benefit. A new trial is underway to test the possible benefit of hypothermia further in a selected group of patients. Clearly, hypothermia should not be utilized in the elderly and its use in younger patients with head injury remains experimental.

In the second patient, the major area of concern was the decision to delay surgery until the patient had clinical evidence of uncal herniation (i.e., third nerve palsy). This in our view is an inappropriate decision that places the patient at excessive risk. An anterior frontotemporal debridement produces little in the way of measurable neurological damage and would have improved the chances of successful functional recovery. To wait until there is evidence of brainstem compression is incorrect because at that point these patients certainly will have sequelae. This is supported by early intervention for intracranial hematomas demonstrating much better outcomes than delayed intervention.[17]

When surgical evacuation is not an option, treatment of traumatic brain injury currently is divided into ICP-targeted, CPP-targeted, and volume-targeted protocols. There are no randomized trials, only detailed analysis of protocols in large groups of likely heterogeneous patient populations. The main characteristics of the therapies are summarized in Table 22-2. For full descriptions of these protocols, the reader is referred to review papers[28,32–34] or a website with fully downloadable files maintained by the Brain Trauma Foundation (www.braintrauma.org). A proposed algorithm for systemic management of severe injury and treatment of intracranial hypertension has been developed by our group (Figure 22-3). This flowchart illustrates a systemic approach to medical management of intracranial hypertension in the severely head-injured patient. It is important in all situations to keep in mind that medical management of elevated ICP is inappropriate in the face of an urgent surgical lesion.

Finally, despite imaginative changes in vehicular design (i.e., airbags and impact design modifications) and road design, patient education (i.e., wearing helmets and safety precautions) is still indispensable to reduce the incidence and severity of head injury.

Major improvement in the outcome of moderate and severe brain injury is likely to be dependent on the identification of effective pharmacological therapies to ameliorate the complex neurochemistry of acute brain injury. The introduction of brain tissue oxygen monitoring, while of significant interest, is not likely to have a substantial impact on patient outcome (further discussion of this topic is presented in Chapter 10). The same is true for microdialysis measurements, which have been quite important in furthering our understanding of the neurochemistry of brain injury. While this technique is likely to provide insight with regard to pharmacological therapy, microdialysis alone is unlikely to have a marked impact on outcome.

Of particular interest is the potential to prevent further expansion of contusions or intracerebral hemorrhages using factor VII. Preliminary discussions

Table 22-2. Targetted Therapies in Traumatic Head Injury

	ICP Target[21]	CPP Target[28,32]	Volume Target[33,34]
Guiding principle	Increased ICP shifts brainstem and causes secondary damage	Perfusion of tissue more important than pressure of tissue	Reduction of cerebral blood volume using arterial and venous vasoconstriction and increase of plasma oncotic pressure
ICP Monitor	Parenchymal	Ventriculostomy	Parenchymal
Hyperventilation	Frequent but brief	Less important	None
Head position	Elevated 30%	Flat	Less emphasis
ICP	<20 mmHg	Less important	<20 mmHg
CPP	60–70 mmHg	≥70 mmHg	Less important
MAP	Optional	Increase with vasopressors	Decrease with metoprolol and clonidine
CBV	Osmotic diuretics	Enhancing cerebral venous drainage	Dihydroergotamine
Fluid balance	Normovolemic	Normovolemic	Balanced or negative
Sedation	Optional	Optional	Imperative

ICP, intracranial pressure; CBV, cerebral blood volume; CPP, cerebral perfusion pressure; MAP, mean arterial blood pressure.

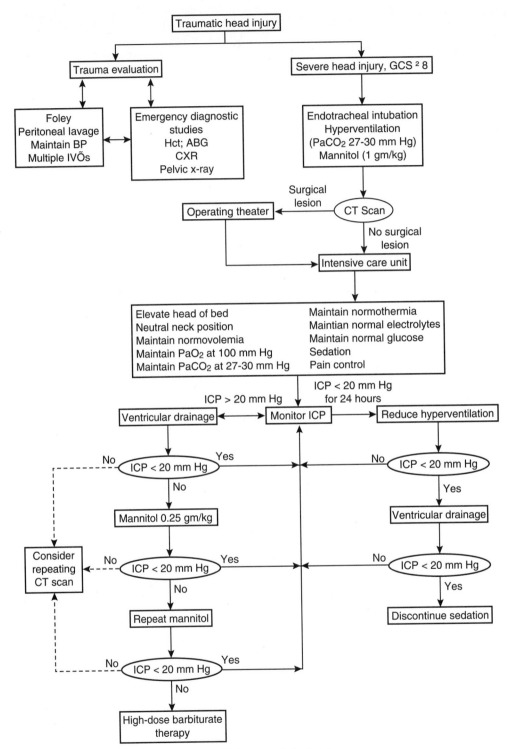

Figure 22-3. Algorithm for treatment of increased ICP in traumatic brain injury.

are underway for the initiation of a clinical trial of this compound. This may be the most dramatic development in the horizon because of the potential prophylactic valve of this sophisticated, genetically engineered hemostatic agent, which can also be used for reversing anticoagulation.[35]

■ The Main Points

- The decision on when to operate on patients with traumatic intraparenchymal hemorrhages is controversial. Early intervention for traumatic intracranial hematomas results in much better outcomes than delayed intervention.
- Cerebral perfusion pressure management alone is unlikely to be beneficial to severely head-injured patients, and the focus should be primarily on reducing the ICP below 20 mmHg.
- The use of induced hypothermia is not warranted at this time given current evidence from a multicenter study.[5]
- The recognition of neurobehavioral sequelae after a relatively trivial injury is very important. Objective assessment and treatment of these cognitive abnormalities should be a priority during the rehabilitation phase.

■ References

1. Klauber MR, Marshall LF, Luerssen TG, Frankowski R, Tabaddor K, Eisenberg HM. Determinants of head injury mortality: importance of the low risk patient. *Neurosurgery* 1989;24:31–36.
2. Brain Trauma Foundation, American Association of Neurological Surgeons, Joint Section on Neurotrauma and Critical Care. Guidelines for the management of severe head injury. *J Neurotrauma* 1996;13:641–734.
3. Bullock R, Chesnut RM, Clifton G, Ghajar J, Marion D, Narayan RK, Newell DW, Pitts LH, Rosner MJ, Wilberger JE. Guidelines for the management of severe head injury. *Eur J Emerg Med* 1996;3:109–127.
4. Marshall LF, Barba D, Toole B, Bowers SA. The oval pupil: clinical significance and relationship to intracranial hypertension. *J Neurosurg* 1983;58:566–568.
5. Clifton GL, Miller ER, Choi SC, Levin HS, McCauley S, Smith KR Jr, Muizelaar JP, Wagner FC Jr, Marion DW, Luerssen TG, Chesnut RM, Schwartz M. Lack of effect of hypothermia after acute brain injury. *N Engl J Med* 2001;344:556–563.
6. Stein SC, Spettell C, Young G, Ross SE. Limitations of neurological assessment in mild head injury. *Brain Inj* 1993;7:425–430.
7. Rose J, Valtonen S, Jennett B. Avoidable factors contributing to death after head injury. *Br Med J* 1977;2:615–618.
8. Teasdale GM, Braakman R, Cohadon F, Dearden M, Jannotti F, Karimi A, Lapierre F, Maas A, Murray G, Ohman J. Persson L, Servadei F, Stochetti N, Trojanowski T, Unterberg A. The European Brain Injury Consortium: Nemo solus satis sapti—Nobody knows enough alone. *Acta Neurochir (Wien)* 1997;139:797–803.
9. Rosner MJ, Rosner SD. Cerebral perfusion pressure management of head injury. In Avezaat CJJ, Van Eijndhoven JHM, Maas AIR, Tans JTJ eds. *Intracranial Pressure VIII*. Berlin, Springer, 1994: 540–543.
10. Wrightson P, Gronwall D. Mild head injury in New Zealand: incidence of injury and persisting symptoms. *NZ Med J* 1998;111:99–101.
11. MacKenzie JD, Siddiqi F, Babb JS, Bagley LJ, Mannon LJ, Sinson GP, Grossman RI. Brain atrophy in mild or moderate traumatic brain injury: a longitudinal quantitative analysis. *AJNR Am J Neuroradiol* 2002;23:1509–1515.
12. McAllister TW, Arciniegas D. Evaluation and treatment of postconcussive symptoms. *NeuroRehabilitation* 2002;17:265–283.
13. Mittenberg W, Canyock EM, Condit D, Patton C. Treatment of post-concussion syndrome following mild head injury. *J Clin Exp Neuropsychol* 2001;23:829–836.
14. Levin HS, Mattis S, Ruff RM, Eisenberg HM, Marshall LF, Tabaddor K, High WM Jr, Frankowski RF. Neurobehavioral outcome following minor head injury: a three-center study. *J Neurosurg* 1987; 66:234–243.
15. Miller JD. Epidemiology of moderate head injury. In Hoff J, Anderson T, Cole T, eds. *Mild to Moderate Head Injury*. Boston, Blackwell Scientific Publications, 1989.
16. Servadei F, Nanni A, Nasi MT, Zappi D, Vergoni G, Giulani G, Arista A. Evolving brain lesions in the first 12 hours after head injury. *Neurosurgery* 1995;37:899–906.
17. Becker DP, Miller JD, Ward JD, Greenberg RP, Young HF, Sakalas R. The outcome from severe head injury with early diagnosis and intensive management. *J Neurosurg* 1977;47:497–502.
18. Oertel M, Kelly DF, McArthur D, Boscardin WJ, Glenn TC, Lee JH, Gravori T, Obukhov D, McBride DQ, Martin NA. Progressive hemorrhage after head trauma: predictors and consequences of the evolving injury. *J Neurosurg* 2002;96:109–116.
19. Rosner MJ, Rosner SD. CPP management. I. Results. In Nagai H, Kamiya K, Ishii S, eds. *Intracranial Pressure IX*. Berlin, Springer, 1994:218–221.

20. Muizelaar JP, Marmarou AM, Ward JD, Kontos HA, Choi SC, Becker DP, Gruemer H, Young HF. Adverse effects of prolonged hyperventilation in patients with severe head injury: a randomized clinical trial. *J Neurosurg* 1991;75:731–739.

21. Marshall LF. Head injury: recent past, present, and future. *Neurosurgery* 2000;47:546–561.

22. Marion DW, Puccio A, Wisniewski SR, Kochanek P, Dixon CE, Bullian L, Carlier P. Effect of hyperventilation on extracellular concentrations of glutamate, lactate, pyruvate, and local cerebral blood flow in patients with severe traumatic brain injury. *Crit Care Med* 2002;30:2619–2625.

23. Imberti R, Bellinzona G, Langer M. Cerebral tissue Po_2 and $SjvO_2$ changes during moderate hyperventilation in patients with severe traumatic brain injury. *J Neurosurg* 2002;96:97–102.

24. Diringer MN, Yundt K, Videen TO, Adams RE, Zazulia AR, Deibert E, Aiyagari V, Dacey RG, Grubb RL, Powers WJ. No reduction in cerebral metabolism as a result of early moderate hyperventilation following severe traumatic brain injury. *J Neurosurg* 2000;92:7–13.

25. Oertel M, Kelly DF, Lee JH, McArthur DL, Glenn TC, Vespa P, Boscardin WJ, Hovda DA, Martin NA. Efficacy of hyperventilation, blood pressure elevation, and metabolic suppression therapy in controlling intracranial pressure after head injury. *J Neurosurg* 2002;97:1045–1053.

26. Cruz J. An additional therapeutic effect of adequate hyperventilation in severe acute brain trauma: normalization of cerebral glucose uptake. *J Neurosurg* 1995;82:379–385.

27. Cruz J, Miner ME, Allen J, Alves WM, Gennarelli TA. Continuous monitoring of cerebral oxygenation in acute brain injury: assessment of cerebral hemodynamic reserve. *Neurosurgery* 1991;29:743–749.

28. Rosner MJ, Rosner SD, Johnson AH. Cerebral perfusion pressure: management protocol and clinical results. *J Neurosurg* 1995;83:949–962.

29. Asgeirsson B, Grände PO, Nordström CH. The Lund concept of post-traumatic brain oedema therapy. *Acta Anaesthesiol Scand* 1995;39:103–106.

30. Juul N, Morris GF, Marshall SB, Marshall LF. Intracranial hypertension and cerebral perfusion pressure: influence on neurological deterioration and outcome in severe head injury—The Executive Committee of the International Selfotel Trial. *J Neurosurg* 2000;92:1–6.

31. Robertson CS, Valadka AB, Hannay HJ, Contant CF, Gopinath SP, Cormio M, Uzura M, Grossman RG. Prevention of secondary ischemic insults after severe head injury. *Crit Care Med* 1999;27:2086–2095.

32. Rosner MJ, Becker DP. Origin and evolution of plateau waves: experimental observations and a theoretical model. *J Neurosurg* 1984;60:321–324.

33. Grände PO, Möller AD, Norström CH, Ungerstedt U. Low-dose prostacyclin in treatment of severe brain trauma evaluated with microdialysis and jugular bulb oxygen measurements. *Acta Anaesthesiol Scand* 2000;44:886–894.

34. Naredi S, Olivercrona M, Lindregren C, Östlund AL, Grände PO, Koskinen LOD. An outcome study of severe traumatic head injury using the "Lund therapy" with low-dose prostacyclin. *Acta Anaesthesiol Scand* 2001;45:402–406.

35. Lin J, Hanigan WC, Tarantino M, Wang J. The use of recombinant activated factor VII to reverse warfarin induced anticoagulation in patients with hemorrhages in the central nervous system: preliminary findings. *J Neurosurgery* 2003;98:737–740.

Chapter 23

Withholding and Withdrawing Life-Sustaining Treatment

James L. Bernat

It is satisfying to rescue a critically ill patient from severe illness by timely and skillful high-technology treatment. Physicians now admit greater numbers of patients to intensive care units (ICUs). But some patients admitted to ICUs have illnesses that have advanced too far to uncover despite maximal intensive treatment. Researchers working in ICUs have developed prognostic scales, such as APACHE III, to attempt to identify prospectively those patients with the greatest probability of successful treatment.[1] But, as the SUPPORT study (discussed later) showed, there are limitations to the statistical predictive powers of such scales. In SUPPORT, using even the most advanced prognostic scale, many critically ill patients admitted to ICUs fell into a middle prognostic range with roughly an equal chance of living and dying.[2] Most such patients and their surrogates wish to continue aggressive, life-sustaining treatment, at least until it becomes clear that the patient cannot survive.[3]

But once it becomes clear that an aggressively treated ICU patient cannot survive despite maximal treatment, the goal of medical care should change from life prolongation to palliation. Surveys have shown that most patients wish to receive high-technology ICU treatment only if such care can help them recover from their illness and regain their baseline functioning.[4] If life-sustaining treatment (LST) cannot help them regain acceptable functioning, most patients and surrogates ultimately refuse it. Such patients should receive palliative care.

Withholding and withdrawing LST is a common component of a palliative care plan because the quality of the patient's remaining life is the primary goal of palliative treatment.[5] As a consequence, competent, hopelessly ill ICU patients, and the families and surrogate decision-makers of incompetent, hopelessly ill ICU patients, frequently decide to withdraw and withhold LST when it can no longer help the patient to recover.

Withholding and withdrawing LST currently represents a common modus of death for patients receiving LST in American ICUs. In several studies, 40–65 percent of all deaths in ICUs resulted from withholding or withdrawing LST.[6] And in a survey of 136 ICUs encompassing 5910 patients, 74 percent of all patients who died first had at least some forms of LST withdrawn.[7]

■ The Patient

The following three case vignettes illustrate some of the real-life aspects of problems encountered in decisions to withdraw support. Most cases of patient or surrogate refusal of LST are appropriate, can be accomplished agreeably, and do not result in disputes. But the opportunity is great for misunderstanding of a patient's wishes in light of the prognosis, or of conflict caused by emotional factors as illustrated in these cases. The hospital ethics committee was asked to consult in each case to facilitate decision-making. Their recommendations are briefly summarized in the comments following each case presentation.

Case 1: "But he filled out a living will"

A 79-year-old man was admitted to the ICU with pneumonia and sepsis. He had chronic obstructive lung disease and mild congestive heart failure. He had been living independently at home with his wife. He had completed a living will that he had placed on file with his physician and attorney. In the ICU, he required ventilator treatment, sedation, and intravenous antibiotics. After several days of sedation and ventilator treatment, his wife asked the attending physician to stop life-sustaining treatment (LST) because he was not improving and because she insisted that he would not want to be maintained "on machines." When told that he likely could recover to his previous state of health she exclaimed "But he filled out a living will" and cited the living will as evidence that he would not wish further LST in this circumstance. But the attending physician did not regard the patient as terminally ill, believed he was still capable of good recovery, and strongly wished to continue his treatment. The dispute was referred to the hospital ethics committee.

Comment

The patient and his wife falsely assumed that they had performed sufficient advance care planning merely by his completion of a living will. She was surprised, frustrated, and angry to learn that the living will was of little use in this situation, largely because the patient was not regarded as terminally ill, and its application was ambiguous. She insisted that she knew "what he meant" when he signed it and that his intention was to prevent receiving the LST that he now was receiving. But the physician explained the limitations of the living will in this circumstance: he was not terminally ill, and the living will directive offered little specific guidance in such a case. The ethics committee later helped clarify the evidence of his prior stated treatment preferences by interviewing family members and friends and listening to their accounts of his

previously expressed preferences for treatment. When he failed to improve over the next 10 days, developed additional organ failures, and was determined to be terminally ill, his physicians agreed to withdraw LST.

Case 2: "She wanted everything possible to be done"

A 62-year-old woman was admitted in coma after cardiopulmonary arrest. She had suffered an out-of-hospital arrest and was resuscitated by emergency medical technicians. After several weeks, she began to open her eyes but remained unresponsive in a vegetative state. She had designated her husband as durable power of attorney for healthcare (DPAHC) but had left no written instructions. She had commented to him on a previous occasion that doctors these days gave up treatment too easily and that if she were hospitalized "she wanted everything possible to be done." Her internist and neurologist discussed treatment options with her husband, and he insisted that she be treated as aggressively as possible, despite her poor prognosis. When she developed renal failure, he insisted that she undergo dialysis. Her physicians thought this decision was inappropriate and asked the ethics committee to consult.

Comment

The ethics committee concurred that her husband as DPAHC was her appropriate surrogate and that he was attempting to reach a substituted judgment on her behalf. They discussed with him what she had meant when she remarked that she wished "everything possible to be done." They reviewed the decision-making process in similar past cases and the normative preferences of patients in surveys reported in the clinical ethics literature. They explained to him that most people who utter this directive mean that they wish to be treated aggressively only if such treatment can plausibly restore their previous function. Most patients do not wish to be treated aggressively if they are consigned to remain in a noncognitive state. He concurred that this was probably what his wife intended to communicate by her statement and agreed to stop LST after she had remained unconscious for 6 weeks.

Case 3: "I couldn't live with myself if we didn't treat her"

A 68-year-old woman was admitted with a large left hemispheric cerebral infarction producing right hemiplegia, global aphasia, and drowsiness. Her husband was her DPAHC. The patient had left supplementary written instructions that she wished to refuse all forms of LST, including artificial hydration and nutrition, if she were ever in a permanent state of incapacity with total dependency requiring full nursing care. Her MRI showed complete infarction of the left middle and anterior cerebral artery territories, resulting from an occlusion of the left internal carotid artery. Her neurologist explained that, should she survive, she would remain permanently hemiplegic and globally aphasic. After 2 weeks without clinical improvement, her physicians discussed with her husband the placement of a feeding gastrostomy tube. Her two daughters vehemently refused the feeding tube based on their support of her clearly stated prior wishes. But her husband, when he learned that she would die without the feeding tube, asked the physicians to insert it and feed her because "I couldn't live with myself if we didn't treat her." The daughters asked for a consultation by the ethics committee.

Comment

The ethics committee met with the husband and daughters. They agreed that he was the appropriate surrogate and discussed the standards of surrogate decision-making. They explained to him that the highest standard of surrogate decision-making is following the clearly expressed wishes of the patient. Even though he was legally empowered to decide on her behalf, he was expected to follow her expressed wishes. They explained that following her wishes permitted her to exert a degree of self-determination, despite her present and future incompetence. They helped him understand that he should not feel guilty about the decision not to insert a feeding tube because the treatment decision was really not his to make. Rather, he was only asked to follow his wife's clearly stated instructions. The daughters were totally supportive of this approach. The husband finally agreed that this course of action was right and the feeding

tube was not inserted. She died in a nursing home 9 days later.

■ The Problem

- On whom should physicians withdraw LST?
- When should LST be withdrawn?
- Who should make the decision?
- How should LST be withdrawn?

■ The Evidence

The locus of medical decision-making in American medicine has undergone an evolution over the past generation from being physician-centered to patient-centered.[8] Patient-centered care is healthcare that is congruent with and responsive to the wants, needs, and preferences of patients.[9] Although many physicians would take umbrage at the suggestion that their care previously had not been centered on the benefit of the patient, traditionally, physicians retained the prerogative to determine what was the best treatment for patients. Patient-centered medicine evolved in the context of the patients' rights and civil rights movements that granted more authority to individuals to make their own decisions about matters affecting them. The growing primacy of the doctrine of informed consent exemplifies this evolution.

In the earlier context of physician-centered medicine, decisions to withhold or withdraw LST were conceptualized as identifying those circumstances in which physicians were ethically and legally permitted to withdraw and withhold LST. Based on prognosis and other factors, physicians decided whether and when to "terminate life-sustaining treatment" on such patients and then ordered continuation or termination of LST. The term "passive euthanasia" was often applied when patients died from their underlying disease as a result of the physician's decision to terminate LST.[10]

By contrast, in today's environment of patient-centered medicine, the same phenomenon is conceptualized as the "refusal of LST" by a competent patient or by the surrogate of an incompetent patient. The contemporary physician's role is not to decide unilaterally to maintain or withdraw LST. Rather, the physician should pronounce the correct diagnosis, communicate the prognosis with and without treatment as accurately as possible, determine the treatment preferences of the competent patient, instruct the surrogates of incompetent patients how to consent or refuse on the patient's behalf, and then work with the patient and surrogate to implement the decision. If patients or surrogates refuse LST, and the patient subsequently dies of the underlying illness, it is misleading and incorrect to refer to such an act as "passive euthanasia."[11] Patients have the ethical and legal right to refuse LST and physicians cannot usually continue LST once patients or their legally authorized surrogates have refused it.

Informed Consent and Refusal

The widespread acceptance of the doctrine of informed consent and refusal represents a seminal advance of medical ethics in the second half of the twentieth century. Despite beneficent motives, physicians cannot conduct courses of diagnostic testing or treatment, except in emergencies, without the consent of a competent patient or the consent of the surrogate decision-maker of an incompetent patient. Informed refusal is implicit in the doctrine of informed consent. Patients and their surrogates may refuse to provide consent once they are knowledgeable about the alternatives and likely outcomes.

There are few circumstances in which physicians are permitted to continue LST in the setting of a patient's explicit informed refusal. The principal one is when a patient's or surrogate's refusal of LST is seriously irrational. For example, it might be regarded as seriously irrational for a young, otherwise healthy patient with Guillain-Barré syndrome, who is expected to recover with appropriate ICU treatment, to refuse positive-pressure ventilator therapy. Refusing ventilator treatment is seriously irrational because the patient who wishes to recover will likely die as a result of this refusal. But in irreversibly, terminally ill patients, it is not usually seriously irrational to refuse treatment because the patient is destined to die soon.

Informed consent and refusal have become established ethical and legal doctrines because of our respect for the autonomy and self-determination of patients. We respect patients' dignity and privacy, and honor their fundamental right to refuse treatment if they wish. Physicians can make a strong treatment recommendation but it is wrong to coerce patients or surrogates into consenting for treatment because coercion deprives patients of self-determination.

Philosophical analyses of consent show that it requires three components to become valid: capacity to make healthcare decisions, adequate information, and freedom from coercion.[12] The capacity to make healthcare decisions has been termed "competence," but here this word is used in its informal clinical sense and not in a strict legal sense. Physicians can assess patients' decision-making capacity at the bedside. To be competent, a patient must be able to understand the information the physician provides, particularly the treatment choices and the probable implications of such treatments.[13] Fully competent patients are permitted to consent or refuse recommended treatments. Incompetent patients require the identification of a surrogate decision-maker to consent or refuse on the patient's behalf.[12]

Patients and surrogates need adequate information to provide valid consent. Most authorities employ the "reasonable person" standard, and ask what information a hypothetically reasonable person would need to know to make a decision. Reasonable people need to know why they need treatment, their treatment choices, and a general understanding of the risks and benefits of the treatment choices. Information sharing is a process during which patients or surrogates can ask questions to clarify their understanding. Risks of treatment should be communicated to the extent that they are common or serious.[12]

For consent to be valid, it requires freedom from coercion by persons or agencies. Although patients' decisions frequently are influenced by the recommendations of family members and friends, their true wishes should be sought. Physicians should make a treatment recommendation, and may make it strongly based on their assessment of what is best for the patient. But physicians should refrain from threats or punishment, such as the refusal to continue to care for the patient, because those activities are coercive.[12] Similarly, physicians should not exaggerate the benefits of their recommended treatment, or the risks of alternative treatments, because these activities are unfairly manipulative.

The physician and competent patient (or the physician and surrogate for the incompetent patient) form a dyad to accomplish shared decision-making. In the shared decision-making model, the physician explains the diagnosis, prognosis, treatment options, likely outcomes with each treatment, and then makes a recommendation for treatment. The patient or surrogate brings the patient's system of values and treatment preferences. Together, they agree on and implement a treatment decision.[14] The inherent tension between patient autonomy and physician paternalism can be settled through the exercise of successful shared decision-making.[15]

Surrogate Decision-Making

Incompetent patients do not lose the right of consent. Rather, the right is transferred to a surrogate decision-maker to exercise on the patient's behalf. Surrogate decision-makers can be appointed formally or informally. Most states have enacted laws of durable power of attorney for healthcare (DPAHC), known in some jurisdictions as "healthcare agent" or "healthcare proxy," that permit competent patients to name a surrogate decision-maker whose authority becomes activated upon the patient's incapacity. Most states endow the DPAHC with the same authority to consent and refuse that the patient has. Physicians should engage the DPAHC of the incompetent patient in the same conversation for consent as the competent patient.

More commonly, however, incompetent patients will not have previously executed a DPAHC appointment. Such incompetent patients have no legally authorized surrogate decision-maker to consent or refuse on their behalf. Some states have enacted healthcare proxy laws that automatically designate a legally authorized surrogate decision-maker from a predetermined list of close relatives, such as a spouse or adult child.[16] But most states have not enacted such laws. The only means to name a legally authorized surrogate in these jurisdictions would be for the physician or family to seek a judicial appointment of a guardian or other surrogate.

It is common practice for physicians to recognize the family unit as an informal surrogate decision-maker for the incompetent patient. This surrogate appointment is valid only if three conditions are fulfilled. First, there must be no disagreement among family members about the treatment plan. Second, the decision must attempt to follow that which the patient would have made on best evidence. And third, the decision must be consistent with good medical practice. Although the family in this setting lacks legal authority, this arrangement works out well in practice.

The principal problem with informal surrogate decision-making is the situation is which members of the immediate family disagree about the treatment plan.[17] Here, physicians, with the assistance of nurses, social workers, chaplains, or the hospital ethics committee, can try to help the family gain consensus on the basis of identifying what the patient would want done. But if no consensus can be reached among the immediate family, physicians should seek judicial appointment of a legally authorized surrogate because it is unclear whose decision the physician should follow.

Surrogate decision-makers require instruction on the criteria they should use to make treatment decisions.[18] There are three general standards for surrogate decision-making: expressed wishes, substituted judgment, and best interests. Surrogates should attempt to apply these standards in this sequential order of priority because this order follows decreasing ethical and legal power.

The *expressed wishes* standard is the most powerful guideline because it respects the self-determination of the patient. This standard asks the surrogate if the patient previously had discussed any expressed wishes for treatment in his or her exact current clinical situation. If so, these directives should be followed. Although ethically and legally the most powerful standard, expressed wishes only rarely can be used in practice because of the unlikelihood that a person could have predicted in advance the particular clinical scenario that later occurs. Looking for and following a patient's advance directives (discussed below) may be useful to follow the standard of expressed wishes.

If the expressed wishes of the incompetent patient remain unknown, the surrogate should be asked to try to predict the precise decision the patient would have made, based on the surrogate's knowledge of the values and preferences of the patient. This process of attempting to reproduce the patient's decision is called *substituted judgment*. The ethical and legal force of substituted judgment is based on the presumption that a surrogate knows the values and preferences of the patient and, by using them, can accurately reproduce the decision the patient would have made. Of course, there are inevitable errors in executing substituted judgments, such as predicting that a patient would want continued LST when they would not, and the reverse error, as have been shown in several studies.[19–21] But attempting to make a substituted judgment is better than not even trying.

Some surrogates have no knowledge whatsoever of the patient's values and preferences and therefore cannot make a substituted judgment. Public guardians and parents of infants are examples in which neither expressed wishes nor substituted judgment standards are possible. In these situations, the surrogate is forced to make a *best interest* determination by weighing the benefits and burdens of the proposed treatment, as seen through the surrogate's eyes. The best interest standard is ethically and legally less powerful than the expressed wishes or substituted judgment standards because its assessment of benefits and burdens relies solely on the surrogate's values and judgment of the patient's quality of life.[22] Assessment of another person's quality of life is notoriously inaccurate because it is subject to numerous biases, the most common of which is for young healthy people to devalue the lives of older and more disabled people.[23] Nevertheless, best interests may be the only standard available in situations where the wishes of the patient remain entirely unknown.

Advance Directives

Surrogate decision-makers should utilize patients' previously completed advance directives. These directives, executed when a patient is competent and intended to take effect when the patient becomes incompetent, are now legal instruments in most states.[24] Advance directives are of two types: the written instructional directive, such as the living will; and the directive that appoints a surrogate decision-maker, such as a DPAHC that often also includes written instructions for the surrogate.[25]

Written instructional directives have advantages and disadvantages. Their principal advantage is in providing a reliable statement of the patient's exact preferences for treatment. Courts regard them as more valid statements of patients' true wishes than patients' previously uttered offhand remarks because of the presumption that patients had more carefully considered written instructions when they composed and signed them. Therefore, written directives usually satisfy the strict "clear and convincing" evidentiary standard prevailing in some jurisdictions.[26]

The disadvantages of written directives result from the vague language in which they usually are framed. Many living wills contain vague statements such as "I wish to forgo life-sustaining therapy if my chance for recovery is hopeless." These directives provide general but not specific advice.[27] When applied to specific situations, they often become ambiguous. For example, what level of function counts as meaningful recovery in the setting of stroke? How long must a patient remain in a poor neurologic state before it is clear that the prognosis for recovery is hopeless? And what therapies are life-sustaining? Do they include artificial hydration and nutrition?

The vagueness of most written directives has led some experts to advocate not even completing a living will.[28] Other experts have tried to minimize this shortcoming by designing lengthy directives that anticipate and discuss treatment preferences in the most common clinical conditions.[29] But lengthy written directives are too complex to be successfully completed by most patients and even obsessively long directives cannot anticipate all clinical contingencies. Further, living wills take effect only when the patient is terminally ill, unlike surrogate appointments that are activated as soon as the patient loses the capacity to make healthcare decisions.

The surrogate appointment, such as DPAHC, is a more flexible and useful directive. The surrogate who knows the values and preferences of the patient can adapt them to unanticipated clinical conditions and use discretion and wisdom to flexibly apply them in the way the patient had intended. It is essential to maximize the value of all directives for the patient to speak in detail with the surrogate and the physician. Advance directives are most useful when they supplement and formalize a clear understanding between the patient and physician about the patient's healthcare goals and preferences. In this way, advance directives can be an important component of advance medical care planning.[30]

Artificial Hydration and Nutrition

A former controversy surrounded the question of whether patients and surrogates should have the right to refuse artificial hydration and nutrition (AHN) along with medical therapies. The controversy historically resulted from the framing of the question as the physician-centered "Should physicians be permitted to terminate AHN on a hopelessly ill patient?" But now that the issue has been correctly framed as the patient-centered concept of a competent patient's or surrogate's "refusal of AHN" and has been given unequivocal legal support, it has lost most of its controversy.

Most authorities in clinical ethics accept that competent patients and the surrogates of incompetent patients generally have a right to refuse AHN along with all other therapies.[31,32] AHN counts as a medical therapy because it requires: (1) a physician's order to receive; (2) surgery to insert a permanent feeding tube; and (3) a nurse to carry out the nutrition and hydration orders. But opponents of this practice point out that, whereas some patients may survive without penicillin or a ventilator, no one can survive without hydration and nutrition. Therefore, they argue that stopping AHN on a patient who cannot swallow is tantamount to killing the patient and is therefore wrong.[33,34]

In the 1990 *Cruzan* decision, the United States Supreme Court asserted a constitutional right for all American citizens to refuse unwanted medical therapies including AHN. The *Cruzan* court ruled that legally authorized surrogates could consent or refuse medical therapies on behalf of incompetent patients, including AHN, once the state's standards of evidence were satisfied clarifying the patient's prior treatment wishes.[35,36] Nearly all state DPAHC statutes permit surrogates to withhold or withdraw AHN, along with other medical therapies. But some DPAHC statutes require the patient's prior specific written instruction that AHN can be stopped in addition to other therapies. Physicians should familiarize themselves with the provisions of surrogate statutes and other relevant law in states in which they practice. The provisions of laws relating to end-of-life care in countries throughout the world have recently been reviewed.[37]

Empirical Studies

Published data permit an evidence-based review of the experience of withdrawing LST by intensivists, neurologists, and other physicians. These studies have recently been critically reviewed.[38] Physicians' willingness to stop LST is a gradual process evolving over time rather than a discrete event.[39] Two longitudinal ICU studies have revealed a growing willingness of physicians to discontinue LST.[40,41] One ICU study of termination of medical treatment found that physicians discontinued therapies roughly in the following order: CPR, vasopressors, ventilators, supplemental oxygen, blood transfusions, antibiotics, antiarrhythmic drugs, dialysis, neurosurgery, intravenous fluids, and total parenteral nutrition.[42]

Another study disclosed the biases that determine which therapies physicians are willing to discontinue and in what circumstances. Physicians had a bias to withdraw therapies: (1) from organs that failed from natural as opposed to iatrogenic causes; (2) that had been started recently, as opposed to those that had been of long duration; (3) that would result in the patient's immediate death rather than in delayed death; and (4) that would result in delayed death when in the presence of the physician's diagnostic uncertainty.[43] Physicians also preferred to withdraw therapies related to their own specialty rather than to other specialties.[44]

Several studies made evidence-based recommendations for the bedside methods used to withdraw LST in the ICU, particularly regarding the judicious use of opiates and benzodiazepines to minimize patient suffering.[45–47] Specifically, both summary extubation and prolonged terminal ventilator weaning were found to be inferior to rapidly dialing down the ventilator volumes as a means of discontinuing ventilatory support.[48]

The largest and most comprehensive study of physicians' practices of withdrawing LST from critically ill and dying patients was the Study to Understand Prognoses and Preferences for Outcomes and Risks of Treatment (SUPPORT).[2] SUPPORT was a 4-year study of over 9000 hospitalized, seriously ill patients whose goals were to measure the quality of end-of-life decision-making, to assess the frequency of unnecessarily painful or prolonged deaths in the hospital, and to attempt to improve the quality of terminal care. Phase I of SUPPORT showed that there were serious deficiencies in the care of critically ill and dying patients: for example, that many patients did not receive DNR orders until 2 days before death; that less than half of physicians knew their patients' resuscitation preferences; and that half of conscious patients suffered pain before they died. Phase II of SUPPORT showed that an intervention by nurses to communicate to physicians the patient's current prognosis failed to influence the physicians in their treatment behaviors. A series of related research reports on withdrawing LST has been published as a result of further analysis of the wealth of data accumulated by SUPPORT.[49–53]

SUPPORT revealed that a major barrier to the willingness of patients, families, and physicians to discontinue LST was the presence of an intermediate prognosis for survival. Many SUPPORT patients were critically ill but not clearly terminally ill. In a typical SUPPORT patient, the prognostic model predicted a 50 percent chance of survival for 6 months. Many of these patients and their families wished them to have aggressive therapy until it was clear that their prognosis was poor. Such a time-limited trial of therapy is frequently appropriate pending further clarification of the prognosis.[3,54]

The process of withdrawal of LST in a neurological-neurosurgical ICU has been reported. Excluding brain-dead patients, 43 percent of dying patients were terminally extubated with a mean duration of survival following extubation of 7.5 hours. Morphine or fentanyl was administered to combat labored breathing in two-thirds of patients. A subsequent survey of surrogate decision-makers revealed that 88 percent were comfortable and satisfied with the process of withdrawing LST.[55]

Implicit in any decision to withhold or withdraw LST is a clear statement of the prognosis. Accurate prognosis can be obtained from properly conducted and reported outcome studies. But physicians using outcome data should be aware to avoid the fallacy of the self-fulfilling prophecy. Many studies purporting to describe the natural history of serious illness contain patients for whom LST was purposely withdrawn based on the perception of a poor prognosis. The bedside decision in each case may have

been ethically appropriate, but inclusion of these patients in the study distorts the natural history of the treated disease. Subsequently relying on such data for prospective determinations of prognosis introduces the fallacy of the self-fulfilling prophecy.

In a critical review, the fallacy of the self-fulfilling prophecy was found to be a common contaminant of many studies reporting prognostic indicators in coma following cardiac arrest.[56] In a study of prognosis in large intracerebral hemorrhage (ICH), this fallacy was also found to be present.[57] Several patients from a large series of patients with large ICH had poor prognoses as calculated by accepted prognostic models. Nevertheless, they were treated aggressively with surgical evacuation and did unexpectedly well, that is, they had much better outcomes than the prognostic model predicted. Physicians should be wary of noncritically relying on outcome studies incorporating the fallacy of the self-fulfilling prophecy when determining prognoses of seriously ill patients.[58]

Cultural issues may be relevant to patient and family decisions to withdraw LST in different countries. For example, the cultural differences in the beliefs and practices of withdrawing LST have been reported from France,[59] Israel,[60] Canada,[61] and the Netherlands.[62] In an attempt to reach international consensus on a unifying set of principles underlying withholding and withdrawing of LST, representatives from 15 countries developed the Appleton international guidelines in 1991.[63] Although these principles have not been ratified by medical societies within the countries of origin, they do comprise a set of generally acceptable, normative guidelines. Similar guidelines had been published earlier by the President's Commission for the Study of Ethical Problems in Medicine and Biomedical and Behavioral Research[64] and the Hastings Center.[65]

Neurologists appear to be unrealistically and inappropriately concerned about legal sanctions and permissions when they are faced with decisions to withdraw LST. For example, in a survey of practicing neurologist members of the American Academy of Neurology, 40 percent of respondents wrongly believed that they needed to consult legal counsel before withdrawing a patient's LST, and 38 percent were wrongly concerned that they might be charged with a crime for withdrawing LST.[66] Surveys of physicians practicing other specialties have disclosed similar legal misconceptions.[67]

In fact, there are few legal constraints on American physicians who withdraw or withhold LST when it follows the valid refusal of LST by competent patients or by the legally authorized surrogates of incompetent patients. Meisel's annually updated monograph thoroughly reviews this topic.[68] The United States Supreme Court in *Cruzan* stated that all citizens possess the right of refusal of all forms of therapy, including LST and AHN.[35] Public prosecutors do not pursue physicians who discontinue LST that has been validly refused, though they may pursue physicians who have committed euthanasia or physician-assisted suicide.[69,70]

■ The Pros and Cons

There remain two controversial issues in patients' and surrogates' decisions to withdraw or withhold LST: (1) whether patients' concomitant depression invalidates their treatment refusal; and (2) the role of the hospital ethics committee in clinical decision-making.

The Role of Depression

The relevance of concomitant depression may become an issue when physicians consider discontinuing LST that has been refused by a competent dying patient. The presence of psychological distress, including depression, is common in dying patients, and has been found to be at least partially responsible for the decisions of some dying patients to terminate further LST.[71] For example, the longer survival of nondepressed patients with amyotrophic lateral sclerosis (ALS) can be at least partially attributed to the greater frequency of refusal of LST by depressed patients.[72]

The question of whether severe depression should invalidate a patient's right to refuse LST remains controversial because of disagreement over the threshold for when patients have become mentally incapacitated, thereby invalidating their treatment refusal.[73,74] For example, physicians

routinely admit severely depressed, suicidal patients and treat them against their will. But is it ever permissible to ignore a severely depressed, dying patient's refusal of LST because the depression is causing the patient to refuse treatment?

There are relatively few instances in which a dying patient's refusal of LST should not be respected, despite concomitant depression. The presence of depression in nondying patients requires greater circumspection. But what remains clear is the duty of physicians to try to optimize the psychological state of critically and terminally ill patients by early recognition and timely treatment of concomitant depression.[75]

The American Academy of Neurology Ethics and Humanities Subcommittee summarized the duties of neurologists who consider honoring the wishes of competent, paralyzed, ventilator-dependent patients with ALS to withdraw ventilator treatment.[76] They emphasized that patients have the right to refuse LST but that certain preconditions should be met before neurologists discontinue LST. The patient should be competent, fully educated about treatment options, and reassured that the neurologist will continue to provide comfort care and will not abandon the patient. Communication should be optimized to permit the patient to fully participate in care decisions. The patient's decision to discontinue LST should be stable over time and not impulsive. Depression should be considered and treated if present. Ideally, the patient's family should agree with and support the decision to discontinue LST.[77]

The Hospital Ethics Committee

Most American hospitals caring for critically ill patients have a functioning hospital ethics committee or similar body. The role of the ethics committee varies among institutions but usually serves an advisory or consultative role to provide assistance to requesting physicians and other parties on the identification and resolution of ethical problems arising in medical practice.[78] The findings or recommendations of hospital ethics committees in nearly all hospitals are nonbinding and purely advisory. The ethical and legal responsibility for the patient rests with the attending physician of record.

Advocates of using hospital ethics committees claim that they can assist medical and nursing staff, families, and patients to reach good decisions by enhancing communication, educating about ethical principles, and helping to elicit and follow patients' preferences.[79] Ethics committees and ethics consultants can work with the principals to help define the problem, identify the reason for the conflict, and assist as mediators in dispute resolution.[80] Their principal role is to protect the best interests and welfare of the patient. The three cases presented earlier illustrate the benefits of ethics committees and consultants in helping resolve disputes over treatment.

Critics of using hospital ethics committees in a clinical role worry that involving a distant and unaccountable committee in clinical decision-making can lead to worsening of patient care, not its betterment.[81] Critics fear that physicians will defer important decisions to a committee that knows nothing about the patient and has no responsibility for the patient. They maintain that attending physicians should not abdicate responsibility for the patient to such a committee. Indeed, some ethics committees probably do act to diffuse responsibility and some are unsuccessful in resolving disputes over treatment.[82]

The proper use of clinical ethics consultants can neutralize some of the concerns of critics of ethics committees.[83] The ethics consultants in many hospitals are clinicians with special training and experience in analyzing, understanding, and resolving ethical issues. The consultant should read the medical record and not rely on second-hand information. The consultant should discuss the case with the principals and help them reach a resolution. Neurologists serving as ethics consultants ("neuroethicists") have a special role in assessing patients with coma, vegetative state, dementia, paralysis, and other neurological conditions.[84] Studies of the impact of ethics consultations generally reveal improvements in the quality of patient care and satisfaction by the principals involved.[85]

The preceding data and arguments can be rendered into a series of practice guidelines for clinicians faced with decisions to withdraw or withhold LST by competent patients or the surrogates of incompetent patients. Following these guidelines can help resolve disputes among families, patients, nurses, and physicians that are common in decisions to limit LST.[86] Readers seeking greater detail on the description and documentation of these guidelines can consult a recent monograph.[87]

■ The Main Points

- *Communicate with the competent patient or the family and surrogate decision-maker of the incompetent patient.* Adequate communication with patients, family members, and the surrogate is essential to be reasonably confident that the physician is following the wishes of the patient. The theme of the communication should be that the hospital staff and family are jointly struggling to do the right thing, namely, to make that decision that the patient would make were he able.
- *Communicate with the hospital staff.* The nursing and ancillary hospital staff, as well as the house staff in teaching hospitals, should clearly understand the treatment plans and goals and how and why they have been chosen. They should be willing to carry out the treatment plan because it is the ethically correct course of action.
- *Document decisions in the medical record.* Notes in the medical record should reflect the reasons the specific treatment plan has been chosen and the process of decision-making. Orders to nurses should be consistent with this plan. The types of therapy to be administered or withheld should be made explicit in a series of orders.
- *Follow hospital bylaws.* Physicians should follow their hospital's bylaws that pertain to termination of treatment decisions.
- *Follow state laws.* Physicians should be knowledgeable and ready to follow applicable state laws pertaining to termination of treatment, including advance directive statutes.
- *Establish the correct diagnosis and prognosis.* Prognosis may not be known precisely but physicians should share their extent of understanding of the prognosis with the patient and surrogate.
- *Identify the patient's preference.* The competent patient can state his or her preferences.

The physician should attempt to discover the incompetent patient's previously expressed wish for treatment or nontreatment. This information may be learned from advance directives or from statements of family members or friends. The decision for treatment of the incompetent patient should be made by a surrogate using the standard of expressed wishes or substituted judgment, or when these are impossible, the standard of best interest.

- *Identify the family's preference.* In the ideal situation, the surrogate and family of the incompetent patient will agree on the treatment plan. It is desirable for the family to have achieved consensus on the grounds that the treatment plan is ethically correct. If consensus cannot be reached, family meetings with physicians, nurses, chaplains, and social workers may help. If the family remains divided despite the best efforts of other professionals and family meetings, the case should be referred to the hospital ethics committee for review. In some cases in which the family is divided and there is no legally authorized surrogate, it may be desirable to refer the matter to court for formal appointment of a legally authorized surrogate.
- *Choose appropriate level of treatment.* Based on the foregoing, the physician and competent patient or the physician and surrogate should choose a level of treatment that is consistent with the previous wishes of the patient. This treatment plan may include provision or withdrawal of LST, medications, and AHN. Orders should be written explicitly describing which therapies will be provided and which will not. Nursing care to maintain dignity and hygiene should always be provided.
- *Provide ideal palliative care.* The patient for whom LST has been discontinued should be kept comfortable and free from suffering by the appropriate and judicious use of opiates, benzodiazepines, or barbiturates.[88,89]
- *Request oversight by the hospital ethics committee.* This step is generally unnecessary for a terminally ill patient. But it may be particularly useful for a nonterminally ill patient for whom withdrawal of LST orders have been written. This review primarily protects the patient by ensuring due process and secondarily

helps the physician by demonstrating that he has followed the proper procedure in his decision. If the committee feels that proper procedures have not been followed, the orders to terminate LST should be suspended until proper procedures are established. In the absence of a functioning hospital ethics committee, another physician can provide the oversight role.
- *Refer to court for judicial review in certain circumstances.* If the preceding guidelines are followed, judicial oversight or formal surrogate appointment should be necessary only rarely. However, it should be considered in the following circumstances: (1) when suggested by the hospital attorney; (2) when there is an intractable substantive disagreement within the family and no formal surrogate has been appointed; (3) when there is evidence or suspicion that a surrogate is deciding for non-altruistic reasons; and (4) in those instances in which the prognosis remains uncertain and there is neither an advance directive nor a surrogate available to guide the physician.

■ References

1. Wagner DP, Knaus WA, Harrell FE, Zimmerman JE, Watts C. Daily prognostic estimates for critically ill adults in intensive care units: results from a prospective, multicenter, inception cohort analysis. *Crit Care Med* 1994;22:1359–1372.
2. SUPPORT Principal Investigators. A controlled trial to improve care for seriously ill hospitalized patients. The Study to Understand Prognoses and Preferences for Outcomes and Risks of Treatment (SUPPORT). *JAMA* 1995;274:1591–1598.
3. Prendergast TJ. The SUPPORT project and improving care for seriously ill patients. *JAMA* 1996;275:1227.
4. Frankl D, Oye RK, Bellamy PE. Attitudes of hospitalized patients toward life support: a survey of 200 medical inpatients. *Am J Med* 1989;86:645–648.
5. Doyle D, Hanks GWC, MacDonald N, eds. *Oxford Textbook of Palliative Medicine*, 2nd ed. New York, Oxford University Press, 1998.
6. Raffin TA. Withdrawing life support: how is the decision made? *JAMA* 1995;273:738–739.
7. Prendergast TJ, Claessens MT, Luce JM. A national survey of end-of-life care for critically ill patients. *Am J Respir Crit Care Med* 1998;158:1163–1167.
8. Bernat JL. Plan ahead: how neurologists can enhance patient-centered medicine. *Neurology* 2001;56:144–145.

9. Laine C, Davidoff F. Patient-centered medicine: a professional evolution. *JAMA* 1996;275:152–156.

10. Hopkins PD. Why does removing machines count as "passive" euthanasia? *Hastings Cent Rep* 1997;27(3): 29–37.

11. Bernat JL. The problem of physician-assisted suicide. *Semin Neurol* 1997;17:271–279.

12. Gert B, Culver CM, Clouser KD. *Bioethics: A Return to Fundamentals.* New York, Oxford University Press, 1997:131–250.

13. Lo B. Assessing decision-making capacity. *Law Med Health Care* 1990;18:193–201.

14. Brock DW. The ideal of shared decision making between physicians and patients. *Kennedy Inst Ethics J* 1991;1:28–47

15. Quill TE, Brody H. Physician recommendation and patient autonomy: finding a balance between physician power and patient choice. *Ann Intern Med* 1996;125: 763–769.

16. Menikoff JA, Sachs GA, Siegler M. Beyond advance directives—health care surrogate laws. *N Engl J Med* 1992;327:1165–1169.

17. Molloy DW, Clarnette RM, Braun EA, et al. Decision making in the incompetent elderly: "the daughter from California syndrome." *J Am Geriatr Soc* 1991;39: 396–399.

18. Buchanan AE, Brock DW. *Deciding for Others: The Ethics of Surrogate Decision Making.* Cambridge, Cambridge University Press, 1989:112–116.

19. Layde PM, Beam CA, Broste SK, et al. Surrogates' predictions of seriously ill patients' resuscitation preferences. *Arch Fam Med* 1995;4:518–523.

20. Sulmasy DP, Terry PB, Weisman CS, et al. The accuracy of substituted judgments in patients with terminal diagnoses. *Ann Intern Med* 1998;128:621–629.

21. Suhl J, Simons P, Reedy T, et al. Myth of substituted judgment: surrogate decision making regarding life support is unreliable. *Arch Intern Med* 1994;154: 90–96.

22. Drane JF, Coulehan JL. The best-interest standard: surrogate decision making and quality of life. *J Clin Ethics* 1995;6:20–29.

23. Uhlmann RF, Pearlman RA. Perceived quality of life and preferences for life-sustaining treatment in older adults. *Arch Intern Med* 1991;151:495–497.

24. Schneiderman LJ, Arras JD. Counseling patients to counsel physicians on future care in the event of patient incompetence. *Ann Intern Med* 1985; 102:693–698.

25. Emanuel L. Advance directives: what have we learned so far? *J Clin Ethics* 1993;4:8–16.

26. Annas GJ. The health care proxy and the living will. *N Engl J Med* 1991;324:1210–1213.

27. Orentlicher D. Advance medical directives. *JAMA* 1990;263:2365–2367.

28. Lynn J. Why I don't have a living will. *Law Med Health Care* 1991;19:101–104.

29. Emanuel LL, Emanuel EJ. The medical directive: a new comprehensive advance care document. *JAMA* 1989;261:3288–3293.

30. Gillick MR. A broader role for advance medical planning. *Ann Intern Med* 1995;123:621–624.

31. Steinbrook R, Lo B. Artificial feeding—solid ground, not a slippery slope. *N Engl J Med* 1988;318: 286–290.

32. Winter SM. Terminal nutrition: framing the debate for the withdrawal of nutritional support in terminally ill patients. *Am J Med* 2000;109:723–726.

33. Siegler M, Weisbard AJ. Against the emerging stream: should fluids and nutritional support be discontinued? *Arch Intern Med* 1985;145:129–131.

34. Rosner F. Why nutrition and hydration should not be withheld from patients. *Chest* 1993;104: 1892–1896.

35. Meisel A. A retrospective on *Cruzan. Law Med Health Care* 1992;20:340–353.

36. White BD, Siegler M, Singer PA, et al. What does *Cruzan* mean to the practicing physician? *Arch Intern Med* 1991;151:925–928.

37. Mendelson D, Jost TS. A comparative study of the law of palliative care and end-of-life treatment. *J Law Med Ethics* 2003;31:130–143.

38. Prendergast TJ, Puntillo KA. Withdrawal of life support: intensive caring at the end of life. *JAMA* 2002;288:2732–2740.

39. Faber-Langendoen K, Bartels DM. Process of forgoing life-sustaining treatment in a university hospital: an empirical study. *Crit Care Med* 1992;20:570–577.

40. Koch KA, Rodefer HD, Wears RL. Changing patterns of terminal care management in an intensive care unit. *Crit Care Med* 1994;22:233–243.

41. Prendergast TJ, Luce JM. Increasing incidence of withholding and withdrawal of life support from the critically ill. *Am J Respir Crit Care Med* 1997; 155:15–20.

42. Smedira NG, Evans BH, Grais LS, et al. Withholding and withdrawal of life support from the critically ill. *N Engl J Med* 1990;322:309–315.

43. Christakis NA, Asch DA. Biases in how physicians choose to withdraw life support. *Lancet* 1993; 342:642–646.

44. Christakis NA, Asch DA. Medical specialists prefer to withdraw familiar technologies when discontinuing life support. *J Gen Intern Med* 1995;10:491–494.

45. Brody H, Campbell ML, Faber-Langendoen K, Ogle KS. Withdrawing intensive life-sustaining treatment—recommendations for compassionate clinical management. *N Engl J Med* 1997;336:652–657.

46. Daily BJ, Thomas DT, Dyer MA. Procedures used in withdrawal of mechanical ventilation. *Am J Crit Care* 1996;5:331–338.

47. Wilson WC, Smedira NG, Fink C, McDowell JA, Luce JM. Ordering and administration of sedatives and analgesics during the withholding and withdrawal of

life support from critically ill patients. *JAMA* 1992; 267:949–953.

48. Gilligan T, Raffin TA. Withdrawing life support: extubation and prolonged terminal weans are inappropriate. *Crit Care Med* 1996;24:352–353.

49. Phillips RS, Wenger NS, Teno J, et al. Choices of seriously ill patients about cardiopulmonary resuscitation: correlates and outcomes. *Am J Med* 1996;100: 128–137.

50. Rosenfeld KE, Wenger NS, Phillips RS, et al. Factors associated with change in resuscitation preference of seriously ill patients. *Arch Intern Med* 1996;156: 1558–1564.

51. Haykim RB, Teno J, Harrell FE Jr, et al. Factors associated with do-not-resuscitate orders: patients' preferences, prognoses, and physicians' judgments. *Ann Intern Med* 1996;125:284–293.

52. Hamel MB, David RB, Teno J, et al. Older age, aggressiveness of care, and survival for seriously ill, hospitalized adults. *Ann Intern Med* 1999;131:721–728.

53. Teno J, Lynn J, Phillips RS, et al. Do formal advance directives affect resuscitation decisions and the use of resources for seriously ill patients? *J Clin Ethics* 1994;5:23–30.

54. Lo B. Improving care near the end of life: why is it so hard? *JAMA* 1995;274:1634–1636.

55. Mayer SA, Kossoff SB. Withdrawal of life support in the neurological intensive care unit. *Neurology* 1999;52:1602–1609.

56. Shewmon DA, DiGiorgio CM. Early prognosis in anoxic coma: reliability and rationale. *Neurol Clin* 1989;7:823–843.

57. Becker KJ, Baxter AB, Cohen WA, et al. Withdrawal of support in intracerebral hemorrhage may lead to self-fulfilling prophecies. *Neurology* 2001;56:766–772.

58. Bernat JL. Ethical aspects of determining and communicating prognosis in critical care. *Neurocrit Care* 2004;1:107–118.

59. Ferrand E, Robert R, Ingrand P, Lemaire F. Withholding and withdrawal of life support in intensive care units in France: a prospective study. *Lancet* 2001;357:9–14.

60. Glick SM. Unlimited human autonomy—a cultural bias? *N Engl J Med* 1997;336:954–956.

61. Cook DJ, Guyatt GH, Jaeschke R, et al. Determinants in Canadian health care workers of the decision to withdraw life support from the critically ill. *JAMA* 1995;273:703–708.

62. Pijenborg L, van der Maas PJ, Kardaun JWPF, Glerum JJ, van Delden JJM, Looman CWN. Withdrawal or withholding of treatment at the end of life: results of a nationwide survey. *Arch Intern Med* 1995;155:286–292.

63. Stanley JM, ed. The Appleton International Conference: developing guidelines for decisions to forgo life-prolonging medical treatment. *J Med Ethics* 1992;18(Suppl):1–22.

64. President's Commission for the Study of Ethical Problems in Medicine and Biomedical and Behavioral Research. *Deciding to Forgo Life-Sustaining Treatment: Ethical, Medical and Legal Issues in Treatment Decisions.* Washington, DC, U.S. Government Printing Office, 1983.

65. Hastings Center. *Guidelines on the Termination of Life-Sustaining Treatment and the Care of the Dying.* Briarcliff Manor, NY, Hastings Center, 1987.

66. Carver AC, Vickrey BG, Bernat JL, Keran C, Ringel SP, Foley KM. End of life care: a survey of U.S. neurologists' attitudes, behavior, and knowledge. *Neurology* 1999;53:284–293.

67. Meisel A, Snyder L, Quill T. Seven legal barriers to end-of-life care: myths, realities, and grains of truth. *JAMA* 2000;284:2495–2501.

68. Meisel A. *The Right To Die,* 2nd ed. New York, John Wiley, 1995.

69. Meisel A, Jernigan JC, Youngner SJ. Prosecutors and end-of-life decision making. *Arch Intern Med* 1999;159:1089–1095.

70. Alpers A. Criminal act or palliative care? Prosecutions involving care of the dying. *J Law Med Ethics* 1998;26:308–331.

71. Chochinov HM, Wilson KG, Enns M, et al. Desire for death in the terminally ill. *Am J Psychiatry* 1995; 152:1185–1191.

72. McDonald ER, Wiedenfeld SA, Hillel A, et al. Survival in amyotrophic lateral sclerosis: the role of psychological factors. *Arch Neurol* 1994;51:17–23.

73. Sullivan MD, Youngner SJ. Depression, competence, and the right to refuse life-sustaining treatment. *Am J Psychiatry* 1994;151:971–978.

74. Ganzini L, Lee MA, Heintz RT, et al. Depression, suicide, and the right to refuse life-sustaining treatment. *J Clin Ethics* 1993;4:337–340.

75. Block SD. Assessing and managing depression in the terminally ill patient. *Ann Intern Med* 2000;132:209–218.

76. American Academy of Neurology Ethics and Humanities Subcommittee. Position statement: certain aspects of the care and management of profoundly and irreversibly paralyzed patients with retained consciousness and cognition. *Neurology* 1993;43: 222–223.

77. Bernat JL, Cranford RE, Kittredge FI Jr, Rosenberg RN. Competent patients with advanced states of permanent paralysis have the right to forgo life-sustaining therapy. *Neurology* 1993;43:224–225.

78. American Medical Association Judicial Council. Guidelines for ethics committees in health care institutions. *JAMA* 1985;253:2698–2699.

79. Ross JW, Glaser JW, Rasinski-Gregory D, et al. *Health Care Ethics Committees: The Next Generation.* Chicago, American Hospital Publishing Corporation, 1993.

80. Orr RD, deLeon D. The role of the clinical ethicist in conflict resolution. *J Clin Ethics* 2000;11:21–30.

81. Fleetwood JE, Arnold RM, Baron RJ. Giving answers or raising questions? The problematic role of institutional ethics committees. *J Med Ethics* 1989;15: 137–142.

82. Lo B. Behind closed doors: promises and pitfalls of ethics committees. *N Engl J Med* 1987;317: 46–50.

83. Aulisio MP, Arnold RM, Youngner SJ. Health care ethics consultation: nature, goals, and competencies. *Ann Intern Med* 2000;133:59–69.

84. Cranford RE. The neurologist as ethics consultant and as a member of the institutional ethics committee: the neuroethicist. *Neurol Clin* 1989;7:697–713.

85. Fox E, Arnold RM. Evaluating outcomes in ethics consultation research. *J Clin Ethics* 1996;7:127–138.

86. Breen CM, Abernethy AP, Abbott KH, Tulsky JA. Conflict associated with decisions to limit life-sustaining treatment in intensive care units. *J Gen Intern Med* 2001;16:283–289.

87. Bernat JL. *Ethical Issues in Neurology*, 2nd ed. Boston, Butterworth-Heinemann, 2002.

88. Doyle D, Hanks GWC, MacDonald N, eds. *Oxford Textbook of Palliative Medicine*, 2nd ed. New York, Oxford University Press, 1998.

89. Carver AC, Foley KM, eds. Palliative care in neurology. *Neurol Clin* 2001;194:789–1044.

Index